Caring for the Vulnerable

THIRD EDITION

Perspectives in Nursing Theory, Practice, and Research

The Pedagogy

Caring for the Vulnerable: Perspectives in Nursing Theory, Practice, and Research, Third Edition drives comprehension through various strategies that meet the learning needs of students, while also generating enthusiasm about the topic. This interactive approach addresses different learning styles, making this the ideal text to ensure mastery of key concepts. The pedagogical aids that appear in most chapters include the following:

CHAPTER OBJECTIVES

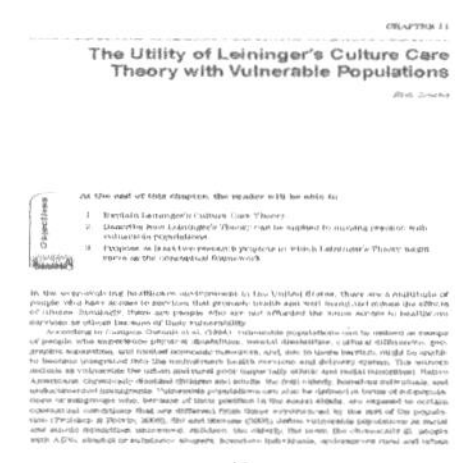
The Utility of Leininger's Culture Care Theory with Vulnerable Populations

These objectives provide instructors and students with a snapshot of the key information they will encounter in each chapter. They serve as a checklist to help guide and focus study. Objectives can also be found on the Companion Website at http://go.jblearning.com/dechesnay.

CHAPTER INTRODUCTORY PARAGRAPHS

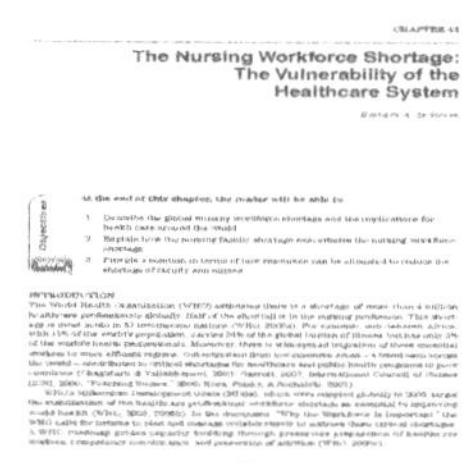
The Nursing Workforce Shortage: The Vulnerability of the Healthcare System

Found at the beginning of each chapter, chapter introductory paragraphs provide an overview of the importance of the chapter's topic. They also help keep students focused as they read.

CASE STUDIES

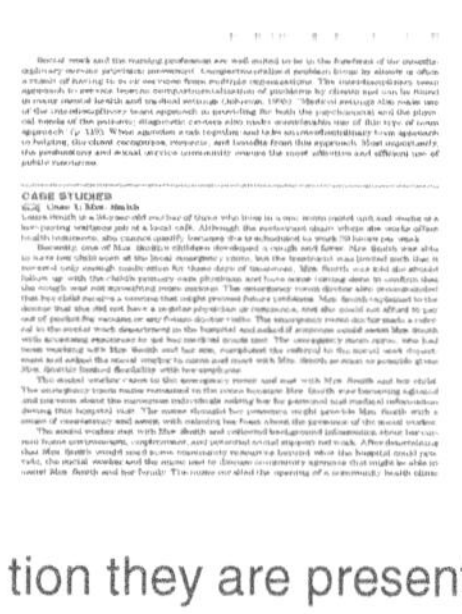

Case studies encourage active learning and promote critical thinking skills in learners. Students can ask questions, analyze the situation they are presented with, and solve problems. Students can also learn how the information in the text applies to everyday practice online at http://go.jblearning.com/dechesnay.

CHAPTER CONCLUSIONS

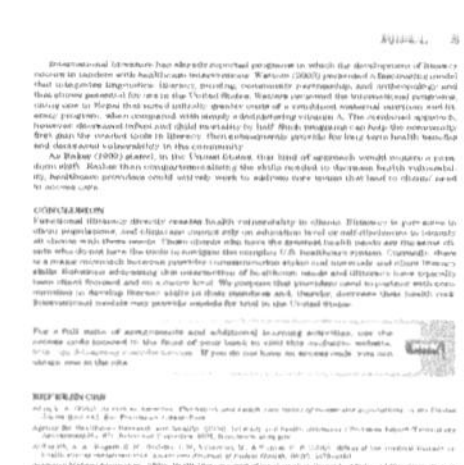

Conclusions are included at the end of each chapter to provide a concise review of material covered in each chapter. These summaries highlight the most important points in the chapter.

Caring for the Vulnerable

THIRD EDITION

Perspectives in Nursing Theory, Practice, and Research

Edited by
Mary de Chesnay, DSN, PMHCNS-BC, FAAN
Professor, WellStar School of Nursing
Kennesaw State University
Kennesaw, Georgia

Barbara A. Anderson, DrPH, RN, CNM, FACNM, FAAN
Professor and Director, Doctor of Nursing Practice
Frontier Nursing University
Hyden, Kentucky

JONES & BARTLETT
LEARNING

World Headquarters
Jones & Bartlett Learning
5 Wall Street
Burlington, MA 01803
978-443-5000
info@jblearning.com
www.jblearning.com

Jones & Bartlett Learning Canada
6339 Ormindale Way
Mississauga, Ontario L5V 1J2
Canada

Jones & Bartlett Learning International
Barb House, Barb Mews
London W6 7PA
United Kingdom

Jones & Bartlett Learning books and products are available through most bookstores and online booksellers. To contact Jones & Bartlett Learning directly, call 800-832-0034, fax 978-443-8000, or visit our website, www.jblearning.com.

Substantial discounts on bulk quantities of Jones & Bartlett Learning publications are available to corporations, professional associations, and other qualified organizations. For details and specific discount information, contact the special sales department at Jones & Bartlett Learning via the above contact information or send an email to specialsales@jblearning.com.

Production Credits
Publisher: Kevin Sullivan
Acquisitions Editor: Amanda Harvey
Editorial Assistant: Sara Bempkins
Associate Production Editor: Sara Fowles
Associate Marketing Manager: Katie Hennessy
V.P., Manufacturing and Inventory Control: Therese Connell
Composition: Laserwords Private Limited, Chennai, India
Cover Design: Scott Moden
Cover Images: (Clockwise from upper left) © psamtik/ShutterStock, Inc.; © prism_68/ShutterStock, Inc.; © Ryan McVay/Photodisc/Getty Images; © Arman Zhenikeyev/ShutterStock, Inc.; © JPagetRFphotos/ShutterStock, Inc.
Printing and Binding: Malloy, Inc.
Cover Printing: Malloy, Inc.

To order this product, use ISBN: 978-1-4496-3592-3

Library of Congress Cataloging-in-Publication Data
Caring for the vulnerable: perspectives in nursing theory, practice, and research/[edited by] Mary de Chesnay, Barbara A. Anderson.
–3rd ed.
p.;cm.
Includes bibliographical references and index.
ISBN 978-1-4496-0398-4 (pbk.)
1. Nursing–Social aspects. 2. Transcultural nursing.
3. Nursing–Cross-cultural studies. 4. Nursing–Philosophy.
I. De Chesnay, Mary. II. Anderson, Barbara A.
[DNLM: 1. Community Health Nursing. 2. Vulnerable Populations. 3. Nursing Theory. 4. Transcultural Nursing. WY 106]
RT86.5.C376 2012
362.17'3–dc22

2011007234

6048
Printed in the United States of America
15 14 13 12 11 10 9 8 7 6 5 4 3 2 1

For my cousin, Sam Surtees, who redefined resilience
when he conquered Guillain-Barré syndrome.
In memory of my brother, John.

MdC

In memory of Father Roger Gillis, S.J., Seattle University,
in appreciation for his friendship for the profession of nursing and
his life commitment to social justice for the vulnerable.

BA

Contents

UNIT III: RESEARCH 183

Preface

For the third edition, the editors have retained material that we consider basic content, yet added new chapters that focus on different vulnerable populations. There are so many nurses dedicated to special groups that we cannot do justice to them all, but we can give new authors a chance to teach us about the people with whom they work most closely. This book was originally written for undergraduates in nursing, but over the years it has been used extensively in graduate education. This edition, therefore, highlights nurse practitioners in two units, "Teaching–Learning" and "Programs," as well as increasing the focus on the advocacy role for nurses. While retaining theoretical models from previous editions, this new edition highlights HIV-infected mothers and vulnerable women who breastfeed. We have also added material on undocumented immigrants, sexual trafficking, and research in global health nursing. Contemporary issues of vulnerability addressed in this edition include nurses in the military, childhood autism, childhood obesity, education on breast cancer, and success at overcoming substance abuse and sexual abuse. Finally the unit titled "Policy Implications" focuses on system-related issues affecting vulnerability and vulnerable populations.

Mary de Chesnay and Barbara A. Anderson

Foreword

"Learn to accept differences" was one of my mother's most dearly held values. In the 1960s, my university nursing program taught me that accepting—even welcoming—differences was not enough. It was crucial to learn more about those differences and gain tools to be of help to diverse populations.

Health professionals have worked to understand vulnerability and gain skills to help those who need assistance because of illness, environmental challenges, homelessness, and impoverishment. Being vulnerable implies being insecure and in danger. Since the Crimean War, nurses have been attentive to protecting the endangered, creating a more healthful environment, and providing support for those in need. Beyond helping, however, lies another challenge. Empowering vulnerable individuals, groups, and communities produces longer-lasting benefits. Florence Nightingale, for example, provided an active role model for advocating for the soldiers that she treated in the fields of war.

The third edition of the award-winning de Chesnay and Anderson book, *Caring for the Vulnerable: Perspectives in Nursing Theory, Practice, and Research*, presents an outstanding road map that enables health professionals to answer six essential questions:

- Who are the vulnerable?
- What are their needs, and which interventions are the best fit for them?
- When is the best time to intervene?
- Where in the culture of the vulnerable is the best place to provide intervention?
- Why has the individual, group, or community become vulnerable and thus in need of intervention?
- How can the vulnerable be best empowered?

There is a danger in assuming that the vulnerable are fragile and unable to manage. Achilles had an endangered heel—yet much of this mythological man was intelligent, strong, and powerful. Disaster can result from doing "for" people in need, and then departing. It is not enough to bandage a heel: More must be done to warn of the risk, and prevent the fatal arrow's flight. The only lasting interventions are those that recognize the strengths of the imperiled and enhance their knowledge and power to manage challenges. Strategies that accomplish empowerment should be the priority. *Caring for the Vulnerable* is a valuable contribution to health professionals' ability to advocate for the vulnerable; enable individuals, groups, and communities to thrive despite challenges; and foster changes that truly reduce risk.

Susan Y. Stevens, DSN, APRN, PMHCNS-BC
Perimeter Adult Learning and Services
Atlanta, Georgia

Contributors

Kathie Aduddell, EdD, MSN, RN
Associate Professor, WellStar School of Nursing
Kennesaw State University
Kennesaw, Georgia

Barbara A. Anderson, DrPH, RN, CNM, FACNM, FAAN
Professor and Director, Doctor of Nursing Practice
Frontier Nursing University
Hyden, Kentucky

David Bennett, PhD, RN
Professor and Associate Dean, WellStar College of Health and Human Services
Kennesaw State University
Kennesaw, Georgia

Charles Bobo, JD, MBA, MSN, RN
Assistant Professor, WellStar School of Nursing
Kennesaw State University
Kennesaw, Georgia

Anne Watson Bongiorno, PhD, RN
Associate Professor
SUNY Plattsburgh
Plattsburgh, New York

Doris M. Boutain, PhD, RN
Associate Professor
University of Washington School of Nursing
Seattle, Washington

Jane Brannan, EdD, RN
Assistant Director, Undergraduate Nursing Programs
Professor, WellStar School of Nursing
Kennesaw State University
Kennesaw, Georgia

Geraldine R. Britton, PhD, RN, FNP
Assistant Professor, Becker School of Nursing
Binghamton University
Binghamton, New York

Ellyn Cavanagh, PhD, RN, APRN
Nurse Practitioner, Child Development
Clinical Faculty, Dartmouth School of Medicine
Lebanon, New Hampshire

Caroline Cogan, MSN, ARNP
St. Luke's Magic Valley Regional Medical Center
Twin Falls, Idaho

Mona M. Counts, PhD, RN, CRNP, FNAP, FAANP
Eloise Ross Eberly Professor
Pennsylvania State University
University Park, Pennsylvania

Kristin Cox, BSN, RN
Alumnus
Kennesaw State University
Kennesaw Georgia

Mary de Chesnay, DSN, PMHCNS-BC, FAAN
Professor, WellStar School of Nursing
Kennesaw State University
Kennesaw, Georgia

Genie Dorman, PhD, APRN, FNP-BC
Professor, WellStar School of Nursing
Kennesaw State University
Kennesaw, Georgia

Janet L. Engstrom, PhD, APN, CNM, WHNP-BC
Professor and Associate Dean for Research
Frontier Nursing University
Hyden, Kentucky

Behice Erci, PhD, RN
Professor
Inonu University
Malaya, Turkey

Janice B. Flynn, DSN, RN
Associate Professor and Associate Director, Undergraduate Nursing Program, WellStar School of Nursing
Kennesaw State University
Kennesaw, Georgia

Terra Grandmason, MSN, ARNP
Family Nurse Practitioner
Yakima Valley Health Center
Yakima, Washington

Rebecca Green, MSN, RN
Valdosta City Schools
Valdosta, Georgia

Sarah Hall Gueldner, DSN, RN, FAAN
Professor
Bolton School of Nursing
Case Western Reserve University
Cleveland, Ohio

Patricia Hart, BSN, MS, PhD
Assistant Professor, WellStar School of Nursing
Kennesaw State University
Kennesaw, Georgia

Annette Jackson, MSN, RN
Gordon College
Barnesville, Georgia

Karen Joines, RN, BSN
Carolinas HealthCare System
Charlotte, North Carolina

Joyce M. Knestrick, PhD, RN, CRNP, FAANP
Professor and Associate Dean for Academic Affairs
Frontier Nursing University
Hyden, Kentucky

Cheryl Ann Lapp, PhD, RN
Professor
University of Wisconsin, Eau Claire
Eau Claire, Wisconsin

Janice Long, MS, RN, PhD
Assistant Professor, WellStar School of Nursing
Kennesaw State University
Kennesaw, Georgia

Margaret McAllister, RN, MHN, BA, MEd, EdD
Professor
University of the Sunshine Coast
Queensland, Australia

Nicole Mareno, BSN, MSN, PhD
Assistant Professor, WellStar School of Nursing
Kennesaw State University
Kennesaw, Georgia

Paula P. Meier, RN, DNSc, FAAN
Professor, Women, Children, and Family Nursing
Professor, Pediatrics
Rush University Medical Center
Chicago, Ilinois

Jeri A. Milstead, PhD, RN
Milstead Innovations
Dublin, Ohio

Patrick J. M. Murphy, PhD
Assistant Professor
Seattle University College of Nursing
Seattle, Washington

Lynda P. Nauright, EdD, RN
Professor, WellStar School of Nursing
Kennesaw State University
Kennesaw, Georgia

Tommie Nelms, RN, MSN, PhD
Interim Director, Professor and Coordinator, DNS Program, WellStar School of Nursing
Kennesaw State University
Kennesaw, Georgia

Ellen Olshansky, DNSc, RN, WHNP-BC, FAAN
Professor and Director, Program in Nursing Science
College of Health Sciences
University of California-Irvine
Irvine, California

Kathryn Osborne, PhD, RN, CNM
Professor
Frontier Nursing University
Hyden, Kentucky

Nataly Pasumansky, DNP, ARBP
Family Nurse Practitioner
Advanced Family Medicine
Seattle, Washington

Heather Payne, BSN, RN
Lakeland Regional Medical Center
Lakeland, Florida

Marilyn Pierce-Bulger, RN, MN, CNM, CFNP
Clinician, Pioneer Consulting
Anchorage, Alaska

Capt. Patricia L. Riley, RN, CNM, MPH, FACNM
Captain, United States Public Health Service
Division of Global HIV/AIDS-Center for Global Health
Centers for Disease Control and Prevention
Atlanta, Georgia

Vanessa Robinson-Dooley, PhD
Dept. of Social Work and Human Services
Kennesaw State University
Kennesaw, Georgia

Lois R. Robley, PhD, MSN, BSN
Professor, WellStar School of Nursing
Kennesaw State University
Kennesaw, Georgia

Susan Y. Stevens, DSN, APRN, PMHCNS-BC
Perimeter Adult Learning and Services
Atlanta, Georgia

Lacie Szekes, BSN, RN
Alumnus
Kennesaw State University
Kennesaw, Georgia

Susan Terwilliger, EdD, RN, PNP-BC
Binghamton University
Binghamton, New York

Jenny Hsin-Chun Tsai, PhD, PMHCNS-BC
Associate Professor
University of Washington
Seattle, Washington

Maile Tuaalii, MPH
Papa Ola Lokahi Native Hawaiian Epidemiology Center
Honolulu, Hawaii

Toni Vezeau, PhD, RNC, IBCLC
Associate Professor, Seattle University College of Nursing
Seattle, Washington

Lisa Marie Walsh
BSN candidate
Kennesaw State University
Kennesaw, Georgia

Capt. Mary Ann White, DSN, RN
Professor, WellStar School of Nursing
Kennesaw State University
Kennesaw, Georgia

Astrid Wilson, DSN, RN
Professor, WellStar School of Nursing
Kennesaw State University
Kennesaw, Georgia

Lynda Law Wilson, PhD, RN, FAAN
Professor
University of Alabama at Birmingham
Birmingham, Alabama

Danuta Wojnar, PhD, RN, Med, IBCLC
Assistant Professor
Seattle University College of Nursing
Seattle, Washington

Suzanne S. Young, BSN, RN
Alumnus
WellStar School of Nursing
Kennesaw State University
Kennesaw, Georgia

Rick Zoucha, PhD, PMHCNS-BC, CTN
Associate Professor
Duquesne University
Pittsburgh, Pennsylvania

Acknowledgments

This book is a reflection of the talents of many people—first among them, both the new and returning contributing authors. These talented scholars represent a small number of the many nurses around the world who practice and write about social justice. That social justice and care for the vulnerable is a universal phenomenon among nurses is reinforced when we attend professional meetings and when we travel to our own fieldwork sites and see social justice in action in some of the poorest communities of the world. It is inspiring to hear these authors speak and an honor to provide a forum for all who read this book to hear about their work.

There are always technical support people who labor quietly behind the scenes of any published work. The editors and staff at Jones & Bartlett Learning made sure the work was published in a timely manner. We are grateful to Amanda Harvey and Sara Bempkins for their diligence and timely assistance. The wonderful staff at Kennesaw State University, especially Cynthia Elery, enabled Mary de Chesnay to complete the book while maintaining a full-time job. In addition, Kathy Rodgers shared her Word skills and offered several shortcuts. My student assistants, Linh Pham and Angela Bostic, developed much of the material for the Instructor Guide, while maintaining a heavy course load.

We thank the wonderful staff at Jones & Bartlett Learning for their diligence at catching missing references and general support and encouragement. In particular, Sara Fowles was a treasure. Amy Sibley and Rachel Shuster are no longer with the company but both were helpful during the early stages of preparing the third edition.

Finally, and perhaps most importantly, the editors would like to thank all of the vulnerable yet resilient people with whom they have worked during their many years of clinical practice and education. Working in every corner of the world, the editors encountered, time and time again, the strength of the human spirit and generosity of nature among people who have no reason to welcome strangers, yet who shared what they had and took the time to teach us about their cultures.

Mary de Chesnay
Barbara A. Anderson

UNIT I

Concepts

Our greatest glory is not in never falling but in getting up when we do.

—Confucius

www.hunch.com

CHAPTER 1

Vulnerable Populations: Vulnerable People

Mary de Chesnay

Objectives

At the end of this chapter, the reader will be able to

1. Distinguish between vulnerability as an individual concept and vulnerable population.
2. Identify at least five populations at risk for health disparities.
3. Discuss how poverty influences vulnerability.

In this chapter, key concepts are introduced to provide a frame of reference for examining healthcare issues related to vulnerability and vulnerable populations. The concepts presented in Unit I, as a whole, form a theoretical perspective on caring for the vulnerable within a cultural context in which nurses consider not only ethnicity as a cultural factor, but also the culture of vulnerability. The goal is to provide culturally competent care.

VULNERABILITY

Vulnerability incorporates two aspects, and it is important to distinguish between them. One is the individual focus, in which individuals are viewed within a system context; the other is an aggregate view of what would be termed "vulnerable populations." Much of the literature on vulnerability is targeted toward the aggregate view, and nurses certainly need to address the needs of groups. Nevertheless, nurses also treat individuals, and this book is concerned with generating ideas about caring for both individuals and groups. It is critical for practitioners to keep in mind that groups are composed of individuals—we should not stereotype individuals in terms of their group characteristics. Yet, working with vulnerable populations is cost-effective because epidemiological patterns can be detected in groups and some standardized interventions can be developed that provide better quality health care to more people.

Vulnerability is a general concept meaning "susceptibility" and has a specific connotation in health care—"at risk for health problems." According to Aday (2001), vulnerable populations are those at risk for poor physical, psychological, or social health. Any person can be at risk statistically by way of having potential for certain illnesses based on genetic predisposition (Scanlon & Lee, 2007). Anyone can also be vulnerable at any given point in time as a result of life circumstances or response to illness or events. However, the notion of a vulnerable population is a public health concept that refers to vulnerability by virtue of status; that is, some groups are at risk at any given point in time relative to other individuals or groups.

To be a member of a vulnerable population does not necessarily mean a person is vulnerable. In fact, many individuals within vulnerable populations would resist the notion that they are vulnerable, because they prefer to focus on their strengths rather than their weaknesses. These people might argue that "vulnerable population" is just another label that healthcare professionals use to promote a system of health care that they, the consumers of care, consider patronizing. It is important to distinguish between a state of vulnerability at any given point in time and a labeling process in which groups of people at risk for certain health conditions are further marginalized.

Some members of society who are not members of the culturally defined vulnerable populations described in this book might be vulnerable only in certain contexts. For example, nurses who work in emergency rooms are vulnerable to violence. Hospital employees and visitors are vulnerable to infections. Teachers in preschool and daycare providers are vulnerable to a host of communicable diseases because of their daily contact with young children. Individuals who work with heavy machinery are at risk for certain injuries. Patients are vulnerable to their nurses, who literally hold their lives in hand.

Other examples of vulnerable groups might include people who pick up hitchhikers, drivers who drink alcohol, people who travel on airplanes during flu season, college students who are cramming for exams, and people who become caught in natural disasters. There is an unfortunate tendency in our culture to judge some vulnerable people as being at fault for their own vulnerability and to blame those who place others at risk. For example, rape victims have been blamed for enticing their attackers. People who pick up hitchhikers might be looked upon as foolish, even though their intentions might have been only kindness and consideration for those stranded by car trouble. Airline passengers who continually sneeze might anger their seatmates, who feel at risk for catching a communicable disease. While it is logical to argue that we should be more cautious about personal protection in societies in which dangers exist in so many contexts, that concept is quite different from blaming the victim. In the final analysis, criminals and predators need to be held accountable for criminal behavior. Victims can be taught self-defense tactics, but they need to be reassured that the crime was not their fault simply because they were in the wrong place at the wrong time.

VULNERABLE POPULATIONS

Who are the vulnerable in terms of health care? Vulnerable populations are those with a greater-than-average risk of developing health problems (Aday, 2001; Sebastian, 1996) by virtue of their marginalized sociocultural status, their limited access to economic resources, or their personal characteristics such as age and gender. For example, members of ethnic minority groups have traditionally been marginalized even when they are highly educated and earning good salaries. Immigrants and the poor (including the working poor) have limited access to health care because of the way health insurance is obtained in the United States. Children, women, and the elderly are vulnerable to a host of healthcare problems—notably violence, but also specific health problems associated with development or aging. Developmental examples might include susceptibility to poor influenza outcomes for children and the elderly, psychological issues of puberty and menopause, osteoporosis and fractures among older women, and Alzheimer's disease.

Bezruchka (2000, 2001), in his provocative work, addressed the correlation between poverty and illness but also asserted that inequalities in wealth distribution are responsible for the state of health of the U.S. population. Bezruchka argued that the economic structure of a country is the single most powerful determinant of the health of its people. He noted that Japan, with its small gap between rich and poor, has a high percentage of smokers but a low percentage of mortality from smoking. Bezruchka advocated redistribution of wealth as a solution to health disparities.

The prescription drug benefit for Medicare recipients highlights Bezruchka's observations about disparities in the United States. Senior citizens are among the most vulnerable in any society, including in the United States, where Medicare is an attempt to address some of their healthcare costs. However, while a philosophy of social justice might be valued by practitioners (Larkin, 2004), the implementation of social justice is usually balanced with cost. In the case of the Medicare prescription drug benefit, the cost is projected to exceed $700 billion over the period 2006–2015 (Gellad, Huskamp, Phillips, & Haas, 2006). The difficulties created by attempting to balance social justice with cost illustrate how difficult it is to implement Bezruchka's ideas in the United States.

CONCEPTS AND THEORIES

Aday (2001) published a framework for studying vulnerable populations that incorporated the World Health Organization's (1948) dimensions of health (physical, psychological, and social) into a model of relationships between individual and community on a variety of policy levels. In Aday's framework, which is still applicable, the variables of access, cost, and quality are critical for understanding the nature of health care for vulnerable populations. Access refers to the ability of people to find, obtain, and pay for health care. Costs can be either direct or indirect: Direct costs are the dollars spent by healthcare facilities to provide care, whereas indirect costs are losses resulting from decreased patient productivity (e.g., absenteeism from work.) Quality refers to the relative inadequacy, adequacy, or superiority of services.

Other authors who have addressed the conceptual basis of vulnerable populations include Sebastian (1996; Sebastian et al., 2002), who focused on marginalization as a factor in resource allocation, and Flaskerud and Winslow (1998), who emphasized resource availability in the broad sense of socioeconomic and environmental resources. Karpati, Galea, Awerbuch, and Levins (2002) argued for an ecological approach to understanding how social context influences health outcomes. Lessick, Woodring, Naber, and Halstead (1992) described the concept of vulnerability in relationship to a person within a system context. Although their study applied the model to maternal–child nursing, the authors argued that the model is appropriate in any clinical settings.

Spiers (2000) argued that epidemiological views of vulnerability are insufficient to explain human experience and offered a new conceptualization based on perceptions that are both etic (externally defined by others) and emic (defined from the point of view of the person). Etic approaches are helpful in understanding the nature of risk in a quantifiable way. Emic approaches enable one to understand the whole of human experience and, in so doing, help people capitalize on their capacity for action.

HEALTH DISPARITIES

In 1998, President Bill Clinton made a commitment to reduce health disparities that disproportionately affect racial and ethnic minorities in the United States by the year 2010. The Department of Health and Human Services selected six areas to target: infant mortality, cancer screening and management, cardiovascular disease, diabetes, human immunodeficiency virus (HIV) infection and acquired immune deficiency syndrome (AIDS), and immunization (National Institutes of Health [NIH], n.d.). Subsequently, the NIH announced a strategic plan for 2002–2006 that committed funding for three major goals related to research, research infrastructure, and public information/community outreach (NIH, 2002). It is clear from the recent healthcare reform actions taken by President Barack Obama that he intends to carry out the mission of improving health care for all. The *Healthy People* objectives are even more important today than when first envisioned.

When Flaskerud et al. (2002) reviewed 79 research reports published in *Nursing Research*, they concluded that although nurse researchers have systematically addressed health disparities, they have tended to ignore certain groups (e.g., indigenous peoples). They also inappropriately lump together as Hispanic members of disparate groups with their own cultural identity (e.g., Puerto Ricans, Mexicans, Cubans, Dominicans).

Aday (2001) emphasized certain groups as vulnerable populations, and the 2010 priorities showcase obvious needs within these groups:

- *High-risk mothers and infants-of-concern.* This population reflects the currently high rates of teenage pregnancy and poor prenatal care, leading to birth-weight problems and infant mortality. Affected groups include very young women, African American women, and poorly educated women, all of whom are less likely than middle-class white women to receive adequate prenatal care due to limited access to services.

- *Chronically ill and disabled persons.* Individuals in this category not only experience higher death rates than comparable middle-class white women as a result of heart disease, cancer, and stroke, but are also subject to prevalent chronic conditions such as hypertension, arthritis, and asthma. The debilitating effects of such chronic diseases lead to lost income resulting from limitations in activities of daily living. African Americans, for example, are more likely to experience ill effects and to die from chronic diseases.
- *Persons living with HIV/AIDS.* In the past decade or so, advances in tracing and treating AIDS have resulted in declines in deaths and increases in the number of people living with HIV/AIDS. This increase is also due, in part, to changes in transmission patterns from largely male homosexual or bisexual contact to transmission through heterosexual contact and sharing needles among intravenous (IV) drug users.
- *Mentally ill and disabled persons.* The population with mental illness is usually defined broadly to include even those individuals with mild anxiety and depression. Prevalence rates are high with age-specific disorders, and severe emotional disorders seriously interfere with activities of daily living and interpersonal relationships.
- *Alcohol and other substance abusers.* The wide array of substances that are abused includes drugs, alcohol, cigarettes, and inhalants (such as glue). Intoxication results in chronic disease, accidents, and, in some cases, criminal activity. Young male adults in their late teens and early twenties are more likely to smoke, drink, and take drugs.
- *Persons exhibiting suicide- or homicide-prone behavior.* Rates of suicide and homicide differ by age, sex, and race, with elderly white and young Native American men being most likely to kill themselves and young African American, Native American, and Hispanic men being most likely to be killed by others.
- *Abusive families.* Children, the elderly, and spouses (overwhelmingly women) are likely targets of violence within the family. Although older children are more likely to be injured, young female children older than 3 years of age are consistently at risk for sexual abuse.
- *Homeless persons.* Because of ongoing problems in identifying this population, it is reasonably certain that the estimated prevalence rates at any given time are low and vary across the country. Generally, more young men are homeless, but all homeless individuals are likely to suffer from chronic diseases and are vulnerable to violence.
- *Immigrants/refugees.* Health care for immigrants, refugees, and temporary residents is complicated by the diversity of languages, health practices, food choices, culturally based definitions of health, and previous experiences with American bureaucracies.

Aday (2001) provided much statistical information for these vulnerable groups, but prevalence rates for specific conditions change periodically. Readers are referred to the website of the National Center for Health Statistics (www.cdc.gov/nchs) for updated information.

Trends in families over the last five decades (the lifetime of the baby boomers) show marked changes in the demographics of families, and these changes in turn affect health disparities. At present, more men and women are delaying marriage, with more people choosing to live together first. Divorce rates are higher, with a concurrent increase in single-parent families.

Out-of-wedlock births have increased, partially due to decreases in marital fertility. There is a sharp and sustained increase in maternal employment (Hofferth, 2003).

INSTITUTE OF MEDICINE STUDY

The U.S. Congress directed the Institute of Medicine (IOM) to study the extent of racial and ethnic differences in health care and to recommend interventions to eliminate health disparities (IOM, 2003). The IOM found consistent evidence of disparities across a wide range of health services and illnesses. Although these racial and ethnic disparities may occur within a wider historical context, they are unacceptable, as the IOM pointed out. It urged a general public acknowledgment of the problem and advocated specific cross-cultural training for health professionals. Other recommendations included specific legal, regulatory, and policy interventions that speak to fairness in access; increases in the number of minority health professionals; and better enforcement of civil rights laws. IOM recommendations with regard to data collection should serve to monitor progress toward the goal of eliminating health disparities based on different treatment for minorities.

VULNERABILITY TO SPECIFIC CONDITIONS OR DISEASES

A large portion of the research that has been done on specific conditions and diseases was generated from psychology data and predates much of the medical and nursing literature on disparities. Researchers on vulnerability to these specific conditions tend to take an individual approach, in that conditions or diseases are treated from the point of view of how a particular individual responds to life stressors and how that response can cause the condition to develop or continue.

Researchers have focused on conditions too numerous to report here, but a search quickly turned up references to alcohol consumption in women and vulnerability to sexual aggression (Testa, Livingston, & Collins, 2000); rape myths and vulnerability to sexual assault (Bohner, Danner, Siebler, & Stamson, 2002); self-esteem and unplanned pregnancy (Smith, Gerrard, & Gibbons, 1997); lung transplantation (Kurz, 2002); coronary angioplasty (Edell-Gustafsson & Hetta, 2001); adjustment to lower limb amputation (Behel, Rybarczyk, Elliott, Nicholas, & Nyenhuis, 2002); reaction to natural disasters (Phifer, 1990); reaction to combat stress (Aldwin, Levensen, & Spiro, 1994; Ruef, Litz, & Schlenger, 2000); homelessness (Morrell-Bellai, Goering, & Boydell, 2000; Shinn, Knickman, & Weitzman, 1991); mental retardation (Nettlebeck, Wison, Potter, & Perry, 2000); anxiety (Calvo & Cano-Vindel, 1997; Strauman, 1992); and suicide (Schotte, Cools, & Payvar, 1990).

Depression

Many authors have focused on cognitive variables in an attempt to explain vulnerability to depression (Alloy & Clements, 1992; Alloy, Whitehouse, & Abramson, 2000; Hayes, Castonguay, & Goldfried, 1996; Ingram & Ritter, 2000). Others have explored gender differences (Bromberger & Mathews, 1996; Soares & Zitek, 2008; Whiffen, 1988). In a major analysis of the existing literature on depression, Hankin and Abramson (2001) explored the development of gender differences in depression. They noted that although both male and female rates of depression rise during middle adolescence, incidence in girls rises more sharply after age 13 or puberty. This model of general depression might account for gender differences based on developmentally specific stressors and implies possible treatment options.

Variables related to attitudes present a third area of focus in the literature (Brown, Hammen, Craske, & Wickens, 1995; Joiner, 1995; Zuroff, Blatt, Bondi, & Pilkonis, 1999). In a study of 75 college students, researchers found that a high level of "perfectionistic achievement attitudes," as indicated on the Dysfunctional Attitude Scale, correlated with a specific stressor (e.g., poorer than expected performance on a college exam) to predict an increase in symptoms of depression (Brown et al., 1995).

Situational factors also produce vulnerability to depression. For example, the stress of providing care to patients with Alzheimer's disease can produce or exacerbate symptoms of depression. In a study of family caregivers of Alzheimer's patients, Neundorfer and colleagues (2006) found that caregivers with prior depressive symptoms were not necessarily more prone to depression than others, but rather that all subjects were more likely to experience depression when the dependency of the patient was high.

Despite the current trend to regulate depression via chemical means, promising evidence suggests that vulnerability to depression can be modified by emotion regulation instruction. Ehring and colleagues (2010) conducted an experiment in which they showed short films with sad content to people with depression as well as a control group. According to the researchers, if subjects were vulnerable to depression, they would spontaneously use dysfunctional emotional regulation strategies, but they were able to use more functional techniques if instructed to do so.

Schizophrenia

Smoking has been observed to be a problem in individuals with schizophrenia, and there is some evidence that smokers have a more serious course of mental illness than nonsmokers. The theory proposed to explain this relationship is that schizophrenic patients smoke as a way to self-medicate (Lohr & Flynn, 1992). In a twin study investigating lifetime prevalence of smoking and nicotine withdrawal, Lyons et al. (2002) found that the association between smoking and schizophrenia may be related to familial vulnerability to schizophrenia.

Other authors have examined the relationship between schizophrenia and personality. This relationship remains largely unexplored, but might provide a new direction in which to search for knowledge about vulnerability to schizophrenia. In their meta-analysis, Berenbaum and Fujita (1994) found a significant relationship between introversion and schizophrenia; they suggested that studies on this link might provide new knowledge about the covariation of schizophrenia with mood disorders, particularly depression. In a thoughtful analysis of the literature on the role of the family in schizophrenia, Wuerker (2000) presented evidence for the biological view, concluding that there is a unique vulnerability to stress in schizophrenic patients and that communication difficulties within families with schizophrenic members may be due to a shared genetic heritage.

Eating Disorders

Acknowledgment of food as a common focus for anxiety has become a way of life. Canadian researchers refer to "food insecurity" to describe the phenomenon of nutritional vulnerability resulting from food scarcity and insufficient access to food by welfare recipients and low-income people who do not qualify for welfare (McIntyre, Glanville, Raine, Dayle, Anderson, & Battaglia, 2003; Tarasuk, 2003). In the United States, eating disorders are often a result of body image problems, which are particularly prevalent in gay men and heterosexual women (Siever, 1994). In a prospective study of gender and behavioral vulnerabilities related to eating disorders, Leon, Fulkerson, Perry, and Early-Zaid (1995) found significant differences among girls in the variables of weight loss, dieting patterns, vomiting, and use of diet pills. They reported a method for predicting the occurrence of eating disorders based on performance scores on risk-factor status tests in early childhood.

HIV/AIDS

In a meta-analysis of 32 HIV/AIDS studies involving 15,440 participants, Gerrard, Gibbons, and Bushman (1996) found empirical evidence to support the commonly known motivational hypothesis. This hypothesis is derived from the Health Belief Model (Becker & Rosenstock, 1987). The authors found that perceived vulnerability was the major force behind prevention behavior in high-risk populations but cautioned that studies were not available for low-risk populations. They also discovered that risk behavior shapes perceptions of vulnerability—that is, people who engage in high-risk behavior tend to see themselves as more likely to contract HIV than those who engage in low-risk behavior.

Evidence that high-risk men tend to relapse into unsafe sex behaviors is provided in a longitudinal study of results of an intervention in which researchers were able to successfully predict relapse behavior (Kelly, St. Lawrence, & Brasfield, 1991). In a gender study on emotional distress predictors, Van Servellen, Aguirre, Sarna, and Brecht (2002) found that although all subjects had scores indicating clinical anxiety levels, HIV-infected women had more symptoms and poorer functioning than HIV-infected men.

In a study that used a vulnerable populations framework, Flaskerud and Lee (2001) considered the role that resource availability plays in the health status of informal female caregivers of people with HIV/AIDS ($n = 36$) and age-related dementias ($n = 40$). Not surprisingly, the caregivers experienced high levels of both physical and mental health problems. However, the use of the vulnerable populations framework explained the finding that the resource variables of income and minority ethnicity made the greatest contribution to understanding health status. In terms of the risk variables, anger was more common in caregivers for HIV-infected patients and was significantly related to depressive mood, which was also common among these caregivers.

Gender differences among HIV-infected people can exacerbate their response to the disease. Murray et al. (2009) interviewed Zambian women infected with HIV about their reasons for taking or not taking antiretroviral drugs. The key informants revealed fears of abandonment by their husbands, a decision to stop the medications when they felt better, choosing instead to die, and fear of having to take medications for the rest of their lives. These women are vulnerable not only to the disease but also to their family's reaction; the barriers to taking medication that could save their lives may be overshadowed by these risks, making them even more vulnerable.

Substance Abuse

In a study of 288 undergraduates, Wild, Hinson, Cunningham, and Bacchiochi (2001) examined the inconsistencies between a person's perceived risk of alcohol-related harm and motivation to reduce that risk. These researchers found a general tendency for people to view themselves as less vulnerable than their peers regardless of their risk status; notably, however, the at-risk group rated themselves more likely to experience harm than the not-at-risk group. The authors concluded that motivational approaches to reducing risk should emphasize not only why people drink but also why they should reduce alcohol consumption. Additional support for the motivational hypothesis—that perceived vulnerability influences prevention behavior—extends to marijuana use (Simons & Carey, 2002) and to early onset of substance abuse among African American children (Wills, Gibbons, Gerrard, & Brody, 2000).

Finally, in a study of family history of psychopathology in families of the offspring of alcoholics, researchers demonstrated that male college student offspring of these families are a heterogeneous group and that the patterns of heterogeneity are related to familial types in relation to vulnerability to alcoholism. Three different family types were identified:

- Low levels of family pathology with moderate levels of alcoholism
- High levels of family antisocial personality and violence with moderate levels of family drug abuse and depression
- High levels of familial depression, mania, anxiety disorder, and alcoholism with moderate levels of familial drug abuse (Finn, Sharkansky, Viken, West, Sandy, & Bufferd, 1997)

Students as a Vulnerable Population

The April 2007 shootings at Virginia Tech highlighted the fact that college students in the United States face a relatively new kind of threat, much as the Columbine tragedy did for high school students. Alienated young people who stalk and kill their classmates, for whatever reasons seem logical to them, represent a new type of terrorist. Yet, the literature has not documented either the experience of these alienated students, nor have we found effective ways of treating and preventing violent behavior among them.

Some attempts have been made to document types of violence toward students. The American College Health Association (ACHA) recently published a white paper on the topic (Carr, 2007). This paper largely focuses on the most frequent types of student-directed violence, such as sexual assault, hazing, suicide, celebratory violence, and racial/gender/sexual orientation–based violence. While spree killings are mentioned, not much attention can be given until more is known about these killers.

Some attention has been given to the relationship between alcohol use and violence. Marcus and Swett (2003) studied precursors to violence among 451 college students at two sites and used the Violence Risk Assessment tool to establish the relationship of patterns related to gender, peer pressure, and alcohol use. Nicholson and colleagues (1998) examined the influence of alcohol use in both sexual and nonsexual violence.

A British study on responding to students' mental health needs illustrates how the previously discussed categories of mental illnesses can be exacerbated in the vulnerable population of college students with mental illnesses. Using surveys and focus groups, Stanley and Manthorpe (2001) assessed college students with mental illnesses and identified many issues related to the problems of providing care to students. The authors noted that high rates of suicide and need for antidepressant medication strained the National Health Service's resources and that colleges varied widely in their ability to provide effective interventions.

While these studies document some issues related to campus violence, they do not go far enough to explain and prevent the types of spree killings students have experienced in the last decade. The threat of copycat attacks has engendered continuing fears among students, parents, and teachers alike. More research is needed on personal characteristics of these young killers, potential interventions, and prevention strategies.

CONCLUSION

A growing body of literature has focused on the concept of vulnerability as a key factor of concern to practitioners who work with clients with many different kinds of presenting problems. Vulnerability may be explored on two levels, in that vulnerability is both an individual concept and a group concept. In public health, the group concept is dominant, and intervention is directed toward aggregates. Other practitioners and researchers focus on individual vulnerabilities to specific conditions or diseases. When working with clients from "vulnerable populations," it is critical to understand that they might not view themselves as vulnerable and may actually resent labels that imply they are not autonomous.

WWW

For a full suite of assignments and additional learning activities, use the access code located in the front of your book to visit this exclusive website: http://go.jblearning.com/dechesnay. If you do not have an access code, you can obtain one at the site.

REFERENCES

Aday, L. (2001). *At risk in America.* San Francisco, CA: Jossey-Bass.

Aldwin, C., Levensen, M., & Spiro, A. (1994). Vulnerability and resilience to combat exposure: Can stress have lifelong effects? *Psychology and Aging, 9*, 34–44.

Alloy, L., & Clements, C. (1992). Illusion of control invulnerability to negative affect and depressive symptoms after laboratory and natural stressors. *Journal of Abnormal Psychology, 101*, 234–245.

Alloy, L., Whitehouse, W., & Abramson, J. (2000). The Temple-Wisconsin Cognitive Vulnerability to Depression Project: Lifetime history of axis I psychopathology in individuals at high and low cognitive risk for depression. *Journal of Abnormal Psychology, 109*, 403–418.

Becker, M., & Rosenstock, I. (1987). Comparing social learning theory and the health belief model. In W. B. Ward (Ed.), *Advances in health education and promotion* (Vol. 2, pp. 245–249). Greenwich, CT: JAI Press.

Behel, J., Rybarczyk, B., Elliott, T., Nicholas, J., & Nyenhuis, D. (2002). The role of perceived vulnerability in adjustment to lower extremity amputation: A preliminary investigation. *Rehabilitation Psychology, 47*(1), 92–105.

Berenbaum, H., & Fujita, F. (1994). Schizophrenia and personality: Exploring the boundaries and connections between vulnerability and outcome. *Journal of Abnormal Psychology, 103*, 148–158.

Bezruchka, S. (2000). Culture and medicine: Is globalization dangerous to our health? *Western Journal of Medicine, 172*, 332–334.

Bezruchka, S. (2001). Societal hierarchy and the health Olympics. *Canadian Medical Association Journal, 164*, 1701–1703.

Bohner, G., Danner, U., Siebler, F., & Stamson, G. (2002). Rape myth acceptance and judgments of vulnerability to sexual assault: An Internet experiment. *Experimental Psychology, 49*, 257–269.

Bromberger, J., & Mathews, K. (1996). A "feminine" model of vulnerability to depressive symptoms: A longitudinal investigation of middle-aged women. *Journal of Personality and Social Psychology, 70*, 591–598.

Brown, G., Hammen, C., Craske, M., & Wickens, T. (1995). Dimensions of dysfunctional attitudes as vulnerabilities to depressive symptoms. *Journal of Abnormal Psychology, 104*, 431–435.

Calvo, M., & Cano-Vindel, A. (1997). The nature of trait anxiety: Cognitive and biological vulnerability. *European Psychologist, 2*, 301–312.

Carr, J. (2007). Campus violence white paper. *Journal of American College Health, 55*(5), 304–319.

Edell-Gustafsson, U., & Hetta, J. (2001). Fragmented sleep and tiredness in males and females one year after percutaneous transluminal coronary angioplasty (PTCA). *Journal of Advanced Nursing, 34*(2), 203–211.

Ehring, J., Tuschen-Caffier, B., Schulke, J., Fischer, S., & Gross, J. (2010). Emotion regulation and vulnerability to depression: Spontaneous versus instructed suppression and reappraisal. *Emotion, 10*(4), 563–572. Doi: 10.1037/a0019010

Finn, P., Sharkansky, E., Viken, R., West, T., Sandy, J., & Bufferd, G. (1997). Heterogeneity in the families of sons of alcoholics: The impact of familial vulnerability type on offspring characteristics. *Journal of Abnormal Psychology, 106*, 26–36.

Flaskerud, J., & Lee, P. (2001). Vulnerability to health problems in female informal caregivers of persons with HIV/AIDS and age-related dementias. *Journal of Advanced Nursing, 33*(1), 60–68.

Flaskerud, J., Lesser, J., Dixon, E., Anderson, N., Conde, F., Kim, S., . . . Koniak-Griffin, D. (2002). Health disparities among vulnerable populations: Evolution of knowledge over five decades in *Nursing Research* publications. *Nursing Research, 51*(2), 74–85.

Flaskerud, J., & Winslow, B. (1998). Conceptualizing vulnerable populations in health-related research. *Nursing Research, 47*(2), 69–78.

Gellad, W., Huskamp, H., Phillips, K., & Haas, J. (2006). How the new Medicare drug benefit could affect vulnerable populations. *Health Affairs, 25*(1), 248–255.

Gerrard, M., Gibbons, F., & Bushman, B. (1996). Relation between perceived vulnerability to HIV and precautionary sexual behavior. *Psychological Bulletin, 119*, 390–409.

Hankin, B., & Abramson, L. (2001). Development of gender differences in depression: An elaborated cognitive vulnerability-transactional stress theory. *Psychological Bulletin, 127*, 773–796.

Hayes, A., Castonguay, L., & Goldfried, M. (1996). Effectiveness of targeting the vulnerability factors of depression in cognitive therapy. *Journal of Consulting and Clinical Psychology, 64*, 623–627.

Hofferth, S. (2003). The American family: Changes and challenges for the 21st century. In H. Wallace, G. Green, & K. Jaros (Eds.). *Health and welfare for families in the 21st century.* (pp. 71–79). Sudbury, MA: Jones and Bartlett.

Ingram, R., & Ritter, J. (2000). Vulnerability to depression: Cognitive reactivity and parental bonding in high-risk individuals. *Journal of Abnormal Psychology, 109*, 588–596.

Institute of Medicine (IOM), National Academy of Sciences. (2003) Unequal treatment: Confronting racial and ethnic disparities in health care. Retrieved February 20, 2004, from www.nap.edu

Joiner, T. (1995). The price of soliciting and receiving negative feedback: Self-verification theory as a vulnerability to depression. *Journal of Abnormal Psychology, 104*, 364–372.

Karpati, A., Galea, S., Awerbuch, T., & Levins, R. (2002). Variability and vulnerability at the ecological level: Implications for understanding the social determinants of health. *American Journal of Public Health, 92*, 1768–1773.

Kelly, J., St. Lawrence, J., & Brasfield, T. (1991). Predictors of vulnerability to AIDS risk behavior relapse. *Journal of Consulting and Clinical Psychology, 59*(1), 163–166.

Kurz, J. M. (2002). Vulnerability of well spouses involved in lung transplantation. *Journal of Family Nursing, 8*, 353–370.

Larkin, H. (2004). Justice implications of a proposed Medicare prescription drug benefit. *Social Work, 49*(3), 406–414.

Leon, G., Fulkerson, J., Perry, C., & Early-Zaid, M. (1995). Prospective analysis of personality and behavioral vulnerabilities and gender influences in the later development of disordered eating. *Journal of Abnormal Psychology, 104*(1), 140–149.

Lessick, M., Woodring, B., Naber, S., & Halstead, L. (1992). Vulnerability: A conceptual model. *Perinatal and Neonatal Nursing, 6*, 1–14.

Lohr, J., & Flynn, K. (1992). Smoking and schizophrenia. *Schizophrenia Research, 8*, 93–102.

Lyons, M., Bar, J., Kremen, W., Toomey, R., Eisen, S., Goldberg, J., . . . Tsuang, M. (2002). Nicotine and familial vulnerability to schizophrenia: A discordant twin study. *Journal of Abnormal Psychology, 111*, 687–693.

Marcus, R., & Swett, B. (2003). Multiple precursor scenarios: Predicting and reducing campus violence. *Journal of Interpersonal Violence, 18*(5), 553–571.

McIntyre, L., Glanville, N., Raine, K., Dayle, J., Anderson, B., & Battaglia, N. (2003). Do low-income lone mothers compromise their nutrition to feed their children? *Canadian Medical Association Journal, 168*(6), 686–691.

Morrell-Bellai, T., Goering, P., & Boydell, K. (2000). Becoming and remaining homeless: Qualitative investigation. *Issues in Mental Health Nursing, 21*, 581–604.

Murray, L., Semrau, K., McCurley, E., Thea, D., Scott, N., Mwiya, M., . . . Bolton, P. (2009). Barriers to acceptance and adherence of antiretroviral therapy in urban Zambian women: A qualitative study. *AIDS Care, 21*(1), 78–86. Doi: 10.1080/09540120802032643

National Institutes of Health (NIH). (n.d.). Addressing health disparities: The NIH program of action. Retrieved December 4, 2003, from http://healthdisparities.nih.gov/whatare.html

National Institutes of Health (NIH). (2002). *Strategic research plan and budget to reduce and ultimately eliminate health disparities.* Washington, DC: US Department of Health and Human Services.

Nettlebeck, T., Wison, C., Potter, R., & Perry, C. (2000). The influence of interpersonal competence on personal vulnerability of persons with mental retardation. *Journal of Interpersonal Violence, 15*(1), 46–62.

Neundorfer, M., McLendon, M., Smyth, K., Strauss, M., & McCallum, T. (2006). Does depression prior to caregiving increase vulnerability to depressive symptoms among caregivers of persons with Alzheimer's disease? *Aging and Mental Health, 10*(6), 606–615.

Nicholson, M., Maney, D., Blair, K., Wamboldt, P., Mahoney, B., & Yuan, J. (1998). Trends in alcohol-related campus violence: Implications for prevention. *Journal of Alcohol and Drug Education, 43*(3), 34–52.

Phifer, J. (1990). Psychological distress and somatic symptoms after natural disaster: Differential vulnerability among older adults. *Psychology and Aging, 5*, 412–420.

Ruef, A., Litz, B., & Schlenger, W. (2000). Hispanic ethnicity and risk for combat-related posttraumatic stress disorder. *Cultural Diversity and Ethnic Minority Psychology, 6*(3), 235–251.

Scanlon, A., & Lee, G. (2007). The use of the term vulnerability in acute care: Why does it differ and what does it mean? *Australian Journal of Advanced Nursing, 24*(3), 54–59.

Schotte, D., Cools, J., & Payvar, S. (1990). Problem-solving deficits in suicidal patients: Trait vulnerability or state phenomenon? *Journal of Consulting and Clinical Psychology, 58*, 562–564.

Sebastian, J. (1996). Vulnerability and vulnerable populations. In M. Stanhope & J. Lancaster (Eds.), *Community health nursing: Promoting health of individuals, aggregates and communities* (4th ed.) (pp. 403–417). St. Louis, MO: Mosby.

Sebastian, J., Bolla, C. D., Aretakis, D., Jones, K. J., Schenk, C., & Napolitano, M. (2002). Vulnerability and selected vulnerable populations. In M. Stanhope & J. Lancaster (Eds.). *Foundations of community health nursing* (pp. 349–364). St. Louis, MO: Mosby.

Shinn, M., Knickman, J., & Weitzman, B. (1991). Social relationships and vulnerability to becoming homeless among poor families. *American Psychologist, 46*, 1180–1187.

Siever, M. (1994). Sexual orientation and gender as factors in socioculturally acquired vulnerability to body dissatisfaction and eating disorders. *Journal of Consulting and Clinical Psychology, 62*(2), 252–260.

Simons, J., & Carey, K. (2002). Risk and vulnerability for marijuana use: Problems and the role of affect dysregulation. *Psychology of Addictive Behaviors, 16*(1), 72–75.

Smith, G., Gerrard, M., & Gibbons, F. (1997). Self-esteem and the relation between risk behavior and perceptions of vulnerability to unplanned pregnancy in college women. *Health Psychology, 16*(2), 137–146.

Soares, C. N., & Zitek, B. (2008). Reproductive hormone sensitivity and risk for depression across the female life cycle: A continuum for vulnerability? Journal *of Psychiatry and Neuroscience, 33*(4), 331–343.

Spiers, J. (2000). New perspectives on vulnerability using etic and emic approaches. *Journal of Advanced Nursing, 31*(3), 715–721.

Stanley, N., & Manthorpe, J. (2001). Responding to students' mental health needs: Impermeable systems and diverse users. *Journal of Mental Health, 10*, 41–52.

Strauman, T. (1992). Self-guides, autobiographical memory, and anxiety and dysphoria: Toward a cognitive model of vulnerability to emotional distress. *Journal of Abnormal Psychology, 101*, 87–95.

Tarasuk, V. (2003). Low income, welfare and nutritional vulnerability. *Canadian Medical Association Journal, 168*, 709–710.

Testa, M., Livingston, J., & Collins, R. (2000). The role of women's alcohol consumption in evaluation of vulnerability to sexual aggression. *Experimental and Clinical Psychopharmacology, 8*(2), 185–191.

Van Servellen, G., Aguirre, M., Sarna, L., & Brecht, M. (2002). Differential predictors of emotional distress in HIV-infected men and women. *Western Journal of Nursing Research, 24*(1), 49–72.

Whiffen, V. (1988). Vulnerability to post-partum depression: A prospective multivariate study. *Journal of Abnormal Psychology, 97*, 467–474.

Wild, T. C., Hinson, R., Cunningham, J., & Bacchiochi, J. (2001). Perceived vulnerability to alcohol-related harm in young adults: Independent effects of risky alcohol use and drinking motives. *Experimental and Clinical Psychopharmacology, 9*, 1064–1297.

Wills, T. A., Gibbons, F., Gerrard, M., & Brody, G. (2000). Protection and vulnerability processes relevant for early onset of substance use: A test among African American children. *Health Psychology, 19*(3), 253–263.

World Health Organization. (1948). Constitution.Geneva, Switzerland.

Wuerker, A. (2000). The family and schizophrenia. *Issues in Mental Health Nursing, 21*, 127–141.

Zuroff, D., Blatt, S., Bondi, C., & Pilkonis, P. (1999). Vulnerability to depression: Reexamining state dependence and relative stability. *Journal of Abnormal Psychology, 108*, 76–89.

CHAPTER 2

Advocacy Role of Providers

Mary de Chesnay and Vanessa Robinson-Dooley

INTRODUCTION

Objectives

At the end of this chapter, the reader will be able to

1. Compare and contrast the concept of advocacy from the points of view of nursing and social work.
2. Identify key features of the role of patient advocate.
3. Provide an analysis of one's own patient cases from the point of view of the social worker or nurse.

People are vulnerable to illness, injury, and psychological trauma in many contexts of their lives and it would seem they should be safe in the arms of their healthcare providers. Nothing could be further from the truth. As healthcare practitioners, we sometimes believe that we know best and, although we often do know best technically, we do not always frame our interventions in consultation with our clients, nor do we consult with one another for the good of the client. The political nature of health care means that we often make decisions for the good of the organization rather than for the good of the patient. An example of this kind of decision making is limiting visiting hours in intensive care units. In the old days, visits by family members were limited to 5 minutes every hour, justified on the basis that staff members were too busy caring for patients to deal with visitors. Now hours are more liberal even though patient acuity levels are higher.

Written by a nurse and a social worker, this chapter describes advocacy as a team effort and demonstrates through case studies how the practitioner can function as an advocate and how a team of healthcare professionals can work together for the good of their clients. The literatures in nursing and social work are reviewed separately because the roles of each professional are distinct in most ways. The case studies bring the two disciplines together to show how the roles can complement each other. We hope that readers will be inspired to look for ways in which to collaborate—to bring the skills and talents of many disciplines together for the sake of the patients, all of whom are vulnerable when they need our services.

REVIEW OF THE NURSING LITERATURE

The Concept of Patient Advocacy

The nursing literature on patient advocacy seems to be divided into conceptualization of advocacy (Hyland, 2002) and role functions of an advocate. Bu and Jewesky (2006) conducted a concept analysis of patient advocacy by using Walker and Avant's (1995) procedure. The concept analysis generated a mid-range theory with three attributes of patient advocacy: safeguarding autonomy, acting on the patient's behalf, and championing social justice. These attributes give recognition to the vulnerability of patients, the need for some protection within the healthcare system while respecting autonomy, and the international recognition of the role of patient advocate.

The attributes described here are consistent with the role of advocate that institutional review boards (IRBs) play in research involving human and animal subjects. The federal regulations for composition of IRBs mandate inclusion of lay members specifically for the purpose of keeping researchers honest by ensuring that investigators consider the needs of the study population and effects of the study on the people who participate. Mmatli (2009) goes even further in his paper on including people with disabilities in evidence-based research, by arguing that such individuals need to be involved not only in designing studies but also in making decisions about application of the research.

In a critical review of the nursing literature on advocacy, Mallik (1997) argued that the literature lacks clarity in the operationalization of the concept of advocacy, suggesting that authors tend to focus more on defending the role of advocate than on explaining it. Historical reasons for justifying the need for the role are explained by cultural shifts in the roles of physicians and patients' rights. Over time, distrust of experts and technology created a climate of fear, resulting in a higher level of participation by patients in decision making about their own care. The result was creation of a Patient's Bill of Rights and the role of patient advocate (Annas, 1988).

Annas also believed that the nurse is in an ideal position to serve as an advocate (Annas & Healey, 1974). Nurses have certainly filled this role quite ably, and there are many examples of nurses taking on healthcare organizations as whistleblowers. Nevertheless, members of other disciplines may also serve as effective advocates. For example, social workers might be even more effective than nurses in this role because they do not act directly in the medical care of patients and do not participate in historical doctor–nurse games. Even so, to claim the role for any one discipline is not only disrespectful to our colleagues in health care, but self-serving and inconsistent with the spirit of advocacy.

In a provocative paper discussing advocacy, Zomorodi and Foley (2009) clarified the thin line between advocacy and paternalism. As healthcare providers who are experts in the treatment of disease, we can easily cross the line between speaking for a patient's right to self-determination and deciding we know what is best for the patient. In fact, this is an occupational hazard for nurses and physicians. Consider the case of a 45-year-old small business owner hospitalized for myocardial infarction. His heart attack comes the day his most trusted employee resigns and the night before a major sales presentation. If he does not get the contract, his business could go under. Because he is the breadwinner, his wife and five children are also at risk if he cannot work. The patient recovers nicely from the acute episode and is in the ICU asking for a phone to make some calls to explain his absence at the meeting. The staff knows that rest and medications are the best treatment and that he should not be upset by anything. They assume that allowing him to talk about business would place him at risk for another heart attack. Unfortunately, denying him the use of the phone causes his anxiety to escalate, which creates a paradoxical effect: His heart rate increases and his blood pressure skyrockets as he sees his life's work destroyed for lack of 10 minutes' access to a phone.

The paternalistic approach is particularly prevalent in settings in which multidisciplinary teams are used to deliver patient care. While nurses tend to use the language of advocacy, physicians often use the language of medical decision making (McGrath, Holewa, & McGrath, 2006). As one physician put it, "Of course, we are a team and I am the captain."

The Role of Patient Advocate

Pullen (1995) makes the case that the role of nurse as advocate is essential to modern health care as a result of paternalism in health care. Paternalism reduces the patient to a passive recipient of care and forces the patient to depend on the integrity and self-regulation of the providers. Yet, patients are often unable to make decisions for themselves without help, either owing to ignorance of their own complex health issues or because of temporary incapacitation. The nurse as advocate can play a major role in helping patients regain autonomy. In the example described earlier, the nurse as advocate might have offered to stay near the monitoring equipment in the nurses' station while the patient made the call to make sure he would be safe.

Just as community-based participatory action research enables communities to generate relevant knowledge to benefit their own people, so patient advocacy groups can benefit healthcare consumers. Lara and Salberg (2009) describe how advocacy groups may play a role in health policy by linking patients and consumer of healthcare services with policy makers. Patients, for their part, have realized that they can serve as their own advocates. As a consequence, they are increasingly educating themselves by searching the Internet for information on their diseases or symptoms and coming to appointments armed with more sophisticated questions for which they demand answers.

Further support for the value of partnerships between patients or consumers and providers comes from a study of 405 patients and 118 nurses in 12 hospital units in Finland. Vaartio, Leino-Kilpi, Suominen, and Puukka (2009) found that patients varied in their acts of advocacy and nurses applied principles of advocacy in a haphazard way when caring for patients with postsurgical pain. They concluded that patients perceived care as being good most of the time but not all of the time, while nurses were quite content with their level of advocacy. The explanation for the patients' perception was that either they were not asked about their preferences or they did not know to ask. At any rate, this lack of participation can be construed as a failure of nurses to provide sufficient information about options for patients and to invite patients to participate more fully in decision making.

In a survey of 5000 medical–surgical nurses registered in the state of Texas, Hanks (2010) found that certain role behaviors were most often cited by the nurses when describing their role as advocates. Education of patients and families emerged as the key response, closely followed by communicating with others on the team and ensuring adequate care. Issues of safety and ensuring that patients' rights were protected were also considered important responsibilities for advocates.

While it is clear that communicating effectively is a key component of effective patient advocacy, little has been done to determine what effective communication in advocacy looks like. In a grounded theory study of 12 nurses at 8 Midwestern hospitals, Martin and Tipton (2007) used the constant comparative method to develop a typology of communication roles that included liaison, feedback remediation, counseling and support, system monitor, troubleshooter, investigator, and group facilitator. An example of the liaison role is communicating with the physician on behalf of patient and family. Feedback remediation includes informing nurses when their behavior toward a patient indicates a less than therapeutic approach. Counseling and support include behaviors such as providing refreshments as well as the traditional counseling activities of listening and problem solving. System monitoring is an important action in terms of environmental issues such as poor room temperature. The troubleshooter makes sure that problems are resolved immediately, sometimes through informal connections such as calling the pharmacy to hurry a prescription. When serious problems occur, the investigator takes action to discover the causes and fix them. Finally, the group facilitator holds meetings with family members, staff, and physicians with families to make difficult decisions such as those involving end-of-life care.

The literature seems clear about role functions and behaviors of nurses who are successful advocates—but how did they get to be so effective? Advocacy is learned behavior, implying the importance of teaching role behaviors to students. In a synthesis of qualitative studies from 1993–2005, MacDonald (2006) found that, while advocacy is a complex concept, it can be studied within the context of relational ethics and, therefore, can be learned. Case studies can help students identify the "authentic" wishes of the patient by helping students to clarify their own values as they learn to help patients clarify theirs.

REVIEW OF THE SOCIAL WORK LITERATURE

Definitions

Advocacy has been defined in numerous ways within the social work literature. It has been called one of the "cornerstone" activities of the profession (Clark, 2007, p. 3). Even though advocacy is often viewed as one of the major roles for the generalist social worker, Dorfman (1996) states that advocacy is also the role of the clinical social worker. The *Encyclopedia of Social Work* defines advocacy as the "act of directly representing, defending, intervening, supporting or recommending a course of action on behalf of one or more individuals, groups, or communities, with the goal of securing or retaining social justice" (Hoefer, 2006, p. 8; Mickelson, 1995, p. 95).

The *Social Work Dictionary* defines advocacy as the "act of directly representing or defending others" (Barker, 1995, p. 11; Hoefer, 2006, p. 8). Both definitions speak to what social workers do in their roles as advocates.

Lens (2004) noted that advocacy could be viewed from the perspective of the activity that the individual is performing. Activities such as brokering, case advocacy, and cause advocacy are all part of social work practice (Lens, 2004). Pierce (1984) defined "class advocacy" as a form of advocacy in which social workers use their training and skills to influence social policies and programs that are created to assist a particular group or potential client. Class advocacy is an activity that is addressed in social workers' professional code of ethics (Brawley, 1997). This form of advocacy focuses on ensuring that clients receive services they are entitled to in the human service arena (Sheafor & Horejsi, 2003). Sosin and Caulum (1983) defined advocacy through "activities" when they sought to conceptualize advocacy by involving the actions of three social actors: the advocate, the client, and the decision maker. This conceptualization resulted in advocacy being defined as the following:

> An attempt, having as greater than zero probability of success, by an individual or group to influence another individual or group to make a decision that would not have been made otherwise and that concerns the welfare or interests of a third party who is in a less powerful status than the decision maker. (p. 13)

Advocacy has also been defined in the literature as an action that is defined by the setting in which it is performed. Schneider and Lester (2000) note that advocacy involves the relationship between the client and a particular system and the social worker working to influence the decision-making process on behalf of the client. Hospitals are a familiar setting for social workers and their advocacy efforts. Advocacy in this setting involves the social worker intervening on behalf of the patient to access needed resources when the organization is not meeting his or her needs (Faust, 2008).

In spite of the varying definitions of advocacy found in the literature, it is clear that the meanings are similar and that advocacy is an important role for the social worker (Gilbert & Specht, 1976; Lynch & Mitchell, 1995; Sosin & Caulum, 1983), both today and historically.

A Brief History of Advocacy and Social Work

Advocacy has been an integral part of the social work profession since its inception. Such advocacy efforts have usually occurred in response to the social needs of the time.

During the Civil War era and World War I, for example, social work focused on responding to the major industrialization changes of this time period. Issues such as working hours, work conditions, and safety became the focus of the advocacy efforts of social workers (Kirst-Ashman & Hull, 2009). The increased migration from rural areas all over the United States to larger cities was fueled by the hopes of prosperity through employment. Individuals came from these rural areas with dreams of finding work in cities, but instead were often met with overcrowded neighborhoods and living conditions that promoted health concerns for many (Kirst-Ashman & Hull, 2009). The settlement house movement of the 1880s represented a response to these poor inner-city living conditions. Settlement houses were places where religious leaders and others moved into neighborhoods to interact with the poor and "advocate for child labor laws, women's suffrage, public housing, and public health" (Smith, 1995, p. 2130).

In contrast to the settlement movement, the Charity Organization Societies (COS) of the early 1900s focused on "curing individuals rather than on empowering communities" (Kirst-Ashman & Hull, 2009, p. 35). Faust (2008) observed that during the early period of the CSO, at the turn of the twentieth century, these "friendly visitors" were concerned with the current social conditions. Although their work sought to address what were perceived as "moral deficiencies" at that time, the ensuing activities, discussions, and work focused on eradicating the wretched conditions that plagued urban cities (Faust, 2008; Miley, O'Melia, M. & DuBois, 2009). As Gilbert and Specht (1976) point out, this attention to therapeutic and clinical interventions prevailed as the major theme of social work from 1935 to 1960.

Although advocacy was a part of the profession long before this time, it became an especially prominent activity of social workers in the 1960s (Gilbert & Specht, 1976). The turbulent 1960s were the period of the civil rights movement, and the pressures for social justice exerted as part of that movement reaffirmed social workers' need to focus on advocacy as a profession (Gilbert & Specht, 1976). "The 1960s produced a new focus on social change versus individual pathology" (Kirst-Ashman & Hull, 2009, p. 36), which required the social work profession to revisit its earlier days of working to empower clients and move beyond therapeutic interventions. In 1969, an Ad Hoc Committee on Advocacy publication included four major papers addressing the need for advocacy-related work in social work (Gilbert & Specht, 1976). The significance of this committee was that it was established by the national organization for the social work profession, the National Association of Social Workers (NASW) Task Force on the Urban Crisis and Public Welfare Problems. "The Ad Hoc Committee of NASW reminded social workers of their social obligation [to advocacy]" (Faust, 2008, p. 293). The National Association of Social Workers (NASW) has, throughout the years, continued to affirm the importance of advocacy for the social work profession. The NASW Code of Ethics (NASW, 1994) details the responsibilities of social workers, including the responsibility to work to "promote general welfare and social justice" (Lynch & Mitchell, 1995, p. 9).

Thus advocacy on behalf of clients has been an important role of social workers for more than 130 years. Advocating on behalf of clients has historically been the responsibility of social workers whether they are working as case workers, general practitioners, researchers, or clinical social workers. Advocacy has come to be something that all social workers are expected to incorporate into their professional role and identity (Gilbert & Specht, 1976, p. 288).

INTERDISCIPLINARY BENEFITS AND APPROACH

In a world where social service organizations have seen their budgets shrink, staff diminished, and ability to provide services cut due to difficult economic times, the interdisciplinary approach to providing services has become even more essential. Working to provide services in an era characterized by limited resources has resulted in clients working with multiple agencies and multiple professions. In this challenging environment, an interdisciplinary team approach to service provision is the best approach.

Social work and the nursing profession are well suited to be in the forefront of the interdisciplinary service provision movement. Compartmentalized problem focus by clients is often a result of having to seek services from multiple organizations. The interdisciplinary team approach to service lessens compartmentalization of problems by clients and can be found in many mental health and medical settings (Johnson, 1995). "Medical settings also make use of the interdisciplinary team approach in providing for both the psychosocial and the physical needs of the patients; diagnostic centers also make considerable use of this type of team approach" (p. 119). When agencies work together and take an interdisciplinary team approach to helping, the client recognizes, respects, and benefits from this approach. Most importantly, the professions and social service community ensure the most effective and efficient use of public resources.

CASE STUDIES

WWW Case 1: Mrs. Smith

Laura Smith is a 24-year-old mother of three who lives in a one-room motel unit and works at a low-paying waitress job at a local café. Although the restaurant chain where she works offers health insurance, she cannot qualify because she is scheduled to work 29 hours per week.

Recently, one of Mrs. Smith's children developed a cough and fever. Mrs. Smith was able to have her child seen at the local emergency room, but the treatment was limited such that it covered only enough medication for three days of treatment. Mrs. Smith was told she should follow up with the child's primary care physician and have some testing done to confirm that the cough was not something more serious. The emergency room doctor also recommended that her child receive a vaccine that might prevent future problems. Mrs. Smith explained to the doctor that she did not have a regular physician or insurance, and she could not afford to pay out of pocket for vaccine or any future doctor visits. The emergency room doctor made a referral to the social work department in the hospital and asked if someone could assist Mrs. Smith with accessing resources to get her medical needs met. The emergency room nurse, who had been working with Mrs. Smith and her son, completed the referral to the social work department and asked the social worker to come and meet with Mrs. Smith as soon as possible given Mrs. Smith's limited flexibility with her employer.

The social worker came to the emergency room and met with Mrs. Smith and her child. The emergency room nurse remained in the room because Mrs. Smith was becoming agitated and nervous about the numerous individuals asking her for personal and medical information during this hospital visit. The nurse thought her presence might provide Mrs. Smith with a sense of consistency and assist with calming her fears about the presence of the social worker.

The social worker met with Mrs. Smith and collected background information about her current home environment, employment, and potential social support network. After determining that Mrs. Smith would need some community resources beyond what the hospital could provide, the social worker and the nurse met to discuss community agencies that might be able to assist Mrs. Smith and her family. The nurse recalled the opening of a community health clinic about one mile from the motel where Mrs. Smith resided. Given the proximity to Mrs. Smith's current home, this was an ideal option for follow-up for her child's medical needs. The social worker agreed to make a call to the clinic to determine if Mrs. Smith might qualify for services.

The social worker was told by the clinic staff that the clinic provided services to families underinsured or uninsured. The clinic also had a sliding-scale policy that it used if families could afford to pay only a small amount. Mrs. Smith was referred to the clinic and received the following services:

1. Mrs. Smith was scheduled to come to the clinic and complete her intake and income assessment paperwork. A social work intern student was assigned to assist her with completing her paperwork.
2. Mrs. Smith's son was seen by the nurse practitioner to evaluate his cough and other symptoms.
3. It was recommended to Mrs. Smith that she be given a brief physical examination, as that she had not been seen by a doctor for several years. Her primary focus had been work and her children, and it was suggested that a physical might provide Mrs. Smith with some knowledge about her own health status. Her physical examination was completed by the nurse practitioner.
4. The social worker at the clinic asked Mrs. Smith if there were any other areas in which she might need assistance. Mrs. Smith stated that she could use some assistance with housing, employment, and food. The social worker and the social work intern provided Mrs. Smith with a contact name and direct number for the local housing authority to determine if she would qualify for assistance with Section 8 housing (housing assistance provided to families meeting federal guidelines). Mrs. Smith was also provided with a referral for a food bank (in the same building as the clinic) so that she would be able to get food after her time at the clinic. Finally, she was referred to an employment support program (provided with an actual contact name and direct number) to assist her with locating full-time employment.
5. The nurse practitioner at the clinic provided Mrs. Smith with a prescription for the medications she needed for her child. The social worker assisted Mrs. Smith with completing prescription assistance paperwork to qualify for prescription assistance from the pharmaceutical company.

WWW Case 2: Mr. Jackson

Marty Jackson is a 35-year-old homeless man who has had repeated incarcerations for alcohol abuse, public drunkenness, and simple assaults when drunk. Mr. Jackson's most recent arrest occurred while he was loitering in a local park in a downtown urban area. Individuals at the park called the police and reported that a man was "harassing" individuals in the park. The police arrived at the park to find Mr. Jackson incoherent and disoriented. The police officer observed that Mr. Jackson had an alcoholic odor and had difficulty walking. The officer also observed that Mr. Jackson had an open wound on his hand that had been hastily wrapped in a soiled bandage.

The police officer transported Mr. Jackson to the local hospital for observation. During the ride in the police car, Mr. Jackson complained that "Marvin" was taking up too much of the backseat and was threatening him with a knife. The only occupants in the vehicle were the police officer and Mr. Jackson. Upon arrival at the hospital, the police officer noted to the intake nurse that Mr. Jackson might be hallucinating and recounted his comments on the ride to the hospital. The intake nurse placed Mr. Jackson in an area of the hospital where he could be observed, and asked the police officer if he could remain with Mr. Jackson until a psychiatric evaluation could be completed.

The nurse then requested a psychiatric consult from the Mental Health Unit in the hospital. The Mental Health Unit used an interdisciplinary approach to service provision, in which patients were seen by a team consisting of a psychiatrist, a psychiatric nurse specialist, a clinical social worker, and a psychologist. A clinical social worker (LCSW) was sent to the emergency room and interviewed Mr. Jackson.

The clinical social worker conducted a bio-psycho-social assessment of Mr. Jackson that included an evaluation of where he posed any harm to himself (suicide) or to others (homicide). The clinical social worker's assessment found that Mr. Jackson was not homicidal or suicidal, but noted that there was a possibility of some mental instability. Mr. Jackson did meet all of the risk markers for alcoholism. He adamantly stated he wanted to stop drinking, but claimed the alcohol subdued his "moments of confusion and voices,"

The clinical social worker called for a consult from another member of the mental health team, the psychiatric nurse. The psychiatric nurse reviewed the initial assessment and assessed Mr. Jackson for any mental health risk. The nurse and clinical social worker met and conferred about their assessment findings and determined that Mr. Jackson had bipolar disorder and needed medication to be able to function without continued intervention by law enforcement. The psychiatric nurse and social worker worked together to create the following treatment plan for Mr. Jackson:

1. Mr. Jackson was given a three-day regimen of medication for bipolar disorder and scheduled for a follow-up consult with the psychiatric team at the county services board. The clinical social worker contacted the mental health worker on the crisis intervention team at the county services board and scheduled an appointment for Mr. Jackson. Initially, the scheduler indicated he could not be seen for at least 3 weeks. The social worker emphasized that Mr. Jackson was an alcoholic and had expressed a desire to stop drinking if he could get some help. The social worker reminded the scheduler that withdrawal from alcohol could have serious medical complications for individuals and Mr. Jackson would need to be seen within 3 days to prevent any serious medical harm. His appointment was scheduled for 3 days from the current day.
2. The psychiatric nurse followed up with the intake nurse to be sure Mr. Jackson had received the needed treatment for his hand wound and to ascertain if he would need any additional medications.
3. The social worker called the local shelter for men dealing with the issue of homelessness to inquire if it had a bed for Mr. Jackson. The shelter intake worker indicated that he would be able to stay at the shelter but would need to remain sober and would

be drug tested. The shelter staff indicated that the program included Alcoholics Anonymous (AA) meetings and residents were required to attend.

4. The psychiatric nurse contacted a colleague (and fellow psychiatric nurse) at a local health clinic to determine if Mr. Jackson would qualify for follow-up services for his wound (physical health) and monitoring until his appointment with the county services board. The community clinic had a partnership with the local men's shelter and agreed to schedule an appointment to follow up with Mr. Jackson the next morning.
5. Mr. Jackson was allowed regain his sobriety in the hospital that evening. Once he was able to travel, he was provided with bus fare to travel to the shelter. The social worker called the shelter to notify the staff there of his impending arrival. The nurse called a few hours later to confirm Mr. Jackson had arrived at the shelter and reviewed his medical and mental health needs with his shelter case worker (with a signed release from the patient).

Implications for Practice

These cases suggest how social work and nursing professionals can work effectively as an interdisciplinary team. The role of the social worker and nurse, in each of the cases, was that of advocate: In each instance, the social worker and nurse sought out resources that would be useful to the client and enhance the client's ability to function in his or her everyday life. The role of advocate played by the professionals in each case scenario was critical to the client's health. The interdisciplinary team worked together to avoid compartmentalizing each client's issues, which ensured the delivery of more effective and efficient services for the client.

WWW

For a full suite of assignments and additional learning activities, use the access code located in the front of your book to visit this exclusive website: http://go.jblearning.com/dechesnay. If you do not have an access code, you can obtain one at the site.

REFERENCES

Annas, G. (1988). The hospital: A human rights wasteland. In G. Annas (Ed.), *Judging medicine.* (pp. 9–29). Clifton, NJ: Human Press.

Annas, G., & Healey, J. (1974). The patients' rights advocate. *Journal of Nursing Administration, 4,* 25–31.

Barker, R. (1995). The social work dictionary (3rd ed.). Washington, DC: NASW Press.

Brawley, E. A. (1997). Teaching social work students to use advocacy skills though mass media. *Journal of Social Work Education, 33*(3), 445–460.

Bu, X., & Jewesky, M. A. (2006). Developing an id-range theory of patient advocacy through concept analysis. *Journal of Advanced Nursing, 57*(1), 101–110. Doi: 10.1111/j.1365-2648.2006.04096.x

Clark, E. J. (2007). Advocacy: Profession's cornerstone. *NASW News, 52*(7), 3.

Dorfman, R. A. (1996). *Clinical social work: Definition, practice, and vision.* New York: Brunner/Mazel.

Faust, J. R. (2008). Clinical social worker as patient advocate in a community mental health center. *Clinical Social Work Journal, 36*, 293–300.

Gilbert, N., & Specht, H. (1976). Advocacy and professional ethics. *Social Work*, 288–293.

Hanks, R. (2010). The medical–surgical nurse perspective of advocate role. *Nursing Forum, 45*(2), 97–107.

Hoefer, R. (2006). *Advocacy practice.* Chicago, IL: Lyceum Books.

Hyland, D. (2002). An exploration of the relationship between patient autonomy and patient advocacy: Implications for nursing practice. *Nursing Ethics, 9*(5), 472–482.

Johnson, L. (1995). Social *work practice: A generalist approach* (5th ed.). Boston, MA: Allyn & Bacon.

Kirst-Ashman, K. K., & Hull, G. Jr. (2009). *Generalist practice with organizations and communities* (4th ed.). Belmont, CA: Brooks/Cole.

Lara, A., & Salberg, L. (2009). Patient advocacy: What is its role? *PACE, 32*(suppl 2), S83–S85.

Lens, V. (2004). Principled negotiation: A new tool for case advocacy. *Social Work, 49*(3), 506– 513.

Lynch, R. & Mitchell, J. (1995) Justice system advocacy: A must for NASW and the social work community. *Social Work, 40*(1), 9–12.

MacDonald, H. (2006). Relational ethics and advocacy in nursing: Literature review. *Journal of Advanced Nursing, 57*(2), 119–126.

Mallik, M. (1997). Advocacy in nursing: A review of the literature. *Journal of Advanced Nursing, 25*, 130–138.

Martin, D., & Tipton, B. (2007). Patient advocacy in the USA: Key communication role functions. *Nursing and Health Sciences, 9*, 185–191. Doi: 10.1111/j.1442-2018.2007.00320.x

McGrath, P., Holewa, H., & McGrath, Z. (2006). Nursing advocacy in an Australian multidisciplinary context: Findings on medico-centrism. *Scandinavian Journal of Caring Science, 20*, 394–402.

Mickelson, J. S. (1995). Advocacy. In R. L. Edwards (Ed.), *Encyclopedia of social work* (pp. 95–100). (19th ed., Vol. 1). Washington, DC: NASW Press.

Miley, K. K., O'Melia, M., & DuBois, B. (2009). *Generalist social work practice: An empowering approach* (6th ed.). Boston, MA: Pearson.

Mmatli, T. (2009). Translating disability-related research into evidence-based advocacy: The role of people with disabilities. *Disability and Rehabilitation, 31*(1), 14–22. Doi: 10.1080/0963828080228037

National Association of Social Workers. (1994). *NASW code of ethics.* Washington, DC: Author.

Pierce, D. (1984). *Policy for the social work practitioner.* New York: Longman.

Pullen, F. (1995). Advocacy: A specialist practitioner role. *British Journal of Nursing, 4*(5), 275– 278.

Schneider, R., & Lester, L. (2000). *Social work advocacy*: A new framework for actionBelmont: Brooks/Cole.

Sheafor, B., & Horejsi, C. R. (2003). *Techniques and guidelines for social work practice* (6th ed.). Boston: Allyn and Bacon.

Smith, R. F. (1995). Settlements and neighborhood center. In *Encyclopedia of social work* (19th ed., Vol. 3, pp. 2129–2135). Washington, DC: NASW Press.

Sosin, M., & Caulum, S. (1983, January–February). Advocacy: A conceptualization for social work practice. *Social Work*, 12–17.

Vaartio, H., Leino-Kilpi, H., Suominen, T., & Puukka, P. (2009). Nursing advocacy in procedural pain care. *Nursing Ethics, 16*(3), 340–362.

Walker, L., & Avant, P. (1995). *Strategies for theory construction in nursing* (3rd ed.). Norwalk, CT: Appleton & Lange.

Zomorodi, M., & Foley, B. J. (2009). The nature of advocacy vs paternalism in nursing: Clarifying the "thin line." *Journal of Advanced Nursing, 65*(8), 1746–1752. Doi: 10.1111/j.1365-2648.2009.05023.x

Cultural Competence and Resilience

Mary de Chesnay, Patricia Hart, and Jane Brannan

Objectives

At the end of this chapter, the reader will be able to

1. Define the term cultural competence, as differentiated from cultural sensitivity.
2. Compare and contrast the models of cultural competence.
3. Analyze the concept of resilience from the points of view of the patient who is resilient and the nurse who is attempting to promote resilience.

www

This chapter examines two key concepts that are particularly useful in caring for people who are vulnerable. *Cultural competence* is a way of providing care that takes into account cultural differences between the nurse and the patient while meeting the health needs of the patient. *Resilience* is both a characteristic and a desired outcome; it is the capacity for transcending obstacles, which is present to some degree in all human beings. A goal of nursing is to enhance resilience. The central idea of the chapter is that the concepts of cultural competence and resilience relate in specific ways that enable nurses to frame care within a cultural context, not just for vulnerable populations but for all clients.

CULTURAL COMPETENCE

Cultural competence is a way of practicing one's profession by being sensitive to the differences in cultures of one's constituents and acting in a way that is respectful of the client's values and traditions while performing those activities or procedures necessary for the client's well-being. In nursing, the outcomes are positive changes in health status or lifestyle changes expected to prevent disease.

A social justice view of cultural competence should take into account what Hall (Hall, 1999; Hall, Stevens, & Meleis, 1994) described as marginalization. Marginalized people experience discrimination, poor access to health care, and resultant illnesses and traumas from environmental dangers or violence that make them vulnerable to a wide range of health problems. In a life history study of successful African American adults, for example, the effect of racism was pronounced; success at overcoming racism emphasizes the importance of culture at reducing health disparities (de Chesnay, 2005). Culturally competent practitioners, then, not only would seem to concern themselves with superficial skills of learning about other cultures, but also would view marginalized patients within a wider system context and intervene within that context.

Historically, nursing has moved from a view of cultural sensitivity (focus on awareness) to one of cultural competence (focus on behavior). In other words, nurses aspire to cultural competence not because the concept is trendy or politically correct as described by Poole (1998), but because nurses are pragmatists who understand that recognizing cultural differences enables them to interact with patients and their families in ways that enable them to heal.

Zoucha (2001) urged that we put aside deep-seated feelings of ethnocentrism and accept the value that every health worldview is equally valid. Locsin (2000) proposed that cultural blurring might be a technique that bridges the gaps in cultural differences by enabling the practitioner to merge the best of both worlds. Cultural competence then becomes a practice with broad appeal in all of the service professions. Teachers, social workers, and physicians all understand the usefulness of this concept as not just politically correct, but good practice (Bonder, Martin, & Miracle, 2001; Dana & Matheson, 1992; Gutierrez & Alvarez, 1996; Leavitt, 2003; Sutton, 2000).

MODELS OF CULTURAL COMPETENCE

As an exciting theoretical development in nursing, several models have been introduced to explore the dimensions of cultural competence. In reference to community health nursing, Kim-Godwin, Clarke, and Barton (2001) constructed a model derived from concept analysis that focuses on the relationship between cultural competence and health outcomes for diverse populations. They suggested that the four dimensions of cultural competence are caring, cultural sensitivity, cultural knowledge, and cultural skills. These authors developed a cultural competence scale that measures all dimensions except caring; items cover both the affective and cognitive domains. When they tested the scale in a sample of 192 senior undergraduate and graduate nursing students, the authors found factors that loaded on two dimensions, sensitivity and skill, explaining 72% of the variance and providing evidence of construct validity.

A second model portrayed cultural competence as a process in which the healthcare provider integrates cultural awareness, cultural knowledge, cultural skill, cultural encounters, and cultural desire (Campinha-Bacote, 2002). This model assumes variations exist both within groups and between groups—an important distinction for those who would treat members of ethnic groups as if they are exactly like everyone else within their group, thereby constructing new stereotypes instead of developing cultural knowledge. Campinha-Bacote (2003, 2005) updated her model to elaborate on several of the key concepts and to suggest the relevance of cultural competence to Christianity and moral reasoning.

Taking a different direction, Purnell (2000, 2002) and Purnell and Paulanka (2003) integrated the concepts of biocultural ecology and workforce issues into his model for cultural competence. Purnell asserted that healthcare providers and recipients of care have a mutual obligation to share information to obtain beneficial outcomes. In this sense, the patient is both a teacher of culture and a client of the provider; the provider, in turn, becomes a teacher of the culture of health care. Derived from many disciplines and including many domains, the Purnell model might be seen as a diagram encompassing the patient within a series of concentric circles that include family, community, and global society.

A third view of cultural competence is that existing models are insufficient and the term itself is limiting. Wells (2000) argued for extending the concept of cultural competence into cultural proficiency. According to this author, cultural competence is not adequate; rather, proficiency is a higher-order concept for institutions in that proficiency indicates mastery of a complex set of skills. The process of moving toward proficiency requires overcoming barriers that are both affective and cognitive. The most serious barrier is the unwillingness to examine one's own assumptions about persons who are different from oneself. Wells would say that the most effective way to develop cultural proficiency is to maintain an open attitude and to interact with people who are different from yourself, allowing them to become your teachers or coaches.

Except for Leininger's (1970, 1995) extensive work, most of the nursing theories do not include cultural competence because they were published long before its emergence as a major concept for nursing. The application of several of the nursing theories to caring for vulnerable populations is discussed elsewhere in Unit II of this book. However, Watson's theory of caring deserves special note. In a theoretical review of Watson's theory, Mendycka (2000) explored the relationship of culture and care, providing a clinical example of how the nurse and the patient become more human through their interaction. In his description of a case of an American Indian who is HIV positive, Mendycka showed how a nurse practitioner trying to treat the patient with a traditional Western medical approach comes into conflict with the patient's cultural belief system. On the one hand, the nurse wants to see the patient more often and suggests pharmacotherapy to prevent progression of the HIV infection to full-blown AIDS. On the other hand, the patient wants to use the healing practices of his tribe: sweat baths, herbs, and prayer. Unless the nurse practitioner can find a way to work with the tribe's medicine man, she is doomed to failure because the patient will place his own cultural belief system above the uncertainties of Western medical practice.

Other authors have recognized the need for institutional change to develop culturally competent models of intervention for the populations served by diverse providers. For example, home care nurses must manage cultural issues with their patients (DiCicco-Bloom & Cohen, 2003). Andrews (1998) applied the process of developing cultural competence to administration in an assessment process leading to organizational change in cultural competence. Holistic nursing, which views patients within a series of contexts, has cultural competence as a core value. In a review of the concept in the holistic nursing literature, however, Barnes, Craig, and

Chambers (2000) found that only 9.6% of the abstracts made reference to concepts of culture or ethnicity; these authors raised the question as to whether the sample sizes were large enough to address cultural differences or whether the researchers lacked awareness of these issues. Finally, authors in psychiatric nursing (Craig, 1999; Kennedy, 1999) and oncology (Kagawa-Singer, 2000) have addressed the need for practitioners to develop cultural competence at both individual and institutional levels.

LEARNING CULTURAL COMPETENCE

Although many methods and ideas for developing cultural competence are described in the literature, there is general agreement on certain precepts—namely, that cultural competence happens on affective, cognitive, and behavioral levels and that self-awareness is a critical indicator of success. Campinha-Bacote (2006) suggests that standardization of nursing curricula might be effective in ensuring that nurses address issues related to cultural competence.

Simulation activities provide a setting in which participants can practice communication and problem solving as well as develop self-awareness (Meltzoff & Lenssen, 2000). Cross-cultural communication exercises for physicians can help them develop the skills needed to overcome barriers in this regard (Shapiro, Hollingshead, & Morrison, 2002).

Immersion programs are powerful learning experiences at all levels because they enable participants to experience different cultures out of their usual safe context. Immersion programs are probably the best way to induce cultural competence, although they are costly and time consuming. There are several examples in the in this book, which also explores in detail how undergraduate students and graduate nursing students can conduct fieldwork that leads to cultural competence. One example of an immersion program used in nutrition studies is a food travel course in which participants learn diverse dietetic preferences and practices (Kuczmarski & Cole, 1999). Another example is a population-based program with the Hutterites of the United States and Canada (Fahrenwald, Boysen, Fischer, & Maurer, 2001).

Didactic materials can be prepared for developing knowledge about groups and are a useful point of reference for practitioners who are under enormous pressure to function with diverse patients in high-acuity settings. An innovative program at the University of Washington used action research as the basis for developing culture clues—a series of documents that enable practitioners to see at a glance the dominant preferences of the diverse cultural groups served by the hospital. These documents cover perception of illness, patterns of kinship and decision making, and comfort with touch. They were written for a variety of cultures, including Korean, Russian, Latino, Albanian, Vietnamese, and African American (Abbot, Short, Dodson, Garcia, Perkins, & Wyant, 2002).

The didactic approach was also used in Sweden, which is becoming more diverse as immigration into the country increases, largely from Eastern Europe and Iraq. The researchers used Leininger's theory to guide development of a curriculum for undergraduate nursing students with specific content areas at all levels (Gebru & Willman, 2003).

Didactic programs are easier and less costly to operate than immersion programs, perhaps because cognitive outcomes are easier to measure than affective outcomes. In one multicultural training course for counseling students, outcomes included development of multicultural knowledge and skill and increased comfort with discussing differing worldviews; the program was less successful at getting participants to examine themselves as racial–cultural beings, however (Tomlinson-Clark, 2000).

RESILIENCE

Resilience is the ability of individuals to bounce back or to cope successfully despite adverse circumstances (Rutter, 1985). The *Merriam-Webster Online Dictionary* (2010) defines resilience as "an ability to recover from or adjust easily to change or misfortune" and the *American Heritage Online Dictionary* (2009) defines it as "the ability to recover quickly from illness, depression, change, or misfortune; buoyancy." Resilience has been referred to as both a personality trait and a dynamic process (Luthar, Cicchetti, & Becker, 2000). Dyer and McGuinness (1996) define resilience as "a global term describing a process whereby people bounce back from adversity and go on with their lives. It is a dynamic process highly influenced by protective factors" (p. 277).

Two recent concept analyses have been conducted for resilience (Earvolino-Ramirez, 2007; Gillespie, Chaboyer, & Wallis, 2007). Both studies used Walker and Avant's (2005) method of inquiry to guide the approach for the concept analysis. In this analytical technique, antecedents are the events or incidents that occur before the occurrence of the concept, whereas consequences are circumstances that result from the concept (Walker & Avant, 2005). Earvolino-Ramirez (2007) found that the main antecedent to resilience is adversity. Gillespie et al. (2007) found that, in addition to adversity, three other antecedents to resilience exist—interpretation of the event as either physically and/or psychologically traumatic, the cognitive ability to interpret adversity, and a realistic worldview rather than a false optimism or depressive attitude. Integration, control, adjustment, growth (Gillespie et al., 2007), effective coping, mastery, and positive adaptation (Earvolino-Ramirez, 2007) were found to be consequences of resilience. Walker and Avant (2005) describe defining attributes as the cluster of characteristics that are most frequently associated with the concept and that are consistently present when the concept occurs. Earvolino-Ramirez (2007) found the defining attributes of resilience to be rebounding/reintegration, high expectancy/self-determination, positive relationships/social support, flex ibility, sense of humor, and self-esteem/self-efficacy, while Gillespie et al. (2007) found them to be self-efficacy, hope, and coping. The importance of conducting concept analyses is to acquire an understanding of the concept so that theoretical models can then be developed to test the concept; the investigation then progresses to research studies that examine the effectiveness of strategies and interventions to help build resilience in vulnerable populations.

Resilience has been studied in numerous vulnerable populations, such as children, older adults, women, and survivors of disasters. Resilience research has also been explored in the nursing profession.

Children

Resilience in children has been studied in many different populations and situations. Research has been conducted of children in poverty (Ahren, 2006; Anthony, 2008; Sanders, Lim, & Sohn, 2008), children with a parent who suffers from mental illness (Fraser & Pakenham, 2008; Mordoch & Hall, 2002), children of divorced parents (Ruschena, Prior, Sanson, & Smart, 2005), children with chronic and terminal illness (Cohen, Biran, Aran, & Gross-Tsur, 2008; Kim & Yoo, 2007; Phipps, 2007), children suffering from child abuse and neglect (Jaffee, Caspi, Moffitt, Polo-Tomas, & Taylor, 2007), and homeless children (Rew, Taylor-Seehafer, Thomas, & Yockey, 2001), to identify but a few populations. Children who are resilient are able to respond to adversity by adapting to their circumstances, coping with and managing major life problems and events, and succeeding despite immeasurable disadvantages in life (Dent & Cameron, 2003).

Family resiliency has been found to comprise a series of complex interactions between risk and protective factors operating at individual (locus of control; emotional regulation; belief systems; self-efficacy; effective coping skills; education, skills, and training; health; temperament; and gender), family (family structure, intimate-partner relationship stability, family cohesion, supportive parent–child interaction, stimulating environment, social support, family of origin influences, stable and adequate income, and adequate housing), and community (involvement in the community, peer acceptance, supportive mentors, safe neighborhoods, access to quality schools and child care, and access to quality health care) levels (Benzies & Mychasiuk, 2009). Risk factors for families may change over time, so different protective factors may be more beneficial at different times resulting in a variety of outcomes. Several intervention programs have been conducted to build resilience in children, such as the Keeping Families Strong program (Riley et al., 2008), Coping and Promoting Strength Program (CAPS) (Ginsburg, 2009), and the Bridge Project (Anthony, Alter, & Jenson, 2009) to name a few.

Women

Resilience has been studied in various situations with women. McGrath, Wiggin, and Caron (2010), for example, found a relationship between body image dissatisfaction and resilience. In their study, college women who had a positive relationship with their parents were more resilient and, therefore, demonstrated less body image dissatisfaction. In a phenomenological study conducted by Singh, Hays, Chung, and Watson (2010), the researchers found resilience strategies used by Asian immigrant women in the United States who survived child sexual abuse. The resilience strategies used by these women included use of silence, sense of hope, South Asian social support, social advocacy, and intentional self-care. These strategies allowed the women to heal and move on in their life.

Kinsel (2005) identified factors that were salient to resilience in older women. Having a social connectedness with family, friends, and the community provided a support mechanism as well as allowing these women to extend themselves to help others. Spiritual grounding was important to the women in providing a higher power to lean on, which gave meaning and purpose to their lives. Resilient older women took a "head-on" approach to adversity to move forward through life challenges (Kinsel, 2005).

Older Adults

Many adults face adversity in their older years, as evidenced by decreasing functional status, declining health, increase stress, poorer living conditions, and experiencing negative life events (Hildon, Montgomery, Blane, Wiggins, & Netuveli, 2010). Protective attributes of more resilient older adults include good-quality relationships, integration in the community, and use of developmental and adaptive coping styles. Older adults who receive support from family, have a broad network of friends (Wells, 2009), and have confiding relationships with others are found to be more resilient than those without these types of relationships (Hildon et al., 2010; Hildon, Smith, Netuveli, & Blane, 2008). Terminally ill older adults facing death demonstrate resilient behaviors by redefining their self, embracing religion and spirituality in times of uncertainty, maintaining social relationships, and defending their independence as the end of their life approaches (Nelson-Becker, 2006).

Cultural values play an important part in how older individuals exhibit resilience as well. Becker and Newsom (2005) found that older African Americans responded to their disabling illness by demonstrating determination, perseverance, and tenacity as resilient behaviors leading to a culturally specific resilience philosophy.

Survivors of Disasters

Several studies have been conducted to explore resilience in survivors of disasters. Bonanno, Bucciarelli, Galea, and Vlahov (2007) examined the role of demographics, resources, and life stress on psychological resilience of individuals in New York City after the September 11, 2001, terrorist attacks. The researchers found that the "prevalence of resilience was uniquely predicted by participant gender, age, race/ethnicity, and education level; by the absence of depression and substance use; by less income loss, social support, and fewer chronic diseases; and by less direct impact of September 11 and fewer recent life stressors, fewer past prior traumatic events, and not having experienced an additional traumatic event since September 11" (p. 676).

Greene (2007) reviewed three case study transcripts of older adult survivors of Hurricane Katrina to identify themes of survivorship that promoted resilience in these older adults. These themes were resolving to live, obtaining food and shelter, choosing survival strategies, keeping family ties, connecting with community, and giving testimony. Kanji, Drummond, and Cameron (2007), in a review of resilience in Afghan children and their families, postulated that protective factors that influenced their survival and abilities to rebuild their lives while still facing a magnitude of challenges included faith in Allah (God), family support, and community support.

Nurses

Factors contributing to the need for resilient behaviors in nurses include challenging workplaces, psychological emptiness, diminishing inner balance, and a sense of dissonance in the workplace (Glass, 2009; Hodges, Keeley, & Troyan, 2008). To date, however, very little research has been conducted on resilience in nurses (Ablett & Jones, 2007; Gillespie, Chaboyer, & Wallis, 2009; Gillespie, Chaboyer, Wallis, & Grimbeck, 2007; Glass, 2009; Hodges et al., 2008; Simoni, Larrabee, Birkimer, Mott, & Gladden, 2004). Characteristics found in resilient nurses include hope, self-efficacy, coping, control, competence, flexibility, adaptability, hardiness, sense of coherence, skill recognition, and nondeficiency focusing. Nurses employed cognitive reframing, grounding connections and work–life balance, critical reflection, and reconciliation as strategies to build resilience (Ablett & Jones, 2007; Glass, 2009; Hodges et al., 2008).

Additional nursing research needs to be conducted on resilience and resilient attributes to enhance the resilience process in vulnerable, diverse populations and situations. Better understanding of how some individuals remain resilience despite facing adversity may lead to successful implementation of strategies and interventions for others. Nurses are in key positions to perform resiliency assessments and intervene to promote well-being and positive outcomes in vulnerable populations (Ahren, 2006).

WWW CASE STUDY

The following example illustrates the relationship of cultural competence and resilience. Although fictional and representing only a small type of population, this case study shows that helping patients to become more resilient is a cross-cultural strategy.

Donna swung her new vehicle into a parking space, grabbed her lunch sack, and trotted upstairs to the cardiovascular rehabilitation unit at Morris Center. Her assignment was already posted, and she noted that she was still working with Mr. Hernandez, a 60-year-old man who had suffered a cerebrovascular accident (CVA, or stroke) and who continued to have hemiparesis on his left side. Donna sighed and prepared for care.

Mr. Hernandez had immigrated to the United States from Cuba 5 years ago and worked for a local food distribution company. His family had been literally swarming around him each day in his room. His wife and grown daughter were there every day. In addition, his two sons, his brother, his elderly mother, and her sister arrived periodically to tend to him. It wasn't so much that they were present frequently (although it did pose a challenge to provide care when weaving among the people); rather, Donna's larger concern was the effect that the family's hovering had on Mr. Hernandez's physical rehabilitation and recovery. Lately, he did not seem to be coping well with his limitations. He seemed depressed, anxious, and fatigued—more so now than when he arrived at the unit two weeks ago.

Donna entered the room and found Mrs. Hernandez shaving her husband. She stated, "Oh my—Mrs. Hernandez, he should do that for himself. Your husband is quite capable of shaving himself. Don't you remember us saying it several days ago, that he must become more independent?" Mrs. Hernandez scurried aside, head bowed, eyes downcast, and mumbling an apology. Donna continued her morning assessment, and provided information to the patient and family about his physical state and the physical therapy he was doing today. But she was annoyed. Didn't they listen? Don't they understand that they were hindering care? Every day Mrs. Hernandez continued to do things for her husband that he could do for himself.

The situation was frustrating. Mr. Hernandez's progress was slower than Donna expected, and she didn't seem to be able to help him deal with his depression. The illness had really hit him hard emotionally. It seemed as if the family was undermining Donna's care—doing everything for the patient and not allowing him to regain his strength.

Later that afternoon, Donna expressed her concerns at a multidisciplinary team meeting. Margarite, the new nurse educator (who was originally from Puerto Rico) spoke up: "I think what you are seeing is very much what is a display of love and concern in this family. Independence and self-care during an illness is not particularly a value for them. The pampering and indulgence by his family are expected by Mr. Hernandez. Maybe we can talk about ways Mrs. Hernandez can still provide care that does not alter his treatment. We also should discuss how we can help Mr. Hernandez deal with the overwhelming concern about how his life has changed with this illness and help him develop some strategies to address his concerns." Donna realized that she had misinterpreted the actions of the Hernandez family by not having a clear understanding of their cultural mores.

Working together, the team made a plan for working with Mr. Hernandez to enhance his coping and resilience. His family priest and counselors at the center began meeting with him and his family. His family also was consulted regarding activities they could do to assist Mr. Hernandez to move forward in his physical development, while still allowing them to care for him. Mrs. Hernandez was asked to help minimally in providing morning care and brought favorite meals from home for him to eat. Other family members accompanied Mr. Hernandez to physical therapy activities during the day to learn how they might help him continue these exercises at home.

Based on Donna's experience working with the Hernandez family, she orchestrated a cultural competency program for the staff working in the rehabilitation hospital. The program focused on caring for patients from various ethnicities and backgrounds to ensure that the staff understood and were sensitive to cultural traditions and relationships within families.

CONCLUSION

Cultural competence is a set of behaviors that transcend mere good intentions. Accepting that cultural differences exist reflects an open mind, which in turn leads to exploring the client's own strengths and adaptive capabilities. Using cultural resources at the client's disposal concurrently with "best practices" in nursing and medicine is not only culturally appropriate, it is also likely to develop resilience. Both cultural competence and resilience have much relevance to nursing practice,

For a full suite of assignments and additional learning activities, use the access code located in the front of your book to visit this exclusive website: http://go.jblearning.com/dechesnay. If you do not have an access code, you can obtain one at the site.

REFERENCES

Abbot, P., Short, E., Dodson, S., Garcia, C., Perkins, J., & Wyant, S. (2002). Improving your cultural awareness with culture clues. *Nurse Practitioner, 27*(2), 44–49.

Ablett, J. R., & Jones, R. S. P. (2007). Resilience and well-being in palliative care staff: A qualitative study of hospice nurses' experience of work. *Psycho-Oncology, 16*(8), 733–740.

Ahren, N. R. (2006). Adolescent resilience: An evolutionary concept analysis. *Journal of Pediatric Nursing, 21*(3), 175–185.

American Nurses' Association. (2001). *Code of ethics for nurses with interpretive statements.* Washington, DC: American Nurses Publishing.

Andrews, M. (1998). A model for cultural change. *Nursing Management, 29*(10), 62–66.

Anthony, E. K. (2008). Cluster profiles of youths living in urban poverty: Factors affecting risk and resilience. *Social Work Research, 32*(1), 6–17.

Anthony, E. K., Alter, C. F., & Jenson, J. M. (2009). Development of a risk and resilience-based out-of-school time program for children and youths. *Social Work, 54*(1), 45–55.

Barnes, D., Craig, K., & Chambers, K. (2000). A review of the concept of culture in holistic nursing literature. *Journal of Holistic Nursing, 18*(3), 207–221.

Becker, G., & Newsom, E. (2005). Resilience in the face of serious illness among chronically ill African Americans in later life. *Journal of Gerontology Series B: Psychological Sciences and Social Sciences, 60B*(4), S214–223.

Benzies, K., & Mychasiuk, R. (2009). Fostering family resiliency: A review of the key protective factors. *Child and Family Social Work, 14*, 103–114. doi:10.1111/j.1365-2206.2008.00586.x

Bonanno, G. A., Galea, S., Bucciarelli, A., & Vlahov, D. (2007). What predicts psychological resilience after disaster? The role of demographics, resources, and life stress. *Journal of Consulting and Clinical Psychology, 75*(5), 671–682.

Bonder, B., Martin, L., & Miracle, A. (2001). Achieving cultural competence: The challenge for clients and healthcare workers in a multicultural society. *Generations, 25*(1), 35–43.

Campinha-Bacote, J. (2002). The process of cultural competence in the delivery of health care services: A model of care. *Journal of Transcultural Nursing, 13*(3), 180–184.

Campinha-Bacote, J. (2003). *The process of cultural competence in the delivery of healthcare services: A culturally competent model of care* (4th ed.). Cincinnati, OH: Transcultural CARE Associates.

Campinha-Bacote, J. (2005). A biblically based model of cultural competence in healthcare delivery. *Journal of Multicultural Nursing and Health, 11*(2), 16–22.

Campinha-Bacote, J. (2006). Cultural competence in nursing curricula: How are we doing 20 years later? *Journal of Nursing Education, 45*(7), 243–244.

Cohen, E., Biran, G., Aran, A., & Gross-Tsur, V. (2008). Locus of control, perceived parenting style, and anxiety in children with cerebral palsy. *Journal of Developmental & Physical Disabilities, 20*(5), 415–423.

Craig, A. B. (1999). Mental health nursing and cultural diversity. *Australian and New Zealand Journal of Mental Health Nursing, 8*, 93–99.

Dana, R., & Matheson, L. (1992). An application of the agency cultural competence checklist to a program serving small and diverse ethnic communities. *Psychosocial Rehabilitation Journal, 15*(4), 101–106.

de Chesnay, M. (2005). "Can't keep me down": Life histories of successful African Americans. In M. de Chesnay (Ed.), *Caring for the vulnerable: Perspectives in nursing theory, practice and research* (pp. 221–234). Sudbury, MA: Jones and Bartlett.

Dent, R. J., & Cameron, R. J. (2003). Developing resilience in children who are in public care: The educational psychological perspective. *Educational Psychology in Practice, 19*(1), 3–20.

DiCicco-Bloom, B., & Cohen, D. (2003). Home care nurses: A study of the occurrence of culturally competent care. *Journal of Transcultural Nursing, 14*(1), 25–31.

Dyer, J. G., & McGuinness, T. M. (1996). Resilience: Analysis of the concept. *Archives of Psychiatric Nursing, 10*(5), 276–282.

Earvolino-Ramirez, M. (2007). Resilience: A concept analysis. *Nursing Forum, 42*(2), 73–82.

Fahrenwald, N., Boysen, R., Fischer, C., & Maurer, R. (2001). Developing cultural competence in the baccalaureate nursing student: A populations-based project with the Hutterites. *Journal of Transcultural Nursing, 12*(1), 48–55.

Fraser, E., & Pakenham, K. I. (2008). Evaluation of a resilience-based intervention for children of parents with mental illness. *Australian & New Zealand Journal of Psychiatry, 42*(12), 1041–1050.

Gebru, K., & Willman, A. (2003). A research-based didactic model for education to promote culturally competent nursing care in Sweden. *Journal of Transcultural Nursing, 14*(1), 55–61.

Gillespie, B. M., Chaboyer, W., & Wallis, M. (2007). Development of a theoretically derived model of resilience through concept analysis. *Contemporary Nurse, 25*(1), 124–135.

Gillespie, B. M., Chaboyer, W., & Wallis, M. (2009). The influence of personal characteristics on the resilience of operating room nurses: A predictor study. *International Journal of Nursing Studies, 46*(7), 968–976.

Gillespie, B. M., Chaboyer, W., Wallis, M., & Grimbeck, P. (2007). Resilience in the operating room: Developing and testing of a resilience model. *Journal of Advanced Nursing, 59(*4), 427–438.

Ginsburg, G. S. (2009). The child anxiety prevention study: Intervention model and primary outcomes. *Journal of Consulting and Clinical Psychology, 77*(3), 580–587.

Glass, N. (2009). An investigation of nurses' and midwives' academic/clinical workplaces. *Holistic Nursing Practice, 23*(3), 158–170.

Greene, R. R. (2007). Reflections of Hurricane Katrina by older adults: Three case studies in resiliency survivorship. *Journal of Human Behavior in the Social Environment, 16*(4), 57–74.

Gutierrez, L., & Alvarez, A. (1996). Multicultural community organizing: A strategy for change. *Social Work, 41*(5), 501–509.

Hall, J. M. (1999). Marginalization revisited: Critical, postmodern and liberation perspectives. *Advances in Nursing Science, 22*(1), 88–102.

Hall, J. M., Stevens, P., & Meleis, A. (1994). Marginalization: A guiding concept for valuing diversity in nursing knowledge development. *Advances in Nursing Science, 16*(4), 23–41.

Hildon, Z., Montgomery, S. M., Blane, D., Wiggins, R. D., & Netuveli, G. (2010). Examining resilience of quality of life in the face of health-related and psychosocial adversity at older ages: What is "right" about the way we age? *Gerontologist, 50*(1), 36–47.

Hildon, Z., Smith, G., Netuveli, G., & Blane, D. (2008). Understanding adversity and resilience at older ages. *Sociology of Health & Illness, 30*(5), 1–15. doi: 10.1111/j.1467-9566.2008.01087.x

Hodges, H. F., Keeley, A. C. & Troyan, P. J. (2008). Professional resilience in baccalaureate prepared acute care nurses: First steps. *Nursing Education Perspectives, 29*(2), 80–89.

Jaffee, S. R., Caspi, A., Moffitt, T. E., Polo-Tomas, M., & Taylor, A. (2007). Individual, family, and neighborhood factors distinguish resilient from non-resilient maltreated children: A cumulative stressors model. *Child Abuse & Neglect, 31*(3), 231–253.

Kagawa-Singer, M. (2000). Addressing issues for early detection and screening in ethnic populations. *Oncology Nursing Forum, 27*(9), 55–61.

Kanji, Z., Drummond, J., & Cameron, B. (2007). Resilience in Afghan children and their families: A review. *Paediatric Nursing, 19*(2), 30–33.

Kennedy, M. (1999). Cultural competence and psychiatric nursing. *Journal of Transcultural Nursing, 10*(1), 11–18.

Kim, D. H., & Yoo, I. Y. (2007). Factors associated with depression and resilience in asthmatic children. *Journal of Asthma, 44*(6), 423–427.

Kim-Godwin, Y. S., Clarke, P., & Barton, L. (2001). A model for the delivery of culturally competent care. *Journal of Advanced Nursing, 35*(6), 918–926.

Kinsel, B. (2005). Resilience as adaptation in older women. *Journal of Women & Aging, 17*(3), 23–39.

Kuczmarski, M., & Cole, R. (1999). Transcultural food habits travel courses: An interdisciplinary approach to teaching cultural diversity. *Topics in Clinical Nutrition, 15*(1), 59–71.

Leavitt, R. L. (2003). Developing cultural competence in a multicultural world: Part II. *Magazine of Physical Therapy, 11*(1), 56–70.

Leininger, M. (1970). *Nursing and anthropology: Two worlds to blend.* New York: John Wiley & Sons.

Leininger, M. (1995). *Transcultural nursing: Concepts, theories, research and practice.* New York: McGraw-Hill.

Locsin, R. (2000). Building bridges: Affirming culture in health and nursing. *Holistic Nursing Practice, 15*(1), 1–4.

Luthar, S., Cicchetti, D., & Becker, B. (2000). The construct of resilience: A critical evaluation and guidelines for future work. *Child Development, 71*(3), 543–562.

McGrath, R. J., Wiggin, J., & Caron, R. M. (2010). The relationship between resilience and body image in college women. *International Journal of Health, 10*(2). Retrieved April 8, 2010, from http://www.ispub.com/journal/the_internet_journal_of_health/volume_10_number_2_12/article_printable/the-relationship-between-resilience-and-body-image-in-college-women.html

Meltzoff, N., & Lenssen, J. (2000). Enhancing cultural competence through simulation activities. *Multicultural Perspectives, 2*(1), 29–35.

Mendycka, B. (2000). Exploring culture in nursing: A theory-driven practice. *Holistic Nursing Practice, 15*(1), 32–41.

Mordoch, E., & Hall, W. A. (2002). Children living with a parent who has a mental illness: A critical analysis of the literature and research implications. *Archives of Psychiatric Nursing, 16*(5), 208–216.

Nelson-Becker, H. B. (2006). Voices of resilience: Older adults in hospice care. *Journal of Social Work in End-of-Life & Palliative Care, 2*(3), 87–106.

Phipps, S. (2007). Adaptive style in children with cancer: Implications for a positive psychology approach. *Journal of Pediatric Psychology, 32*(9), 1055–1066.

Poole, D. (1998). Politically correct or culturally competent? *Health and Social Work, 23*(3), 163–167.

Purnell, L. (2000). A description of the Purnell model for cultural competence. *Journal of Transcultural Nursing, 11*(1), 40–46.

Purnell, L. (2002). The Purnell model for cultural competence. *Journal of Transcultural Nursing, 13*(3), 193–196.

Purnell, L., & Paulanka, B. (2003). *Transcultural health care: A culturally competent approach* (2nd ed.). Philadelphia: F. A. Davis.

Resilience. (2009). *The American heritage dictionary of the English language*, (4th ed.). Retrieved April 12, 2010, from http://dictionary.reference.com/browse/resilience

Resilience. (2010). *In Merriam-Webster online dictionary.* Retrieved April 12, 2010, from http://www.merriam-webster.com/dictionary/resilience

Rew, L., Taylor-Seehafer, M., Thomas, N. Y., & Yockey, R. D. (2001). Correlates of resilience in homeless adolescents. *Journal of Nursing Scholarship, 33*(1), 33–43.

Riley, A. W., Valdez, C. R., Barrueco, S., Mills, C., Beardslee, W., Sandler, I., & Rawal, P. (2008). Development of a family-based program to reduce risk and promote resilience among families affected by maternal depression: Theoretical basis and program description. *Clinical Child and Family Psychology Review, 11*(1–2), 12–29.

Ruschena, E., Prior, M., Sanson, A., & Smart, D. (2005). A longitudinal study of adolescent adjustment following family transitions. *Journal of Child Psychology and Psychiatry, and Allied Disciplines, 46*(4), 353–363.

Rutter, M. (1985). Resilience in the face of adversity: Protective factors and resistance to psychiatric disorder. *British Journal of Psychiatry, 147*, 598–611.

Sanders, A. E., Lim, S., & Sohn, W. (2008). Resilience to urban poverty: Theoretical and empirical considerations for population health. *American Journal of Public Health, 98*(6), 1101–1106.

Shapiro, J., Hollingshead, J., & Morrison, E. (2002). Primary care resident, faculty and patient views of barriers to cultural competence and the skills needed to overcome them. *Medical Education, 36*, 749–759.

Simoni, P. S., Larrabee, J. H., Birkhimer, T. L., Mott, C. L., & Gladden, S. D. (2004). Influence of interpretive styles of stress resiliency on registered nurse empowerment. *Nursing Administration Quarterly, 28*(3), 221–22.

Singh, A. A., Hays, D. G., Chung, Y. B., & Watson, L. (2010). South Asian immigrant women who have survived child sexual abuse: resilience and healing. *Violence Against Women, 16*(4), 444–458.

Sutton, M. (2000). Cultural competence. *Family Practice Management, 7*(9), 58–61.

Tomlinson-Clark, S. (2000). Assessing outcomes in a multicultural training course: A qualitative study. *Counseling Psychology Quarterly, 13*(2), 221–232.

Walker, L., & Avant, K. (2005). *Strategies for theory construction in nursing* (4th ed.). Upper Saddle River, NJ: Pearson Prentice Hall.

Wells, M. (2000). Beyond cultural competence: A model for individual and institutional cultural development. *Journal of Community Health Nursing, 17*(4), 189–200.

Wells, M. (2009). Resilience in rural community-dwelling older adults. *Journal of Rural Health, 25*(4), 415–419.

Zoucha, R. (2001). President's message. *Journal of Transcultural Nursing, 12*(2). Academic Journal

CHAPTER 4

Social Justice in Nursing: A Review of the Literature

Doris M. Boutain

Objectives

At the end of this chapter, the reader will be able to

1. Define social justice for nursing.
2. Compare and contrast the types of justice found in the nursing literature.
3. Present a concise statement of the state of the art of social justice as a concept for further development in nursing scholarship.

This chapter explores how social justice was conceptualized in the nursing literature over the years 1990–2009. Analysis of this literature reveals that various authors ascribe to social, distributive, and market views of justice. Most authors, however, do not explicitly attend to the differences among these concepts. The three predominant models of justice are reviewed here first, and then a framework for how nurses can focus on injustice awareness, amelioration, and transformation as forms of social justice is presented. The multiple methods of promoting a social justice agenda, from consciousness raising to the re-creation of social policies, are also delineated. Recognizing the many ways to promote social justice can have a transformational impact on how nurses teach, research, and practice.

Although social justice is not a new concept, the nursing literature lacks a coherent and complex understanding of its implications for studying societal health (Drevdahl, Kneipp, Canales, & Dorcy, 2001; Liaschenko, 1999). Social justice is often mentioned only briefly, as an afterthought to elaborate discussions about ethics. When ethics is defined in the forefront, the concept of social justice often recedes to the background, appearing fleetingly in the conclusion section of articles. Inattention to the subtle variations in how social justice is conceived can inadvertently result in nursing practice, research, and education that are antithetical to a social justice agenda.

LITERATURE SEARCH METHODOLOGY

A search of the Cumulative Index of Nursing and Allied Health (CINAHL) literature from the years 1990 to 2009 revealed a total of 396 publications, including journal articles ($n = 373$), dissertations ($n = 14$), book chapters ($n = 8$), and a pamphlet ($n = 1$) categorized with the key terms "social justice and nursing" as major words in the subject heading. A major word is a term ascribed by the manuscript authors to classify the main focus of their work. Of all the works reviewed, eight journal articles offered continuing education credits.

Journal articles using the major words of "social justice and nursing" form the major basis of this review. Although all articles were reviewed, only selected articles that emphasize uncommon points are included in the reference list to limit the chapter's length. The literature reviewed in the sections about views of justice in nursing education, research, and practice is limited to published journal articles written in English-language journals in the stated time frame. Publications from nursing, sociology, social work, philosophy, public health, and religious studies supplement the literature analysis in the sections about the literature review critique and implications.

Defining Justice in Nursing

The ethical principle of justice was referenced frequently in the nursing literature surveyed. More than half of the publications retrieved equated justice with what is fair or what is deserved or "giving to others what is their due" (Lamke, 1996, p. 55). Authors discussed ethics, which is primarily viewed as a framework for understanding how values, duties, principles, and obligations inform people's sense of societal fairness, as the basis for moral decision making (Aroskar, 1995; Harper, 1994). The notion that two orientations to ethics exist was also highlighted in the literature (Mathes, 2004, 2005). Specifically, ethics can be defined by a care orientation or by a justice orientation. For example, ethics can be defined by universal truths (justice orientation) or in relationship to caring for others in context (care orientation) (Mathes, 2004, 2005).

Although many authors mentioned justice, few articles actually defined justice beyond notions of ethical fairness (Drevdahl, 1999; Drevdahl et al., 2001; Harris, 2005; Kneipp & Snider, 2001; Liaschenko, 1999; Thorne, 1999; Vonthron Good & Rodrigues-Fisher, 1993) or ethical relationship formation (Myhrvold, 2003). Only one article examined the theoretical connection between social justice and spirituality (Pesut, Fowler, Reimer-Kirkham, Taylor, & Sawatzky, 2009). Liaschenko (1999) outlined the relationship between personal values and justice in an effort to describe how justice can guide nursing practice. Vonthron Good and Rodrigues-Fisher (1993) considered how justice was useful in assessing whether vulnerability is compromised or protected in research. Exploring the philosophical underpinning of justice, Drevdahl et al. (2001) compared the concepts of social justice, distributive justice, and market justice. Like other scholars (Sellers & Haag, 1992), they posited that most nurses neither consider the distinction among concepts related to justice (Drevdahl et al., 2001) nor distinguish between social justice and social analysis (Stys, 2008). A few authors broaden the discussion of ethics to globalization (Falk-Rafael, 2006) or structural inequality (Sistrom & Hale, 2006) as having implications for social justice.

Without an intricate understanding of the different views of justice, nurses may limit their problem-solving abilities when attempting to understand how unjust social conditions influence health status, access, and delivery. Although concepts such as care (Boersma, 2006) and culture (Jackson, 2003) are not mutually exclusive to a justice ideology, inattention to the distinctions between care and justice may result in limited theoretical analysis and thus action. A review of the American Nurses Association's *Code of Ethics with Interpretive Statements, Nursing's Social Policy Statement* and *Nursing: Scope and Standards of Practice*, for example, revealed inconsistent and superficial conceptualizations of social justice (Bekemeier & Butterfield, 2005). These points were also a cause for debate in review of the Canadian Nurses Association's (CNA) 2002 Revised Code of Ethics (Hubert, 2004; Kikuchi, 2004). The disjunctions between practice, policy, and politics of justice, however, have a long history in nursing (Murphy, Canales, Norton, & DeFilippis, 2005). For this reason, it is important to explore the most prominent forms of justice in nursing literature today.

Social, Distributive, and Market Justice

Social, distributive, and market justice are the most common forms of justice referenced in the nursing literature. Social justice is often defined as a concern for "the equitable distribution of benefits and burdens in society" (Redman & Clark, 2002). Social justice is also—albeit less often—defined as changing social relationships and institutions to promote equitable relationships (Drevdahl et al., 2001). Distributive justice is discussed in reference to the equal distribution of goods and services in society (Schroeder & Ward, 1998; Silva & Ruth, 2003). Market justice posits that people are entitled only to those goods and services that they acquire according to guidelines of entitlement (Young, 1990).

Although these forms of justice may appear similar at first glance, there are distinct differences between them (Beauchamp, 1986; Whitehead, 1992). Social justice is concerned with making equitable the balance between societal benefits and burdens. It posits that social rights exist, but that collateral responsibilities come with those rights (Lebacqz, 1986). Social beings are to both give and receive, using equity as a framework for relating to one another. Equity, derived from the Greek word *epiky*, means that persons must conduct themselves with reasonableness and moderation when exercising their rights (Whitehead, 1992). Distributive justice involves equality more than equity; this concept is used most often to discuss the allocation or distribution of goods and services in society (Young, 1990). Equality focuses on giving the same access and resources to different groups (Sellers & Haag, 1992).

Social justice advocates explore social relationships, including how those relationships form the basis for the allocation of goods and services (Young, 1990). Social justice focuses on equity because many theories of social justice assert that "equal" does not mean "just" (Lebacqz, 1986). Thus the concepts of social and distributive justice are somewhat parallel, yet have different primary foci of study (Drevdahl et al., 2001).

Market justice is also viewed as a form of justice in nursing (Drevdahl, 2002). It is based on honoring the rights of those who have earned entitlement to those privileges. Market justice permits inequality as long as those inequalities result from a fair market system. That is, only those who earn rights can receive their entitled privileges in a market system. Those who earn no rights do not have secured privileges.

Critics of the market justice agenda note that using the word "market" as an adjective for "justice" is itself an oxymoron (Beauchamp, 1986). "Justice" is a word most often used to discuss fairness, equity, or the process of deliberation. The term "market" is most often concerned with the balance between monetary value and goods allocation. Thus, according to these critics, the two terms do not work together when discussing equity. Simply "applying the word 'justice' to 'market' does not bring the concept into the realm of justice" (Drevdahl et al., 2001, p. 24). Social justice is not a parallel model to market justice; rather, it is antithetical to a market model (Beauchamp, 1986). These two ways of viewing the world, therefore, diametrically oppose each other and simultaneously coexist.

An example may clarify the difference between social, distributive, and market justice. Using a social justice framework, everyone in the United States would be entitled to health care as needed if health care was deemed a right of citizenship. Health care, using a social justice view, is a moral obligation and a right of citizenship. A distributive justice framework would give a certain level of health care to everyone as a result of citizenship. The leveling of health care is needed to make sure that enough health care services are available for all citizens to receive at least minimal benefit. Within a distributive justice model, health is a right of citizens but not necessarily a moral responsibility. Persons can receive health care as a result of how much they can pay for those services in a market system. The focus of a market system is not on moral or citizenship rights, but rather on making sure that those citizens who want the good of health care, for example, can pay for those services.

All forms of justice, although somewhat distinct, may coexist to varying degrees. For example, some healthcare services in the United States are given as needed, such as the care given to children who are orphaned. In other cases, minimal health care is given, such as the medical and dental benefits associated with Medicaid. Persons who can afford more treatment or faster treatment may get those services as well if they can pay a particular price; an example is healthcare clinics that are designed to give expanded services if clients pay certain access fees. Although these three forms of justice are noted in the nursing literature to varying degrees, seldom is it discussed how these views of justice guide nursing education, research, or practice.

Views of Justice in Nursing Education Articles

Most manuscripts about nursing education and justice focus on the clinical preparation of undergraduate students to meet the needs of a culturally diverse population (Herman & Sassatelli, 2002; Leuning, 2001; Redman & Clark, 2002; Scanlan, Care, & Gessler, 2001). Other publications proclaim the need for a global consciousness (Leuning, 2001; Messias, 2001), critical thinking (Pereira, 2006), culturally sensitive evidence-based practice (McMurray, 2004), and human rights education (Fitzpatrick, 2003) among nurses as the starting point for justice awareness. Also present in the nursing literature are curricular considerations (Fahrenwald, Bassett, Tschetter, Carson, White, & Winterboer, 2005; MacIntosh & Wexler, 2005; Myrick, 2005; Vickers, 2008), teaching models (Bond, Mandleco, & Warnick, 2004; Boutain, 2005; Fahrenwald, 2003; Leuning, 2001), clinical evaluation frameworks (Boutain, 2008), case examples (Thompson, 1991), and service-learning experiences (Herman & Sassatelli, 2002; Redman & Clark, 2002) that use justice as a framework to educate undergraduate students. A limited number of articles focus on teaching justice content in general (Abrams, 2009) or in graduate education (Shattell, Hogan, & Hernandez, 2006). Only one article was found exploring how teaching social justice affects faculty directly (Fahrenwald, Taylor, Kneipp, & Canales, 2007). Few articles use social justice as a theoretical framework for educational scholarship (Kirkham, Hofwegen, & Harwood, 2005; Moule, 2003) or as a means to understand how to conduct educational research in nursing (Comer, 2009).

Although some nurse educators discuss the practical application of justice principles, few distinguish between the use of social justice and distributive justice concepts. For instance, authors may define social justice using distributive justice principles of equality (Thompson, 1991) or as working with vulnerable populations (Redman & Clark, 2002). One manuscript introduces justice in terms of contractual justice, meaning the fair and honest contract between equals (Oddi & Oddi, 2000). In one instance, the term "social justice" was used but never defined (Herman & Sassatelli, 2002). Rarely is social justice used as a framework to critique nursing education models (Sellers & Haag, 1992) and student–faculty relationships (Oddi & Oddi, 2000; Scanlan et al., 2001).

Views of Justice in Nursing Research Articles

Most articles about justice and nursing research focus on the protection of vulnerable populations or working with those who are marginalized in society (Alderson, 2001; Dreseden, McElmurry, & McCreary, 2003; Guenter, Majumdar, Willms, Travers, Browne, & Robinson, 2005; Lamke, 1996; McKane, 2000; Mill & Ogilvie, 2002; Rew, Taylor-Seehafer, & Thomas, 2000; Thomas, 2004; Vonthron Good & Rodrigues-Fisher, 1993). Nurses (Alexis & Vydelingum, 2004; Giddings, 2005a, 2005b; Mantler, Armstrong-Stassen, Horsburgh, & Cameron, 2006; Spence Laschinger, 2004) and nursing students (Grant, Giddings, & Beale, 2005) were study participants in six research studies assessing issues of justice in nursing practice accounts. Nevertheless, few articles explicitly state and define how social justice was used as a theoretical research framework (Blondeau, Lavoie, Valois, Keyserlingk, Hebert, & Martineau, 2000; Clark, Barton, & Brown, 2002; Giddings, 2005a, 2005b; Grant et al., 2005), as a measurement parameter for understanding concepts related to nursing (Altun, 2002), or as an outcome of a particular methodological approach (Sullivan-Bolyai, Bova, & Harper, 2005). Messias, McDowell, and Estrada (2009), for example, highlight how social justice is useful to consider while practicing language interpreting.

In the last decade, however, more researchers have begun identifying how the concept of social justice was used in the research process (Guo & Phillips, 2006; Mohammed, 2006; Racine, 2002; Tee & Lathlean, 2004; Peterson, Trapp, Fanale, & Kaur, 2003) in the United States and globally (Bathum, 2007). Overall, social justice is infrequently defined as a framework for guide nursing research, as a theory to develop research instruments to assess values (Weis & Schank, 2009), or as a way to measure justice concepts in practice (Rodwell, Noblet, Demir, & Steane, 2009). A growing number of research articles do state the social justice implications for the research area studied (Andrews & Heath, 2003; Lynam et al., 2003).

Views of Justice in Nursing Practice Articles

Articles about how justice relates to nursing practice focus on how ethics is useful in making moral judgments about care of individuals or populations (Baisch, 2009; Bell, 2003; Hildebrandt & Ford, 2009; Lawson, 2005; MacKinnon, 2009; McMurray, 2006; Peter & Morgan, 2001; Phillips & Phillips, 2006; Pieper & Dacher, 2004; Purdy & Wadhwani, 2006; Stinson, Godkin, & Robinson, 2004; Turkoski, 2005; Williams, 2004). In the last decade, a growing number of articles have begun to focus on using justice as a concept to guide nursing administration and leadership (Curtin & Arnold, 2005a, 2005b; Williams, 2006), nursing practice (Bell & Hulbert, 2008; Falk-Rafael, 2005; Sutton, 2003), and healthcare management (Williams, 2005). Crock (2009) is one of few authors to focus on how nursing practice is increasingly connected to and lured by organized power in other disciplines.

Justice is often defined as treating people fairly (Aroskar, 1995) in clinical practice. Other authors view justice not just as related to fairness but also as a social obligation for nurses to understand how practice is influenced by assumptions and social inequalities that guide the design of health care and society (Benner, 2005; Drevdahl, 2002; Ervin & Bell, 2004; Leung, 2002; Ludwick & Silva, 2003; Russell, 2002). Most authors agree that discussions of justice are needed to assess how the work of individual nurses and the profession at large contribute to the formation of a just healthcare system and society (Haddad, 2002; Schroeder & Ward, 1998).

Despite the recognition that exploring justice is needed, most articles on this topic do not define justice beyond notions about fairness. Alternatively, if justice is defined more elaborately in relationship to nursing practice, authors often use a distributive justice framework (Schroeder & Ward, 1998; Silva & Ruth, 2003). Authors using a distributive justice viewpoint assert that "all humans are born with equal opportunities and equal political agency and efficacy" (Schroeder & Ward, 1998, p. 230). The belief that persons are equal forms the basis for the even allocation of goods and services. A main limitation of the distributive view of justice is the lack of acknowledgment that social groups are often regarded unequally on the basis of gender, class, and race; thus the allocation of goods and services is also unequal in U.S. society (Young, 1990). Even fewer authors use social justice as a lens through which to view how nurses practice in unjust healthcare settings (Anderson, Rodney, Reimer-Kirkham, Browne, Khan, & Lynam, 2009).

Acknowledging the limitations of the distributive paradigm, a few authors explore the practice of nurses as embedded in the concept of the just state (Harper, 1994; Kikuchi & Simmons, 1999). The just state is concerned with how laws, public institutions, and communities act to limit or promote social inequalities in society. This view of the just state most closely parallels the concept of social justice.

SOCIAL JUSTICE: DEFINITIONAL LIMITATIONS IN THE NURSING LITERATURE

The main concern with definitions of social justice in nursing is that injustice is viewed as a personal act, and justice is seen as an individual response to that act (Liaschenko, 1999; Olsen, 1993). The individualization of social justice is historically related to how nurses conceive the person as the primary site of, and remedy to, unjust conditions (Allen, 1996). Rarely is it highlighted how injustice nationally or globally (Austin, 2001) is created by power imbalances in the distribution of wealth, resources, and access. Moreover, seldom is it noted how unequal distribution of resources and access influences healthcare delivery, health status, and health actualization or achievement of optimal health.

Often the articles about health and social justice in nursing limit the focus to underrepresented, vulnerable, or people of color populations (Herman & Sassatelli, 2002; Redman & Clark, 2002). In the last decade, however, more focus has been directed toward the practices of nurses in terms of enabling or limiting justice. Nevertheless, nursing literature rarely addresses how inequitable conditions contribute to diminished health actualization in majority groups as well. Deaton and Lubotsky (2003), for example, determined that death rates in U.S. states with more income inequality were higher for all groups than the corresponding rates in states with more equal income distributions. After considering the racial and ethnic composition of those states, it remained unclear why the mortality of the majority group of white Americans was related to racial composition and income inequality (Deaton & Lubotsky, 2003). There is also a tendency to compare health indicators of people of color to white Americans, even though white Americans as a population may not experience the best health outcomes nationally or globally. In part, this bias exists because of the lack of research into how inequality contributes to poor health outcomes for both minority and majority members of society. Despite this consideration, some literature suggests that injustice lessens the presence of optimal health for all (Kawachi & Kennedy, 1999; Subramanian, Blakely, & Kawachi, 2003). Even on a global level, poor environments foster poor health locally and nationally (World Health Organization, 1997).

Considerations such as this remain underdocumented in the nursing literature for several reasons. Most nurses have a limited view of social justice (Drevdahl, 2002) and inadequate social policies to guide their depth of thinking about social justice (Bekemeier & Butterfield, 2005; Kikuchi, 2004). When justice is defined in relationship to individual equality and fairness, the social dimensions of justice and injustice are also minimized. What is fair, however, does not necessary need to be equal, or vice versa (Thorne, 1999). Given the historic disadvantages encountered by underrepresented groups in the United States, for instance, to give equal treatment would not remedy current or past ills.

Social justice asserts that vulnerable persons should be protected from harm and promoted to achieve full status in society. The dynamics of being perceived as privileged or vulnerable require further exploration. Particularly relevant would be an investigation of how nurses themselves are influenced by privilege as they espouse their role as social justice advocates. One question becomes critical in this kind of research: Can nurses really promote a social justice agenda when that promotion will result in the critique and dismantlement of their own advantage?

Social justice critique means, for example, that one must recognize the social factors that construe persons as privileged or vulnerable at different points in time. A social justice agenda necessitates transforming systems that promote subordination or disadvantage in the long term and the immediate conditions that limit self-actualization in the short term

(Kirkham & Anderson, 2002). It requires a consistent focus on understanding how concepts are developed to limit or promote justice (Lutz & Bowers, 2003). The focus on multiple simultaneous sites of social justice action is needed to begin to address the short- and long-term oppressive situations that create social injustice and limit access to health care. A multifocal approach to social justice is needed but as yet has not been fully articulated in the nursing literature.

ALTERNATIVE VIEWS OF SOCIAL JUSTICE

Definitions of social justice vary across disciplines and over time. Theories about social justice are espoused in philosophy (Young, 1990), public health science (Beauchamp, 1986), and religious studies (Lebacquz, 1986). The use of social justice by nurses as a research framework gained momentum in the early 1990s with the application of womanist, feminist, and social critical theories (Boutain, 1999) and in the late 1990s with the use of postcolonial perspectives (Kirkham & Anderson, 2002). Authors who use critical theories to critique nursing education, research, and practice help guide the nursing profession toward a social justice agenda (Boutain, 1999). Unfortunately, many of these works were not developed to give explicit attention to the multiple ways to understand social justice as a concept.

One useful framework for nurses to consider is based on the work of Holland (1983). He argues that to be effective in promoting justice, scholars must think of addressing injustice on many fronts. Specifically, scholars must deal with the antecedents of injustice, the processes of injustice, and the results of injustice in society. These stages of injustice creation and re-creation will help focus nursing on points of intervention. Nurses can then address social justice in terms of social justice awareness, amelioration, or transformation.

SOCIAL JUSTICE AWARENESS, AMELIORATION, AND TRANSFORMATION

Social justice awareness entails exploring how one perceives others as vulnerable or privileged. Awareness involves asking critical questions about how systems of domination and oppression foster categorizations such as "vulnerability" and "privilege." An example may be helpful in understanding social justice awareness.

Homelessness is a major health and social concern. A focus on social justice awareness may involve conducting a self-interview and client interview on how housing influences health. Think about how health is related to housing. Write down your thoughts prior to interviewing clients with and without a home. Talk with clients who have homes and those who do not. Ask them about how having or not having a home influences their health. Record their thoughts.

Conduct a literature review on housing, home ownership, and health. Questions to consider include these: How does having a home relate to health? What is the health status of those who have homes? What is the health status of those who do not have homes? Compare your initial thoughts to the knowledge gained in the interview and review of relevant literature. You may discover that your awareness of the relationship between housing and health increases.

Social justice awareness is an ongoing process. To alter the analogy described by Lebacquz (1986), injustice is like a proverbial elephant standing right next to you. You cannot appreciate the entire view, and you may not fully recognize how you are affected by or are affecting the elephant. You must continue to move, sensing each part of the elephant at different angles and with different senses. Social justice awareness is temporal and dependent on your frame of reference. Being aware is a start, but it is not enough.

Social justice amelioration involves addressing the immediate results or antecedents to unjust conditions. To continue with the example of health and homelessness, amelioration entails a direct attempt to address the situation of the clients who are homeless. How that situation is addressed, however, is often to treat the most immediately seen concerns of a person experiencing homelessness. Getting grants to provide temporary shelter, food, clothing, or health care to the homeless, for example, is an illustration of social justice amelioration. In the short term, amelioration remedies urgent or semi-urgent concerns—but it does not really change the conditions that will create others as homeless over and over again.

Social justice transformation also involves critically deliberating about the conditions of home dwelling and homelessness in relationship to health. Who are the people most likely to have homes? Which conditions were present that allowed them to have homes? Who are the people most likely to be homeless? Which conditions led them to become known as homeless? How does housing relate to health services allocation, current health status, or future health attainment? Social justice transformation advocates seek to answer these questions as part of their attempts to change or develop just housing and health policies. Their aim is to eliminate or limit the conditions that result in homeless. Social justice transformation is devoted to redressing unjust conditions by changing the structures that foster those unjust situations. Transformation focuses individual actions toward long-range systematic solutions to unjust situations.

The work of Iris Young (1990) is helpful in further understanding social justice transformation. She argues that distributive justice (similar to social justice amelioration) is based on a false system of distributing services and rights to those who are already marginalized. Thus the rendering of service re-creates the system of privilege by allowing those who give the services (the privileged) to remain in a position of power over those who receive those services (the needy). In the short term, this strategy addresses the needs of the most vulnerable; in the long term, however, the system does not change because those privileged few in power maintain their positions. Young believes it is most helpful to restructure systems so that certain services, such as homeless shelters, are no longer needed or are needed only infrequently. System restructuring is accomplished by recognizing, confronting, and diminishing entrenched inequalities associated with gender, class, and racial inequalities in society (Young, 1990).

CONCLUSION

A social justice agenda recognizes that social groups are not treated equally in society. Social justice gives moral privilege to the needs of the most vulnerable group in an effort to promote justice within the society at large. As vulnerability among persons is eliminated or minimized, the moral agency of those privileged can be simultaneously elevated. This view of social justice is not clearly articulated in the literature on nursing education, research, and practice, however.

Discussions about social justice remain conceptually limited in the majority of published works in nursing. Without a more complex and nuanced view of social justice, nurses are less able to fully utilize this concept as a framework to redress unjust conditions in healthcare delivery and health attainment. Social justice is regarded as central to the nursing profession, despite the need to critically revisit discussions about this concept. Nurses can contribute much to understanding how the interdisciplinary concept of social justice is useful in promoting just health and social relationships in society.

ACKNOWLEDGMENTS

Manuscript support for the first edition of this chapter was provided by grants from the National Institute of Child Health and Human Development (HD-41682); the National Institute of Nursing Research (F31 NR07249-01); and the Centers for Disease Control and Prevention (U48/CCU009654-06). Support for the second edition of the chapter was provided by National Institute of Child Health and Human Development (HD-41682), an Intramural Award from the University of Washington School of Nursing, and Community Award the March of Dimes. Support for the third edition of this chapter was funded by an Intramural Award from the University of Washington School of Nursing. The author wishes to thank Joseph Fletcher III.

WWW

For a full suite of assignments and additional learning activities, use the access code located in the front of your book to visit this exclusive website: http://go.jblearning.com/dechesnay. If you do not have an access code, you can obtain one at the site.

REFERENCES

Abrams, S. (2009). Education at the margins and beyond borders. *Public Health Nursing, 26*(6), 487–488.

Alderson, P. (2001). Prenatal screening, ethics, and Down's syndrome: A literature review. *Nursing Ethics, 8*, 360–374.

Alexis, O., & Vydelingum, V. (2004). The lived experience of overseas black and minority ethnic nurses in the NHS in the south of England. *Diversity in Health and Social Care, 1*(1), 13–20.

Allen, D. (1996). Knowledge, politics, culture, and gender: A discourse perspective. *Canadian Journal of Nursing Research, 28*, 95–102.

Altun, I. (2002). Burnout and nurses' personal and professional values. *Nursing Ethics, 9*, 269–278.

Anderson, J., Rodney, P., Reimer-Kirkham, S., Browne, A., Khan, K., & Lynam, M. (2009). Inequalities in health and healthcare viewed through the ethical lens. *Advances in Nursing Science, 32*(4), 282–294.

Andrews, J., & Heath, J. (2003). Women and the global tobacco epidemic: Nurses call to action. *International Council of Nurses, 50*, 215–228.

Aroskar, M. (1995). Envisioning nursing as a moral community. *Nursing Outlook, 43*, 134–138.

Austin, W. (2001). Nursing ethics in an era of globalization. *Advances in Nursing Science, 24*, 1–18.

Baisch, M. (2009). Community health: An evolutionary concept analysis. *Journal of Advanced Nursing, 65*(10), 2464–2476.

Bathum, M. (2007). Global health research to promote social justice: A critical perspective. *Advances in Nursing Science, 30*(4), 303–314.

Beauchamp, D. (1986). Public health as social justice. In T. Mappes & J. Zembaty (Eds.), *Biomedical ethics* (pp. 585–593). New York: McGraw-Hill.

Bekemeier, B., & Butterfield, P. (2005). Unreconciled inconsistencies: A critical review of the concept of social justice in three national nursing documents. *Advances in Nursing Science, 28*(2), 152–162.

Bell, S. (2003). Community health nursing, wound care, and . . . ethics? *Journal of Wound, Ostomy and Continence Nurses Society, 30*(5), 259–265.

Bell, S. E., & Hulbert, J. (2008). Translating social justice into clinical nurse specialist practice. *Journal for Advanced Nursing Practice, 22*(6), 293–301.

Benner, P. (2005). Honoring the good behind the rights and justice in healthcare when more than justice is needed. *American Journal of Critical Care, 14*(2), 152–156.

Blondeau, D., Lavoie, M., Valois, P., Keyserlingk, E., Hebert, M., & Martineau, I. (2000). The attitude of Canadian nurses towards advance directives. *Nursing Ethics, 7*, 399–411.

Boersma, R. (2006). Integrating the ethics of care and justice—or are they mutually exclusive? *International Journal for Human Caring, 10*(2), 21.

Bond, A., Mandleco, B., & Warnick, M. (2004). At the heart of nursing: Stories reflect the professional values in AACN's *Essentials* document. *Nurse Educator, 29*(2), 84–88.

Boutain, D. (1999). Critical nursing scholarship: Exploring critical social theory with African-American studies. *Advances in Nursing Science, 21*, 37–47.

Boutain, D. (2005). Social justice as a framework for professional nursing. *Journal of Nursing Education, 44*(9), 404–408.

Boutain, D. (2008). Social justice as a framework for undergraduate community health clinical experiences in the United States. *International Journal of Nursing Education Scholarship, 5*(1), 13.

Clark, L., Barton, J., & Brown, N. (2002). Assessment of community contamination: A critical approach. *Public Health Nursing, 19*, 354–365.

Comer, S. (2009). The ethics of conducting educational research on your own students. *Journal of Nursing, 13*(4), 100–105.

Crock, E. (2009). Ethics of pharmaceutical company relationships with the nursing profession: No free lunch or no more pens? *Contemporary Nurse: A Journal for the Australian Nursing Profession, 33*(2), 202–209.

Curtin, L., & Arnold, L. (2005a). A framework for analysis: Part I. *Nursing Administration Quarterly, 29*(2), 183–187.

Curtin, L., & Arnold, L. (2005b). A framework for analysis: Part II. *Nursing Administration Quarterly, 29*(3), 288–291.

Deaton, A., & Lubotsky, D. (2003). Mortality, inequality and race in American cities and states. *Social Science and Medicine, 56*, 1139–1153.

Dresden, E., McElmurry, B., & McCreary, L. (2003). Approaching ethical reasoning in nursing research through a communitarian perspective. *Journal of Professional Nursing, 19*(5), 295–304.

Drevdahl, D. (1999). Sailing beyond: Nursing theory and the person. *Advances in Nursing Science, 21*(4), 1–13.

Drevdahl, D. (2002). Social justice or market justice? The paradoxes of public health partnerships with managed care. *Public Health Nursing, 19*(3), 161–169.

Drevdahl, D., Kneipp, S., Canales, M., & Dorcy, K. (2001). Reinvesting in social justice: A capital idea for public health nursing. *Advances in Nursing Science, 24*, 19–31.

Ervin, N., & Bell, S. (2004, Spring/Summer). Social justice issues related to uneven distribution of resources. *Journal of the New York State Nurses Association*, 8–13.

Fahrenwald, N. (2003). Teaching social justice. *Nurse Educator, 28*(5), 222–226.

Fahrenwald, N., Bassett, S., Tschetter, L., Carson, P., White, L., & Winterboer, V. (2005). Teaching core nursing values. *Journal of Professional Nursing, 21*(1), 46–51.

Fahrenwald, N., Taylor, J., Kneipp, S., & Canales, M. (2007). Academic freedom and academic duty to teach social justice: A perspective and pedagogy for public health nursing faculty. *Public Health Nursing, 24*(2), 190–197.

Falk-Rafael, A. (2005). Advancing nursing theory through theory-guided practice: The emergence of a critical caring perspective. *Advances in Nursing Science, 28*(1), 38–49.

Falk-Rafael, A. (2006). Globalization and global health: Toward nursing praxis in the global community. *Advances in Nursing Science, 29*(1), 2–14.

Fitzpatrick, J. (2003). From the editor: Social justice, human rights, and nursing education. *Nurse Educator, 28*(5), 222–226.

Giddings, L. (2005a). Health disparities, social injustice, and the culture of nursing. *Nursing Research, 54*(5), 304–312.

Giddings, L. (2005b). A theoretical model of social consciousness. *Advances in Nursing Science, 28*(3), 224–239.

Grant, B. M., Giddings, L., & Beale, J. (2005). Vulnerable bodies: Competing discourses of intimate bodily care. *Journal of Nursing Education, 44*(11), 498–503.

Guenter, D., Majumdar, B., Willms, D., Travers, R., Browne, G., & Robinson, G. (2005). Community-based HIV education and prevention workers respond to a changing environment. *Journal of the Association of Nurses in AIDS Care, 16*(1), 29–36.

Guo, G., & Phillips, L. (2006). Key informants' perceptions of health for elders at the U.S.–Mexico border. *Public Health Nursing, 23*(3), 224–233.

Haddad, A. (2002). Fairness, respect, and foreign nurses. *RN, 65*(7), 25–28.

Harper, J. (1994). For-profit entities and continuing education: A nursing perspective. *Nursing Outlook, 42*, 217–222.

Harris, G. (2005). Ethical issues in community care. *Journal of Community Nursing, 19*(11), 12–16.

Herman, C., & Sassatelli, J. (2002). DARING to reach the heartland: A collaborative faith-based partnership in nursing education. *Journal of Nursing Education, 41*(10), 443–445.

Hildebrandt, E., & Forde, S. (2009). Justice and impoverished women: The ethical implications of work-based welfare. *Policy, Politics, & Nursing Practice, 10*(4), 295–302.

Holland, J. (1983). *Social analysis: Linking faith and justice.* Maryknoll, NY: Orbis Books.

Hubert, J. (2004). Continuing the dialogue: A response to Kikuchi's critique of the 2002 CNA Code of Ethics. *Canadian Journal of Nursing Leadership, 17*(4), 10–13.

Jackson, D. (2003). Epilogue: Culture, health and social justice. *Contemporary Nurse, 15*(3), 347–348.

Kawachi, I., & Kennedy, B. (1999). Income inequality and health: Pathways and mechanisms. *Health Services Research, 34*(1 Pt 2), 215–227.

Kikuchi, J. (2004). 2002 CNA Code of Ethics: Some recommendations. *Canadian Journal of Nursing Leadership, 17*(3), 28–33.

Kikuchi, J., & Simmons, H. (1999). Practical nursing judgment: A moderate realist conception. *Scholarly Inquiry in Nursing Practice, 13*(1), 43–55.

Kirkham, S., & Anderson, J. (2002). Postcolonial nursing scholarship: From epistemology to method. *Advances in Nursing Science, 25*(1), 1–17.

Kirkham, S., Hofwegen, L., & Harwood, C. (2005). Narratives of social justice: Learning in innovative clinical settings. *International Journal of Nursing Education Scholarship, 2*(1), Article 28.

Kneipp, S., & Snider, M. (2001). Social justice in a market model world. *Journal of Professional Nursing, 17*(3), 113.

Lamke, C. (1996). Distributive justice and HIV disease in intensive care. *Critical Care Nursing Quarterly, 19*(1), 55–64.

Lawson, L. (2005). Furthering the search for truth and justice. *Journal of Forensic Nursing, 1*(4), 149–150.

Lebacqz, K. (1986). *Six theories of justice.* Minneapolis, MN: Augsburg.

Leung, W. (2002). Why the professional–client ethic is inadequate in mental health care. *Nursing Ethics, 9*(1), 51–60.

Leuning, C. (2001). Advancing a global perspective: The world as classroom. *Nursing Science Quarterly, 14*(4), 298–303.

Liaschenko, J. (1999). Can justice coexist with the supremacy of personal values in nursing practice? *Western Journal of Nursing Research, 21*(1), 35–50.

Ludwick, R., & Silva, M. (2000, August). Nursing around the world: Cultural values and ethical conflicts. *Online Journal of Issues in Nursing.* Retrieved January 25, 2007, from http://www.nursingworld.org/#jin/ethical/ethics_4.htm

Lutz, B., & Bowers, B. (2003). Understanding how disability is defined and conceptualized in the literature. *Rehabilitation Nursing, 28*(3), 74–78.

Lynam, M., Henderson, A., Browne, A., Smye, V., Semeniuk, P., Blue, C., & Singh, S. (2003). Healthcare restructuring with a view and efficiency: Reflections on unintended consequences. *Canadian Journal of Nursing Leadership, 16*(1), 112–140.

MacIntosh, J., & Wexler, E. (2005). Interprovincial Partnership in Nursing Education. *Canadian Nurse, 101*(4), 17–20.

MacKinnon, C. (2009). Applying feminist, multicultural, and social justice theory to diverse women who function as caregivers in end-of-life and palliative home care. *Palliative & Supportive Care, 7*(4), 501–512.

Mantler, J., Armstrong-Stassen, M., Horsburgh, M., & Cameron, S. (2006). Reactions of hospital staff nurses to recruitment incentives. *Western Journal of Nursing Research, 28*(1), 70–84.

Mathes, M. (2005). Ethical decision making and nursing. *Dermatology Nursing, 17*(6), 444–458.

Mathes, M. (2004). Ethical decision making and nursing. *Medsurg Nursing, 13*(6), 429–431.

McKane, M. (2000). Research, ethics and the data protection legislation. *Nursing Standard, 2*(14), 36–41.

McMurray, A. (2004). Culturally sensitive evidence-based practice. *Collegian, 11*(4), 14–18.

McMurray, A. (2006). Peace, love and equality: Nurses, interpersonal violence and social justice. *Contemporary Nurse, 21*(2), vii–x.

Messias, D. (2001). Globalization, nursing, and health for all. *Journal of Nursing Scholarship, 33*(1), 9–11.

Messias, D., McDowell, L., & Estrada, R. (2009). Language interpreting as social justice work: Perspectives of formal and informal healthcare interpreters. *Advances in Nursing Science, 32*(2), 128–143.

Mill, J., & Ogilvie, L. (2002). Ethical decision making in international nursing research. *Qualitative Health Research, 12*(6), 807–815.

Mohammed, S. (2006). Moving beyond the "exotic": Applying postcolonial theory in health research. *Advances in Nursing Science, 29*(2), 98–109.

Moule, P. (2003). ICT: A social justice approach to exploring user issues? *Nurse Education Today, 23*, 530–536.

Murphy, N., Canales, M., Norton, S., & DeFilippis, J. (2005). Striving for congruence: The interconnection between values, practice, and political action. *Policy, Politics, & Nursing, 6*(1), 20–29.

Myhrvold, T. (2003). The exclusion of the other: Challenges to the ethics of closeness. *Nursing Philosophy, 4*, 33–43.

Myrick, F. (2005). Educating nurses for the knowledge economy. *International Journal of Nursing Education Scholarship, 2*(1), Article 20.

Oddi, L., & Oddi, S. (2000). Student–faculty joint authorship: Ethical and legal concerns. *Journal of Professional Nursing, 16*(4), 219–227.

Olsen, D. (1993). Populations vulnerable to the ethics of caring. *Journal of Advanced Nursing, 18*, 1696–1700.

Pereira, A. (2006). Critical thinking, *Dynamics, 17*(3), 4–5.

Pesut, B., Fowler, M., Reimer-Kirkham, S., Taylor, E., & Sawatzky, R. (2009). Particularizing spirituality in points of tension: Enriching the discourse. *Nursing Inquiry, 16*(4), 337–346.

Peter, E., & Morgan, K. (2001). Explorations of a trust approach to nursing ethics. *Nursing Inquiry, 8*, 3–10.

Phillips, L., & Phillips, W. (2006). Better reproductive healthcare for women with disabilities: A role for nursing leadership. *Advances in Nursing Science, 29*(2), 134–151.

Pieper, B., & Dacher, J. (2004). Looking backward toward our future: Creating the nexus between community health nursing and palliative care. *Journal of the New York State Nurses Association, 35*(1), 20–24.

Purdy, I., & Wadhwani, R. (2006). Embracing bioethics in neonatal intensive care. Part II: Case histories in neonatal ethics. *Neonatal Network, 25*(1), 43–53.

Racine, L. (2002). Implementing a postcolonial feminist perspective in nursing research related to non-Western populations. *Nursing Inquiry, 10*(2), 91–102.

Redman, R., & Clark, L. (2002). Service-learning as a model for integrating social justice in the nursing curriculum. *Journal of Nursing Education, 41*, 446–449.

Rew, L., Taylor-Seehafer, M., & Thomas, N. (2000). Without parental consent: Conducting research with homeless adolescents. *Journal of the Society of Pediatric Nurses, 5*, 131–138.

Rodwell, J., Noblet, A., Demir, D., & Steane, P. (2009). Supervisors are central to work characteristics affecting nurse outcomes. *Journal of Nursing Scholarship, 41*(93), 310–319.

Russell, K. (2002) Silent voices. *Public Health Nursing, 19*(4), 233–234.

Scanlan, J., Care, W., & Gessler, S. (2001). Dealing with unsafe students in clinical practice. *Nurse Educator, 26*(1), 23–27.

Schroeder, C., & Ward, D. (1998). Women, welfare, and work: One view of the debate. *Nursing Outlook, 46*(5), 226–232.

Sellers, S., & Haag, B. (1992). Achieving equity in nursing education. *Nursing & Health Care, 13*(3), 134–137.

Shattell, M., Hogan, B., & Hernandez, A. (2006). The interpretive research group as an alternative to the interpersonal process recording. *Nurse Educator, 31*(4), 178–182.

Silva, M., & Ruth, L. (2003). Ethics and terrorism: September 11, 2001 and its aftermath. *Online Journal of Issues in Nursing, 8*(1), 21–24.

Sistrom, M., & Hale, P. (2006). Integrative review of population health, income, social capital and structural inequality. *Journal of Multicultural Nursing & Health, 12*(2), 21–27.

Spence Laschinger, H. (2004). Hospital nurses' perceptions of respect and organizational justice. *Journal of Nursing Administration, 34*(7/8), 354–364.

Stys, J. (2008). Social analysis formation for nurse educators. *Nursing Education Perspectives, 29*(6), 366–369.

Stinson, C., Godkin, J., & Robinson, R. (2004). *Dimensions of Critical Care Nursing, 23*(1), 38–43.

Subramanian, S., Blakely, T., & Kawachi, I. (2003). Income inequality as a public health concern: Where do we stand? *Health Services Research, 38*, 153–167.

Sullivan-Bolyai, S., Bova, C., & Harper, D. (2005). Developing and refining interventions in persons with health disparities: The use of the qualitative description. *Nursing Outlook, 53*, 127–133.

Sutton, J. (2003). The ethics of theatre nurse practice under the microscope. *British Journal of Perioperative Nursing, 13*(10), 405–408.

Tee, S., & Lathlean, J. (2004). The ethics of conducting a co-operative inquiry with vulnerable people. *Journal of Advanced Nursing, 47*(5), 536–543.

Thomas, S. (2004). School connectedness, anger behaviors, and relationship of violent and nonviolent American youth. *Perspectives in Psychiatric Care, 40*(40), 135–148.

Thompson, D. (1991). Ethical case analysis using a hospital bill. *Nurse Educator, 16*(4), 20–23.

Thorne, S. (1999). Are egalitarian relationships a desirable ideal in nursing? *Western Journal of Nursing Research, 21*(1), 16–34.

Turkoski, B. (2005). Culturally sensitive healthcare. *Home Healthcare Nurse, 23*(6), 355–358.

Vickers, D. (2008). Social justice: A concept for undergraduate nursing curricula? *Southern Online Journal of Nursing Research, 8*(1), 18.

Vonthron Good, B., & Rodrigues-Fisher, L. (1993). Vulnerability: An ethical consideration in research with older adults. *Western Journal of Nursing Research, 15*(6), 780–783.

Weis, D., & Schank, M. (2009). Development and psychometric evaluation of the Nurses Professional Values Scale—Revised. *Journal of Nursing Measurement, 17*(3), 221–231.

Whitehead, M. (1992). The concepts and principles of equity and health. *International Journal of Health Services, 22*(3), 429–445.

Williams, A. (2004). Nursing, health and human rights: A framework for international collaboration. *Association of Nurses in AIDS Care, 15*(3), 75–77.

Williams, A. (2005). Thinking about equity in health care. *Journal of Nursing Management, 13*, 397–402.

Williams, L. (2006). The fair factor in matters of trust. *Nursing Administration Quarterly, 30*(1), 30–37.

World Health Organization. (1997). *Health and environments in sustainable development: Five years after the Earth Summit.* Geneva, Switzerland: Author.

Young, I. (1990). *Justice and the politics of difference.* Princeton, NJ: Princeton University Press.

CHAPTER 5

Low Literacy and Vulnerable Clients

Toni Vezeau

Objectives

At the end of this chapter, the reader will be able to

1. Describe the current status of health literacy in the United States.
2. Explain how health literacy affects vulnerability.
3. Provide solutions that health care providers might implement to reverse the negative effects of health illiteracy.

WWW

Effective health care requires skills on the part of both providers and clients. Providers must have a strong knowledge base and successful communication skills that match the needs of their clients. Clients must be able to take in information, make sense of it, apply it to their own situations, and retain the information for future use. These skills are the hallmarks of literacy. Without literacy as a base client skill, there is little chance that healthcare interactions will meet their intended goals. This chapter presents literacy as a primary driver of vulnerability in health care. The discussion explores the current status of literacy skills in the United States, client and provider aspects of the problem, and recommendations for current practice.

WHAT IS THE STATUS OF LITERACY IN THE UNITED STATES?

The National Adult Literacy Survey (NALS), conducted in 1992, defined literacy as the use of printed information to maneuver in society, meet one's goals, and develop one's knowledge and abilities (Kirsch, Jungeblut, Jenkins, & Kolstad, 1993). Doak, Doak, and Root (2001) modified this definition to include comprehension and retention of verbal and gestural information.

The 1992 NALS remains the largest study on adult literacy carried out in the United States ($n = 26{,}000$). This study went far beyond establishing the reading grade level of participants and tested their performance in three areas (Figure 5–1):

1. Prose literacy: printed word in connected sentences and passages; implies skill in finding information and integrating information from several sections of the text.
2. Document literacy: structured prose in arrays of columns and rows, lists, and maps; implies skill in locating information, repeating the search as often as needed, and integrating information.
3. Quantitative literacy: information displayed in graphs, charts, and in numerical form; in addition to locating information, this skill implies that one can infer and apply the needed arithmetic.

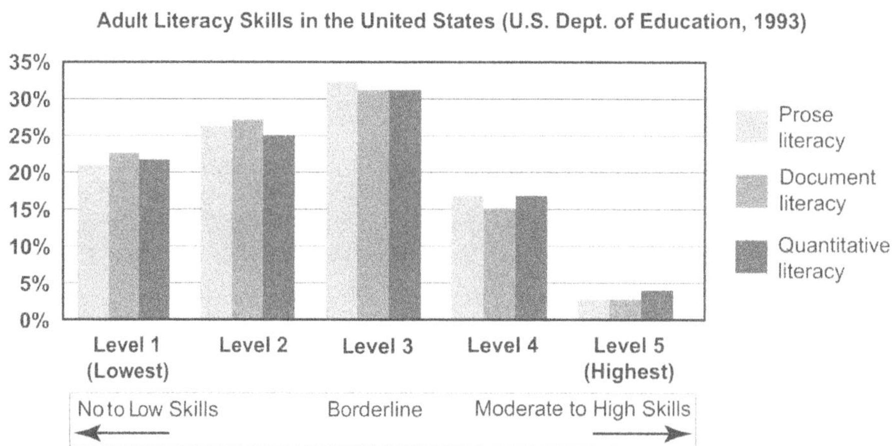

Figure 5–1 Adult literacy skills in the United States.
Source: Adapted from US Department of Education, Office of Educational Research and Improvement, National Center for Educational Statistics, 1993.

Participants were tested on a wide variety of tasks encountered at work, home, and community activities, such as signing a mock Social Security card and filling out personal information on a simple job application.

The original NALS data suggested that one-fourth to one-third of American adults are functionally illiterate and approximately an equal number have marginal literacy skills that disallow full functioning in society. Essentially, half of the adult population in the United States has poor to nonexistent skills in reading, listening, and computation. Minor proportions of the NALS survey were learning disabled (5%) and spoke English as a second language, if at all (15%). However, most were white and born in America. Although education correlated with literacy, generally those adults who had a tenth-grade education read at the seventh- to eighth-grade level. Participants receiving Medicaid had an average of a fifth-grade reading level. One-third of the NALS sample demonstrated basic functionality in understanding and using written information. Only 20% of the sample demonstrated a level of proficiency in handling information to perform complex reading and computation tasks. When these data were recomputed using 2003 data and released in 2006 (National Center for Education Statistics, 2006), the results showed a slightly worsening trend.

The NALS data suggested that certain groups fared much worse in their literacy skills than the general population. Of those adults who tested at the lowest reading level,

- 41% to 44% were poor
- 33% were older than age 65 years
- 25% were immigrants
- 62% did not finish high school (disproportionately represented by Hispanic, African American, and Asian Pacific participants)
- 12% had physical, mental, or health conditions that disallowed participation in work or school settings
- 75% of the subfunctional group had a mental health problem

Participants in the lowest literacy level had difficulty with performing usual tasks of daily living based on printed information and in performing complex tasks that required following directions and computation. Interestingly, members of the group considered to have no or minimal functional literacy did not acknowledge themselves as vulnerable, related to their illiteracy. This group noted that they could read "adequately to very well," and fewer than 25% of these participants stated that they received help with information from family and friends.

A meta-analysis of U.S. studies on literacy in 2005 (Paasche-Orlow, Parker, Gazmararian, Neilsen-Bohlman, & Rudd, 2005) reviewed literature from January 1963 through January 2004 and, based on a pool of 85 articles, essentially validated the same prevalence rates mentioned earlier, with one exception: These findings did not show gender to be associated with literacy. The authors concluded that limited literacy is highly prevalent, negatively affects health, and is consistently associated with education, ethnicity, and age. Could it be true that persons with low literacy are not vulnerable in American society?

WHAT IS THE RELATIONSHIP BETWEEN LITERACY AND HEALTH VULNERABILITY?

Kirsch et al. (1993) discussed literacy as currency in the United States, because those with less literacy are much less likely to meet the needs of daily living and to pursue life goals. From this perspective, illiteracy has the potential to create health risks and exacerbate existing health conditions.

Literacy as a Predictor of Vulnerability

Aday's (2001) model of vulnerability and health posits that although all humans are vulnerable to illness, certain segments of the community are much more vulnerable to ill health in terms of initial susceptibility and in their response. Illiteracy is related to each of Aday's (2001) predictors of vulnerability. Persons with poor reading skills who are unable to perform basic literacy functions, such as reading a bus schedule or following directions in completing a task, generally have low social status outside of their immediate social ties. For example, low social status is often associated with low-paying jobs that offer no or minimal healthcare insurance. Low status also can affect a provider's perception of client abilities, creating care that is "edited" based, at times, on misperceptions (Aday, 2001).

Social Status

Social status has been correlated with poor health (Duncan, Daly, McDonough, & Williams, 2002), in that persons with low status are more likely to use disproportionately more healthcare services, receive substandard care and less information about their illness, and be presented with fewer options. Kirsch et al. (1993) identified that persons with low literacy have much greater difficulty in accessing what Aday (2001) calls human capital (e.g., jobs, schools, income, and housing) than those persons with functional literacy skills. Similarly, NALS data are congruent with Aday's third driver of vulnerability, lack of social capital, in that persons who are illiterate are more likely to be single or divorced, live in single-parent homes, and be loosely connected to their own communities.

Access to Care

Additionally, Aday (2001) addresses relationships of vulnerability to access to health care, cost of care, and quality of care. Accessing care in the United States most often requires complex language skills that are applied to the following tasks:

- Identifying and evaluating possible providers of care
- Negotiating appropriate entry points into the system
- Contacting and communicating needs to obtain an appointment
- Successfully traveling to and finding the actual site of care
- Interpreting written materials and relating to clock and calendar skills

Access to care is seriously challenged when clients have low literacy skills.

Consequences of Vulnerability

Quality of Care

The literature published in the last decade documents well how illiteracy has affected the cost of care and the quality of care (Agency for Healthcare Research and Quality, 2004; Baker et al., 2002; Institute of Medicine [IOM], 2003). Illiteracy is a significant component of client adherence to care regimens and hospitalizations in numerous health contexts—for example, pregnancy, diabetes, AIDS, asthma, sexually transmitted diseases, women's health, rural residents, immigrants, mental health, advanced age, cardiac surgery, rheumatoid arthritis, prostate cancer, psychiatric clients, older adults, cardiac surgical clients, and payer status.

Without exception, the populations just cited have high prevalence of illiteracy, in proportions that mirror the findings from the NALS data. Studies have shown that persons with literacy problems do not understand instructions and demonstrate less comprehension of their illness or condition.

Costs

Healthy People 2010 (U.S. Department of Health and Human Services, 2000) noted that the consequences of illiteracy include both poorer health outcomes and increased healthcare costs; in fact, costs of health care may be as much as four times greater for those clients who read at or below the second-grade level than for the general populace. Baker et al. (2002) reported that clients with documented low literacy had a 52% higher risk of hospital admission compared with those with functional literacy, even after controlling for age, social and economic factors, and self-reported health. In another study, client illiteracy was the highest predictor of poor asthma knowledge and ineffective use of metered-dose inhalers (Williams, Baker, Honig, Lee, & Nowlan, 1998).

Acknowledging the pervasive influence of illiteracy on the quality of care in the United States, the IOM has identified literacy as one of the top three areas that cut across all other priorities for improvement in the nation's health. As noted by the IOM, literacy is required for self-management and collaborative care, the other two priority cross-cutting areas.

REDEFINING THE FOCUS

Since the mid-1990s, the medical literature has used a new term—"health literacy"—to address the literacy problem. The Ad Hoc Committee on Health Literacy for the Council on Scientific Affairs of the American Medical Association (1999) defined an individual's functional health literacy as "the ability to read and comprehend prescription bottles, appointment slips, and other essential health-related materials required to successfully function as a patient." To this definition, the National Health Education Standards added the understanding of basic health information, ability to effectively handle the healthcare system, and understand consent forms (Williams, 2000). "Health literacy" has now become the preferred term when referring to this intersection of health concerns and literacy skills. Williams is articulate in describing the complexity of this nexus, which requires listening, analytical, decision-making, computation, and application skills.

International healthcare work has addressed health literacy in these terms for a much longer time; related literature exists from the 1960s onward. Interestingly, the issues discussed in international literature correspond well to current Western health literature. Watters (2003) summarized well the healthcare implications of no or low literacy in international work: increased use of health systems and costs, late entry into care secondary to poor interpretation of symptoms, poor participation in preventive care, shame over literacy status eliminating self-identification of needs to care providers, self-administration medication errors related to literacy errors, and inconsistent shows at appointments. Each of these health concerns related to literacy has been documented in the United States as well (American Medical Association, 1999; Baker, 1999; Kripalani, Henderson, Chiu, Robertson, Kohm, & Jacobson, 2006).

After being long silent on this issue, The Joint Commission's National Patient Safety Goals now include systematic approaches to address low-literacy clients by focusing on organizational strategies and policy development (Murphy-Knoll, 2007).

In summary, research has supported Aday's (2001) theoretical work on health vulnerability. It is clear that—as yet without exception—literacy strongly influences the health of individuals and populations. The problems with literacy, however, are jointly owned and created by clients and providers. It is important to understand specific literacy problems of clients and to consider how providers have contributed to these problems.

HOW DOES ILLITERACY SPECIFICALLY INCREASE HEALTH RISKS OF CLIENTS?

Clients with no or low literacy cannot read or interpret pamphlets, directions on prescribed or over-the-counter medications, or diet instructions. A mismatch of vocabulary and skill is just one of the problems. Comprehension of graphics and pictures pose additional and, for many clients, insurmountable challenges (Doak et al., 2001).

Literacy is a complex skill requiring much more than the simple reading of words. It has many components, such as decoding, comprehension, and retention of information. In addition, the development of literacy involves a series of stages. Finally, literacy is not a "free-standing skill," but rather involves integration of related life skills to navigate the healthcare system, effectively perform self-care, and make healthcare decisions.

Health and health care add unique aspects to the concern for client literacy. The effects of health and health care on literacy skills can be either temporary or sustained. Such situations as anesthesia due to surgery, blood loss, or acute pain may temporarily impair one's decoding, comprehension, and recall skills. Moreover, sustained medical conditions can interfere with mentation, cognition, and attention on a longer-term basis. Delayed mental development; neurological conditions, such as Alzheimer's disease; cerebral vascular accidents; and psychological disorders, such as depression or anxiety, may affect literacy skills and the ability of the client to interact effectively with providers. Understandably, clients who have sensory impairments are likely to have literacy difficulty. Visual difficulties were noted in 20% of the NALS sample that tested in the lowest level of literacy (Kirsch et al., 1993).

Medications may also negatively affect clients' abilities to effectively use their literacy skills, increasing risk for the client. Drug categories such as opiates, anticonvulsants, antidepressives, glucocorticosteroids, some antihypertensives, and thyroid and ovarian hormones are but a few medications that are known to affect information processing.

Providers need to appreciate how certain therapies and health conditions affect the client's ability to use the literacy skills he or she has. For those clients with low literacy skills, the health situations noted provide serious challenges to a client's ability to use healthcare information.

HOW DO HEALTHCARE PROVIDERS INFLUENCE THE LITERACY PROBLEM?

Clients come to providers with their unique characteristics and abilities related to health literacy. In the past, providers, in their listening, speaking, and written interactions with clients, generally have ignored the literacy variable in care and, in most cases, increased the literacy challenge for their clients (Doak et al., 2001; Hohn, 1998). A review of the literature reveals several threads addressing how providers have influenced health literacy: readability of client health education text, measurement of clients' reading levels in specific healthcare settings, and client–provider communications.

Readability of Written Healthcare Education Materials

Since 1988, the literature has documented that the readability of written healthcare instructions, booklets, and informed consent forms has not matched the skills of clients in a general care population (Cutilli, 2007; Doak et al., 2001; Forbis & Aligne, 2002). Health educational materials have been tested but often only a few at a time. When Doak et al. (2001) evaluated 1234 health education materials, they found that more than half were written at or above the tenth-grade level. It is important to remember that education levels of clients do not generally match their reading skill levels. Specifically, reading skills average four to five grades lower when tested when compared with level of educational attainment (Cutilli, 2007). Thus the news is even more dire: If a client population has a mean of tenth-grade education, most educational materials in current use would outstrip the client skill level (Doak et al., 2001) (Figure 5–2). Studies have documented discharge instructions and client educational materials to be written well above a ninth-grade level of difficulty (Gannon & Hildebrandt, 2002). Recent studies have confirmed that the readability level of even commercially produced materials that are targeted to lower-literacy populations is far above the skill level of most clients (Cutilli, 2007; Sanders, Federico, Klass, Abrams, & Dreyer, 2009)

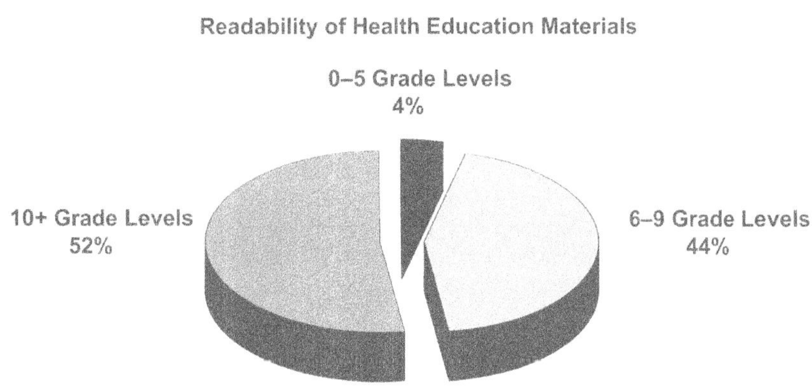

Figure 5–2 Readability of health education materials.
Source: Adapted from Doak, Doak, & Root, 2001. Readability levels of 1234 healthcare materials.

Consent forms, contracts, and commonly used self-report diagnostic tools are consistently documented as having a readability level higher than a ninth-grade level. For example, clients who read at a sixth-grade level or lower did not demonstrate comprehension of 54% of the items on the Beck Depression scale; good readers experienced difficulty with one-third of the items (Sentell & Ratcliff-Baird, 2003). Similarly, in a study of 1014 adults completing the Baltimore STD and Behavior Survey, 28% of the adults read at or lower than the eighth-grade level; this group showed a high error rate in comprehending survey items. The error rate in item comprehension decreased significantly as the literacy level increased ($p < 0.0001$) (Al-Tayyib, Rogers, Gribble, Villarroel, & Turner, 2002).

Studies investigating the literacy challenge of informed consent have consistently rated forms above the twelfth-grade level and noted that institutional review boards typically do not take reading difficulty of consent forms into account (Raich, Plomer, & Coyne, 2001). When institutional review boards do act on this matter, the effect is generally to lower the reading level by one grade (Raich et al., 2001).

Clients with no or low literacy who are given materials that directly affect their understanding of their health condition, who sign written forms that direct care, or who are tested using self-report tools are vulnerable to a host of negative consequences, including inadequate understanding of healthcare instructions, agreeing to procedures they do not fully understand, and faulty diagnosis.

Provider–Client Interactions and Communication

Interactions with low-literacy clients are just beginning to be studied. Provider–client interactions are influenced by perceptions of both client and provider. Both U.S. Census Bureau literacy data and NALS data indicate that persons with low literacy state to others that they read well enough to meet their needs. For healthcare providers, it is important to understand that such clients generally do not self-identify or discuss their literacy status because of the stigma associated with illiteracy (Doak et al., 2001; Parikh, Parker, Nurss, Baker, & Williams, 1996; Safeer & Keenan, 2005). Not only do low-literacy clients not admit to difficulties with literacy to their care providers, but they may also hide their need for help from their spouses and families (Parikh et al., 1996).

Stigma and Shame

Stigma is both self-imposed in the form of shame and evident in how providers interact with clients. When Baker et al. (1996) interviewed clients who tested as having no to low literacy, they found that participants in the study held a deep sense of shame, which was exacerbated when healthcare providers became distressed or irritated when clients had difficulty in filling out forms or reading instructions. Study participants stated that accessing care is daunting because of problems with registration and forms. In many cases, these clients avoided seeking care because of poor interactions with their care providers. Low literacy has been found to inhibit client questions, and it may be a major factor in overall participation in a healthcare encounter (Arthur, Geiser, Arriola, & Kripalani, 2009; Katz, Jacobson, & Kripalani, 2007).

Myths and Misidentification

Providers are generally not knowledgeable about illiteracy and interact differentially with clients who admit to literacy problems (Doak et al., 2001; Schillinger et al., 2003). Few providers have had any formal training in identification of and approaches to low-literacy clients (Jukkala,

Deupree & Graham, 2009; Schlicting, Quinn, Heuer, Schaefer, Drum, & Chin, 2007). As a consequence, there are a number of common myths held by providers (Doak et al., 2001, p. 6):

- "Illiterates are dumb and learn slowly if at all."
- "Most illiterates are poor, immigrants, or minorities."
- "Years of schooling are a good measure of literacy level."

Research refutes each of these myths (Doak et al., 2001). A person's measurement of intelligence does not correlate strongly with literacy skills; the correlation with income level is better. In terms of raw numbers, most persons with illiteracy in the United States are white native-born Americans in all areas of society; minorities and foreign-born groups in the United States have disproportionately high percentages of persons with no to minimal literacy. Years of schooling show the amount of education the person was exposed to, not the skill level achieved.

Incorrectly, providers may believe they can identify which clients need extra support related to their literacy needs. Bass, Wilson, Griffith, and Barnett (2002) conducted a study to see whether medical residents could correctly identify persons with low literacy out of a pool of 182 clients. The residents identified 90% of the clients as having no literacy problem. Of this client group, 36% tested as functionally illiterate. Only 3 of 182 clients were thought to have literacy problems when they did not test as such. Schlichting et al. (2007) found that the typical provider in their survey of 803 primary care providers could identify 41% and 43% of low-literacy English-speaking and Spanish-speaking clients, respectively.

Only recently have nurses been studied, with similar results. In one study, bachelor's degree–prepared nurses could identify the risks and consequences of low literacy, but could not identify elderly clients as an important low-literacy population and could not identify interventions for working with low-literacy clients (Cormier & Kotrlik, 2009).This study suggests that providers seriously underestimate the literacy problem in their client group.

Inattention to Literacy Needs

Another study observed senior physicians interacting during several outpatient visits with 74 diabetic clients who spoke only English and tested as having no or low literacy (Schillinger et al., 2003). Even when made aware of the literacy needs of their clients, provider use of language was assessed as being well above the literacy level of their clients. The physicians in 80% of encounters did not test their clients' comprehension and recall. Those clients whose physicians did test for understanding and short-term recall had significantly greater glycemic control.

Rootman and Ronson (2005, p. 62) stated the following:

> [W]e are mired in a state of denial over literacy. The immensity of the issue has paralyzed our public institutions, which seem to spend as much energy holding strategy sessions or denying responsibility as they do actually supporting programs of proven success. . . . It's hardly a promising time for a major national crusade against anything—especially poor literacy, which has no quick fix.

HOW CAN PROVIDERS DECREASE THE HEALTH RISK DUE TO ILLITERACY?

The literature reports a variety of approaches to decrease vulnerability of clients related to literacy problems. Currently, many websites, developed by private and public agencies, exist as clearinghouses to guide clinicians on preferred approaches to working with low-literacy clients (Table 5–1).

Table 5–1 Helpful Websites on Health Literacy

- National Adult Literacy Survey (Full Report)
  http://nces.ed.gov/pubs93/93275.pdf
- National Center for Education Statistics
  http://nces.ed.gov/naal/health.asp
- National Institute for Literacy
  http://www.nifl.gov
- National Cancer Institute, Clear & Simple: Developing Effective Print Materials for Low-Literate Readers
  http://www.nci.nih.gov/cancerinformation/clearandsimple
- U.S. Census Bureau Website (Education Statistics)
  http://www.census.gov/population/www/index.html
- Empowerment Health Education in Adult Literacy: A Guide for Public Health and Adult Literacy Practitioners, Policy Makers and Funders (White Paper by Marcia Hohn, NIFL)
  http://www.nifl.gov/nifl/fellowship/reports/hohn/HOHN.HTM
- Center for Health Care Strategies: Fact Sheets on Literacy
  http://www.chcs.org/usr_doc/Health_Literacy_Fact_Sheets.pdf
- Partnership for Clear Health Communication (Health Literacy Bibliography, 183 citations)
  http://www.askme3.org/pdfs/bibliography.pdf
- Pfizer Clear Health Communication: Corporate Initiative on Health Literacy
  http://www.pfizerhealthliteracy.com
- Health Literacy Consulting: Corporation Information on Multiple Types of Client Communication
  http://www.healthliteracy.com/articles.asp
- Healthy People 2010—Health Communication
  http://www.healthypeople.gov/Document/HTML/Volume1/11HealthCom.htm#_Toc490471353

Identification

Many studies have emphasized a personal approach in discretely asking about literacy status (Feifer, 2003; Nutbeam, 2008). Nevertheless, given the breadth of the literacy problem and the reading demand placed on clients in the United States, a systematic approach to address literacy in a client population is indicated. It is now recommended that as part of routine primary care, literacy should be a measured baseline, comparable with many baselines obtained in the course of quality health care.

A first step in intervention for low literacy is to identify those clients with literacy deficits. It has been thoroughly validated in research that physicians tend to overestimate clients' literacy levels (Powell & Kripalani, 2005). One study compared physicians who screened for literacy issues with their clients and physicians who did not. It was found that physicians overestimated 62% of the time and voiced more dissatisfaction with the client visit (Seligman et al., 2005). In contrast, other researchers have found that residents have increased comfort and skill in working with low-literacy clients after completing a training program (Rosenthal, Werner, & Dubin, 2004).

A few researchers have identified some tools to efficiently screen clients:

- The Rapid Estimate of Adult Literacy in Medicine (REALM) is a 2-minute test that measures a client's recognition and ability to pronounce common healthcare words (Davis, Long, & Jackson, 1993).
- The Test of Functional Health Literacy in Adults (TOFHLA) uses hospital-written materials to test both reading comprehension and basic computational skills. This test takes much longer to administer, approximately 20 to 25 minutes. A shortened version of this test (S-TOFHLA) takes 10 to 15 minutes to administer. These tests may be useful to assess individual clients with specific needs. Recent testing suggests that using just three of the S-TOFHLA 16 questions was effective in identifying low-literacy clients ("How often do you have someone help you read hospital materials?" "How confident are you filling out medical forms by yourself?" "How often do you have problems learning about your medical condition because of difficulty understanding written information?") (Chew, Bradley, & Boyko, 2004).
- The Newest Vital Sign is a nutrition label that is accompanied by six questions; it takes 3 minutes to give to a client and broadly screens for low literacy (Johnson & Weiss, 2008; Weiss et al., 2005).
- The most recently introduced test, the Single Item Literacy Screener (SILS; Morris, MacLean, Chew, & Littenberg, 2006), was used to evaluate 999 adults with diabetes, 169 of whom had low literacy. SILS asks, "How often do you need to have someone help you when you read instructions, pamphlets, or other written material from your doctor or pharmacy?" The sensitivity of this test was reported to be 54%, and specificity was 83%. Similarly, a one-question screen ("How confident are you filling out forms by yourself?") was found to be the best predictor of low literacy and as good as more time-consuming formal evaluations of literacy (Chew et al., 2008).

Although it takes time and other resources to obtain literacy measures, recent research suggests that this effort may be as simple as asking a single question. Proper identification of client literacy levels can give clear guidance in effective client education.

Within those systems that do not routinely screen clients, asking blunt questions regarding reading abilities may not yield accurate responses. As discussed earlier, clients with low literacy generally do not disclose their difficulties related to reading. They may deliberately conceal their literacy problems or, in some cases, may be unaware of their level of difficulty. Schultz (2002) and Doak et al. (2001) have identified several potential indicators of literacy problems: reading text upside down, difficulty orienting to a brochure, excuses for not reading in front of others (e.g., forgot glasses), mispronouncing words (for English speakers), reluctance to ask questions, missed appointments, difficulty following verbal instructions, relying on family members to fill out forms, and tiring quickly when reading text. When such client behaviors are noticed, it is important for the provider to explore the underlying issues.Perhaps one of most important themes in current research in this area is that providers who had training in identification of and clinical approaches to low-literacy clients were much more successful in their assessment of literacy status (Jukkala et al., 2009; Schlichting et al., 2007).

Education Strategies

Low-literacy clients may learn better when multiple modes are used to deliver information, such as audiovisual materials, pictographs, and small-group classes, if they are thoughtfully constructed and pretested (Hahn & Cella, 2003; Houts, Wismer, Egeth, Loscalzo, & Zabora, 2001; Oermann, Webb, & Ashare, 2003). At the same time, it is important to understand that changing the mode of communication by itself does not decrease the literacy demand of the message—the decoding, comprehension, and recall components remain the same. However, if there is careful use of language, appropriate use of pictographs and vignettes, client control over the pacing of the information, and provider follow-up to assess comprehension and to individualize the message, then these strategies can prove successful (Doak et al., 2001; Hahn & Cella, 2003; Houts et al., 2001).

Such a combination of strategies is now being tested. DeWalt et al. (2006) included picture-based educational materials, training sessions, a digital scale, and frequent telephone follow-up in a heart-failure management program and found that it reduced hospitalization and death.

Readability of Written Materials

Readability of written materials for healthcare can be vastly improved. Indeed, both the IOM (2003) and *Healthy People 2010* (U.S. Department of Health and Human Services, 2000) list evidence-based health communication as a high-priority item for the improvement of health care. Multiple tools exist that can be used to assess the reading level of materials (Doak et al., 2001); SMOG, FOG, Flesch, and Fry are among the most frequently used of these readability tools. The formulae employed in these measures are simple, and calculations can be done often by hand or by using widely available software programs, taking only a few minutes (National Cancer Institute, 2003).

The means used to assess the reading demand of text have encountered much criticism in recent years. The tools noted previously evaluate aspects of reading demand, such as word familiarity, length of sentences, punctuation, and number of prepositional words. More recently, new formulae have been introduced that address multiple other variables that affect readability. The Singh Readability Assessment Instrument, for example, includes handwriting or typography that is legible, interest level of the text, and style of writing when evaluating material's reading demand (Singh, 2003).

Given the expense and importance of written materials in today's healthcare environment for vulnerable clients, written materials need to be tested in a systematic fashion (National Cancer Institute, 2003) before their use with actual patient populations. Given the alarming findings based on the NALS data, all systems of health care need to systematize how written materials are evaluated before their dissemination (IOM, 2003; U.S. Department of Health and Human Services, 2000).

English as a Second Language Clients

Addressing the needs of English as a second language (ESL) clients is very complex. Providers generally have taken shortcuts in providing simple English or translated pamphlets that are far above the skill level of such clients—an especially critical shortcoming given that these individuals tend to have significantly longer hospital stays than English-speaking patients (Schillinger & Chen, 2004). Clients with limited English proficiency, even if skilled in their primary language, may be more likely to have children with a fair to poor health status (Flores, Abreu, & Tomany-Korman, 2005). Tools to measure literacy in languages other than English have just begun to be introduced (Lee, Bender, Ruiz, & Cho, 2006). Such development is particularly important because research suggests that a significant number of clients who report proficiency in English in healthcare settings actually have very limited English literacy (Zun, Sadoun, & Downey, 2006).

Use of Computers and the Internet

A number of studies have suggested that technology can be used to address the learning needs of low-literacy clients. One primary drawback, however, is that the reading level of most health-related information (83%) in both English and Spanish on the Internet has been found to require a twelfth-grade reading level or higher to ensure adequate comprehension (Berland et al., 2001). Friedman, Hoffman-Goetz, and Arocha (2004) found that cancer-related information was often written at a college level. This finding was validated in a 2006 study of websites providing colorectal cancer information: Not only did the material have a high reading level, but access and skills in the use of such technology represented barriers for those with low literacy.

One study reported a high level of client satisfaction with using the Internet to obtain health care information, but also found that low-literacy users greatly overestimated their reading skill in relation to access and comprehension of such information (Birru et al., 2004). Three-fourths of the low-literacy subjects in this investigation did not look past the first page on Google search retrievals, stating that the first page always gives them what they need. Seligman et al. (2005) found similar results in a study of diabetic patients with limited literacy. Specifically, the Internet education strategy alone did not result in significant changes in weight, hypertension, knowledge, and self-efficacy. Programs that had an adaptive component so that each user used a tailored educational approach yielded more positive results (Nebel et al., 2004).

IMPROVING LITERACY THROUGH HEALTH CARE

Potential strategies to address illiteracy in health care focus on ways to identify and work with individual clients so that providers' styles of oral and written communication fit with their clients' skill levels. However, these approaches may essentially be skirting the core issue related to client vulnerability.

As reviewed in this chapter, literacy problems themselves create health risks. By using methods that ignore or accommodate the literacy deficit, providers essentially perpetuate the illiteracy problem. This approach, in which providers address the consequences of such core problems as illiteracy, perpetuates the predominant tertiary care focus in the current system of health care. Literacy affects the lives of our clients in foundational ways: the creation of social stigma and prejudicial attitudes; the ability to navigate within complex systems throughout society, including and beyond health care; housing; and money management. Literacy is a core driver of vulnerability in the United States and needs to be addressed as a foundational aspect of health care.

Healthy People 2010 and the IOM state that providers need to improve their communication skills related to literacy needs to improve the quality of health care. In addition, healthcare providers can and should improve their clients' health by increasing their literacy. As David Baker, a researcher in health literacy, has stated (Marwick, 1997) how critical is the need to find better ways of communicating with people to change their learning capabilities in order to achieve health literacy.

The literature review for this chapter found few clinical intervention recommendations that spoke to the need to directly improve client literacy skills. Miles and Davis (1995) recommended that healthcare providers need to partner with community-wide agencies, such as the schools and neighborhood settings where the opportunity to become literate initially foundered. In 2005, Parker evaluated more community approaches to improve literacy by working with libraries to address the long-term nature of low literacy and interventions. Uniquely, she asserted that proper design of all healthcare information—whether written, verbal, or electronic—aligned with the Plain Language Initiative of the National Institutes of Health is a necessary first step.

Improvements in provider sensitivity and skills in working with low-literacy clients are also required. Providers must be aware of their tendency to overestimate literacy levels, especially in individuals with altered health states. Alternative approaches, such as use of pictures, can be useful. Slowing down, bringing other family members into the discussion, and consistent evaluation of learning of all clients are needed. Use of therapeutic relationships and meaningful interactions can change outcomes dramatically. Paasche-Orlow, Reikert, et al. (2005), for example, studied a "teach to goal" strategy that used a multiple-method and multiple-encounter approach that emphasized effective evaluation of learning. Even with well-planned, focused, and simplified instruction, fully one-third of the clients were unable to demonstrate comprehension of instructions on first evaluation. The authors note that this approach is very time intensive, but the outcomes were significantly different than the more typical single-encounter, single-method approach in health care.

International literature has already reported programs in which the development of literacy occurs in tandem with healthcare interventions. Watters (2003) presented a fascinating model that integrates linguistics, literacy, nursing, community partnership, and anthropology and that shows potential for use in the United States. Watters reviewed the international programs, citing one in Nepal that noted initially greater costs of a combined maternal nutrition and literacy program, when compared with simply administering vitamin A. The combined approach, however, decreased infant and child mortality by half. Such programs can help the community first gain the needed tools in literacy, then subsequently provide for long-term health benefits and decreased vulnerability in the community.

As Baker (1999) stated, in the United States, this kind of approach would require a paradigm shift. Rather than compartmentalizing the skills needed to decrease health vulnerability, healthcare providers could actively work to address core issues that lead to clients' need to access care.

CONCLUSION

Functional illiteracy directly creates health vulnerability in clients. Illiteracy is pervasive in client populations, and clinicians cannot rely on education level or self-disclosure to identify all clients with these needs. Those clients who have the greatest health needs are the same clients who do not have the tools to navigate the complex U.S. healthcare system. Currently, there is a major mismatch between provider communication styles and materials and client literacy skills. Solutions addressing this intersection of healthcare needs and illiteracy have typically been client focused and on a micro level. We propose that providers need to partner with communities to develop literacy skills in their members and, thereby, decrease their health risk. International models may provide models for trial in the United States.

For a full suite of assignments and additional learning activities, use the access code located in the front of your book to visit this exclusive website: http://go.jblearning.com/dechesnay. If you do not have an access code, you can obtain one at the site.

REFERENCES

Aday, L. A. (2001). *At risk in America: The health and health care needs of vulnerable populations in the United States* (2nd ed.). San Francisco: Jossey-Bass.

Agency for Healthcare Research and Quality. (2004). Literacy and health outcomes (Evidence Report/Technology Assessment No. 87). Retrieved December 2006, from www.ahrq.gov

Al-Tayyib, A. A., Rogers, S. M., Gribble, J. N., Villarroel, M., & Turner, C. F. (2002). Effect of low medical literacy on health survey measurements. *American Journal of Public Health, 92*(9), 1478–1480.

American Medical Association. (1999). Health literacy report of the Council on Scientific Affairs. Ad Hoc Committee on Health Literacy for the Council on Scientific Affairs. *Journal of the American Medical Association, 10*(6), 552–557.

Arthur, S. A., Geiser, H. R., Arriola, K. R., & Kripalani, S. (2009). Health literacy and control in the medical encounter: A mixed-method analysis. *Journal of the National Medical Association, 101*(7), 677–683.

Baker, D. (1999). Reading between the lines: Deciphering the connections between literacy and health. *Journal of General Internal Medicine, 14*, 315–317.

Baker, D. W., Gazmararian, J. A., Williams, M. V., Scott, T., Parker, R. M., Green, D., . . . Peel, J. (2002). Functional health literacy and the risk of hospital admission among Medicare managed care enrollees. *American Journal of Public Health, 92*(8), 1278–1283.

Baker, D. W., Parker, R. M., Williams, M. V., Pitkin, K., Parikh, N. S., Coates, W., . . . Imara, M. (1996). The health care experience of patients with low literacy. *Archives of Family Medicine, 5*(6), 329–334.

Bass, P. F. 3rd, Wilson, J. F., Griffith, C. H., & Barnett, D. R. (2002). Residents' ability to identify patients with low literacy skills. *Academic Medicine, 77*(10), 1039–1041.

Berland, G. K., Elliott, M. N., Morales, L. S., Algazy, J. I., Kravitz, R. L., Broder, M. S., . . . McGlynn, E. A. (2001). Health information on the Internet: Accessibility, quality, and readability in English and Spanish. *Journal of the American Medical Association, 285*(20), 2612–2621.

Birru, B. A., Monaco, V. M., Drew, L., Njie, V., Bierria, B. A., Detlefsen, E., & Steinman, R. A. (2004). Internet usage by low-literacy adults seeking health information: An observational analysis. *Journal of Medical Internet Research, 6*(3), e25.

Chew, L. D., Bradley, K. A., & Boyko, E. J. (2004). Brief questions to identify patients with inadequate health literacy. *Family Medicine, 36*(8), 588–594.

Chew, L. D., Griffin, J. M., Partin, M., Noorbaloochi, S., Grill, J., Snyder, A., . . . Vanryn, M. (2008). Validation of screening questions for limited health literacy in a large VA outpatient population. *Journal of General Internal Medicine, 23*(5), 561–566.

Cormier, C., & Kotrlik, J. (2009). Health literacy knowledge and experience of senior baccalaureate nursing students. *Journal of Nursing Education, 48*(5), 237–248.

Cutilli, C. (2007). Health literacy in geriatric patients: An integrative review of the literature. *Orthopaedic Nursing, 26*(1), 43–48.

Davis, T. C., Long, S.W., Jackson, R. H., Mayeaux, E. J., George, R. B., Murphy, P. W., . . . Crouch, M. A. (1993). Rapid Estimate of Adult Literacy in Medicine: A Shortened Screening Instrument. *Family Medicine, 1993*(25), 391–395.

DeWalt, D. A., Malone, R. M., Bryant, M. E., Kosnar, M. C., Corr, K. E., Rothman, R. L., . . . Pignone, M. P. (2006). A heart failure self-management program for patients of all literacy levels: A randomized, controlled trial. *BMC Health Services Research, 6*, 6–30.

Doak, C. C., Doak, L. G., & Root, J. H. (2001). *Teaching patients with low literacy skills* (2nd ed.). Philadelphia: Lippincott.

Duncan, G. J., Daly, M. C., McDonough, P., & Williams, D. (2002). Optimal indicators of socioeconomic status for health research. *American Journal of Public Health, 92*(7), 1151–1158.

Feifer, R. (2003). How a few simple words improve patients' health. *Managed Care Quarterly, 11*(2), 29–31.

Flores, G., Abreu, M., & Tomany-Korman, S. C. (2005). Limited English proficiency, primary language at home, and disparities in children's health care: How language barriers are measured matters. *Public Health Reports, 120*(4), 418–430.

Forbis, S., & Aligne, C. (2002). Poor readability of asthma management plans found in national guidelines, *Pediatrics, 109*, e52.

Freidman, D. B., Hoffman-Goetz, L., & Arocha, J. F. (2004). Readability of cancer information on the Internet. *Journal of Cancer Education, 19*(2), 117–122.

Gannon, W., & Hildebrandt, E. (2002). A winning combination: Women, literacy, and participation in health care. *Health Care of Women International, 23*(6–7), 754–760.

Hahn, E. A., & Cella, D. (2003). Health outcomes assessment in vulnerable populations: Measurement challenges and recommendations. *Archives of Physical Medicine and Rehabilitation, 84*(4 suppl 2), S35–S42.

Hohn, M. D. (1998). Empowerment health education in adult literature: A guide for public health and adult literacy practitioners, policy makers, and funders. Retrieved August 22, 2007, from http://www.nifl.gov/nifl/fellowship/reports/hohn/HOHN.HTM

Houts, P. S., Wismer, J. T., Egeth, H. E., Loscalzo, M. J., & Zabora, J. R. (2001). Using pictographs to enhance recall of spoken medical instruction. *Patient Education and Counseling, 43*(3), 231–242.

Institute of Medicine (IOM). (2003). *Priority areas for national action: Transforming health care quality.* Washington, DC: National Academies Press.

Johnson, K., & Weiss, B. (2008). How long does it take to assess literacy skills in clinical practice? *Journal of the American Board of Family Medicine, 21*(3), 211–214.

Jukkala, A., Deupree, J., & Graham. (2009). Knowledge of limited health literacy at an academic health center. *Journal of Continuing Education in Nursing, 40*(7), 298–302.

Katz, M., Jacobson, E., & Kripalani, S. (2007). Patient literacy and question-asking behavior during the medical encounter: A mixed-methods analysis. *Journal of General Internal Medicine, 22*(6), 782–786.

Kirsch, I. S., Jungeblut, A., Jenkins, L., & Kolstad, A. (1993). Executive summary of adult literacy in America: A first look at the results of the National Adult Literacy Survey. Retrieved August 22, 2007, from http://nces.ed.gov/pubs93/93275.pdf

Kripalani, S., Henderson, L., Chiu, E., Robertson, R., Kohm, P., & Jacobson, T. (2006). Predictors of medication self-management skill in a low-literacy population. *Journal of General Internal Medicine, 21*(8), 852–856.

Lee, S. Y., Bender, D. E., Ruiz, R. E., & Cho, Y. I. (2006). Development of an easy-to-use Spanish health literacy test. *Health Services Research, 41*(4 Pt 1), 1392–1412.

Marwick, D. (1997). Patients' lack of literacy may contribute to billions of dollars in higher hospital costs. *Journal of the American Medical Association, 278*(12), 971–972.

Miles, S., & Davis, T. (1995). Patients who can't read: Implications for the health care system. *Journal of the American Medical Association, 274*(21), 1677–1682.

Morris, N. S., MacLean, C. D., Chew, L. D., & Littenberg, B. (2006). The Single Item Literacy Screener: Evaluation of a brief instrument to identify limited reading ability. *BMC Family Practice, 7*(21), 107.

Murphy-Knoll, L. (2007). Low health literacy puts patients at risk. *Journal of Nursing Care Quality, 22*(3), 205–209.

National Cancer Institute. (2003). Clear and simple: Developing effective print materials for low-literate clients. Retrieved August 22, 2007, from http://www.nci.nih.gov/cancerinformation/clearandsimple

National Center for Education Statistics. (2006). National assessment of adult literacy. Retrieved August 22, 2007, from http://nces.ed.gov/NAAL/index.asp?file=AssessmentOf/HealthLiteracy/HealthLiteracyResults.asp&PageID=158

Nebel, I. T., Klemm, T., Fasshauer, M., Muller, J., Verlohren, H. J., Klaiberg, A., & Paschke, R. (2004). Comparative analysis of conventional and an adaptive computer-based hypoglycaemia education programs. *Patient Education and Counseling, 53*(3), 315–318.

Nutbeam, D. (2008). The evolving concept of health literacy. *Social Science & Medicine, 6*(8), 2072–2078.

Oermann, M. H., Webb, S. A., & Ashare, J. A. (2003). Outcomes of videotape instruction in clinic waiting area. *Orthopedic Nursing, 22*(2), 102–105.

Paasche-Orlow, M., Parker, R., Gazmararian, J., Neilsen-Bohlman, L., & Rudd, R. R. (2005). The prevalence of limited health literacy. *Journal of General Internal Medicine, 20,* 175–184.

Paasche-Orlow, M., Reikert, K. A., Bilderback, A., Chanmugam, A., Hill, P., Rand, C., . . . Krishnan, J. A. (2005). Tailored education may reduce health literacy disparities in asthma self-management. *American Journal of Respiratory and Critical Care Medicine, 172*(8), 980–986.

Parikh, N. S., Parker, R. M., Nurss, J. R., Baker, D. W., & Williams, M. V. (1996). Shame and health literacy: The unspoken connection. *Patient Education and Counseling, 27*(1), 33–39.

Parker, R. (2005). Library outreach: Overcoming health literacy challenges. *Journal of the Medical Library Association, 93*(3), S81–S85.

Powell, C., & Kripalani, S. (2005). Resident recognition of low literacy as a risk factor in hospital readmission. *Journal of General Internal Medicine, 20*(11), 1042–1044.

Raich, P. C., Plomer, K. D., & Coyne, C. A. (2001). Literacy, comprehension, and informed consent in clinical research. *Cancer Investigation, 19*(4), 437–445.

Rootman, I., & Ronson, B. (2005). Literacy and health research in Canada: Where have we been and where have we gone? *Canadian Journal of Public Health, 96*(suppl 2), S62–S77.

Rosenthal, M. S., Werner, M. J., & Dubin, N. H. (2004). The effect of a literacy training program on family medicine residents. *Family Medicine, 36*(8), 582–587.

Safeer, R. S., & Keenan, J. (2005). Health literacy: The gap between physicians and patients. *American Family Physician, 72*(3), 463–468.

Sanders, L. M., Federico, S., Klass, P., Abrams, M. A., & Dreyer, B. (2009). Literacy and child health. *Archives of Pediatric and Adolescent Medicine, 163*(2), 131–140.

Schillinger, D., & Chen, A. (2004). Literacy and language: Disentangling measures of access. *Journal of General Internal Medicine, 19*, 288–290.

Schillinger, D., Piette, J., Grumbach, K., Wang, F., Willson, C., Daher, C., . . . Bindman, A. B. (2003). Physician communication with diabetic patients who have low literacy. *Archives of Internal Medicine, 163*(1), 83–90.

Schlichting, J., Quinn, M., Heuer, L., Schaefer, C., Drum, M., & Chin, M. (2007). Provider perceptions of limited health literacy in community health centers. *Patient Education and Counseling, 69*(1), 114–120.

Schultz, M. (2002). Low literacy skills needn't hinder care. *RN, 65*(4), 45–48.

Seligman, H. K., Wang, F. F., Palacios, J. L., Wilson, C. L., Haher, C., Piette, J. D., & Schillinger, D. (2005). Physician notification of their diabetes patients' limited health literacy: A randomized controlled study. *Journal of General Internal Medicine, 20*, 1001–1007.

Sentell, T., & Ratcliff-Baird, B. (2003). Literacy and comprehension of Beck Depression Inventory response alternatives. *Community Mental Health Journal, 39*(4), 323–331.

Singh, J. (2003). Research briefs reading grade level and readability of printed cancer education materials. *Oncology Nursing Forum, 30*(5), 867–870.

U.S. Department of Health and Human Services. (2000). *Healthy people 2010: Understanding and improving health.* Washington, DC: National Academies Press.

Watters, E. K. (2003). Literacy for health: An interdisciplinary model. *Journal of Transcultural Nursing, 14*(1), 48–54.

Weiss, B. D., Mays, M. Z., Martz, W., Castro, K. M., DeWalt, D., Pignone, M., . . . Hale, F. A. (2005). Quick assessment of literacy in primary health care: The Newest Vital Sign. *Annals of Family Medicine, 31*(6), 514–522.

Williams, M. V. (2000). Definition of "health literacy." Message posted to National Institute for Literacy list server. Retrieved August 23, 2007, from http://www.nifl.gov/nifl-health/2000/0439.html

Williams, M. V., Baker, D., Honig, E. G., Lee, T. M., & Nowlan, A. (1998). Inadequate literacy as a barrier to asthma knowledge and self-care. *Chest, 114*, 1008–1015.

Zun, L. S., Sadoun, T. A., & Downey, L. (2006). English-language competency of self-declared English-speaking Hispanic patients using written tests of health literacy. *Journal of the National Medical Association, 98*(6), 912–919.

UNIT II

Nursing Theories

Theory helps us bear our ignorance of the facts.

—George Santayana
www.quotegarden.com

CHAPTER 6

Nursing Theories Applied to Vulnerable Populations: Examples from Turkey

Behice Erci

Objectives

At the end of this chapter, the reader will be able to

1. Identify the key concepts of the theories discussed in this chapter.
2. Compare and contrast the application of theories with the same patient for each example given.
3. Explain how the application of the theories might differ with patients from cultures other than Turkey.

Nursing must continue to develop distinctive, if not unique, knowledge if it is to take its place as a legitimate professional discipline. Within the last 25 years, nurse theorists have made extensive contributions in defining the essence of nursing practice and in delineating the role nurses play in supporting the health and well-being of clients (Villarruel, Bishop, Simpson, Jemmott, & Fawcett, 2001).

This chapter describes the areas in which nursing models and theories guide nursing practice related to vulnerable populations. Nine nursing theories are presented, with detailed clinical examples being offered for several of those theories believed to be more applicable. Readers are referred to the primary sources for complete description and explanation of the theoretical concepts. In addition, this chapter briefly reviews such prior discussion concerning the theory–practice split, including the major concerns regarding theory's contribution to practice in the design of instruction (or lack there of) as well as proposals and progress made by scholars to address those concerns. We suggest, however, that the gap between theory and practice has yet to be satisfactorily resolved and that an alternative way of thinking about this long-standing problem, and about theory per se, can improve attempts to generate usable theoretical understanding. As we explicate this alternative perspective, we will suggest several of its implications for future theorizing and inquiry in the field (Yanchar & South, 2009).

The Importance of Theories in Advanced Nursing Practice

The dilemma for nurse educators is how best to prepare nurses for advanced practice roles. Is nursing theory important? Does it contribute to clinical practice? Which theories form sound foundations for advanced practice? Theories exist to challenge existing practice, create new approaches to practice, and remodel the structure of rules and principles. Furthermore, theories should ultimately improve nursing practice. Usually, this goal is achieved by using theory or portions of theory to guide practice.

Defining the scope of advanced practice requires that the role of nurses be perceived as unique. For nursing practice to be viewed as professional, it is essential that practice is based on theory. Theory and theoretical frameworks are intended to provide guidance and rationale for professional practice, but as advanced practice roles evolve in nursing, the incorporation of nursing theory becomes problematic. Some critics have suggested that the wide variety of definitions and concepts discussed in most nursing theories do not explain or predict anything and, therefore, cannot practically be applied to clinical situations and are of little use to nurses in advanced practice.

OREM'S SELF-CARE DEFICIT THEORY

Orem's self-care theory (Berbiglia, 1997; Orem, 1995) links patient assessments with nursing diagnosis, expected patient outcomes, discharge planning, quality assurance, clinical research, and external agency reports. This theory includes three subtheories:

- The *theory of self-care deficit* details how individuals can benefit from nursing because they are subject to health-related or self-derived limitations.
- The *theory of self-care* states that care is a learned behavior that purposely regulates human structural integrity, functioning, and development.
- The *theory of nursing systems* describes how nurses use their abilities to prescribe, design, and provide nursing care.

Application to Vulnerable Populations

To provide nursing care, Orem identifies operations that are specifically professional-technological, including diagnostic, prescriptive, treatment, or regulatory and case management. The application of Orem's theory to nursing practice is relevant as a framework in a variety of settings, including acute care units, ambulatory clinics, community health programs, high-rise senior centers, nursing homes, hospices, and rehabilitation centers. The theory is applied to patients with specific diseases or conditions, including adolescents with chronic disease, alcoholics, the chronically ill, patients who have undergone head and neck surgery, patients with rheumatoid arthritis, and patients with cardiac conditions (Conway, McMillan, & Solman, 2006; Taylor, Geden, Issaramalai, & Wongvatunyu, 2000). The theory is also applied to selected age groups, including the aged, children, coronary care, prenatal and postnatal care, and mothers with newborns.

Example

Yeliz is 29 years old, married, and 5 months pregnant. She has anemia, is underweight, and is under the care of a primary healthcare center. Complete data have been compiled from this client's records and a home visit. The nurses are concerned that Yeliz's self-care requisites (or requirements) are not being met—specifically, food, healthy activity, and rest. Yeliz requires assistance in food preparation but can eat on her own. Her priority diagnoses are inadequate food intake, low activity level, and fatigue due to inadequate rest.

Diagnostic and Prescriptive Operations

All three of these priority diagnoses are related to preventing health deterioration. In this client's case, the self-care deficit theory of nursing proposes a supportive educational nursing system that is designed to individualize her care. The individualization of the nursing system is accomplished through the overlay of basic conditioning factors and developmental self-care requisites (or requirements for life and health) on the therapeutic self-care demands (those processes necessary to maintain life or health). The expected outcome is health status maintenance, health promotion, and prevention of further health deterioration through the strengthening of the self-care agency. Unless expected outcomes are provided, the nursing system design will change.

Regulatory Operations

The self-care deficit theory of nursing is especially useful with this client. It shifts the focus away from disease and toward the strengths and weaknesses of the self-care agent. It is evident that this client does seek to prevent or manage the conditions threatening her health, yet she requires assistance in this area. The most significant self-care deficit is in the area of nutrition. Guided by the theory, the nurse analyzed the self-care agency from the perspective of the basic conditioning factors. Cultural variety should be considered in reaching for the expected outcome.

Data collection for Yeliz in terms of her self-care requisites led to the following proposed outcomes: maintenance of the healthy environment, ability of the client to feed herself, and discussion of her condition and medical regimen with the home health nurse and aide and the client's family. The nursing diagnosis showed a potential for anemic complications such as falls and decreased mobility. Methods of help and intervention included teaching, guiding, and providing and maintaining direction in an environment that supported personal development. Self-care agency is inadequate and implies the necessity to gain better understanding of the cause and subsequent prevention of problems. The nursing diagnosis is "potential for exacerbation and increased disability related to knowledge deficits concerning problems." Teaching, guiding, and directing are methods of helping. For the nursing diagnosis, "inability to maintain ideal body weight related to cultural attitudes toward eating and weight gain and meal preparation by aide," the methods of helping are to provide and maintain an environment that supports personal development.

ROY'S ADAPTATION MODEL

Roy drew upon expanded insights in relating spirituality and science to present a new definition of adaptation and related scientific and philosophical assumptions (Connerley, Ristau, Lindberg, & McFarland, 1999; Lopes, Pagliuca, & Araujo, 2006). Roy believes that adaptation involves human response to stimuli within the system. According to Roy, a person's response may be either adaptive or ineffective during interaction with the environment (Ducharme, Ricard, Duquette, Levesque, & Lachance, 1998; Roy, 1997). Her philosophical stance articulates that nurses see persons as coextensive with their physical and social environments. Furthermore, nurse scholars take a value-based stance rooted in beliefs and hopes about the human person, and they develop a discipline that participates in enhancing the well-being of persons and of the earth. Roy views persons and groups as adaptive systems, for which cognator and regulator subsystems act to maintain adaptation in the four modes: physiological–physical, self-concept–group identity, role function, and interdependence.

Application to Vulnerable Populations

Roy used a problem-solving approach for gathering data, identifying the capacities and needs of the human adaptive system, selecting and implementing approaches for nursing care, and evaluating the outcome of the care provided. This approach includes assessment of behavior and stimuli and is consistent with the nursing process of assessment, diagnosis, planning, implementation, and evaluation.

Example

Hasan is a 35-year-old man who was recently admitted to the oncology nursing unit for evaluation after undergoing surgery for class IV prostate cancer. He has smoked approximately two packs of cigarettes per day for the past 9 years. Hasan is married and lives with his wife. He has done well after surgery except for being unable to completely empty his urinary bladder. Hasan is having continued postoperative pain. When he goes home, it will be necessary for him to perform intermittent self-catheterization. His home medications are an antibiotic and an analgesic as needed. In addition, he will be receiving radiation therapy on an outpatient basis.

Hasan is extremely tearful. He expresses great concern over his future. He believes that this illness is a punishment for his past life.

Physiological Adaptive Mode

This client's health problems are complex. It is impossible to develop interventions for all of his health problems within this chapter. Therefore only representative examples are given. The physiological adaptive mode refers to the basic and complex biological processes necessary to maintain life.

Assessment of Behavior

Postoperatively, the patient is unable to completely empty his urinary bladder. He states that he is "numb" and unable to tell when he needs to void. Catheterization for residual urine reveals that he is retaining 300 mL of urine after voiding. As a consequence, this patient needs to perform intermittent self-catheterization at home. Unsanitary conditions at Hasan's home place him at high risk for developing a urinary tract infection. He states that he is scared about performing self-catheterization.

Assessment of Stimuli

In this phase of the nursing process, the nurse searches for the stimuli responsible for certain observed behaviors. After the stimuli are identified, they are classified as focal, contextual, or residual. The focal stimulus for Hasan's urinary retention is his disease process. Contextual stimuli include tissue trauma resulting from surgery and radiation therapy. Anxiety is a residual stimulus. Infection is a potential problem.

The focal stimulus is the need for intermittent self-catheterization. Contextual stimuli include altered skin integrity related to surgical incision, poor understanding of aseptic principles, and unsanitary conditions at Hasan's home.

Nursing Diagnosis

From the assessment of behaviors and the assessment of stimuli, the following nursing diagnoses are made:

- Altered elimination: urinary retention related to surgical trauma, radiation therapy, and anxiety
- Potential for infection related to intermittent self-catheterization, altered skin integrity resulting from surgical incision, poor understanding of aseptic principles, and unsanitary conditions at the client's home

Goal Setting

Goals are set mutually between the nurse and the client for each of the nursing diagnoses. The goals are (1) complete urinary elimination every 4 hours as evidenced by correct demonstration of the procedure for intermittent self-catheterization and (2) continued absence of signs of infection of the surgical incision and urinary tract.

Implementation

To help the client attain these goals, the following nursing interventions were implemented:

- To address the issue of incomplete elimination, the client is taught the importance of performing intermittent self-catheterization every 4 hours to prevent damage to the urinary bladder. He is taught to assess his abdomen for bladder distention and the proper procedure for intermittent self-catheterization. He is instructed to keep a record of the exact time and amount of voiding and catheterizations. In addition, the client is taught relaxation techniques to facilitate voiding so it will not be necessary for him to catheterize himself as often.
- To address the potential for infection, the client is taught the importance of washing hands before touching the surgical incision or doing incision care. After the procedure for incision care is demonstrated by the nursing staff, the client is asked to perform a return

demonstration. After the intermittent self-catheterization procedure is explained and demonstrated, the client is asked to perform a return demonstration.

Evaluation
An evaluation of the client's adaptive level is performed each shift.

Self-Concept Adaptive Mode
Assessment of Behavior
The client is extremely tearful and expresses great concern over his future. Exploration of the client's tearfulness revealed that the client is afraid of dying. Also, the client has not asked the nurse any questions about sexuality. His hesitancy to introduce the subject may be related to his cultural background. In this case, the nurse introduces the topic. Salient findings are as follows: (1) the client recently learned of his diagnosis of prostate cancer, (2) he has undergone a recent operation, (3) he is receiving radiation therapy in the hospital and this therapy will continue when he leaves the hospital, and (4) the client has a lack of information about the impact of prostate cancer and chemotherapy on sexuality.

Assessment of Stimuli
The client is an adult, is married, and has a fifth-grade education. He is in an emotionally distant and sometimes abusive relationship. Being diagnosed with prostate cancer at an early age has resulted in a maturational crisis for the client, which is further complicated by the fact that several of his relatives have died of cancer. It is important for the nurse to assess coping strategies. One coping strategy that is mentioned is that the client is frequently tearful.

Nursing Diagnosis
The following nursing diagnoses are made:

- Fear and anxiety of dying related to medical diagnosis and witnessing other family members' deaths as a result of cancer
- Spiritual distress related to severe life-threatening illness and perception of the moral–ethical–spiritual self
- Sexual dysfunction related to the disease process, need for radiation therapy at home, weakness, fatigue, pain, anxiety, and a lack of information about the impact of prostate cancer and chemotherapy on sexuality
- Grieving related to body image disturbance, lack of self-ideal, and potential for premature death

Goal Setting
To help the client achieve adaptation in the self-concept adaptive mode, the following goals are set:

- Decrease fear and anxiety of dying, as evidenced by less tearfulness, relaxed facial expression, relaxed body movements, verbalization of new coping strategies, and fewer verbalizations of fear and anxiety

- Decrease spiritual distress, as evidenced by verbalization of positive feelings about the value and meaning of his life, and less tearfulness
- Resume sexual relationship that is satisfying to both partners, as evidenced by verbalization of self as sexually capable and acceptable, and verbalization of alternative methods of sexual expression during the first 10 weeks after surgery
- Progression through the grieving process as evidenced by verbalization of feelings regarding body image, self-ideal, and potential for premature death

Implementation

The following nursing interventions are implemented to help achieve these goals in the self-concept adaptive mode.

- Fear and anxiety of dying related to the medical diagnosis and witnessing other family members' deaths as a result of cancer

Although the client's prognosis appeared to be good, he remained fearful of dying. Time is taken to sit with the client, make eye contact, and actively listen. The client is asked to share an extremely difficult experience he encountered in the past. He is asked how he coped with that experience. Once his present coping strategies are assessed, new coping strategies are suggested.

In addition, the client is encouraged to express his feelings openly. After allowing the client adequate time to express his feelings, truthful and realistic hope based on the client's medical history is offered. A cancer support group meets each week in the hospital where the client is a patient. The client is given a schedule of the meeting times and topics. He and his partner are encouraged to attend the cancer support group meetings.

- Spiritual distress related to severe life-threatening illness and perception of the moral–ethical–spiritual self

The client is encouraged to express his feelings openly about his illness. It is suggested that times of illness are good times to renew spiritual ties. The client is supported in positive aspects of his life.

- Sexual dysfunction related to the disease process, need for radiation therapy at home, weakness, fatigue, pain, anxiety, and a lack of information about the impact of prostate cancer and chemotherapy on sexuality

A complete sexual assessment is conducted to evaluate the perceived adequacy of the client's sexual relationship and to elicit concerns or issues about sexuality before his diagnosis with prostate cancer. A private conversation is initiated with the client to gain an understanding of his sexual concerns resulting from his therapy and his beliefs about the effects of prostate cancer in regard to sexual functioning. The client is instructed regarding possible changes in sexual functioning, such as a temporary inability to achieve or sustain an erection, which may last for several months.

- Grieving related to body image disturbance, loss of self-ideal, and potential for premature death

The client's perceptions regarding the impact of the diagnosis of prostate cancer on his body image, self-ideal, roles, and his future are explored. Hasan is encouraged to verbally acknowledge the losses he is experiencing. He is observed to determine which stage of the grief process he currently experiences. The grieving process is explained to the client and to his family, and they are assured that grieving is a normal process. The nursing staff should offer realistic reassurance about the client prognosis. The client is encouraged to attend the cancer support group so he can talk to others who better understand his grief.

Evaluation
Behavior change is expected.

KING'S GENERAL SYSTEMS FRAMEWORK THEORY

The focus of King's (1997) theory is on individuals whose interactions in groups within social systems influence behavior within the systems (Sieloff, 2006). In other words, the perceptions that people experience as a result of their surroundings influence their own behavior. King's theory is system based. Concepts of self-growth and development and body image are important (Frey & Norris, 1997; Sieloff, 2006). King's conceptual system provides a comprehensive view of three dynamic interacting systems—personal, interpersonal, and social. Her theory of goal attainment has been used as the basis for practice, education, research, and administration, examples of which are presented here (King, 1997). According to this theory, the goal of nursing is to help individuals maintain their health so they can function in their roles.

Application to Vulnerable Populations

It is within the nurse–client interpersonal system that the traditional steps of the nursing process are carried out. Nurse and client meet in some situation, perceive each other, make judgments about the other, take some mental action, and react to each one's perceptions of the other. Because these behaviors cannot be directly observed, one can only draw inferences from them. The next step in the process is interaction that can be directly observed. When interactions lead to transactions, goal attainment behaviors are exhibited. An assumption underlying the interaction process is that of reciprocally contingent behavior in which the behavior of one person influences the behavior of the other, and vice versa (Sieloff, 2006).

Example

Elif is 50 years old and has heart failure. She is married and lives with her husband. She describes him as emotionally distant and abusive at times. Elif is having continued cardiac pain and palpitation. She will be receiving cardiac therapy on an outpatient basis. Elif is extremely tearful and anxious, and she expresses great concern over her future.

Within King's framework, Elif is conceptualized as a personal system in interaction with other systems. Many of these interactions influence her health. In addition, her recent diagnosis of heart failure influences her health. Together Elif and the nurse communicate, engage in mutual goal setting, and make decisions about the means to achieve goals.

Nursing care for Elif begins with assessment, which includes collection, interpretation, and verification of data. Sources of data include Elif herself—primarily, her perceptions, behavior, and past experiences. In addition, the nurse uses knowledge of concepts in the systems framework; critical thinking skills; the ability to use the nursing process; and medical knowledge about the treatment and prognosis of heart failure. Care should cover the full range of nursing practice: maintenance and restoration of health, care of the sick, and promotion of health.

The nurse forms an interpersonal system with Elif. The transaction process includes perception, judgments, mental actions, and reactions of both individuals. The nurse assesses and applies her knowledge of concepts and processes. Critical concepts are perception, self-coping, interaction, role, stress, power, and decision making. The nurse's perception serves as a basis for gathering and interpreting information. Elif's perceptions influence her thoughts and actions and are assessed through verbal and nonverbal behaviors. Because perceptual accuracy is important to the interaction process, the nurse analyzes her own perceptions and her interpretation of Elif's perceptions collaboratively with Elif. It is expected that perceptions might be influenced by her emotional state, stress, or pain.

According to King, self is the conception of who and what one is; it includes one's subjective totality of attitudes, values, experiences, commitments, and awareness of individual existence. Elif reveals important information about herself. She is tearful and expresses fear and concern. Her past behavior provides some basis for her present feelings, in that Elif has not taken actions to promote and maintain her own health. Clearly, her feelings about herself and the situation are psychological stressors.

Elif has physical and interpersonal stressors as well. The physical stressors are a result of her illness. Cardiac function, pain, and palpitation are identified as immediate problems. In the interpersonal system, Elif identifies a distant and abusive relationship with her husband. She is experiencing a major lack of emotional support during this very difficult time. Her husband's inability to provide basic emotional support is likely to change Elif's physical status.

An additional stressor is Elif's living situation. It is also possible that the lack of personal and perhaps family space contributes to stress. Coping with personal and interpersonal stressors is likely to influence both health and illness outcomes. Elif may need additional resources to help her cope with the immediate situation and the future.

Communication is the key to establishing mutuality and trust between Elif and the nurse, which are key components needed to establish patient priorities and move the interaction process toward goal setting. Elif is expected to participate in identifying goals. However, direction from the nurse will likely be necessary because of Elif's overwhelming needs and lack of resources.

Nurses can find direction for assisting patients in identifying goals based on the assumptions that underlie King's systems framework. They assist patients to adjust to changes in their health status. Decisions about goals must be based on the capabilities, limitations, and priorities of the patient, as well as the unique situation. In this case, the immediate goals seem to be control of cardiac pain and palpitation, although this needs validation by Elif.

The first nursing action is to perform a psychological assessment and provide crisis intervention. Other important goals and actions will be directed toward mobilizing resources, especially support from Elif's husband. However, it is possible that nursing goals and client goals may be incongruent. Continuous analysis, synthesis, and validation are critical to keep this process on track.

In addition to decisions about goals, Elif is expected to be involved in decisions about actions to meet goals. Involving Elif in decision making may be a challenge because of her sense of powerlessness over the illness, treatment, and ability to contribute to family functioning. Yet empowering Elif is likely to increase her sense of self, which in turn can reduce her level of stress, improve her coping ability, change her perceptions, and lead to positive changes in her physical state.

Goal attainment needs ongoing evaluation. For Elif, follow-up on pain, palpitation, and cardiac function after discharge is necessary. An option might be to arrange for in-home nursing services. Having a professional in the home would also contribute to further assessment of the family, validation of progress toward goals, and modifications in plans to achieve goals. According to King, if transactions are agreed upon and carried out, goals will be attained. Goal attainment can improve or maintain health, control illness, or lead to a peaceful death. If goals are not attained, the nurse needs to reexamine the nursing process, critical thinking process, and transaction process.

LEININGER'S THEORY OF CULTURE CARE

Leininger's interest in the cultural dimensions of human care and caring led to the development of her theory (Leininger, 1995). This author subscribed to the central tenet that "care is the essence of nursing and the central, dominant, and unifying focus of nursing" (McFarland, 2006, p. 472). The unique focus of Leininger's theory is care, which she believes to be inextricably linked with culture. She defines culture as "the learned, shared, and transmitted values, beliefs, norms, and life ways of a particular group that guides their thinking, decisions, and actions in patterned ways" (Leininger, 1991, p. 47). The ultimate purpose of care is to provide culturally congruent care to people of different or similar cultures to "maintain or regain their well-being and health or face death in a culturally appropriate way" (Leininger, 1991, p. 39).

Example

A group of Iraqi refugees fled to a city in southeastern Turkey to seek refuge from political unrest, persecution, and extreme poverty. Providing culturally congruent nursing care to this group of people is difficult because of differences in language, which in turn leads to difficulty in understanding the lifeways of this group. The children have diarrhea, and it is difficult for the nurse to observe, interview, and collect data related to cultural practices that might explain the diarrhea. The nurse helps the group to preserve favorable health and caring lifestyles related to their poverty and diarrhea. The nurse assists group members in accomplishing cultural adaptation, negotiation, or adjustment to the refugees' health and lifestyles. To do so, the nurse can reconstruct or alter designs to help clients change their health or life patterns in ways that are meaningful to them.

WATSON'S THEORY OF HUMAN CARING

The caring model or theory can also be considered a philosophical and moral–ethical foundation for professional nursing and part of the central focus for nursing at the disciplinary level. Watson's model of caring is both art and science; it offers a framework that embraces and intersects with art, science, humanities, spirituality, and new dimensions of mind–body–spirit. Key concepts in this theory include nursing, person, health, human care, and environment. Watson's theory has particular relevance to nursing ethics (Watson, 2005).

Application to Vulnerable Populations

Watson emphasizes that it is possible to read, study, learn about, even teach and research the caring theory; however, to truly "get it," one has to personally experience it. Thus the model is both an invitation and an opportunity to interact with the ideas, to experiment with them, and to grow through their application. If one chooses to use the caring perspective as theory, model, philosophy, ethic, or ethos for transforming self and practice or self and system, then asking a variety of questions related to one's view of caring and what it means to be human might help in clarifying the theory's application (McCance, McKenna, & Boore, 1999; Watson, 1996; Watson & Smith, 2002).

Example

Nesim is 60 years old, is married, and lives with his family. His primary diagnosis is hypertension. Under older models of care, this patient might be convinced that he would simply overcome his hypertension—that it would "go away." In the Watson model, however, the nurse should aim to sustain a helping–trusting, authentic, caring relationship to develop the capacity of the patient to problem solve and to teach him and his family proper care of his condition. The nurse educates the patient about hypertension and about improving self-health, thereby enabling and authenticating the deep belief system of the patient. The nurse is supportive of the expression of both positive and negative feelings by the patient. Nesim improves as the nurse creates a healing environment at all levels (physical as well as nonphysical).

The patient should be assisted in the creative use of self and all ways of knowing as part of the caring process. The nurse must engage Nesim in the artistry of caring-healing practices that are "human care essentials," and that facilitate alignment of mind–body–spirit, wholeness, and unity of being in all aspects of care (Watson, 1996, p. 157). The patient should be followed to evaluate the medical and dietary treatment of hypertension.

ROGERS' SCIENCE OF UNITARY HUMAN BEINGS

Rogers formulated a theory to describe humans and the life process in humans (Daily, Maupin, Murray, Satterly, Schnell, & Wallace, 1994; Rogers, 1992, 1994). Over the ensuing years, four critical elements emerged that are basic to the proposed system: energy fields, open systems, pattern, and pandimensionality (Rogers, 1992). The final concept, pandimensionality, was previously known as multidimensionality and four-dimensionality. Although Rogers never updated her work, the theory still provides much that is useful (Malinski, 2006).

Application to Vulnerable Populations

Within Rogers' model, the critical-thinking process can be divided into three components: pattern appraisal, mutual patterning, and evaluation. The critical-thinking process begins with a comprehensive pattern appraisal. The life process possesses its own unity and is inseparable from the environment; thus a holistic appraisal requires the identification of patterns that reflect the whole. Pattern appraisal is a comprehensive assessment.

Knowledge gained in the appraisal process occurs via cognitive input, sensory input, intuition, and language. The nurse gains a great deal of appraisal knowledge during the interview with the client by using the feeling or sensing level of knowing. Often described as instinctual, such intuitive knowledge is best realized through reflection. Reflection, in turn, assists in appraising patterns. Manifestations of patterns are not static, but rather partial perceptions of the synthesis of the past, present, and future. These perceptions provide the basis for intuitive knowing. Manifestation, patterns, and rhythms are an indication of evolutionary emergence of the human field. Pattern appraisal and rhythm identification, along with reflection, provide the content for appraisal validation with the patient.

Once the client and the nurse have reached a consensus with respect to the appraisal, then nursing action centers on mutual patterning of the client's human–environmental field. The goal of the nursing action is to bring about and promote symphonic interaction between human and environment. This interaction is intended to strengthen the coherence and integrity of the human field and to "direct and redirect patterning of the human and environmental fields" (Rogers, 1992, p. 122). Patterning activities can be devised with respect to the initial pattern appraisal.

The evaluation process is ongoing and fluid as the nurse reflects on his or her intuitive knowing. During the evaluation phase, the nurse repeats the pattern appraisal process to determine the level of dissonance perceived. These perceptions are then shared with the client and his or her family and friends. Further mutual patterning is directed by the perceptions found during the evaluation process. This process continues as long as the nurse–client relationship continues (Bultmeier, 1997).

Example

Ayse is a 32-year-old woman who was recently admitted to the infection nursing unit for evaluation after experiencing urinary infection and late-stage AIDS. Her weight is 58 kilograms, down from her usual weight of 80 kilograms. She has smoked approximately one pack of cigarettes per day for the past 16 years. Ayse has two children; she is married and lives with her husband in conditions that she describes as less than sanitary. She describes her husband as emotionally distant and abusive at times. She is having continued pain and nausea. It will be necessary for her to perform intermittent self-catheterization at home. Her home medications are an antibiotic, an analgesic, and an antiemetic. She will soon be receiving radiation therapy on an outpatient basis.

Ayse is extremely tearful. She expresses great concern over her future and the future of her two children. She believes that this illness is a punishment for her past life.

Within the Rogerian model, the process of caring for Ayse begins with pattern appraisal, which is seen as the most important component of the nursing process. The nurse must engage in caring–healing practices that are human care essentials. The purpose is to potentiate alignment, followed by engagement in mutual patterning and evaluation.

Pattern Appraisal

The history provides a major portion of the pattern appraisal. Ayse has a pattern of smoking, which has been associated with poor health. This visible rhythmical pattern is a manifestation of evolution toward dissonance. In addition, Ayse has a pattern manifestation that has been labeled AIDS. This emergent pattern manifests as dissonant. Ayse has a low educational level, which is relevant as patterning activities are introduced. The nurse has reported that Ayse has a manifestation of fear; she reports the fear of dealing with her life after this illness, and the nurse senses this manifestation of fear. Ayse's self-knowledge links the illness to her personal belief of "being punished" for past mistakes. History and focusing on the "relative present" to explore the pattern of punishment is imperative. It is important that the nurse appraise the environment of the hospital and of the others who share her existence.

The pain and fear are dissonant manifestations. Dissonance can be perceived in many aspects of Ayse's appraisal: her unsanitary living conditions, her relationship with her husband, the manifestations of AIDS, weight loss, pain, nausea, and tobacco use. Likewise, dissonance is conceptualized as fear and is manifested in the emotional distance that Ayse feels.

On completion of the pattern appraisal, the nurse presents the analysis to the patient. Emphasis can be placed on areas in which dissonance and harmony are noted in the personal and environmental field manifestations. Consensus needs to be reached with Ayse before patterning activities can be suggested and implemented.

Mutual Patterning

Patterning can be approached from many directions, but is always mutual between nurse and patient. Medications are patterning modalities, for example, and Ayse is receiving medications. Decisions are made in conjunction with Ayse regarding the use of the medications and the patterning that emerges with the introduction of these modalities. Personal knowledge regarding the medications empowers Ayse to be a vital agent in the selection of modalities. She possesses freedom and involvement in these decisions. Options include therapeutic touch, humor, meditation, visualization, and imagery.

Therapeutic touch can be introduced to Ayse, particularly to reduce her pain. Touch in combination with medications provides patterning that Ayse can direct. The nurse can introduce the process of touch to Ayse's husband and teach him how to incorporate touch into her care. Another option would be to teach Ayse how to center her energy and channel it to the area that is experiencing pain.

Patterning directed at the manifestation of Ayse's fear is critical. Options to alter her current pattern include imagery, music, light, and meditation. Fear is manifested as her apprehension about self-catheterization, for example. Emphasis needs to be placed on having Ayse direct how, where, when, and with whom the self-catheterization is taught. Establishing a rhythm to the catheterization schedule that is harmonious with Ayse's life would reduce dissonance. Patterning of nutrition and catheterization based on the pattern appraisal can assist in empowering Ayse to learn self-catheterization. A rhythm will evolve that is harmonious with Ayse and her energy field rhythm and that empower Ayse to direct this phase of her treatment.

Human–environment patterning needs to involve the other individuals who share Ayse's environment, including her husband and children. Options relate to increased communication and sanitation patterns. The nurse talks with the family and Ayse to determine what Ayse would prefer to change in her environment to improve sanitation. Options are introduced that allow pattern evolution to be integral with her environment in way that is not perceived as dissonant.

Evaluation

The evaluation process centers on the perceptions of dissonance that exist after the mutual patterning activities are implemented, to determine whether they were successful. Specific emphasis is placed on emergent patterns of dissonance that are still evident. Manifestations of pain, fear, and tension with family members are appraised. The nurse continually evaluates the amount of dissonance that is apparent with respect to Ayse as he or she cares for her. A summary of the dissonance or harmony that the nurse perceives is then shared with Ayse, and mutual patterning is modified or instituted as indicated based on the evaluation.

ROPER, LOGAN, AND TIERNEY'S MODEL OF NURSING

In the United Kingdom, the model of nursing used most predominantly is that developed by Roper, Logan, and Tierney (2002), which bases its principles on a model of living. This model consists of five components: activities of daily living, life span, dependence–independence continuum, factors influencing activities of daily living, and individuality in living. Roper, Logan, and Tierney suggest that these five components are as applicable to a model of living as they are to a model of nursing. Their work has applicability to a variety of clinical situations (Mooney & O'Brien, 2006; Timmins, 2006).

Example

Hatice is 55 years old. She has difficult respiration and constipation. She cannot do her own cleaning.

First, considering 12 activities of daily living and affecting factors, the nurse collects data about the client and sets nursing diagnoses, goals, and activities.

Diagnosis: Difficult breathing
Goal setting: Effective breathing

Activity: The nurse monitors Hatice's breathing patterns and respirations and ensures that her room is clean and at a normal temperature.

Diagnosis: Constipation
Goal setting: Normal defecation
Activity: The nurse provides warm water for the client every morning and encourages appropriate exercise. After these activities, the nurse should evaluate the results.

PEPLAU'S INTERPERSONAL MODEL

Pearson et al. (2005, p. 179) describe Hildegard Peplau as "one of the earliest American theorists to recognize and respond to the need for changes in nursing practice," Peplau's primary area of interest was psychiatric nursing, but her work can be applied to other fields as well (Pearson et al., 2005).

Peplau's interpersonal relations model relates to the meta-paradigm of the discipline of nursing (Forchuk, 1993) and includes four concepts—the view of the person, health, nursing, and environment. This model describes the individual as a system with physiological, psychological, and social component. The individual is viewed an unstable system for which equilibrium is a desirable state but occurs only through death. This perspective is supported by Peplau's statement that "man is an organism that lives in an unstable equilibrium (i.e., physiological, psychological, and social fluidity) and life is the process of striving in the direction of stable equilibrium (i.e., a fixed pattern that is never reached except in death)" (Peplau, 1992, p. 82). Despite the fact that her model was developed some years ago, Peplau's work continues to have high applicability (McCamant, 2006; Moraes, Lopes, & Brage, 2006; Stockmann, 2005; Vandemark, 2006).

Application to Vulnerable Populations

The interpersonal relationship between the nurse and the client as described by Peplau (1992) has four clearly discernible phases: orientation, identification, exploitation, and resolution. These phases are interlocking and require overlapping roles and functions as the nurse and the client learn to work together to resolve difficulties in relation to health problems.

During the orientation phase of the relationship, the client and the nurse come together as strangers meeting for the first time. At this stage, the development of trust and empowerment of the client are primary considerations. This is best achieved by encouraging the client to participate in identifying the problem and allowing the client to be an active participant. By asking for and receiving help, the client will feel more at ease expressing needs, knowing that the nurse will take care of those needs. Once orientation has been accomplished, the relationship is ready to enter the next phase.

During the identification phase of the relationship, the client, in partnership with the nurse, identifies problems. Once the client has identified the nurse as a person willing and able to provide the necessary help, the main problem and other related problems can then be worked on, in the context of the nurse–client relationship. Throughout the identification phase, both the nurse and the client must clarify each other's perceptions and expectations, as these considerations affect the ability of both to identify problems and the necessary solutions. When clarity of perceptions and expectations is achieved, the client will learn how to make use of the nurse–client relationship. In turn, the nurse will establish a trusting relationship. Once identification has occurred, the relationship enters the next phase.

During the exploitation phase, the client takes full advantage of all available services. The degree to which these services are used reflects the needs and interests of the client. During this time, the client begins to feel like an integral part of the helping environment and starts to take control of the situation by using the help available from the services offered. In other words, the client begins to develop responsibility and become more independent. From this sense of self-determination, the client develops an inner strength that allows him or her to face new challenges. This point is best described by Peplau: "Exploiting what a situation offers gives rise to new differentiations of the problem and to the development and improvement of skill in interpersonal relations" (Peplau, 1992, pp. 41–42).

As the relationship passes through all the aforementioned phases and the needs of the client have been met, the relationship passes to closure—that is, the resolution phase.

The strength of Peplau's model derives from its focus on the nurse–client relationship. This emphasis allows for the nurse and the client to work together as partners in problem solving. Peplau's model encourages and supports empowerment of the client by encouraging the client to accept responsibility for well-being. The focus on the partnership of the nurse and the client and the emphasis on meeting the identified needs of the client make this model ideal for short-term crisis intervention. Although it is often applied to getting sick people well, the model is also appropriate for health promotion. Indeed, its clear focus on the nurse–client relationship provides a foundation for many types of interactions between the nurse and the client that can enhance health.

Example

Tarkan is a 46-year-old married man who is scheduled to undergo a heart operation next week. He has had a few hospitalizations and is anxious about the operation.

The first phase of Peplau's model is orientation. Because this client has previously been cared for at the hospital, he is familiar with the layout of the facility as well as the general rules and regulations of the facility. Thus orientation is quickly established.

In the next phase of the relationship (identification), the nurse and Tarkan identify problems that require attention, including his feelings about the operation and potential to die as a result. The nurse determines that the client is experiencing mixed emotions about the operation because he understands it is necessary. The nurse then identifies that this client requires additional support because he has been relatively stable for a time, yet now requires an operation.

In the third phase (exploitation), Tarkan quickly begins making use of the available resources and services at his disposal and talks with the nurse about his fears and hopes. He expresses feelings of mixed emotions, and the nurse comforts him by reminding him that his feelings are normal. In turn, he expresses relief.

Because the client had been hospitalized twice within a one-year period, the client is provided with information on services that can be accessed to assist him further should the need arise. With the client making full use of the available services, the nurse–client relationship then enters the final phase, resolution. During resolution, the client becomes less dependent on the nurse for one-on-one interactions and no longer seeks further assistance.

NEUMAN'S HEALTHCARE SYSTEMS MODEL

The Neuman healthcare systems model (Neuman, 1995) is related here to the meta-paradigm of the discipline of nursing. As in other models of nursing, the major concepts are the person, health, nursing, and the environment. Neuman, however, uses a systems approach to explain how these elements interact in ways that provide nurses with guidance to intervene with patients, families, or communities. Her view of health seems to be that of a continuum rather than a dichotomy of health versus illness (Freese, 2006). Not much is found in the current nursing literature on Neuman's model, as newer models have developed. Nevertheless, her legacy should be honored. For example, this model has been successfully used in the examination of anxiety (August-Brady, 2000).

Example

Dilek is a 25-year-old woman experiencing violence from her husband and auditory and visual hallucinations. An intrapersonal stressor for Dilek is the limited effectiveness of her current medication regimen in relieving her acute symptoms, including difficulty sleeping. Other interpersonal and extrapersonal stressors are also exacerbating her distress. The interpersonal stressors include a strained relationship with her husband related to the charges brought against him for sexual and physical abuse. The extrapersonal stressor comprises inadequate community resources that could help her stay in her home. Once the stressors have been identified, a determination of the level of prevention required to strengthen the flexible line of defense is made.

In Dilek's situation, the identified stressors have penetrated the line of defense, so the goal is to prevent further regression. This is a tertiary level of intervention—in this case, focused on maintaining and supporting the existing strengths of the client. Such an intervention is best achieved through intensive conversations of the nurse with the client to emphasize her existing strengths. Dilek is encouraged to express her mixed feelings of relief and sadness about her relationship with her husband, and her feelings are validated as normal. The alleviation of her psychiatric symptoms is achieved without alteration to her established medication regimen.

The primary level of intervention is aimed at health promotion. One of the identified stressors is inadequate community resources. The client attends the local mental health center on a regular basis, but these appointments take place only once a month. The client should be provided with information about crisis centers, emergency support, and grief counseling. The nurse follows up to ensure that the client makes contact with these resources to strengthen the flexible line of defense.

CONCLUSION

This chapter reviewed some of the major nursing theories. Although the examples presented here are from Turkey, the elements of these models are global and timeless.

For a full suite of assignments and additional learning activities, use the access code located in the front of your book to visit this exclusive website: http://go.jblearning.com/dechesnay. If you do not have an access code, you can obtain one at the site.

REFERENCES

August-Brady, M. (2000). Prevention as intervention. *Journal of Advanced Nursing, 31*(6), 1304–1308.

Berbiglia, V. A. (1997). Orem's self-care deficit theory in nursing practice. In M. Alligood & A. Marriner-Tomey (Eds.), *Nursing theory utilization and application* (pp. 255–282). St. Louis, MO: Mosby-Year Book.

Bultmeier, K. (1997). Rogers' science of unitary human being in nursing practice. In M. Alligood & A. Marriner-Tomey (Eds.), *Nursing theory utilization and application* (pp. 283–306). St. Louis, MO: Mosby-Year Book.

Connerley, K., Ristau, S., Lindberg, C., & McFarland, M. (1999). The Roy model in nursing practice. In *The Roy adaptation model* (2nd ed., pp. 515–534). Stamford, CT: Appleton & Lange.

Conway, J., McMillan, M., & Solman, A. (2006). Enhancing cardiac rehabilitation nursing through aligning practice to theory: Implications for nursing education. *Journal of Continuing Education in Nursing 37*(5), 233–238.

Daily, L. S., Maupin, J. S., Murray, C. A., Satterly, M. C., Schnell, D. L., & Wallace, T. L. (1994). Martha E. Roger: Unitary human beings. In A. Marriner-Tomey (Ed.), *Nursing theorists and their work* (3rd ed., pp. 211–230). St. Louis, MO: C. V. Mosby.

Ducharme, F., Ricard, N., Duquette, A., Levesque, L., & Lachance, L. (1998). Empirical testing of a longitudinal model derived from the Roy adaptation model. *Nursing Science Quarterly, 11*(4), 149–159.

Forchuk, C. (1993). *Hildegarde E. Peplau: Interpersonal nursing theory.* Newbury Park, CA: Sage.

Freese, B.T. (2006). Betty Neuman: Systems model. In A.M. Tomey & M. R. Alligood (Eds.), *Nursing theorists and their work* (pp. 318–334). St. Louis, MO: Mosby.

Frey, M. A., & Norris, D. (1997). King's system framework and theory in nursing practice. In M. Alligood & A. Marriner-Tomey (Eds.), *Nursing theory utilization and application* (pp. 181–206). St. Louis, MO: Mosby-Year Book.

King, I. M. (1997). King's theory of goal attainment in practice. *Nursing Science Quarterly, 10*(4), 180–185

Leininger, M. M. (1991). *Culture care diversity and universality: A theory of nursing.* New York: National League of Nursing Press.

Leininger, M. M. (1995). *Transcultural nursing: Concepts, theories, research and practice* (2nd ed.). New York: McGraw-Hill.

Lopes, M. V. O., Pagliuca, L. M. F., & Araujo, T. L. (2006). Historical evolution of the concept environment proposed in the Roy adaptation model. *Rev Latino-am Enfermagem, 14*(2), 259–265.

Malinski, V. (2006). Rogerian science-based nursing theories. *Nursing Science Quarterly, 19*(1), 7–12.

McCamant, K. (2006). Humanistic nursing, interpersonal relations theory and the empathy–altruism hypothesis. *Nursing Science Quarterly, 19*(4), 334–338.

McCance, T., McKenna, H., & Boore, J. (1999). Caring: Theoretical perspectives of relevance to nursing. *Journal of Advanced Nursing, 30*, 1388–1395.

McFarland, M. (2006). Madeleine Leininger: Culture care theory of diversity and universality. In A. M. Tomey & M. R. Alligood (Eds.), *Nursing theorists and their work* (pp. 472–496). St. Louis, MO: Mosby.

Mooney, M., & O'Brien, F. (2006). Developing a plan of care using the Roper, Logan and Tierney model. *British Journal of Nursing, 15*(16), 887–892.

Moraes, L., Lopes, M., & Brage, V. (2006). Analysis of the functional components of Peplau's theory and its confluence with the group reference. *Acta Paulista de Enfermagen, 19*(2), 228–233.

Neuman, B. (1995). *The Neuman systems model* (3rd. ed.). Stamford, CT: Appleton & Lange.

Orem, D. E. (1995). *Nursing concepts of practice* (5th ed.). St. Louis, MO: Mosby.

Pearson, A., Vaughan, B., & Fitzgerald, M. (2005). The self-care models for nursing. In *Nursing models for practice* (3rd ed., pp. 103–122). Philadelphia, PA: Butterworth-Heinemann, Elsevier.

Peplau, H. E. (1992). *Interpersonal relations in nursing*. New York: Springer.

Rogers, M. E. (1992). Window on science of unitary human beings. In M. O'Toole (Ed.), *Miller-Keane encyclopedia and dictionary of medicine, nursing and allied health* (p. 1339). Philadelphia: W. B. Saunders.

Rogers, M. E. (1994). The science of unitary human beings: Current perspectives. *Nursing Science Quarterly, 7*(1), 33–35.

Roper, N., Logan, W., & Tierney, A. (2002). *The elements of nursing* (4th ed.). Edinburgh: Churchill Livingstone.

Roy, C. (1997). Future of the Roy model: Challenge to redefine adaptation. *Nursing Science Quarterly, 10*(1), 42–48.

Sieloff, C. L. (2006). Imogene King: Interacting systems of goal attainment. In A. M. Tomey & M. R. Alligood (Eds.), *Nursing theorists and their work* (pp. 297–318). St. Louis, MO: Mosby.

Stockmann, C. (2005). A literature review of the progress of the psychiatric nurse–patient relationship as described by Peplau. *Issues in Mental Health Nursing, 26*, 911–919.

Taylor, S. G., Geden, E., Issaramalai, S., & Wongvatunyu, S. (2000). Orem's self-care deficit nursing theory: Its philosophic foundation and the state of the science. *Nursing Science Quarterly, 13*(2), 104–108.

Timmins, F. (2006). Conceptual models used by nurses working in coronary care units: A discussion paper. *European Journal of Cardiovascular Nursing, 5*(4), 253–257.

Vandemark, L. (2006). Awareness of self and expanding consciousness: Using nursing theories to prepare nurse therapists. *Issues in Mental Health Nursing, 27*(6), 605–615.

Villarruel, A. M., Bishop, T. L., Simpson, E. M., Jemmott, L. S., & Fawcett, J. (2001). Borrowed theories, shared theories, and the advancement of nursing knowledge. *Nursing Science Quarterly, 14*(2), 158–163.

Watson, J. (1996). Watson's theory of transpersonal caring. In P. H. Walker & B. Neuman (Eds.), *Blueprint for use of nursing models: Education, research, practice, and administration* (pp. 141–184). New York: NLN Press.

Watson, J. (2005). Caring science: Belonging before being as ethical cosmology. *Nursing Science Quarterly, 18*(4), 304–305.

Watson, J., & Smith, M. (2002). Caring science and the science of unitary human beings: A trans-theoretical discourse for nursing knowledge development. *Journal of Advanced Nursing, 37*, 452.

Yanchar, S. C., & South J. B. (2009). Beyond the theory–practice split in instructional design: The current situation and future directions. In M. Orey et al. (Eds.), *Educational media and technology yearbook*. New York: Springer Science-Business Media. Doi: 10.1007/978-0-387-09675-9 6

Culturally Competent Care for South Pacific Islanders

Karen Joines and Mary de Chesnay

Objectives

At the end of this chapter, the reader will be able to

1. Give some examples of how Samoans view health and health care.
2. Explain how Watson's theory can be applied to improve health care for the Samoan population.
3. Discuss the dangers of ignoring spirituality when providing health care to Samoans.

WWW

This chapter discusses how Samoan beliefs might be considered in designing culturally competent nursing interventions for Samoan patients using Watson's theory of human care. Although the focus here is on Samoans in America, the same principles also apply to Samoans who have settled in other countries. The principles of providing culturally competent care are relevant globally as world immigration patterns challenge nurses in many countries to meet the needs of their newest citizens.

Emigrating from the South Pacific during the past few decades, Samoans have contributed to the cultural diversity of the United States, particularly along the West Coast. Americans often view the territories of the Pacific Islands in terms of exotic tourism to this tropical paradise. In reality, many Samoans in their native land live in impoverished conditions; while they might view their homeland as paradise, they are limited in the degree to which they can advance economically. According to McGrath (2000), more than 60% of American Samoans have moved to the continental United States in recent decades in search of better educational and economic opportunities.

Dietary patterns are particularly relevant to nursing practice among Samoan immigrants, particularly those who move to New Zealand and the United States, because the high-fat, low-fiber diet of many Samoans is related to increased risk of cardiovascular disease. In a New Zealand study, Galanis et al. (1999) found that there are differences in dietary patterns among western Samoans and those from American Samoa, with westerners tending toward a diet high in fat (primarily from coconut cream). American Samoans tended to eat more processed foods and had diet containing higher levels of cholesterol, protein, and sodium.

Similarly, diabetes is of concern to Samoans. To address this problem, a unique partnership among Pacific Islanders has led to the development of coalitions to educate people about the risks of the disease. For example, Braun et al. (2003) described a training program in the South Pacific. Among the outcomes of this project for American Samoa has been the creation of community-building efforts to sponsor programs in diabetes awareness, education, and screening. Ideally, such programs will facilitate prevention of diabetes and early intervention in persons who show signs of developing it.

Fritsch (1992) identified the need for nurses of the South Pacific to take the lead in efforts to improve the health of their people. In a speech to the South Pacific Nurses Forum, she urged nurses to become actively involved in formulating health policy. As both nurses and Samoans, these professionals are in a particularly powerful position to develop policy for Samoans. For example, researchers in preventing suicide argue that Western models of health promotion and suicide prevention are not appropriate for Pacific Islanders and argue that resilience strategies must be culturally relevant—that is, "developed by the people for the people" (Stewart-Withers & O'Brien, 2006, p. 209). Despite Western influence and governance, Samoans retain their culture and traditions and maintain political power at the tribal level.

Samoan views on health often conflict with those held by practitioners in the U.S. healthcare delivery system. Thus, to provide appropriate care to Samoans, American healthcare providers must learn how to integrate Samoan culture into care plans in a culturally competent way. In particular, three beliefs primarily influence Samoan health perceptions and practices: (1) a holistic view of self, (2) collective involvement, and (3) spirituality. Although Samoans' views on health are different from Americans' views, it is not impossible to incorporate Samoan beliefs into quality health care. Watson's theory of human care provides direction for how nurses might design interventions that are culturally based (Watson, 2002, 2005; Watson & Smith, 2002).

WATSON'S THEORY OF HUMAN CARE

Watson's theory of human care is one of many models and theories created to help nurses understand how culture influences well-being. Watson described a central focus of her theory as addressing the meaning of illness, health and caring, as cited in Bernick, 2004. With this focus at the forefront of their practice, nurses create healing environments for their patients that reach deep facets of the human experience, encompassing the soul, mind, and body. Watson identified 10 carative factors as aiding nurses in using the theory in nursing practice:

1. Humanistic–altruistic system of values
2. Faith–hope
3. Sensitivity to self and to others

4. Helping–trusting, human care relationship
5. Expressing positive and negative feelings
6. Creative problem-solving caring processes
7. Transpersonal teaching–learning
8. Supportive, protective, and/or corrective mental, physical, societal, and spiritual environment
9. Human needs assistance
10. Existential–phenomenological–spiritual forces (as cited in Bernick, 2004)

Using the 10 carative factors, the healing-caring model serves as an appropriate guideline in creating culturally competent interventions because of its inherent focus on what is meaningful to the individual. In applying Watson's theory, the work of Mendyka is particularly relevant.

Mendyka (2000) explored Watson's theory in a case study in which he provided a strong rationale for the applicability of Watson's work to culturally competent practice, based on three reasons. First, Watson utilized a phenomenological approach to understand what health and illness mean to the patient. When nurses work with clients of a different ethnicity or culture, it is essential for the nurse to understand their perceptions and meanings of health and illness prior to performing any care or teaching. Without a basic understanding of the client's culture, the client and nurse may experience cultural conflict and confusion, and the client may not return for care. Second, Watson's theory involves an intersubjective process that teaches the nurse how to identify with himself or herself and with others by engaging with clients in their experiences. This promotes an environment in which a therapeutic relationship can develop; it also assists nurses in developing care plans in concert with patients and families rather than for them. Third, the goal of Watson's theory is to establish holistic harmony within mind, body, and soul.

In particular, the third aspect of holism is relevant to Samoans and has been discussed in regard to other cultures. Erci (2005), in reviewing Watson's theory, noted that the healing environment is key. The fact that Erci applied the theory to a patient from Turkey reinforces the universality of the model. Irish nurses also validated the theory in terms of individual healing processes that are strengthened through authentic relationships defined by caring practices (McCance, McKenna, & Boore, 1999).

Because Samoans view care holistically and value collective family involvement, Watson's theory provides a useful basis for health interventions with Samoans:

- Develop a helping and trusting relationship with the patient (carative factor 4)
- Develop a capacity to problem-solve with the patient and family (carative factor 6)
- Educate, enable, and empower the client while authenticating his or her beliefs (carative factors 3, 7, and 10)
- Create a healing environment on all levels to reach harmony (carative factor 8)

These interventions capture the essence of Watson's theory and are consistent with Samoan beliefs. Indeed, one might argue that Watson's principles are universal.

SAMOAN PERCEPTIONS OF HEALTH AND TRADITIONAL TREATMENTS

One of the issues related to providing culturally competent care to populations from small countries or isolated regions of the world is that data-based literature is not available to guide practice. As more studies are conducted, the state of the art of literature will evolve and more sophisticated approaches can be designed. One key study was conducted by a team of Samoan and Japanese nurses and involved qualitative interviews with Samoan caregivers and family members. The philosophy underlying the research was to develop culturally based ways in which nurses could conduct workshops to help caregivers of Samoan elderly provide better care and relieve their own stress (Mulatilo, Taupau, & Enoka, 2000).

Holistic View of Self

The Samoan concept of self is holistic, in that each person has three parts—physical, mental, and spiritual—that together make the person complete. Based on this belief in holism, Samoans assert that a person is healthy when all elements are in balance and harmony. When a patient is not well in one part, all other parts are affected. Therefore, when illness affects a person, Samoans believe treatment should be aimed at all three parts, with the goal of reaching harmony and balance (Tamasese, Peteru, Waldegrave, & Bush, 2005). The family is key to successful intervention with Samoan patients (Mulatilo et al., 2000).

Rather than focusing on cures, traditional Samoan healing emphasizes achieving balance and wellness. Traditional remedies use medicinal plants in a variety of ways. For example, Samoans boil leaves or bark to create a drinkable tea and cook roots into a healing meal. In addition to plants, Samoans use oils, massage, and hot and cool applications as treatments (Rogers, n.d.; Saau, 1996). Thus a common approach used by elderly Samoan women to heal headaches includes heating tea leaves with water and massaging them into the forehead (Saau, 1996).

Contrast with Western Medicine

Holistic views regarding health and treatment are in sharp contrast with traditional U.S. health care, which is aimed primarily at curing physical ailments and disease. Conventional treatments focus on alleviating biological or physical symptoms using modern technologies and treatments established through scientific research. To accommodate their beliefs when they reside in the United States, many Samoans continue to practice traditional healing as adjuncts to American treatments, rather than as replacements for them (Rogers, n.d.).

Issues Contributing to Vulnerability

Many Samoans attempt to find traditional healers who have knowledge of ancient healing practices. In Seattle, few Samoan healers are available to elderly clients; as a result, many families perform traditional healing practices to the best of their knowledge with the supplies that are available to them (Saau, 1996). This practice may cause emotional stress and feelings of cultural isolation if they attempt to create the remedies themselves and feel unsuccessful and limited by resource constraints. The homemade remedies may also be harmful if the client is not fully knowledgeable of which plants to use and how to use them properly. In addition, elderly Samoans may feel alienated or not respected by U.S. healthcare providers who discourage their traditional practices. As a result, many choose not to access American health care.

Interventions

In applying Watson's theory, several carative factors are used. Carative factor 3 is utilized when nurses approach elderly Samoans in a nonjudgmental and unbiased manner. Beginning with a comprehensive assessment, the nurse converses with the client to elicit the client's perspective on the meaning of the ailment, utilizing carative factor 10 to discover the patient's phenomenological beliefs regarding health. By asking for information concerning his or her perceptions and cultural practices, the nurse conveys genuine appreciation and interest in the client's priorities. Thus a door opens in the nurse–patient relationship that enables the nurse to establish trust (carative factor 4). Demonstrating respect is critical to success in working with vulnerable clients (de Chesnay, Wharton, & Pamp, 2005).

Several practical interventions may be used to achieve a trusting and partnering relationship with culturally diverse patients. When assessing alternative health treatments, the nurse should ask clients about their health practices and assess the knowledge they have regarding the treatment being used (Which plant is used? How is it used?). Efficacy and safety are two important topics to address when confronted with a client who uses complementary and alternative medicine. It is important not to diminish the meaning of the client's experience by making judgments about cultural healing methods. Rather, the more effective approach is to encourage the client to use complementary healing methods as supplementary treatments to conventional treatments. Safety is a concern when patients use combinations of treatments. If the nurse does not know whether a specific practice is safe, he or she will have to research the treatment and discuss it with the healthcare team. While teaching, the nurse should authenticate the client's beliefs and avoid discounting them.

It is essential that the nurse document and inform the physician regarding all alternative treatments, which will have the additional benefit of developing a positive relationship between the physician and the client. The nurse can advocate for the patient's needs by creating a care plan that integrates a holistic approach. By asking the cultural questions and conducting a thorough, meaningful assessment of the client's perspective, the nurse will foster appreciation of the client's cultural identity, enhance the client's sense of control, and achieve partnership in care.

Collective Involvement

Samoans believe that every human exists in the context of an interrelated network of family and community and that the interdependence and harmony created within the relationships contribute to health and well-being (Tamasese et al., 2005). They believe each relationship is defined by specific roles and responsibilities. If a person cannot fulfill his or her roles, disharmony occurs within the relationship. This disharmony can impair the health of the individual (Management Science for Health [MSH], n.d.). Therefore, when illness affects a person, a key element of healing involves reconnecting and strengthening those relationships that are unbalanced. One method for doing so is a ritual called *ho'oponopono*, which includes a method of family counseling, conflict resolution, self-reflection, and a formal session of apology and forgiveness (MSH, n.d.).

Because Samoan patients maintain an existence within a collective context, families are included in all aspects of health care, including the decision-making process. McLaughlin and Braun (1998) conducted a study on healthcare decision-making processes within Samoan families and discovered the following principles regarding the elderly and decision making. Samoans do not prefer to have a choice in major healthcare decisions because they rely on a physician's paternalistic judgment to decide the best course of action. If they must make a decision, the Samoan family collectively decides on the best course of action. In addition, elderly patients often do not want physicians to inform them if they have a terminal illness because the family prefers to be informed first to protect the patient from troubling information regarding his or her health.

Contrast with Western Medicine

The Samoan value of collective involvement comes in direct conflict with values in Western health care, primarily the values of personal autonomy, self-reliance, and independence. In the United States, there is a strong focus on protecting an individual's right to privacy, right to refuse treatment, and right to autonomous choice. Based on these values, it is unethical and illegal for a physician to perform or provide treatments to a client without informed consent, even if the client requests otherwise (Lundy & Janes, 2001). U.S. healthcare providers do acknowledge the effects that relationships have on a patient's health and claim to practice family-centered care, but always within the parameters of individualism.

Issues Contributing to Vulnerability

The difference in how decisions are made can delay treatment and create a frustrating experience for both the Samoan family and the healthcare providers. If a Samoan experiences resistance from physicians in allowing the family to make the decision, he or she may choose not to participate in any treatment. Language barriers, unclear communication, and lack of knowledge of U.S. health policy can all contribute to the conflicts between Samoans and healthcare providers. Most importantly, in situations in which the client is most vulnerable, such as in an incapacitated state, his or her preference to have the family make decisions will not be honored without legal recourse. If no durable power of attorney has been established, the family will not have authority to decide what is in the best interests of the patient.

Interventions

As highlighted in Watson's theory of human care, nurses must strive to develop a capacity to problem-solve with the patient and family (Erci, 2005; Mendyka, 2000). In utilizing carative factor 6 while working with Samoans, essential tasks for the nurse are to maintain flexibility, establish a partnership, ensure clear communications, and ensure appropriate legal action. Partnership with the family is an essential aspect of providing care to elderly Samoans. Therefore, it is critical to use a true family-centered approach while creating the care plan. The nurse should view the family as a positive influence and include them in the treatment strategy. Family members, in turn, can help keep the patient adherent with treatment and can increase the patient's resilience by providing support and encouragement. The nurse can provide education and information to all members of the family. To do so, however, the nurse must ensure that all information is handled with confidentiality unless otherwise permitted by the patient. Therefore, it is important to determine who is legally permitted to receive the information without formal permission by the patient. Having the family elect a spokesperson can streamline the communication process.

Conflict may arise if the client is asked directly to make a decision among treatment options. The nurse should discuss all options with the family and allow adequate time for them to make a decision. If the patient does not want to know the diagnosis, but wishes to receive treatment, the nurse can discuss the importance of informed consent with the family. Their involvement will make the process easier for the client to cope. Prior to planning health teaching, the nurse must assess the need for an interpreter, as this step indicates to the client and family that the nurse values their involvement and wishes to make it easier for them to participate.

The most difficult conflict may arise in situations where the patient is incapacitated and the family wishes to make all decisions regarding end-of-life treatments. The nurse can assist in preventing ethical and legal conflicts by providing information to the patient (while he or she is competent) and the family on advance directives. By explaining the role of a durable power of attorney, the nurse ensures that the patient has the option of legally designating a person to serve as a surrogate decision maker in end-of-life decisions. This step will ensure that the patient and family are prepared, and adequate preparation will prevent insult to the family, who would otherwise have limited decision-making authority in which treatments their family member would receive.

Spirituality and Health

Religion and spirituality are highly valued in Samoan culture. Faith in God permeates all areas of life, including perceptions of health. Samoans believe that deceased family members exist as spirits, actively influencing and participating in their lives. If unresolved conflict existed while the family member was alive, the deceased person can return as a spirit to "curse" an individual (Saau, 1996). For this reason, many Samoans assert that two forms of illness exist: one that involves "Samoan spirits" and another identified as "European illnesses" (Rogers, n.d.). They base their healthcare decisions on the belief that traditional Samoan healers can treat spiritual illnesses, and American doctors can treat European illnesses (Rogers, n.d.). In addition, Samoans believe that through prayer intervention, God manifests His healing powers by granting positive outcomes of medical treatment (traditional or Western) (Saau, 1996). Furthermore, medical treatment can be effective only if the family has faith that God can manifest His healing powers through the treatment. They ultimately believe that everything occurs in accordance with God's will; thus there is a strong belief in fate (Saau, 1996).

Contrast with Western Medicine

Western healthcare providers do not generally view spiritual conflicts as causative factors for disease and illness. The "superstitions" described by the client are often undervalued and ignored as the medical team focuses on finding biological and physical causes for the illness. For example, while nursing curricula addresses spirituality to some extent, nurse educators do not fully explore what this means in practice and how nurses might use spiritual techniques with patients. In fact, many settings seem to have a cultural norm in which prayer and spiritual comfort are to be provided only by the chaplain.

Even so, prayer is a recognized source of strength among many healthcare providers, and studies have been conducted in which a key finding is that prayer is associated with better patient outcomes (DiJoseph & Cavendish, 2005; Meraviglia, 2006; Tracy et al., 2005; Tzeng & Yin, 2006). In particular, the DiJoseph and Cavendish (2005) paper draws the connection of prayer to nursing theories, including Watson.

Many nurses and physicians do not utilize prayer as an effective method for treatment for a variety of reasons. In some cases, they have not received formal training that prepares them to provide spiritual care. They may not view spiritual care as an important aspect of nursing or medical care. They may have their own spiritual conflicts and not be comfortable talking with others about issues of spirituality. In addition, time constraints, the need to focus on technology, or misdiagnosis of spiritual issues as manifestations of anxiety and depression may cause healthcare providers to ignore this aspect of care (E. Weeg, personal communication, 2007).

Issues Contributing to Vulnerability

Many Samoans may be reluctant to use Western healthcare providers because of the lack of spiritual acknowledgment and appreciation in treatment modalities. In addition, Samoans may underutilize treatment that may be beneficial if they believe they have a Samoan illness that can only be healed through traditional methods. In these cases, Samoans may delay seeking treatment, with their illnesses then being complicated by the wait to determine whether it is a Samoan or European illness.

Interventions

It is important for nurses to wait to discuss spiritual practices until after they have established rapport with patients, because Samoan clients may view spirituality as a sensitive topic and may be reluctant to share information. The nurse should explain the purpose of gathering the information so that the patient is aware that the nurse values spiritual needs and wants to incorporate these needs into the care plan. The client will be more open to the discussion if the nurse is honest, nonjudgmental, and respectful.

The nurse should assess what the client perceives to be the cause and meaning of the illness, and whether the illness is "Samoan" or "European," followed by an assessment of the spiritual practices in which the patient participates (carative factor 10). In addition, providing clients with an opportunity to disclose their spiritual journey or experience may help them reflect on the impact their spirituality has on the meaning of past and present life experiences. Identifying and validating their spiritual practices and beliefs as strengths that promote positive coping methods will convey that the nurse is open to ideas held by the client (carative factor 5). Nurses can also assist in connecting patients with spiritual resources, such as chaplains. Christian Samoans might appreciate knowing the chaplain and visiting the chapel, but it should not be assumed that all Samoans will want to see the chaplain.

At any rate, the nurse should not dismiss the importance of spiritual care, because it is a primary strength in Samoan life that provides clients with hope. Meeting the spiritual needs of patients promotes resilience. For elderly Samoans who maintain spiritual practices developed over a lifetime, it is critical to respect their need to pray in their own way (carative factor 8).

WWW CASE STUDY

A young Samoan woman was admitted with encephalopathy of unknown etiology to a local Seattle hospital. Although she remained physically recognizable, her incoherent speech and violent attacks were a shock to her family and friends. The healthcare team conducted many tests to reach a diagnosis, but could not find a cause for her behavior. Because the doctors had no physical explanation for the behavior, the Samoan family members diagnosed her with a spiritual curse: The young woman had been possessed by the spirits of several deceased family members. The woman's grandmother made a homemade lotion with native plants and oils. In an emotional routine, the family rubbed this lotion on the woman's body, surrounding her in a tight circle of prayer for more than two hours. On several occasions, they called out to the deceased family members, asking them to remove themselves from the woman's body.

This case study is an example of two cultures and perspectives meeting in a hospital setting: Samoan tradition and American health care. The situation in the case study is not uncommon, especially in regional or inner-city hospitals. The following discussion is aimed at providing the acute care nurse with practical interventions to handle the situation described in the case study with culturally competent care.

In the acute care setting, the goal for nursing personnel is to develop collaboration and partnership with the patient and family so that the healthcare, spiritual, and cultural needs of the patient are met. This is not to say that the nurse is responsible only for managing his or her basic nursing tasks; rather, the nurse serves as the mediator and the connector between the healthcare team and the patient and family, and is responsible for overseeing that the patient is having his or her holistic needs met.

To begin a collaborative relationship with the patient and family, the nurse coming on shift must first establish rapport. Establishing rapport is a process of communication laced with veracity and compassion. Upon entering the room, it may be as simple as asking, "How are you doing?", or as complex as asking, "How do you interpret your daughters behavior?" In this case study, the nurse should take the time to address the family's feelings regarding the tests being performed. He or she should save up 10 to 15 minutes to sit down and speak with the family and address their frustrations and questions, keeping in mind that it is most important to listen and not to speak. At this point, the nurse could find out the family's perspective on what the illness means to them and whether any cultural beliefs reflect their understanding on how it is caused and treated (if this information is not known). If the nurse encounters a time constraint, he or she can suggest that the family come back together so that the nurse can gather more information or determine whether they would prefer to meet with a multi-faith chaplain who could get more information for the healthcare team. When mentioning the request for a chaplain, the nurse should explain that a multi-faith chaplain is used to provide spiritual support and to gather information that can be passed to the healthcare team so that team members can provide the best care for the patient in accordance with her cultural and spiritual needs.

After establishing rapport, the nurse can assess the patient's holistic needs by communicating with the family, "How can we support her cultural and spiritual needs?" Nursing personnel should discuss the plan of care with the family and develop a schedule, highlighting the need for clustering care to ensure the family has privacy. Ideally, the nurse involved in this case study will have been aware of the spiritual routine prior to its occurrence so that maximal time and privacy is given to the patient and her family. If the ritual is performed without the nurse's knowledge and he or she happens to interrupt the routine, the nurse must prioritize the care tasks that need to be performed to interrupt as little as possible, if at all.

SUMMARY

This chapter has focused on the nurse's pivotal role in promoting the integration of cultural diversity and holistic care into care plans for Samoans. Watson's theory of human care may be applied to the process of forming culturally competent interventions. The primary interventions include conducting thorough and meaningful assessments to evaluate the patient's perspectives, developing a trusting relationship, and collaborating with the patient and family to integrate their beliefs and practices into the care plan. In particular, spiritual practices need to be incorporated into the care plan.

Many issues are involved in providing effective care for the elderly within this population, but healthcare workers are always most effective if they have an appreciation for cultural diversity and ways in which they can integrate their cultural sensitivity in practice. While it might appear that these techniques would automatically be useful with clients who are not Samoan, it is important to stress that the specific techniques are based on what the literature says about Samoan culture and should be validated with individuals and families. The world is becoming increasingly smaller and more diverse. Our healthcare systems should reflect a caring orientation that reflects competence in nursing with diverse vulnerable populations.

ACKNOWLEDGMENT

The authors are indebted to Eileen Weeg, a nurse expert in spirituality, for her helpful comments regarding the draft of this chapter.

WWW

For a full suite of assignments and additional learning activities, use the access code located in the front of your book to visit this exclusive website: http://go.jblearning.com/dechesnay. If you do not have an access code, you can obtain one at the site.

REFERENCES

Bernick, L. (2004). Caring for older adults: Practice guided by Watson's caring-healing model. *Nursing Science Quarterly, 17*(2), 128–134.

Braun, K., Ichiho, H., Kuhaulua, R., Aitaoto, N., Tsark, J., Spegal, R., & Lamb, B. (2003, November). Empowerment through community building: Diabetes today in the Pacific. *Journal of Public Health Management Practice* (suppl), S19–S25.

De Chesnay, M., Wharton, R., & Pamp, C. (2005). Cultural competence, resilience and advocacy. In M. de Chesnay (Ed.), *Caring for the vulnerable* (pp. 45–60). Sudbury, MA: Jones and Bartlett.

DiJoseph, J. & Cavendish, R. (2005). Expanding the dialogue on prayer relevant to holistic care. *Holistic Nursing Practice, 19*(4), 147–155.

Erci, B. (2005). Nursing theories applied to vulnerable populations: Examples from Turkey. In M. de Chesnay (Ed.), *Caring for the vulnerable* (pp. 45–60). Sudbury, MA: Jones and Bartlett.

Fritsch, K. L. (1992). South Pacific nursing education: Visions of the future. *International Nursing Review, 39*(1), 19.

Galanis, D., McGarvey, S., Quested, C., Sio, B., & Amuli, S. A. (1999). Dietary intake of modernizing Samoans: Implications for risk of cardiovascular disease. *Journal of the American Dietetic Association, 99*(2), 184–191.

Lundy, K. S., & Janes, S. (2001). *Community health nursing: Caring for the public's health.* Sudbury, MA: Jones and Bartlett.

Management Science for Health (MSH). (n.d.). The provider's guide to quality and culture: Pacific Islanders. Retrieved June 9, 2006, from http://erc.msh.org/mainpage.cfm?file=5.4.8.htm&module=provider&language=English&ggroup=culture.

McCance, T., McKenna, H., & Boore, J. (1999). Caring: Theoretical perspectives of relevance to nursing. *Journal of Advanced Nursing, 30*(6), 1388–1395.

McGrath, B. B. (2002). Seattle fa'a Samoa. *The Contemporary Pacific, 14*, 307–340. Retrieved February 26, 2006, from *Project Muse: Scholarly Journals Online.*

McLaughlin, L. A., & Braun, K. L. (1998). Asian and Pacific Islander cultural values: Considerations for health care decision-making. *Health and Social Work, 2*, 116–126.

Mendyka, B. (2000). Exploring culture in nursing: A theory-driven practice. *Holistic Nursing Practice, 15*(1), 32–41.

Meraviglio, M. (2006). Effects of spirituality on breast cancer survivors. *Oncology Nursing Forum, 33(1)*, 1–7.

Mulatilo, M., Taupau, T., & Enoka, I. (2000). Teaching families to be caregivers for the elderly. *Nursing and Health Sciences 2*, 51–58.

Rogers, N. (n.d.). Creating balance: Samoa struggles to find and equilibrium between ancient healing techniques and modern medical practices. *A Broad View Magazine: South Pacific Region.* Retrieved February 26, 2006, from http://www.abroadviewmagazine.com/regions/so_pac/creat_bal.html

Saau, L. (1996). *Voices of the Samoan community.* Retrieved February 26, 2006, from http://www.xculture.org/resource/library/download/samoan.pdf

Stewart-Withers, R. R., & O'Brien, A. P. (2006). Suicide prevention and social capital: A Samoan perspective. *Health Sociology Review, 15*, 209–220.

Tamasese, K., Peteru, C., Waldegrave, C., & Bush, A. (2005). Ole taeao afua, the new morning: A qualitative investigation into Samoan perspectives on mental health and culturally appropriate services. *Australian and New Zealand Journal of Psychiatry, 39*, 300–309.

Tracy, M., Lindquist, R., Savik, K., Watanuki, S., Sendelbach, S., Kreitzer, M., & Berman, B. (2005). Use of complementary and alternative therapies: A national survey of critical care nurses. *American Journal of Critical Care, 14*(5), 404–416.

Tzeng, H., & Yin, C. (2006). Learning to respect a patient's spiritual needs concerning an infectious disease. *Nursing Ethics, 13*(1), 17–28.

Watson, J. (2002). Intentionality and caring-healing consciousness: A practice of transpersonal nursing. *Holistic Nursing Practice, 16*(4), 12–19.

Watson, J. (2005). Caring science: Belonging before being as ethical cosmology. *Nursing Science Quarterly, 18*(4), 304–305.

Watson, J., & Smith, M. C. (2002). Caring science and the science of unitary human beings: A trans-theoretical discourse for nursing knowledge development. *Journal of Advanced Nursing, 37*(5), 452–461.

CHAPTER 8

Theories of Mothering and HIV-Infected Mothers

Tommie Nelms

Objectives

At the end of this chapter, the reader will be able to

1. Define "mothering" from the author's perspective.
2. Describe the process of theory building the author presented.
3. Compare and contrast the special considerations of mothering for women who disclose HIV/AIDS.

WWW

Mothering is said to be a continuous struggle requiring superordinate efforts against great odds (Ruddick, 1995). Even in the best of circumstances, mothering is fraught with self-doubt, fatigue, and overwhelming emotion as women try to comply with their own and others' perceptions of the "good mother." What must mothering and motherhood be like for women who are infected with HIV, and how do their experiences fit within current theories of mothering?

This chapter presents an emergent fit of data (Artinian, 1988) from the author's previous research investigating mothering issues faced by HIV-infected women (Nelms, 2005; Nelms & Zeigler, 2008). It begins with an overview of theoretical frameworks of mothering and motherhood espoused by Sara Ruddick (1995) and Toni Morrison as proposed by Andrea O'Reilly in her book, *Toni Morrison and Motherhood: A Politics of the Heart* (2004). Research findings are situated within Ruddick and Morrison's maternal frameworks. The chapter concludes with the author's demonstration that the mothering experienced by HIV-infected women is similar to the kind of mothering required of black women portrayed by Toni Morrison in her body of work.

In *Maternal Thinking: Toward a Politics of Peace* (1995), maternal theorist Sara Ruddick argues that out of the maternal necessity for thinking and thoughtfulness, a distinctive discipline or practice of mothering develops. "Practices are collective human activities distinguished by the aims that identify them and by the consequent demands made on practitioners committed to those aims" (Ruddick, 1995, p. 13). For something to be considered a practice, its aims or goals must be so central or "constitutive" that in the absence of the aims there would be no practice. To engage in a practice, persons must be committed to meeting its demands. Practices are created as persons pursue certain goals and make sense of (think about) the pursuits.

According to Ruddick, there are three demands of motherwork: preservation, growth, and social acceptance. Mothers who are committed to these demands use preservative love, nurturance, and training to meet these demands of mothering. As Ruddick says, "In a mother's day, the demands of preservation, growth, and acceptability are intertwined. Yet a reflective mother can separately identify each demand, partly because they are often in conflict" (1995, p. 23). The preservation and protection of the lives of their children are the first constitutive demands of maternal practice. For Ruddick, preservation and protection of children do not require enthusiasm or even love; they simply require mothers to see the child's vulnerability and respond to it with care, rather than abuse, indifference, or flight.

Nurturance of emotional and intellectual growth—which according to Ruddick is "complex, gradual, and subject to distinctive kinds of distortion or inhibition" (p. 83)—is the second demand that structures maternal thinking. Ruddick believes that *all* children are complex beings who "grow in complex ways, undergoing radical qualitative as well as quantitative change from childhood to adulthood" (p. 19), which demands nurturance. Children have complicated lives, with minds and psyches that need maternal attention.

Training and social acceptability of children is the third demand of maternal practice. Social groups require mothers to shape their children's growth in "acceptable" ways. While the demand for acceptability does not change, what counts as acceptable varies greatly within and among groups and cultures. A mother's group is that set of people from whom the mother seeks approval for her children; the mother would consider it a failure if her children did not meet with their approval. Mothers want their children to grow into people whom they and those closest to them "delightedly appreciate." Such a demand gives an urgency to mothers' daily lives that is sometimes exhilarating and at other times painful. There is general agreement that children cannot naturally develop in socially acceptable ways without help and, therefore, must be trained to meet these expectations. The training strategies used by mothers may be persuasive, manipulative, educative, abusive, seductive, or respectful, and are typically a mix of these approaches.

For Ruddick, maternal practice consists of mothers' engagement with the demands to protect, nurture, and train their children that produce a specific kind of thought or maternal thinking that is a cluster of attitudes, beliefs, and values (O'Reilly, p. 28). According to Ruddick, maternal thought requires many responses from mothers—that is, many ways of seeing and dealing with the world. Humility, cheerfulness, and acceptance of ambiguity are some of the attitudes mothers develop in response to motherwork. Because so much of motherwork is beyond the control of the mother, humility and acceptance of ambiguity are required by mothers in response to recognition "of the limits of one's actions and the unpredictability of the consequences of one's work" (1995, p. 72). Cheerfulness is what Ruddick calls the response of mothers to respect chance, limit, and imperfection while still working to keep children safe. For Ruddick, mothers are no more or less wonderful than other people. Mothers often speak of the contradictions of mothering: They speak of failure as often as success, and almost always recount their *struggles* to protect, nurture, and train their children.

In the preface of her book, *Toni Morrison and Motherhood: A Politics of the Heart* (2004), white feminist writer and mothering expert Andrea O'Reilly says that while she found mothering to be the most difficult work she ever undertook, she never felt oppressed or disempowered by motherhood as Toni Morrison's work has portrayed it. O'Reilly calls Toni Morrison a maternal theorist who presents perspectives of black motherhood that are different from the traditional views of Anglo-American motherhood such as that espoused by Ruddick. Morrison portrays motherhood with its dimensions of motherwork, motherlove, and motherline as a "political enterprise with social consequences" (O'Reilly, 2004, p. 23). Morrison's views of black motherhood regarding both maternal identity and role are radically different from the motherhood practiced and prescribed in the dominant culture. Mothers of children from the dominant culture, unlike black mothers, do not have to concern themselves with sociocultural acceptance of their children. While mothers of the dominant culture may be concerned with the sexism their daughters will encounter, they do not have to concern themselves with bringing their children into a racist world.

In terms of maternal identity, Morrison views motherhood as the site of power for black women; thus the maternal role is concerned with the empowerment of children. Motherwork, according to Morrison, concerns how mothers, raising black children in a racist and sexist world, can best protect their children, teach their children how to protect themselves, challenge racism, and, in the case of daughters, the sexism that seeks to harm them (O'Reilly, 2004).

According to black feminist Patricia Hill Collins (1991), black womanhood is controlled by images of black women that are constructed by the dominant culture. The four controlling images that Collins examines are the mammy, the matriarch, the welfare mother, and the Jezebel. These images of black women prevent black women from forming or articulating self-defined images. Morrison's views of black motherhood, however, enable black women to resist the negative cultural images by "rearticulating the power that is inherent in black women's everyday experiences of motherhood" (O'Reilly, 2004, p. 3).

Black women raise children in a society that is at best indifferent to the needs of black children and the concerns of black mothers. The focus for black mothers, in practice and thought, is how to preserve, protect, and empower black children so that they may resist those practices that seek to harm them and grow into whole and complete adults. As a consequence, black mothers require power to do the important work of mothering and are accorded this power through the value that African American culture places on mothering. According to O'Reilly (2004), African American culture offers black mothers a tradition of valuing motherhood that is different from the value of motherhood seen in the dominant culture. Black mothers and grandmothers are considered the "guardians of the generations," who are charged with the responsibility for providing education, social and political awareness, and unconditional love, nurturance, socialization, and value to their children and the children within their communities (p. 9). In the dominant culture, these responsibilities fall to fathers as well as to mothers.

The power that comes to African American motherhood is derived in part from the culture's matrifocality, which resides in the fact that black women view the pinnacle of womanhood as being a mother rather than as being a wife (O'Reilly, 2004). As such, power comes to black women through the construction of a homeplace where the dignity that is denied to them by the outside public world can be restored. According to bell hooks (1990), a homeplace is a safe place where black people can affirm one another, thereby healing the wounds inflicted by racism; it is a place where they have the opportunity to grow and develop, to nurture their spirits. Thus it is within the homeplace that black children who are seen as inferior, unworthy, and unlovable by dominant culture can receive powerful maternal love to counteract public world perspectives. The notion that minority children are empowered within the home by mothers who teach resistance and give knowledge differs from the dominant discourse on mothering that portrays home as politically neutral and nurturance as no more than the natural calling of mothers.

Morrison has described motherhood as "the most liberating thing that ever happened to me" (O'Reilly, 2004, p. 19). She calls motherhood "liberating" because the things her children demanded of her were unlike things that "others" demanded of her, and were things she could live up to—to be a good manager, have a sense of humor, and deliver something that someone could use. As Morrison has said, "The person that was in me that I liked best was the one my children seemed to want" (p. 20). This notion of mothering has been called "a freeing and generative experience" and stands in contrast to the white Western image of the mother, which assumes that mothers are all-giving, ever-present, self-sacrificing, and never destroyed or overwhelmed by the demands of their children (Bassin, Honey, & Kaplan, 1994).

Morrison's notions of motherhood as liberating and the source of her better self came from what she termed "the ancient properties" and traditional black values, which she called "the funk" (O'Reilly, 2004, p. 20). Ancient properties, according to Morrison, are seen when looking back at the strengths of black women, not when gazing forward. Although concepts of the black mammy are traditionally considered in negative terms, Morrison notes that black mammies could nurse, heal, and chop wood—all terrific things that were the full and complete manifestations of the ancient properties that represent maternal identity. Traditional black values or funk, for Morrison, represent "the funkiness of passion, the funkiness of nature, the funkiness of a wide range of emotions" (p. 24).

For Morrison, as for Ruddick, the practices of preservation and nurturance are the primary aspects of motherwork. Morrison also supports the notion of training children to make them acceptable to their social group. For Morrison, however, the notion of training is expanded to include the African American maternal custom of cultural bearing whereby children are raised in accordance with the values, beliefs, and customs of traditional African American culture, particularly the values of funk and ancient proprieties. In each of the practices of motherwork—preservation, nurturance, and cultural bearing—"Morrison is concerned with protecting children from the hurts of racist, and for daughters, sexist culture, and with teaching children how to protect themselves so they may be empowered to survive and resist the racist and patriarchal culture in which they live and to develop a strong and authentic identity as a black person" (O'Reilly, 2004, p. 29). Nurturing from black mothers is required to protect black children from racism by loving them so that they can learn to love themselves in a culture that considers them unworthy of love. Through cultural bearing, the history of blacks and images of blacks are transmitted. The cultural bearings *of* blacks *by* blacks serve as a substitute for the controlling images of blacks set forth by the dominant culture and give children a way to develop an authentic sense of black personhood.

Morrison adds a fourth maternal aim related to nurturance, termed *healing* by O'Reilly (2004). With healing, the focus is restoration of adults who never received protection, nurturance, and cultural bearing as children and, therefore, grew into adults who were psychologically wounded by racism and/or sexism. Morrison argues that African American maternal practices create self-defined identities that are key to survival and resistance for African American people. "Whether it is expressed as resistance against racism's dehumanization of her children or resistance against the mother's own oppression in the patriarchal institution of motherhood, nurturance is viewed as essential for the empowerment of children" (O'Reilly, 2004, p. 34). Morrison believes that her reformulation of motherwork as a political enterprise counters the master narratives of motherhood within the dominant culture. For her, "motherhood is a cultural construction that varies from time and place; there is no one essential or universal experience of motherhood" (p. 29).

MOTHERING WITH HIV/AIDS

Living with a diagnosis of HIV/AIDS pervades and infuses one's life in much the same way that race and gender do. For mothers, a diagnosis of HIV is a life-altering experience that deeply influences maternal identity, maternal role, and maternal thinking. Previous research with HIV-infected mothers revealed that living and mothering with a diagnosis of HIV was a *burden* for women in a number of ways (Nelms, 2005). One factor that greatly enhanced the burden of mothering with HIV was the stigma associated with a diagnosis of HIV/AIDS. While mothers with breast cancer or ovarian cancer are burdened with a life-threatening disease process that may eventually take their lives like HIV/AIDS, a diagnosis of cancer is not associated with stigma or "spoiled identity," nor does a "courtesy stigma" extend to family and associates of persons with cancer (Goffman, 1963).

Data from previous phenomenological inquiries into the end-of-life and mothering issues experienced by HIV-infected women (Nelms, 2005; Nelms & Zeigler, 2008) consisted of in-depth, open-ended, face-to-face interviews with 16 HIV-infected mothers living in north Texas: two Hispanic, two African American, two African, one Jamaican, and nine Caucasian. All of the women were clients within a comprehensive AIDS service organization (ASO).

Approval for this study was received from the institutional review board (IRB) at Texas Woman's University, Denton, Texas. Audiotaped interviews were conducted by the author and transcribed verbatim by a paid transcriptionist. In the interest of the self-disclosure, which is congruent with the original research methodology, I want to disclose that I am a white middle-class woman who has two grown sons. I am a nurse academician and feminist and have been a student of mothering informally all my life and formally since becoming a labor and delivery nurse in 1970. I do not have HIV.

The women who participated in the study were between the ages of 23 and 54 and had been diagnosed with HIV for 2 to 18 years at the time of the interviews. They were low- to middle-income, working-class women, with between one and seven children each, for a total of 42 children. The children ranged in age from 20 months to young adult, with the majority being in their teens and preteens. At the time of the interviews, half the women were married and half were not. Of the eight who were not married, three had never married, four were divorced, and one was an AIDS widow.

In the initial study, data were analyzed to identify common themes and patterns revealed by the HIV-infected mothers. For the presentation in this chapter, an emergent fit (Artinian, 1988) of the previous data was conducted, whereby the data were reexamined and interpreted against a background of the practices of mothering described by maternal theorists Sara Ruddick (1995) and Toni Morrison (O'Reilly, 2004). Both theorists note that mothers practice preservation, nurturance, and social acceptance of their children, but for Morrison there are special ways these practices operate for black mothers given their need to protect their children from racist, and for daughters, sexist culture. The similarities and differences of Ruddick's and Morrison's practices of mothering for HIV-infected mothers are presented along with supporting interview data. Pseudonyms are used to identify the mothers' words.

The HIV-infected mothers were extremely conscious of the maternal practices of preservation and protection of their children. Their primary protective functions were their attempts to protect their children from motherlessness; for many of the study participants, this meant protecting their children from knowledge of the mother's diagnosis (Nelms, 2005; Nelms & Zeigler, 2008). Of the 16 women, only five had disclosed their diagnosis to all or some of their (older) children. Eleven of the women said they had not or "would not" disclose this information to their children. A couple of women with older school-age children said their children "might" know about the diagnosis, although there had been no mention of it by the children or the mother.

The mothers clearly recognized the vulnerability of their children and believed their children's vulnerability was greatly enhanced by having a mother with a stigmatized life-threatening illness like HIV. They knew that the loss of one's mother made children even more vulnerable. Indeed, for many, just the knowledge that one's mother had a life-threatening illness was more than they could bear for their children to know. Unlike Morrison's recommendations for black mothers, however, the HIV-infected mothers had no cultural traditions or ancient properties upon which to build acceptance of their children and no positive motherline of a culture of HIV to pass along to their children, thereby ensuring the development of a strong self-hood associated with being the child of an HIV-positive mother.

For Morrison, the empowerment of children comes from the maternal nurturance they receive. A diagnosis of HIV seriously limited the practices of nurturance of their children for the HIV-infected mothers. All of the mothers in the study acknowledged the lack of energy they had for nurturing their children because of their diagnosis. Their lack of energy was attributable to both physical and emotional reactions to their disease process, as well as side effects and reactions to the drugs they were required to take. Barbara had experienced a problem with depression since being diagnosed: "It's hard just to get up every day." According to Jane, her diagnosis made her too tired to be the kind of mother she wanted to be; she felt she was cheating her second child out of the good mothering she deserved. Jane felt bad because she did not do the things with her second daughter that she had done with her first daughter, such as play dates and birthday parties. Yolanda said she felt bad when her health caused her to be in bed for a few days. She knew that her two young sons worried when she was too tired or sick to care for them like she wanted to: "It's almost impossible being a mother and being this sick; it kills me to be with the kids and not be able to take care of them like I want to." She said her boys often asked her what was wrong with her, but she did not tell them the truth because she felt they were too young to know.

While Ruddick acknowledged that much of mothering is beyond the control of mothers and, therefore, requires mothers to be comfortable with ambiguity and imperfection, for these mothers there was added ambiguity and imperfection in their mothering. For all of the study participants, their major source of ambiguity was the uncertain future for themselves and their children. At the same time, they also expressed other ambiguities and imperfections about their mothering due to HIV. Anne said HIV "took attention away" from her mothering. She believed she was not as strict with her children as she should have been. Her children were adolescents, and she believed they needed more supervision than she was giving them. Anne also noted that having HIV had taken away her "confidence to be an outgoing person"—something she felt could have benefited her children's lives. This woman did not even have the confidence to take short day trips to visit relatives for fear that a health-related mishap would take place. Jane struggled to determine how much housework her 10-year-old daughter should help her with. She believed it was the mother's job to do the housework, but her lack of energy prevented her from maintaining the house in the way that she wanted. Jane and her husband argued because he thought the daughter was old enough to help out with household chores, but Jane thought she was too young to have to begin such activities.

Another source of ambiguity for most of the women was the issue of who would look after their children if they became too ill or died of HIV/AIDS. Although all of the mothers acknowledged their mothering was not as good as they wanted it to be, most echoed Jane's thoughts when she said that "no one else would be *good enough* to mother" their children if they died. The four women with husbands who were not infected with HIV were somewhat less concerned about the child care after death issue, and some of the mothers had arranged with their mothers, mothers-in-law, grandmothers, or sisters to care for their children if necessary. For women like Jane and Donna, whose husbands were also infected with HIV, there was concern about the abilities of relatives to parent satisfactorily and the question of whether anyone would love their children and care for them like they would want.

For many of the women, having HIV prevented them from giving their children the powerful love that Morrison indicates is essential from black mothers to counteract the inferior, unworthy, and unlovable views held by the dominant culture of black children. Sara had come to the United States from Africa three years before her daughter was able to join her. Sara sadly shared that when her daughter finally joined her in America, despite her happiness at seeing her child, she "held back love" from her daughter because of her diagnosis and the knowledge they would both be hurt if she let herself get too close to her daughter and then eventually died of AIDS. Donna learned of her diagnosis during her first pregnancy. She said she regretted that HIV had kept her from enjoying her baby and "wished she could go back and enjoy" her baby's first year.

According to Ruddick (1995), many mothers find that the central challenge to mothering lies in training a child to be the kind of person whom others accept and whom the mothers themselves can actively appreciate. According to Morrison, black mothers have to be concerned with "others'" notions of social acceptability of their children in a way that mothers of the dominant culture do not. Some of the HIV-infected mothers in the study expressed concerns about guiding their children to ensure the children's social acceptability. Some told of their intentions to prevent their children from making the same mistakes that led to the mother's diagnosis. Barbara's son was approaching adolescence and she was planning to talk to him about drug, alcohol, and sexual responsibility so he "will be careful." Donna wanted to teach her stepchildren that "you need to know who you are sleeping with because if you don't this [HIV] is what can happen to you." Jane caught her oldest daughter in a lie and worried that her daughter would take an irresponsible path similar to the one that led Jane to become HIV positive. She had counseled her daughter about always being honest and listening to her mother's guidance, although she did not tell her daughter the reason she was so concerned about her behavior.

Both Ruddick and Morrison speak of the contradictions of mothering. In contrast to the negative implications of a diagnosis of HIV, a number of the mothers in the study said that having HIV heightened their mothering in certain ways. Many of the mothers said having HIV made them take better care of themselves so they could stay as healthy as possible and live as long as they could for their children. As Lucille said of her three children, "I have to stay healthy because I have to raise those kids." Most spoke of future goals they hoped to live to see their children accomplish, such as "get married and be loved for who and what they are" or graduate from high school or college.

Morrison speaks of the notion of mothering as a liberating practice and one that makes women their best selves. For all of the mothers in the study, HIV brought mothering to the forefront for them; it was something they no longer took for granted, as they might have done without the diagnosis. Some interviewees spoke of how their diagnosis had liberated them as mothers. For Jane, having HIV made her pay more attention to her mothering, although she often noticed things about her mothering that she did not like. According to Patricia, having HIV caused her to "stay caught up with saying 'I love you' and what needs to be said" to her children.

A number of the mothers talked about ways that being HIV infected made them "a better self." Patricia noted that she and her sons had learned a lot from her HIV and were better people because of her diagnosis, in spite of the chaos it brought to their lives when she first learned her diagnosis. She had become a more "accepting and nonjudgmental" person as a result of having

HIV. For Barbara, having HIV meant that "you pay more attention to things." This mother stated that HIV had opened her "eyes to a lot" and made her "stop and look at life." Before having HIV, Barbara "used to put things off," but recently she had decided to return to school and finish her business degree. Yolanda said she was a more compassionate person and thanked "God for even a miserable day that I get." According to Sara, she became a more spiritual and prayerful person as a result of HIV.

For Morrison, mothering was liberating because she came to realize that what she liked best about herself was what her children seemed to want from her. Unfortunately for the HIV-infected mothers, most did not express a great deal that they liked about themselves as mothers, although they all reported efforts to do things for their children that their children requested of them. Ruth said it was positive that her children "kept her moving" because of "the cooking, ironing, and washing their cars." She felt bad, however, when she and her children did not get along or when she fussed at them in front of their friends. Ruth's greatest fear was that her children's most lasting memories of her would be as a stressed-out, grouchy mother, rather than as a loving mother.

Ruddick (1995) notes that mothers are beset by the multiple temptations of passivity. Indeed, when mothers are despairing or powerless, silenced and silent, their humility may well degenerate into passivity (1995, p. 73). The HIV-infected mothers in this study clearly expressed despair and feelings of powerlessness that tempted them into passivity from time to time. As Yolanda said, "You want to do so much for your kids you aren't able to." Angie felt bad when she was "moody and didn't do for" her son. The HIV-infected mothers also recognized the importance of being authentically cheerful and seeing their children hopefully (Ruddick, 1995, p. 74). Sally said her biggest issue was trying to keep her children happy. Monica said of her sons, "They're my strength; they're my fight to get well." Ruth hoped she and her family (husband, son, and daughter) could take a vacation together in the future, which for her represented a time for relaxation and enhanced family well-being.

CONCLUSIONS

For these HIV-infected women, mothering was more like the mothering described by Toni Morrison. The stigma of their diagnosis of HIV became a stand-in for the racism and sexism that Morrison says makes African American mothering different from mothering in the dominant culture. In fact, Nancy Scheper-Hughes (1993) equates stigma to the "murderous racism that pervades the United States, the West, and the world." According to Scheper-Hughes, stigma is "undesired difference . . . everything that makes us turn away from another human being in fear, disgust, anger, pity, or loathing." Stigmatizing for Scheper-Hughes is the "most anti-social of human acts, for it consigns the victim to a living death on the margins of human interaction" (p. 373).

What the HIV-infected mothers in the study lacked that black mothers have access to, however, is what Morrison calls the ancient properties and traditions, the funk, of the black culture upon which black children can build strong identities and authentic personhood. For

HIV-infected mothers, there are no ancient properties or traditions of a culture of HIV, there is only "undesired difference" that makes others turn away "in fear, disgust, anger, pity, or loathing." In addition to the stigma that the HIV-infected mothers felt made them undesirably different, most believed their stigma would attach to their children and make the children undesirably different and, therefore, unacceptable.

Ironically, within Morrison's many novels, the profound importance of mothering and motherhood are not demonstrated by whole, self-affirmed, authentic black mothers and children, but rather by children and mothers who experience the agonizing suffering and profound devastation from *not receiving*, or in the case of the mothers *not being able to give*, maternal preservation, nurturance, and cultural bearing (O'Reilly, 2004). These HIV-infected mothers sensed the sentiment of loss or absence that pervades Morrison's work; the appreciation or understanding of something only when that something or someone is lost or absent. While all said they worked to maintain their health so that they could live as long as possible and not leave their children motherless, the lack of energy and the mental and emotional distractions of their diagnosis prevented them from providing their children with the protection and nurturance they believed their children required, thereby causing their children to experience an absence of mothering or an absence of what the mothers perceived to be good mothering.

For Morrison, mothering is a potential site of empowerment of children. While the HIV-infected women did not directly address the empowerment of their children, all of them had clearly bought into the contemporary notion of "sensitive mothering," defined as child-centered care that is characterized by flexibility, spontaneity, democracy, affection, nurturance, and playfulness, as opposed to previous notions of stern, rigid, authoritative, "children should be seen and not heard" parenting. The HIV-infected mothers seemed to believe that being a good mother would empower their children; conversely, most believed that having a mother stigmatized by a diagnosis of HIV would disempower their children and spoil the child's identity, just as it had the mother's. For these mothers, the idealized figure of the Good Mother cast a long shadow on the reality of their lives and caused them to fear and fantasize about the Bad Mother (Ruddick, 1995, p. 31). A diagnosis of HIV was considered a failure as a mother. Good Mothers are not HIV positive, they thought—only Bad Mothers are.

The HIV-infected mothers were clearly not living the white Western image of the "ever-bountiful, ever-giving, self-sacrificing, never destroyed or overwhelmed by their children" kind of motherhood (Bassin et al., 1994). In contrast to the dominant discourse on mothering, the politics of HIV/AIDS had invaded these mothers' homes and lives, so that nurturance of their children was more of a struggle than a "natural calling." The HIV-infected mothers were living the kind of mothering described by Morrison that requires greater effort to ensure the protection, nurturance, and acceptability of one's children. For the four black HIV-infected mothers, their burden was further compounded by the challenges inherent in being a black mother.

To meet the extra challenges of black motherhood, Morrison advocates strategies whereby black mothers can empower their children. One strategy discussed throughout her work is nurturance through powerful love, which Morrison believes inoculates children against racist and sexist ideologies. Another strategy is a parent's strong sense of self, which is passed along to children and thus nurtures self-love in the children. For Morrison, mothers must find and share what she calls the *beloved* in themselves so their children can, in turn, find the *beloved* within themselves (O'Reilly, 2004). The HIV-infected mothers wanted their children to see the best in them and did not want to be remembered as bad mothers. Most, however, seemed to feel that HIV had extinguished or "covered over" the *beloved* in them and made it harder for them to help their children find their *beloved.* For one mother who vowed to "never tell" her children her diagnosis, her greatest hope was that when she died, her children would value her efforts to be a good mother and not judge her for her diagnosis.

Morrison has also advocated education about racism and sexism, along with work to withstand and fight those dominant forces as a strategy for black mothers. Of the five HIV-infected mothers who had disclosed their diagnosis to all or some of their children, only two spoke of knowingly educating themselves and their children about their diagnosis and treatments. While several mothers told of plans to instruct their children in safe social and sexual behaviors at some point in the future, they did not say whether self-disclosure of their HIV diagnosis would be part of the "talk." Some of the mothers said they knew their children had learned about HIV/AIDS at school, a fact that made them even more fearful of disclosing their diagnosis to the children because of the attitudes that may have accompanied the children's lessons.

Within the black culture, another strategy used to insulate black families from the criticism and devaluation by the dominant culture is creation of what bell hooks (1990) called a homeplace, a space where blacks can be among themselves and affirm their true identities and traditions. All of the HIV-infected mothers considered the ASO where they received health care and various social services to be a homeplace. For many, the nurses, counselors, and case managers of the ASO were some of the only people who knew of their diagnosis, and were among the few individuals with whom they could openly and honestly share their experiences of being HIV positive. In fact, several of the mothers specifically spoke of efforts to consciously withhold information about their burdens of mothering with HIV with outside healthcare providers for fear they would be reported to social services and have their children taken away from them. Many of the women attended regularly scheduled women's support groups and weekend retreats sponsored by the ASO. They shared stories of supporting and learning from each other in the ASO activities. Several of the mothers had gained the strength and courage to disclose their diagnosis to friends and family by listening to the disclosure stories of other women. One of the mothers regularly brought her three school-age children with her to parties sponsored by the ASO at Thanksgiving and Christmas. Given the stigma of HIV/AIDS, ASOs are one of the few true homeplaces for HIV-infected individuals and a space where any ancient properties, cultural bearings, and HIV traditions, if such exist, can be created, maintained, and shared.

Ruddick (1995) has also recommended mothering strategies for the empowerment of children. She advocates that mothers use the strategy of telling children about themselves through the use of compassionate stories or maternal narratives. According to Ruddick, such stories allow children to see their mother's love and generosity, allow them to learn to forgive themselves as the mother forgave them (1995, p. 100). Ruddick also seems to advocate the kind of mothering where both the mother and her children would benefit from the mother's disclosure of her HIV status to her children. As she said, "Children are vulnerable . . . they will be capable of protesting maternal failure only if they trust their mother not to turn on them or—surrendering to guilt—on themselves" (p. 119). For the most part, these HIV-infected mothers had surrendered to their guilt, and most had not or would not forgive themselves for their diagnosis and its implications for their mothering. To some extent, all of the mothers saw themselves as maternal failures because of HIV.

Perhaps it is the children of parents with HIV who hold the key to helping diminish or eliminate the stigma of HIV/AIDS through the receipt of what Ruddick calls attentive love, which "implies and rewards a faith that love will not be destroyed by knowledge" (p. 119). Most of these mothers lacked the faith that the knowledge of their diagnosis would not destroy their children's love for them. Just as black mothers cannot hide their race or gender from their children, so knowledge of the mother's diagnosis of HIV holds the potential to liberate mothers and empower children to bear witness to their mothers' struggles to be a good mother in the face of a life-changing disease process. Without that knowledge, what may be needed by children of HIV-infected women is the healing that Morrison says is required when the mother or adequate practices of mothering are absent.

FINAL THOUGHTS

These and other mothers may take comfort in Ruddick's notion that in spite of the fact that mothers are often overwhelmed tending to their children's survival, preoccupied with their own projects, or simply exhausted and confused, "children survive nonetheless" (1995, p. 21). According to Ruddick, it is exceedingly difficult to predict what will actually damage children; damage is almost never attributable to maternal "failure" alone, but at most to maternal fallibility in a complicated and troubling family and world" (p. 36). Morrison, in contrast, has predicted that without the best features of black motherlove, the racism and sexism of the "complicated and troubling world" will damage black children. HIV-infected mothers are just hoping their diagnosis will not cause their children to see them as maternal failures.

Regardless of the mother and the kind of mothering children receive, no one ever considers the mother–child relationship anything other than exceedingly profound and phenomenally life defining. Mothers are said to be irreplaceable (Davidman, 2000) and children without mothers, regardless their age, race, or gender, think often about what their mothers would think of them and their activities. Anything that can be done by nurses to illuminate and enhance the mothering relationship for all mothers and their children should be attempted. A broad understanding of maternal theory, thought, and experience is a good place to begin.

WWW

For a full suite of assignments and additional learning activities, use the access code located in the front of your book to visit this exclusive website: http://go.jblearning.com/dechesnay. If you do not have an access code, you can obtain one at the site.

REFERENCES

Artinian, B. (1988). Qualitative modes of inquiry. *Western Journal of Nursing Research, 10*(2), 138–49.

Bassin, D., Honey, M., & Kaplan, M. (Eds.). (1994). *Representations of motherhood.* New Haven, CT: Yale University Press.

Collins, P. H. (1991). *Black feminist thought: Knowledge, consciousness, and the politics of empowerment.* New York: Routledge.

Davidman, L. (2000). *Motherloss.* Berkeley, CA: University of California Press.

Goffman, E. (1963). *Stigma.* New York: Simon and Schuster.

hooks, b. (1990). *Yearning: Race, gender, and cultural politics.* Boston: South End.

Nelms, T. (2005). Burden: The phenomenon of mothering with HIV. *Journal of the Association of Nurses in AIDS Care, 16*(4), 3–13.

Nelms, T., & Zeigler, V. (2008). A study to develop a disclosure to children intervention for HIV-infected women. *Journal of the Association of Nurses in AIDS Care, 19*(6), 461–469.

O'Reilly, A. (2004). *Toni Morrison and motherhood: A politics of the heart.* New York: State University of New York Press.

Ruddick, S. (1995). *Maternal thinking: Toward a politics of peace.* Boston: Beacon Press.

Scheper-Hughes, N. (1993). *Death without weeping.* Berkeley, CA: University of California Press.

CHAPTER 9

Giving Voice to Vulnerable Populations: Rogerian Theory

Sarah Hall Gueldner, Geraldine R. Britton, and Susan Terwilliger

Objectives

At the end of this chapter, the reader will be able to

1. Explain Rogers' perspective on vulnerability.
2. Describe the characteristics of vulnerability.
3. Define "well-being" from the perspective of the research on Rogers' theory described by the authors.

The human condition of vulnerability is a concept of vital concern to nurses, in that a large portion of nursing practice is spent either helping individuals who find themselves in a vulnerable position or helping them avoid vulnerability. Nursing, however, has been slow in developing theoretical constructs of vulnerability within a nursing perspective (Spiers, 2000). Traditional definitions of vulnerability are framed within an epidemiological approach to identify individuals and groups at risk for harm. Groups most often labeled as vulnerable include the elderly, children, the poor, people with disability or chronic illness, people from minority cultures, and captive populations such as prisoners and refugees (Saunders & Valente, 1992). Labels of vulnerability are customarily applied in relation to socioeconomic, minority, or other stigmatizing status (Demi & Warren, 1995) and reflect a tendency to blame the victim for his or her status rather than the prevailing social structures. The generally accepted marker for vulnerability has been the inability to function independently in accord with the values of a particular society. Fortunately, there is growing dialogue about vulnerability from the perspective of the person experiencing it—a view that is more congruent with the philosophical stance of nursing (Morse, 1997; Spiers, 2000).

The Rogerian conceptual system (Rogers, 1992), which focuses on the person as integral with and inseparable from his or her environment, holds considerable relevance as an innovative nursing framework to use in addressing the problem of vulnerability. Accordingly, the remainder of this chapter is directed toward application of the theoretical base of Rogerian nursing science to the human condition of vulnerability. Because persons who are vulnerable are at greater risk for not being heard, the last section of the chapter describes the Wellbeing Picture Scale (WPS), a 10-item innovative picture-based tool that offers a menu of paired pictures rather than words, giving people who may not be able to read English text an alternative, more user-friendly way of expressing their sense of well-being.

A ROGERIAN PERSPECTIVE OF VULNERABILITY

According to Martha Rogers, energy fields are the fundamental unit of everything, both living and nonliving. These fields are without boundary and dynamic, changing continuously. Two energy fields are identified: the human field and the environmental field. Rogers emphasized that humans and environments do not *have* energy fields; rather, they *are* energy fields. Likewise, she insisted that the human field is unitary and cannot be reduced to a biological field, a physical field, or a psychosocial field. As postulated by Rogers, human and environmental fields flow together in a constant mutual process that is unitary rather than separate. Within this worldview, humans are energy fields that exist in constant mutual process with their immediate and extended environmental energy field, which includes, and cannot be separated from, other living and nonliving fields. She also postulated that both human and environmental energy patterns change continually during this process. The inseparability of the human energy field from its immediate and extended environmental energy field is perhaps the most central feature of the Rogerian conceptual system.

Phillips and Bramlett (1994) assert that the mutual human–environmental field process can be harmonious or dissonant. Resonant with Rogers' science, these researchers posit vulnerability as an emergent condition that arises when there is dissonance within the mutual human–environmental field process. This view is consistent with Rogerian scholar Barrett's (1990) theory of power, which associates power with individuals' knowing participation in change within their mutual human–environmental process for the betterment of the whole, including themselves. These authors perceive vulnerability as the opposite condition of power—as a condition that may occur when an individual is unable or does not choose to participate in an informed and purposeful way in change. Persons in this situation essentially have no voice and may be intentionally or unintentionally left behind in a compromised position. Within this line of thinking, an individual's sense of dissonance or disharmony within the mutual human–environmental field process would be viewed as a manifestation of vulnerability, placing individuals or groups at risk. Barrett developed a text-based tool, Power as Knowing Participation in Change (PKPC), to measure this concept; a subscale of the tool addresses awareness as an essential feature of knowing participation.

Lack of knowing participation may be associated with a number of scenarios. Individuals may be uninformed or misinformed about situations involving their unique human–environmental field process, or they may be unable to participate due to one or more specific circumstances such as illness (e.g., stroke or dementia) or injury (e.g., hip fracture). Common situations that may limit or prevent knowing participation include compromised vision or hearing, aphasia, difficulty with mobility, and confusion or dementia. Other circumstances that may limit knowing participation include any situation that hinders a person from engaging in sufficient communication within the community; examples might include lack of transportation or limited language facility. Insufficient means or the inability to move about freely may diminish presence, making it more difficult, if not impossible, to be "at the table" to achieve representation. Stigmatized individuals or groups such as single mothers, persons who are homeless, and persons perceived as unattractive or different are also at risk for a lack of information or misinformation that may lead to inappropriate participation based on misjudgment. Indeed, information may even be withheld intentionally if participation is not welcome.

Parse's (2003) theory of community becoming, which is also an extension of Rogers' nursing science, is particularly applicable to the theoretical tenet of vulnerability. Parse defines community in terms of the relational experience of being "in community," describing it as a resource that is dynamic and continuously changing to represent the good of the individual to achieve the best for all. According to her definition, community is not a location or a group of people who have similar interests; rather, community is the human connectedness with the universe, including connectedness with what she terms "yet-to-be possibles." This view represents a paradigm shift, wherein vulnerability is an emergent characteristic of the community in the process that occurs when an individual or group becomes disconnected from the group and, therefore, from needed resources. Parse describes a nontraditional model of health service for individuals and families who have become disconnected from resources in this way. This process involves developing a vision of possibilities and inviting others to capture this vision, thereby energizing the community to build partnerships to overcome the disconnect.

Within this conceptualization, vulnerability arises as an emergent characteristic when connectedness is compromised by a lack of communication or flawed communication that leads to exclusion from resources. Vulnerability might be seen as an unfortunate estrangement from the process of community. Within this view, persons who are at particular risk for vulnerability are those who for some reason are unable to call enough attention to their needs to garner the support of their community.

Based on Parse's (1997) "human becoming" perspective, this author's view of nursing practice also differs from traditional nursing practice in that the nurse does not offer standardized professional advice or opinions stemming from the nurse's own value system. Rather, according to Parse, nursing involves a "true presence with and respect for the other," wherein the nurse dwells with the person or family to enhance their perceived "possibles." Parse points out that it is essential to go with vulnerable persons to where they are rather than to attempt to judge, change, or control these individuals. It is in dwelling with the individual in discussion that meanings emerge, and it is in this process of illuminating meaning that possibilities for transcendence are seen.

In Parse's words:

> The nurse in true presence with person or family is not a guide or a beacon, but rather an inspiring attentive presence that calls the other to shed light on the meaning moments of his or her life. It is the person or family in the presence of the nurse that illuminates the meaning and mobilizes the capacity to transcend and move beyond. The person is coauthor of his or her own health . . . choosing rhythmical patterns of relating while reaching for personal hopes and dreams. (Parse, 1997, p. 40)

She continues:

> True presence is a special way of *being with* in which the nurse bears witness to the person's or family's own living of value priorities. True presence is an interpersonal art grounded in a strong knowledge base "reflecting the belief that each person knows *the way* somewhere within self." (Parse, 1997, p. 40)

Certainly, nowhere is it more important to respect the person as he or she is than when working with vulnerable individuals.

Parse describes a humanitarian model of nursing practice based on true presence and profound respect. Use of this model enables people to find actions that increase their ability to knowingly participate in change to improve their position, thereby becoming less vulnerable. Parse refers to this process as the search for the possible beyond the now.

Unfortunately, even in this overall positive system, some persons are likely to find themselves in vulnerable circumstances. Some individuals and groups (such as young children) are placed at risk because they cannot speak for themselves and depend on others to advocate for them. Likewise, sick or frail members of the community may be too weak or impaired to participate knowingly (or sufficiently) in the change process to advance their betterment. They may not be mobile enough, think clearly enough, or be articulate enough to capture community attention and garner the resources they need.

Individuals or families at special risk for vulnerability include those with the following characteristics:

- Have energy-draining illnesses or conditions such as stroke, heart attack, cancer, or depression
- Are not included in the dominant culture
- Have compromised language facility, making them at greater risk for being unheard
- Are out of their familiar turf (i.e., new in the community and do not know the "rules" or avenues for help)
- Are unable to comprehend information (i.e., never learned to read, have diminished vision or hearing, are unconscious or have dementia, or are unable to comprehend English)
- Have illness or injury that limits independence (i.e., broken hips that make it more difficult to stay physically connected with the community)

- Lack the ability to access services needed for everyday life (i.e., means for obtaining food, place to live, health services)
- Are in a position of diminished visibility (e.g., live in a remote area or are homebound, becoming disconnected from community notice)

Viewed from Parse's theory of community becoming, the approach to overcoming vulnerability is a matter of reconnecting the person or group to the community. This bonding sometimes happens naturally through family and friends or through social institutions and/or programs such as churches and civic organizations. In other cases, it may take the focused attention and time of individuals, such as nurses, to help the person or family as they gain insight about the possibilities that are available to them.

GIVING VOICE: AN APPLICATION OF ROGERIAN NURSING SCIENCE

To address the lack of voice that is so intricately associated with the experience of vulnerability, this section describes a simple picture tool, the WPS, developed within the Rogerian conceptual system to amplify the voice of persons who otherwise might not be heard (Gueldner et al., 2005).

The WPS is a 10-item non–language-based pictorial scale that measures general sense of well-being as a reflection of the mutual human–environmental field process. It was originally designed as an easy-to-administer tool for use with the broadest possible range of adult populations, including persons who have limited formal education, do not speak English as their first language, may not be able to see well, or may be too sick or frail to respond to lengthier or more complex measures. Ten pairs of 1-inch drawings depicting a sense of high or low well-being are arranged at opposite ends of a seven-choice, unnumbered, semantic differential scale. The 10 items included are eyes open and closed, shoes sitting still and running, a butterfly opposite a turtle, a candle lit and not lit, a faucet running full and dripping, puzzle pieces together and separated, a pencil sharp and dull, the sun full and partially cloud covered, balloons inflated and partially deflated, and a lion and a mouse. Individuals are asked to view each of the 10 picture pairs and mark the point along the scale between the pictures to indicate which they feel most like—for example, a lighted candle or an unlit candle. The brief instructions for the WPS are translated and administered in Taiwanese, Japanese, Korean, Egyptian, and Spanish.

Psychometric properties for the WPS tool were established in a sample of 1027 individuals in the United States, Taiwan, and Japan; the sample was 56% Asian, 34% white, and 10% African American or Hispanic. The overall Cronbach's alpha was found to be 0.8795 across the three countries. Five of the 10 items were completely consistent across countries (puzzle, balloon, sun, eyes, and lion), and all others were consistent across two of the three countries.

CONCEPTUAL FORMULATION OF WELL-BEING

Rogers maintained that "the purpose of nursing is to promote health and well-being for all persons wherever they are" (1992, p. 258). According to Hills (1998), well-being is generally defined as a relative sense of harmony and satisfaction in one's life. Smith (1981) and Todaro-Franceschi (1999) have defined health as movement toward self-fulfillment or realization of one's potential, a view that is congruent with Parse's (1997) theory of human becoming. Newman (1994) does not distinguish health from well-being, but singularly defines it as a manifestation of expanding consciousness that may occur during, but is not separate from, the experience of illness. This view is supported by the work of Hills (1998), who demonstrated a relationship between well-being and awareness.

Conceptually, the WPS assesses the energy field in regard to four characteristics judged to be associated with well-being: frequency of movement (i.e., intensity) within the energy field, awareness of oneself as energy, action emanating from the energy field, and power as knowing participation in change within the mutual human–environmental energy field process.

Frequency

The term *frequency* denotes the intensity of motion within the energy field(s). It is postulated that higher frequency is associated with a greater sense of well-being and that it is experienced as a sense of vitality.

Awareness

Awareness refers to the sense an individual has of his or her potential for change within the mutual human–environmental field. It signals readiness for moving toward one's potential and is postulated to be positively associated with a sense of well-being. The concept of awareness is congruent with Newman's (1994) theory of health as expanding consciousness and Parse's (1997) theory of human becoming (unfolding). Barrett (1990) included a subscale of awareness in her PKPC tool, and Hills (1998) discussed enlightenment as a manifestation of expanded awareness, higher level field motion, and well-being. Awareness is postulated to be a positive manifestation of the dynamics of the mutual human–environmental field process.

Action

Action is conceptualized as an emergent of the "continuous mutual human–environmental field process" (Rogers, 1992), reflecting the frequency of the human energy field. It is viewed as an expression of field energy associated with well-being. Examples of action include activities associated with daily living, such as preparing food, eating, personal grooming, participating in social events, exercising, or doing chores, as well as actively engaging in innovative thinking or the creation of art forms.

Power

As described by Barrett (1990), *power* is the capacity of an individual to engage knowingly in change. Barrett defined it as the degree to which an individual is able to express energy as power to create desired change within his or her human–environmental energy field process. When power is prominent, a person is expected to possess a sense of confidence; conversely powerlessness is associated with a sense of vulnerability. Power might also be conceptualized as the capacity of an individual to commute the three aforementioned conditions (energy expressed as frequency, awareness, and action) into an emergent sense of well-being.

WPS DEVELOPMENT

The more than 10 years of developmental work and field testing of early versions of the WPS revealed a correlation with several other tools designed to measure aspects of well-being within the Rogerian framework (Gueldner, Bramlett, Johnston, & Guillory, 1996). Johnston (1994), in a sample of nursing home residents and community-dwelling elders, reported a highly significant correlation ($r = 0.6647$) between the WPS tool and her Human Field Image Metaphor Scale, which uses two- or three-word metaphors to measure image. Gueldner et al. (1996) found an even greater correlation ($r = 0.7841$) between the WPS and Barrett's (1990) PKPC tool, which measures an individual's capacity for awareness, choices, freedom to act intentionally, and involvement to bring about harmony in the human–environmental field process.

Davis (1989), in a matched sample of 30 men 19–51 years of age who had been hospitalized for traumatic injuries and 30 non-injured men, demonstrated positive significant correlations between the score on the WPS and scores on the PKPC tool ($p = 0.002$) and Rosenberg's self-esteem scale ($p = 0.02$).

Hindman (1993), in a sample of 40 nursing home residents and 40 community-dwelling older adults, demonstrated a significant correlation ($p = 0.001$) between the mean score on the WPS and humor as measured by the Situational Humor Response Questionnaire. She also found that the mean score was higher for the community-dwelling group of older adults ($p = 0.001$) than for their counterparts who lived in nursing homes, and that individuals who perceived their income as adequate scored higher ($p = 0.05$) than those who perceived their income to be less than adequate. Older participants scored lower ($p = 0.05$) on the WPS.

Hills (1998), in a study of 874 mothers of 6-month-old infants, found that mothers who scored higher on the picture tool also reported higher levels of awareness ($p = 0.001$) as measured by the awareness subscale of Barrett's (1990) PKPC tool and well-being ($p < 0.001$) as measured by Cantril's Ladder for Well-Being.

Gueldner et al. (2005) administered the WPS and the Geriatric Depression Scale (GDS) to 215 community-dwelling older adults (64% female and 36% male; 55 to 97 years old) who were attending lunch events at six senior centers in upstate New York. These researchers reported a significant negative correlation ($p < -0.01$) between the WPS and the GDS. One-fifth of the study participants (20%) scored above the cut-off point of 5 (indicating concern for depression) on the GDS; 10% scored above 8 on the GDS, and three individuals scored an alarming 13–14 on the GDS. These findings support the ability of the more user-friendly WPS to screen for depression in community-dwelling elders.

USE OF THE WPS WITH CHILDREN

Because of their dependent status, children are at particular risk for vulnerability. Their voices may not be heard, but others tend to speak for them. Thus the developers of the WPS believe that this tool holds promise for giving voice to children as well as to adults. The WPS has been used by two researchers to measure well-being in children.

Abbate (1990) used the early 18-item version of the tool as a pre- and post-test measure of well-being in eight school-aged children (aged 5 to 16 years) with cerebral palsy who participated in a 10-week therapeutic horsemanship program. The mean of the pre-test scores was 82.75; the mean of the post-test scores was 86.38. The scores of four children increased over the 10-week period, the score of one child did not change, and the scores of three children decreased. All of the children in the study had already been riding horses for several years, leading Abbate to suggest that some of the children may have already achieved the most significant gains from their participation in the riding program before the study began. Abbate noted that even the most impaired children seemed comfortable and confident in placing their mark along the seven-point scoring line between the picture pairs (the younger ones used crayons), supporting this tool's utility with children. This investigation was the first study to use the WPS tool with children, and the sample was small. Nevertheless, its findings provided impetus and direction for developing a children's version of the instrument.

Terwilliger (2008; Terwilliger, Gueldner, & Bronstein, in press) modified the format of the 10-item WPS for use with a sample of 19 fourth- and fifth-grade elementary school children (13 girls and 6 boys; 53% white, 37% black, and 10% Hispanic) who were judged by the school nurse as being overweight or at risk for depression. The primary purpose of this study was to test the capacity of a 4-month-long after-school physical activity program to decrease childhood overweight and depression. Overweight was determined based on waist circumference and actual weight by height, and depression was identified via the Childhood Depression Inventory, Long Version (CDI-LV).

The scoring mechanism for the WPS was simplified for use with these children. The original seven-point Likert scale between each pair of pictures was reconfigured and abbreviated to four boxes; two boxes were placed closer to the picture on the left of the page and the other two boxes were placed closer to the picture pair on the right side of the page. For each item, the investigator asked the children to point to the picture they "felt most like." The children were then asked to place a mark in one of the two boxes to indicate whether they felt "a little bit" like the picture they had chosen or "a lot" like it. The investigator repeated each item and pointed out the designated boxes as many times as necessary if the child seemed to have difficulty understanding the scoring instructions. The scoring mechanism was adjusted so that the children's scores retained the range from 7 to 70, with higher scores indicating a higher sense of well-being.

The scores for the WPS-CV in this sample of children ranged from 22 to 70, with a mean score of 58. No statistically significant difference was found between the WPS-CV pre-intervention and post-intervention scores, which is not surprising given the small sample size. Nevertheless, a score of 50 or less on the WPS-CV pinpointed the two students whose CDI-LV responses indicated suicidal intent, and use of a score of 60 or less as a cut-off point would have identified all but one of the students found to be at risk for depression. These findings lend support for the further testing of the WPS-CV in at-risk children.

In summary, work by Gueldner et al. (1996), Hills (1998), and Johnston (1994) confirmed a high correlation between scores on the WPS and other measures of well-being developed within the Rogerian conceptual system. Additionally, the work of Davis (1989), Hills (1998), and Hindman (1993) demonstrated a high correlation between the WPS tool and a number of established measures of well-being developed by other disciplines. Although both were limited in sample size, the studies of Abbate (1990) and Terwilliger (2008) demonstrated the potential utility of this tool in children.

CONCLUSION

Based on these findings, the WPS is offered as a general measure of well-being mediated through frequency, awareness, action, and power emanating within an individual's mutual human–environmental field process. This instrument is seen as having the potential to give voice to those who are too sick or weak to participate in studies that require lengthy or complex measures of well-being. A secondary purpose of the tool rests in its potential for use as an easy-to-administer clinical indicator of well-being across a wide sector of clinical settings. Based on the work of Abbate (1990) and Terwilliger (2008; Terwilliger et al., in press), a children's version of the tool has been developed and tested, and is offered as a measure of well-being in children. A growing number of studies have also demonstrated its ability to give voice to persons within international populations who may have difficulty reading English text.

For a full suite of assignments and additional learning activities, use the access code located in the front of your book to visit this exclusive website: http://go.jblearning.com/dechesnay. If you do not have an access code, you can obtain one at the site.

REFERENCES

Abbate, M. F. (1990). *The relationship of therapeutic horsemanship and human field motion in children with cerebral palsy.* Unpublished master's thesis, Georgia State University, Atlanta, GA.

Barrett, E. A. M. (1990). A measure of power as knowing participation in change. In O. L. Strickland & C. F. Waltz (Eds.), *The measurement of nursing outcomes: Measuring client self-care and coping skills* (pp. 159–180). (Vol. 4). New York: Springer.

Davis, A. E. (1989). *The relationship between the phenomenon of traumatic injury and the patterns of power, human field motion, esteem and risk taking.* Unpublished doctoral dissertation, Georgia State University, Atlanta, GA.

Demi, A. S., & Warren, N. A. (1995). Issues in conducting research with vulnerable families. *Western Journal of Nursing Research, 17,* 188–202.

Gueldner, S. H., Bramlett, M. H., Johnston, L. W., & Guillory, J. A. (1996). Index of Field Energy. *Rogerian Nursing Science News, 8*(4), 6.

Gueldner, S. H., Michel, Y., Bramlett, M. H., Liu, C. F., Johnston, L. W., & Endo, E. (2005). The Wellbeing Picture Scale: A refined version of the Index of Field Energy. *Nursing Science Quarterly, 18*(1), 42–50.

Hills, R. (1998). *Maternal field patterning of awareness, wakefulness, human field motion and well-being in mothers with 6 month old infants: A Rogerian science perspective.* Unpublished doctoral dissertation, Wayne State University, Detroit, MI.

Hindman, M. (1993). *Humor and field energy in older adults.* Unpublished doctoral dissertation, Medical College of Georgia, Augusta, GA.

Johnston, L. W. (1994). Psychometric analysis of Johnston's Human Field Image Metaphor Scale. *Visions: Journal of Rogerian Nursing Science, 2*, 7–11.

Morse, J. M. (1997). Responding to threats to integrity of self. *Advances in Nursing Science, 19*, 21–36.

Newman, M. A. (1994). *Health as expanding consciousness.* New York: National League for Nursing.

Parse, R. R. (1997). The human becoming theory: The was, is, and will be. *Nursing Science Quarterly, 10*(1), 32–38.

Parse, R. R. (2003). *Community: A human becoming perspective.* Sudbury, MA: Jones and Bartlett.

Phillips, B. B., & Bramlett, M. H. (1994). Integrated awareness: A key to the pattern of mutual process. *Visions, 2*, 7–12.

Rogers, M. E. (1992). Nursing science and the space age. *Nursing Science Quarterly, 5*, 27–34.

Saunders, J. M., & Valente, S. M. (1992). Overview. *Western Journal of Nursing Research, 14*, 700–702.

Smith, J. A. (1981). The idea of health: A philosophical inquiry. *Advances in Nursing Science, 4*, 43–49.

Spiers, J. (2000). New perspectives on vulnerability using emic and etic approaches. *Journal of Advanced Nursing, 31*, 715–721.

Terwilliger, S. (2008). *A study of children enrolled in a school-based physical activity program with attention to overweight and depression.* Unpublished doctoral dissertation, Binghamton University, Binghamton, NY.

Terwilliger, S., Gueldner, S.H., & Bronstein, L. (In press). A preliminary evaluation of the Well-Being Picture Scale–Children's Version (WPS-CV) in a sample of fourth and fifth graders, *Nursing Science Quarterly.*

Todaro-Franceschi, V. (1999). *The enigma of energy.* New York: Crossroad.

CHAPTER 10

Application of the Barnard Parent/Caregiver–Child Interaction Model to Care of Premature Infants

Danuta Wojnar

Objectives

At the end of this chapter, the reader will be able to

1. Explain key components of the Barnard Interaction Model.
2. Evaluate the usefulness of the Barnard Model in terms of its applicability to nursing practice.
3. Apply the Barnard Interaction Model to research with pre-term infants.

www

Parent–infant interaction is the context in which most infants initially experience the world. Under normal circumstances, it is within the parent–infant relationship that the infant learns about the environment. It is the parent who teaches the infant basic principles of communication while mediating the amount of sensory input the infant receives. In the United States, more than 10% of infants are born prematurely (less than 37 weeks' gestation) (Centers for Disease Control and Prevention [CDC], 2010). The vast majority of premature infants require hospitalization in the newborn intensive care unit (NICU) (Hamilton, Minino, Martin, Kochanek, Strobino, & Guyer., 2007; Leversen et al., 2010). Highly specialized care available in the NICU enhances preterm infants' chance for survival. Even so, complications of prematurity ranging from acute to chronic illness (Guzzetta et al., 2006; Simpson, Ye, Hellmann, & Tomlinson, 2010), to developmental delays (Casey, Whiteside-Mansell, Barrett, Bradley, & Gargus, 2006; Lype, Prasad, Nair, Geetha, & Kailas, 2008), to deprivation of quality parent–child interactions (Als, 1997; Barnard, 1997; Lindrea & Stainton, 2000; Mackley Locke, Spear, & Joseph, 2010; Obeidat, Bond, & Callister, 2009) pose serious threats to long-term child development outcomes.

The purpose of this chapter is to discuss the Barnard (1976) Parent/Caregiver–Child Interaction Model as a framework for delivering relationship-based, developmentally supportive interventions to preterm infants and their parents. Examples are provided from research and practice that demonstrate clinical applicability of the Barnard model.

THE BARNARD PARENT/CAREGIVER–CHILD INTERACTION MODEL

In the early 1970s, Dr. Kathryn Barnard was contracted by the U.S. Public Health Service to study ways of measuring the health and caregiving environments of infants and young children (Barnard, 1994). Prior to Barnard's work, research findings had indicated that the primary focus of caregiving in the early months of an infant's life is to establish routines and positive patterns of interaction to support the infant's optimal growth and development (Brazelton, 1973; Sameroff & Chandler, 1975). Barnard's research with mothers and infants indicated that all dimensions of child development—physical, emotional, intellectual, and social development—interact in complex ways. In turn, deficit in one of the domains affects the others.

Another insight Barnard and her research team gained from this work was that infants and young children undergo behavioral changes and internal reorganization in response to their caregiving and environmental stimuli, suggesting that one cannot understand early child development without taking into consideration interactions between the child, caregiver, and environment (Barnard, 1994; Jolley, Elmore, Barnard, & Carr, 2007; Tsai, Barnard, Lentz, & Thomas, 2010). As a result of Barnard's early work, she developed the Parent/Caregiver–Child Interaction Model to depict strengths and weaknesses in interactions between infants and parents/caregivers and to direct behavior-specific interventions to foster children's social–emotional and cognitive growth and development (Barnard, 1976).

The Parent/Caregiver–Child Interaction Model uses the language of systems and developmental theories in its introduction of ideas. Barnard (1994) calls the elements of her model "an interactive system" (p. 6). In contrast to reductionist theories, system theory focuses on understanding how the parts of the system are arranged, what they do, how they are related, how as a whole they interact with the environment, and how they evolve and acquire new properties (von Bertalanffy, 1968).

An influence of developmental theory is also evident in Barnard's model. According to developmental theory, learning occurs when individuals interact with their environment. The learner actively constructs understanding from processing his or her behavior and making meaning of every new experience (Rowe, 1966). Barnard (1994, p. 6) asserts that it is within the interactive system with the environment that the child's emotional, intellectual, and physical needs are either met or not met.

The Barnard model expands on existing knowledge by focusing on the parent/caregiver–child environment interactive process, reflecting the fact that infants and young children influence the parent and the environment, while simultaneously depending on parents to mediate their life experiences and create learning opportunities. The central focus of this model is to assess the child's health in the context of interpersonal interaction and adaptation that occurs between the child and the caregiver in any given environment.

MAJOR CONCEPTS AND DEFINITIONS

The integral component of the Barnard Parent/Caregiver–Child Interaction Model is the interactive system consisting of the parent/caregiver, the child, and the environment (Barnard, 1994). The concepts in Barnard's model are directly observable and include the infant's behaviors, the parent/caregiver's behaviors, and the parent/caregiver's and child's environment.

Parent/Caregiver Behavior

The parent/caregiver refers to the child's mother, father, or primary caregiver. The Barnard model takes into account this person's characteristics, including psychosocial skills, concern about the child, physical and mental health, expectations of the child, parenting style, and ability to adapt to new situations (Barnard, 1994):

- *Sensitivity to cues* refers to the caregiver's ability to accurately interpret and respond sensitively to the infants' needs and wants.
- *Alleviation of distress* refers to the effectiveness of the parent/caregiver in responding to the infant's distress, which depends on the ability to recognize that the distress has occurred and a repertoire of soothing actions to calm the child.
- *Social–emotional growth fostering* refers to the ability to initiate age-appropriate affectionate play and to provide appropriate verbal and nonverbal reinforcement for desirable child behavior.

Infant/Child Behavior

- *Clarity of cues* refers to the infant's ability to communicate his or her needs and wants through changes in facial expressions, alertness, fussiness, and body posture, to name a few. Cues that are inconsistent can cause difficulties in the parent/caregiver's adaptation process (Barnard, 1994).
- The responsiveness to the parent/caregiver refers to the child's ability to reciprocate the caregiver's efforts such as smiling, rocking, or soothing activities.

The lack of the child responsiveness to the caregiver's efforts is assumed to make the parental adaptation to the child difficult or even impossible (Barnard, 1994).

The Environment

The *environment* refers to the environment of both the parent/caregiver and the child. The characteristics of the environment include both the animate (people) and inanimate (physical environment of the family, including objects, sounds, and visual and tactile stimulation) elements (Barnard, 1994).

Schematic Representation

Barnard (1976) depicted the parent/caregiver–child interactive system in a diagram in which arrows move in circular motion from the child to the parent/caregiver and from the parent/caregiver to the child. A break in each arrow signals interference in the adaptive process, which can be caused by the caregiver, the infant, or the environment.

Propositions

The Barnard Parent/Caregiver–Child Interaction Model is based on 10 theoretical propositions:

1. In the child health assessment, the goal is to identify problems at a point before they develop and when intervention would be most effective.
2. Social–environmental factors are important for determining child health outcomes.
3. The parent/caregiver–infant interaction provides information that reflects the nature of the child's ongoing environment.
4. Each parent brings to caregiving a basic personality and skill level that is the foundation upon which caregiving skill is built. The enactment of caregiving depends on these characteristics as well as on the characteristics of the child and environment.
5. Through interaction, caregivers and children modify each other's behavior. That is, the caregiver's behavior influences the child and, in turn, the child influences the caregiver, so that both are changed.
6. The adaptation process of the parent/caregiver and child is more modifiable than the child's and the parent/caregivers' characteristics; therefore, intervention should be aimed at supporting the parent's sensitivity and responsiveness to the infant's needs.
7. An important way to promote learning is to respond to child-initiated behaviors and to reinforce the child's attempts to try new things.
8. A major task for the helping professions is to promote a positive early learning environment that includes a nurturing relationship.
9. Assessing the child's social environment, including the quality of parent/caregiver–child interaction, is important in any comprehensive child health assessment model.
10. Assessing the child's physical environment is equally important in any child health assessment model (Barnard, 1994).

EVALUATION OF THE BARNARD MODEL

According to Meleis (2007), evaluation is the cornerstone of further theory development, education, research, practice, administration, and the daily decision-making process. The criteria used to evaluate Barnard's model include clarity, consistency, simplicity/complexity, usefulness, and generalizability. Meleis (2007) states that "precision of boundaries, a communication of a sense of orderliness, vividness, and consistency through theory" (p. 262) are indicators of a theoretical model's clarity. Although Barnard (1976) did not clearly define theoretical concepts in her model, she described them and, therefore, implied their definitions. The concepts in the Barnard model are interconnected and form an interactive system. Because of the ongoing interaction, they influence one another and acquire new properties. The model articulates only some concepts consistent with the core domains of nursing as proposed by Meleis (2007). For example, Barnard clearly addresses the concept of environment (the physical and social environment of the child) and the client (parent/caregiver and the child), the interaction (between the parent–child dyad and environment). Health is treated indirectly (interactive system provides the basis for assessing optimal child growth and development).

Client transitions, nursing therapeutics, and health are not articulated and require further development.

Simplicity of a theory refers to whether a theory includes a minimal number of concepts. On the other hand, complexity refers to the explanations and relationships among variables (Chinn & Kramer, 2008; Meleis, 2007). The appropriateness of the level of complexity within a theory depends on the nature of the concepts and relationships they are set to explain or predict (Meleis, 2007). At first glance, the Barnard model seems to be a relatively simple and elegant framework, which relates to the parent–child interaction and its important elements. However, the many propositions made by Barnard about the nature of relationships between the parent/caregiver, the child and the environment imply high-level abstraction and complexity. According to Meleis (2007), the consistency of a theoretical model depends on the level of congruency and the fit between different components of theory; for example, the fit between assumptions and concept definitions, the fit between concept definitions and their use in propositions, and the fit between concepts and exemplars (Meleis, 2007).

The theoretical basis of the Barnard model may be assessed using the Nursing Child Assessment Satellite Training (NCAST) Feeding and Teaching Scales (Barnard, 1994). Barnard's team and others tested these scales for reliability; they were established as reliable by studies of internal consistency and test–retest procedures (Barnard, 1994). The validity of the scales to evaluate the quality of parent/caregiver–child interaction has also been assessed (Barnard, 1994). Researchers, nurses and other clinicians interested in using the scales to assess parent–child interaction are required to receive certification by NCAST Programs at the University of Washington and to achieve reliability of at least 85% in using these scales.

RESEARCH APPLICATIONS WITH PRETERM INFANTS

The application of the Barnard model in practice has been discussed widely in the interdisciplinary (Shonkoff & Meisels, 2000; Shonkoff & Philips, 2002; Zeanah, 2009) and nursing (Margolis et al., 2001; Marriner Tomey, 2006; Sumner & Spietz, 1994) literatures. A considerable amount of research has been conducted over the past 20 years to assess and test parent/caregiver–child interaction. Using prospective, longitudinal designs, researchers have consistently demonstrated important links between the quality of parent/caregiver–child interaction, environmental influences, and child development outcomes (Banerjee & Tamis-Lemonda, 2007; Diehl, 1997; Farel, Freeman, Keenan, & Huber, 1991; Leitch, 1999; Lewis & Coates, 1980; Nakamura, Stewart, & Tatarka, 2000; Schiffman, Omar, & McKelvey, 2003; Starling Washington, Reifsnider, Bishop, Domingeaux Ethington, & Ruffin, 2010).

Fewer published studies have tested early NICU interventions designed to prevent the development of negative parent–infant interaction trajectories or to reduce hospital length of stay. In one of the earliest intervention studies, Parker, Zahr, Cole, and Brecht (1992) examined the efficacy of maternal education, training, and support related to premature infants' behavioral and developmental functioning. Random assignment of participants was made to the intervention ($n = 26$) and control ($n = 15$) groups. Follow-up assessment took place at 4 and 8 months to determine the quality of infant stimulation in home environment. No statistically significant differences either in maternal affective behavior or in infant social behavior were noted between the groups. However, mothers in the intervention group scored significantly higher on the quality of the stimulation value of the child's home environment using the Home Observation for Measurement of the Environment (HOME) Inventory.

Likewise, Harrison, Sherrod, Dunn, and Olivet (1991) reported encouraging findings from a pilot intervention study that sought to measure the effectiveness of teaching parents about preterm infants' cues. The participants were assigned to two intervention groups and one control group. Mothers in the first intervention group ($n = 10$) received demonstration as well as verbal and written instruction that focused on understanding preterm infants' cues. Members of the second intervention group ($n = 10$) received brief instruction about mothers' assessment of infant behavior and were asked to rate their infants' behavior. The control group ($n = 10$) received routine NICU care and support. A feeding episode was scored approximately 6 weeks after discharge using the Barnard Feeding Scale (Barnard, 1976). The total highest parent score was reported for the mothers who received the most intense preparation.

In a subsequent study, Lawhon (1994) provided individualized interventions that focused on enhancing parental and newborn competence in interaction to parents and their infants born prior to 32 weeks' gestation. At approximately 1 month after discharge, a trained observer rated feeding interaction using Barnard's NCAST Feeding Scale. The scores in the intervention group were comparable to the scores previously reported for full-term infants, suggesting that the intervention designed for the study was quite effective.

Most recent investigations have focused on two areas: (1) testing early NICU interventions with parents to prevent the development of negative parent–infant interaction trajectories to reduce hospital length of stay and (2) reducing parenting stress after preterm birth. Using randomized controlled design, a Norwegian team (Kaarsen, Roning, Ulvund, & Dahl, 2006) tested the effects of an early-intervention program on parenting stress after a preterm birth until 1 year corrected age, using a sample of 140 infants and their parents. The intervention consisted of 8 sessions given shortly before discharge and 4 home visits by specially trained nurses focusing on the infant's unique characteristics, temperament, and developmental potential and the interaction between the infant and the parents. Seventy-one infants were included in the preterm intervention group, and 69 were included in the preterm control group. Fathers and mothers in the intervention group reported consistently lower scores related to distractibility and hyperactivity behavior, and higher scores on parenting competence; the attachment subscales matched those of the preterm control group. There were no differences in mean summary stress scores between the mothers and fathers in the two groups at 12 months, suggesting that parenting programs may reduce the level of stress among both mothers and fathers of preterm infants to a level comparable to that of parents of peers infants.

Melnyk et al. (2006) investigated the efficacy of an educational–behavioral intervention program called Creating Opportunities for Parent Empowerment (COPE) that was designed to enhance parent–infant interactions and parent mental health outcomes for the ultimate purpose of improving child developmental and behavior outcomes. A sample of 260 families participated in the intervention from 2001 to 2004 in 2 NICUs in the northeast United States. Parents completed self-administered instruments during the hospitalization period, within 7 days after infant discharge, and at 2 months' corrected age. Blinded observers rated parent–infant interactions in the NICU. All participants received 4 intervention sessions of audio-taped and written materials. Parents in the COPE program received information and behavioral activities about the appearance and behavioral characteristics of preterm infants and ways to best parent them. The comparison intervention contained information regarding hospital services and policies.

Mothers who participated in the COPE program reported significantly less stress in the NICU and less depression and anxiety at 2 months' corrected infant age than did the comparison mothers. Blinded observers also rated mothers and fathers in the COPE program as more positive in interactions with their infants. In addition, mothers and fathers reported stronger beliefs about their parental role and the expected behaviors and characteristics for their infants during hospitalization. Infants in the COPE program had a 3.8-day shorter NICU length of stay (mean: 31.86 days versus 35.63 days) and 3.9-day shorter total hospital length of stay (mean: 35.29 days versus 39.19 days) than did comparison infants, suggesting that a reproducible educational–behavioral intervention program for parents that begins soon after the infant's admission to the NICU can improve parents' mental health outcomes, enhance parent–infant interaction, and reduce hospital length of stay.

Most recently, Melnyk (2010) and her research team have focused on translating the evidence-based NICU COPE program for parents of premature infants into clinical practice. In the latest study, the research participants included 81 (45%) out of 180 nurses from a 55-bed NICU of a large hospital located in the Southwest region of the United States. The nurses completed the evidence-based practice (EBP) beliefs and EBP implementation scales at baseline and 6 months after an educational offering that consisted of a full-day workshop on COPE and EBP and introduction of the COPE intervention into the unit. Nurses employed in the two pods in which COPE was being implemented reported higher EBP beliefs and greater EBP implementation compared to nurses who did not receive COPE education. The authors reported that having an EBP mentor was instrumental in the delivery of the COPE program to the parents. The authors concluded that translating effective data-based interventions into clinical practice is urgently needed to develop a culture supportive of EBP.

Collectively, the lessons learned from the intervention studies with preterm infants and their parents indicate that relatively simple interventions can be a powerful way of improving the quality of parent–child interaction as well as parent and child outcomes. Findings also suggest that the parent–child interaction can be modified to meet the preterm infants' capacity to interact, and that this therapeutic aim can be an integral part of everyday clinical practice in NICUs. It appears that the most effective interventions involve multiple parent teaching modalities and time points. Lastly, strategies to accelerate the translation of efficacious interventions such as routine use of NCAST Feeding and Teaching Scales or evidence-based programs such as COPE into clinical practice with preterm infants are needed to create a culture that supports evidence-based care in a variety of healthcare settings.

BARNARD MODEL: PRACTICE APPLICATION TO PRETERM INFANTS

The usefulness of Barnard's model has been demonstrated in research, education, and clinical practice. Barnard's (1976) original research led to the development of the NCAST Feeding and Teaching Scales, which have since been standardized for use with several ethnic groups and infant age groups. These outcome measures are now used as a key assessment tool of parent–infant feeding and teaching interactions in more than 10 countries by over 10,000 researchers and health professionals, and produce reliable results in 85% or more cases. Barnard's model has an international appeal among educators and appears in maternity nursing courses at the baccalaureate, master's, and doctoral levels. It has also been used as a framework for nursing practice with childbearing families (e.g., Early Head Start programs in Washington, and public health services across the United States).

One specific application of Barnard's model in clinical practice focuses on facilitating the parent–infant interaction that occurs during feeding. For example, during the past decade, nurses at the IWK Health Center in Halifax, Nova Scotia, have effectively used Barnard's principles to provide individualized guidance for parents who are learning to interact with both term and preterm newborns. In the NICU, caregivers routinely discuss the strengths and gaps in feeding interaction using the model as a framework for feedback after feeding. Specific NCAST Feeding Scale items are used in an effort to help mothers recognize infant cues that would signal them to respond in ways that promote more effective feeding. Staff nurses encourage mothers to pay attention to sustained eye contact, their facial expressions, gentle talking and stroking, and recognition of satiation cues, such as a slowdown in feeding. They are encouraged to maintain a relaxed posture, and to note disengagement cues, such as crying, back arching, or falling asleep, as a signal to terminate the feeding. Recognizing that the preterm infant's cues are not as clear as in the term infant's signals, the teaching strategies may require focusing on one cluster of cues at a time and setting small, measurable goals to promote positive parent–child relationship and positive feeding interactions in the future.

CONCLUSIONS AND FUTURE DIRECTIONS

Barnard's Parent/Caregiver–Child Interaction Model has been used in education, research, and clinical practice for more than two decades. The results of the research review and evaluation of the model suggest that it effectively describes child development within the context of the infant's interaction with both the caregiver and the environment. The process of model development is consistent with the inductive form of logic in that the theorist formulates concepts and relationships based on existing theory, research, and clinical observations. Barnard provides evidence of the applicability of her model in health education, research, and clinical practice. The model has been used internationally as a theoretical framework for maternity nursing practice. The NCAST Feeding and Teaching Scales to assess parent/caregiver–child interactions in clinical practice and research have a high level of precision and reliability. The information presented in this chapter suggests that the Barnard model offers a useful framework for designing and testing clinical interventions with preterm infants and their parents. Intervention research findings suggest that timing of the clinical interventions should occur early in the parent–child relationship and be sustained over time for maximal effects.

Although Barnard's model is limited to early child development within the context of relationships with caregiver and environment, it is applicable to all disciplines that are concerned with parent–child relationships. There has been no effort to refine or test the model in recent years. In its current state, the model does not fulfill the criteria for theories set forth by Meleis (2007). However, in spite of its limitations, the Barnard model does offer an excellent framework for use in clinical practice and research with preterm infants and their parents.

For a full suite of assignments and additional learning activities, use the access code located in the front of your book to visit this exclusive website: http://go.jblearning.com/dechesnay. If you do not have an access code, you can obtain one at the site.

REFERENCES

Als, H. (1997). Earliest intervention for preterm infants in newborn intensive care unit. In M. J. Guralnick (Ed.), *The effectiveness of early intervention* (pp. 23–47). Baltimore: Brooks.

Banerjee, P. N., & Tamis-Lemonda, C. S. (2007). Infants' persistence and mothers' teaching as predictors of toddlers' cognitive development. *Infant Behavior and Development, 30*(3), 479–491.

Barnard, K. E. (1976). The Barnard model. In G. Sumner & A. Spietz (Eds.), *NCAST caregiver/parent–child interaction feeding manual* (pp. 8–14). Seattle: NCAST Publications, University of Washington School of Nursing.

Barnard, K. E. (1994). Development of feeding and teaching scales. In G. Sumner & A. Spietz (Eds.), *NCAST caregiver/parent–child interaction feeding manual* (pp. 3–7). Seattle: NCAST Publications, University of Washington School of Nursing.

Barnard, K. E. (1997). Influencing parent–child interaction for children at risk. In M. J. Guralnick (Ed.), *The effectiveness of early intervention* (pp. 249–271). Baltimore: Brooks.

Brazelton, T. B. (1973). Neonatal Behavioral Assessment Scale. *Clinics in Developmental Medicine, 50*. London, UK: Spastics International Medical Publications.

Casey, P. H., Whiteside-Mansell, L., Barrett, K., Bradley, R. H., & Gargus, R. (2006). Impact of prenatal and/or postnatal growth problems in low birth weight preterm infants on school age outcomes: An 8-year longitudinal evaluation. *Pediatrics, 118*(3), 1078–1086.

Centers for Disease Control and Prevention (CDC). (2010). Retrieved October 16, 2010, from http://www.cdc.gov/reproductivehealth/maternalinfanthealth/PBP.htm

Chinn, P. L, & Kramer, M. K. (2008). *Integrated theory and knowledge development in nursing* (7th ed.). St. Louis, MO: Mosby.

Diehl, K. (1997). Adolescent mothers: What produces positive mother–infant interaction? *American Journal of Maternal Child Nursing, 22*, 89–95.

Farrel, A. M., Freeman, V. A., Keenan, N. L., & Huber, C. J. (1991). Interaction between high-risk infants and their mothers: The NCAST as an assessment tool. *Research in Nursing and Health, 14*(2), 109–118.

Guzetta, A., Mazotti, S., Tinelli, F., Bancale, A., Ferretti, G., Battini, R., . . . Cloni, G. (2006). Early assessment of visual information processing and neurological outcome for preterm infants. *Neuropediatrics, 37*(5), 278–285.

Hamilton, B. E., Minino, A. M., Martin, J. A., Kochanek, K. D., Strobino, D. M., & Guyer, B. (2007). Annual summary of vital statistics: 2005. *Pediatrics, 11*(20), 345–360.

Harrison, L., Sherrod, R. A., Dunn, L., & Olivet, L. (1991). Effects of hospital based instruction on interactions between parents and preterm infants. *Neonatal Network, 9*, 27–33.

Jolley, S. N., Elmore, S., Barnard, K. E., & Carr, D. B. (2007). Dysregulation of the hypothalamic–pituitary–adrenal axis in postpartum depression. *Biological Research in Nursing, 8*(3), 210–222.

Kaarsen, P. I., Ronning, J. A., Ulvund, S. E., & Dahl, L. B. (2006). A randomized, controlled trial of the effectiveness of an early intervention program in reducing parenting stress after preterm birth. *Pediatrics, 118*(1), e9–e19.

Lawhon, G. (1994). *Facilitation of parenting within the newborn intensive care unit.* Unpublished doctoral dissertation, University of Washington, Seattle, WA.

Leitch, D. B. (1999). Mother–infant: Achieving synchrony. *Nursing Research, 48*, 55–58.

Leversen, K. T., Sommerfelt, K., Rønnestad, A., Kaaresen, P. I., Farstad, T., Skranes, J., . . . Markestad, T. (2010). Predicting neurosensory disabilities at two years of age in a national cohort of extremely premature infants. *Early Human Development, 86*(9), 581–586.

Lewis, M., & Coates, D. L. (1980). Mother–infant interaction and cognitive development in 12-week-old infants. *Infant Behavior and Development, 3*, 95–105.

Lindrea, K. B., & Stainton, C. M. (2000). Infant massage outcomes. *Journal of Maternal Child Nursing, 25*, 95–98.

Lype, M., Prasad, M., Nair, P. M., Geetha, S., & Kailas, L. (2008). The newborn with seizures: A follow-up study. *Indian Pediatrics, 45*(9), 749–752.

Mackley, A. B., Locke, R. G., Spear, M. L., & Joseph, R. (2010). Forgotten parent: NICU paternal emotional response. *Advances in Neonatal Care, 10*(4), 200–2003.

Margolis, P. A., Stevens, R., Bordley, W. C., Stuart, J., Harlan, C., Keyes-Elstein, L., & Wisseh, S. (2001). From concept to application: The impact of a community-wide intervention to improve the delivery of preventive services to children. *Pediatrics, 108*(3), E42.

Marriner Tomey, A. (2006). Nursing theorists of historical significance. In A. Marriner Tomey & M. Raile Alligood (Eds.), *Nursing theorists and their work* (6th ed., pp. 62–64). St. Louis, MO: Mosby.

Meleis, A. I. (2007). *Theoretical nursing: Development and progress* (4th ed.). Philadelphia: Lippincott, Williams & Wilkins.

Melnyk, B. M., Feinstein, N. F., Alpert-Gillis, L., Fairbanks, E., Crean, H. F., Sinkin, R. A., . . . Gross, S. J. (2006). Reducing premature infants' length of stay and improving parents' mental health outcomes with Creating Opportunities for Parent Empowerment (COPE) neonatal intensive care unit program: A randomized, controlled trial. *Pediatrics, 118*(5), e1414–e1427.

Melnyk, B. M., Bullock, T., McGrath, J., Kelly, S., Jacobson, D., & Baba, L. (2010). Translating the evidence-based NICU COPE Program for Parents of Premature Infants into Clinical Practice: Impact on nurses' EBP and lessons learned. *Journal of Perinatal and Neonatal Nursing, 24*(1), 74–80.

Nakamura, W. M., Stewart, K. B., & Tatarka, M. E. (2000). Assessing father–infant interactions using the NCAST teaching scale: A pilot study. *American Journal of Occupational Therapy, 54*(1), 44–51.

Obeidat, H. M., Bond, E. A., & Callister, L. C. (2009). The parental experience of having an infant in the newborn intensive care unit. *Journal of Perinatal Education, 18*(3), 23–29.

Parker, S. J., Zahr, L. K., Cole, J. G., & Brecht, M. L. (1992). Outcome after developmental intervention in the neonatal intensive care unit for mothers of preterm infants with low socioeconomic status. *Journal of Pediatrics, 120*, 780–785.

Rowe, G. P. (1966). The developmental conceptual framework to the study of the family. In F. I. Nye & F. M. Berardo (Eds.), *Emerging conceptual frameworks in family analyses* (pp. 198–222). New York: Praeger.

Sameroff, A. J., & Chandler, M. J. (1975). Reproductive risk and the continuum of caretaker casualty. In F. D. Horowitz (Ed.), *Review of child development research* (pp. 187–245). Chicago: University of Chicago Press.

Schiffman, R. F., Omar, M. A., & McKelvey, L. M. (2003). Mother–infant interaction in low-income families. *American Journal of Maternal Child Nursing, 28*(4), 246–251.

Shonkoff, J., & Meisels, S. J. (2000). *Handbook of early childhood intervention.* Cambridge, UK: Cambridge University Press.

Shonkoff, J., & Phillips, D. (2002). *From neurons to neighborhoods: The science of early childhood development.* Washington, DC: National Academy Press.

Simpson, C. D., Ye, X. Y., Hellmann, J., & Tomlinson, C. (2010, November 15). Trends in cause specific mortality at a Canadian Outborn NICU. *Pediatrics* [Epub ahead of print].

Starling Washington, P., Reifsnider, E. L., Bishop, S., Domingeaux Ethington, M. E., & Ruffin, R. (2010). Changes in family variables among normal and overweight preschoolers. *Issues in Comprehensive Pediatric Nursing, 33*(1), 20–38.

Sumner, G., & Spietz, A. (Eds.). (1994). *NCAST caregiver/parent–child interaction teaching manual* (pp. 3–6). Seattle, WA: NCAST Publications, University of Washington School of Nursing.

Tsai, S. Y., Barnard, K. E., Lentz, M. J., & Thomas, K. A. (2010, August 26). Mother–infant activity synchrony as a correlate of the emergence of circadian rhythm. *Biological Research in Nursing* [Epub ahead of print].

von Bertalanffy, L. (1968). *General system theory: Foundations, development application.* New York: George Braziller.

Zeanah, C. J. (2009). *Handbook of infant mental health* (3rd ed.). New York: Guilford Press.

CHAPTER 11

The Utility of Leininger's Culture Care Theory with Vulnerable Populations

Rick Zoucha

Objectives

WWW

At the end of this chapter, the reader will be able to

1. Explain Leininger's Culture Care Theory.
2. Describe how Leininger's Theory can be applied to nursing practice with vulnerable populations.
3. Propose at least two research projects in which Leininger's Theory might serve as the conceptual framework.

In the ever-evolving healthcare environment in the United States, there are a multitude of people who have access to services that promote health and well-being and reduce the effects of illness. Similarly, there are people who are not afforded the same access to healthcare services as others because of their vulnerability.

According to Campos-Outcalt et al. (1994), vulnerable populations can be defined as groups of people who experience physical disabilities, mental disabilities, cultural differences, geographic separation, and limited economic resources, and, due to these barriers, might be unable to become integrated into the mainstream health services and delivery system. The authors include as vulnerable the urban and rural poor (especially ethnic and racial minorities), Native Americans, chronically disabled children and adults, the frail elderly, homeless individuals, and undocumented immigrants. Vulnerable populations can also be defined in terms of subpopulations or subgroups who, because of their position in the social strata, are exposed to certain contextual conditions that are different from those experienced by the rest of the population (Frohlich & Potvin, 2008). Shi and Stevens (2005) define vulnerable populations as racial and ethnic minorities, uninsured, children, the elderly, the poor, the chronically ill, people with AIDS, alcohol or substance abusers, homeless individuals, underserved rural and urban groups, people who do not speak English or have difficulties in communicating in healthcare settings, those who are poorly educated or illiterate, low-income individuals, and members of minority groups. In addition, persons who are victims of violence are at risk of being vulnerable (Zoucha, 2006).

Leininger (1996a) contends that, regardless of economic, political, and even genetic differences, everyone has a culture. This chapter discusses Leininger's culture care theory and the utility of the theory in working with vulnerable populations defined by their cultural differences in the research and practice settings.

LEININGER'S THEORY OF CULTURAL CARE DIVERSITY AND UNIVERSALITY

Leininger defines care as "those assistive, supportive and enabling experiences or ideas towards others with evident or anticipated needs to ameliorate or improve human conditions or lifeways" (Leininger & McFarland, 2006, p. 12). Leininger (1996b) further describes culture as learned values, beliefs, rules of behavior, and lifestyle practices of a particular group of people. Andrews and Boyle (2008) determined that culture has four basic characteristics: Culture is learned, shared, dynamic, and able to adapt to specific conditions. Culture involves all types of behavior that are socially acquired and transmitted by means such as customs, techniques, beliefs, institutions, and material objects (Locke, 1998). According to Leininger (1991b) and Andrews and Boyle (1999), humans exist within a culture, and culture is viewed as a universal phenomenon.

Leininger has combined the concept of culture and an ethical orientation of caring to develop a theory appropriate for nursing practice, research, and education (Zoucha & Husted, 2000). She also contends that individuals, families, and communities must be viewed in the context of culture (Zoucha & Husted, 2002).

Leininger's theory of culture care diversity and universality (Leininger & McFarland, 2006) is the product of more than 50 years of research and development, during which she studied more than 60 cultures and identified 172 care constructs for use by nursing and other healthcare professionals. The sunrise model (Leininger & McFarland, 2002) depicts Leininger's theory as having seven cultural and social structure dimensions: (1) technological, (2) religious and philosophical, (3) kinship and social, (4) political and legal, (5) economic, (6) educational factors, and (7) cultural values, beliefs, and lifeways. The theory describes diverse healthcare systems as ranging from folk beliefs and practices to nursing and other heathcare professional systems often utilized by people around the world.

Leininger describes two systems of caring that exist in every culture she studied (Leininger & McFarland, 2006). The first system of caring is generic and is considered the oldest form of caring or nurturing. Generic caring consists of culturally derived interpersonal practices, and is considered essential for health, growth, and survival of humans (Reynolds & Leininger, 1993). Generic caring is often referred to as folk practices and defined culturally (Leininger, 1996b).

The second type of caring is considered therapeutic, cognitively learned, practiced, and transmitted through formal and informal means of professional education such as schools of nursing, medicine, and dentistry (Leininger & McFarland, 2006). Professional learning can and does include concepts and techniques to enhance professional practices, as well as interpersonal communication techniques and holistic aspects of care. Historically, professional care has not always included ideas about folk care, because such beliefs may not have been valued by nurses and other healthcare professionals (Leininger & McFarland, 2002).

In her theory, Leininger contends that if professional and generic care practices do not fit together, this discordance might affect client/patient recovery, health, and well-being, and result in care that is not culturally congruent with the beliefs of the person, family, or community (Leininger & McFarland, 2006). To provide culturally congruent care, Leininger asserts that professionals must link and synthesize generic and professional care knowledge to benefit the client (Leininger & McFarland, 2002). This link is a bridge, where a bridge is appropriate, between the professional and folk healthcare systems.

According to this theory (Clarke, McFarland, Andrews, & Leininger, 2009). three predictive modes of care may be derived from and based on the use of generic (emic) care knowledge and professional (etic) care knowledge obtained from research and experience using the sunrise model. The three modes of action are (1) cultural care preservation/maintenance, (2) cultural care accommodation/negotiation, and (3) cultural care repatterning/restructuring.

Cultural care preservation/maintenance refers to assistive, supportive, facilitative, or enabling professional actions and decisions that help individuals, families, and communities from a particular culture to retain and preserve care values so that they can maintain well-being, recover from illness, or face possible handicap or death (Leininger & McFarland, 2006). Leininger describes cultural care accommodation/negotiation as assistive, facilitative, or enabling creative professional actions and potential decisions that can help individuals, families, and communities of a particular culture to adapt to, or to negotiate with, others for the purpose of satisfying healthcare outcomes with professional caregivers (Leininger & McFarland, 2002). Cultural care repatterning/restructuring is described as the assistive, supportive, facilitative, and enabling activities by nurses and other healthcare professionals that promote actions and decisions that may help the person, family, or community change, or modify behaviors affecting their lifeways to achieve a new and different health pattern. This repatterning/restructuring (Leininger, 2002b) is done while respecting the individual's, family's, and community's cultural values and beliefs while still providing and promoting a healthier lifeway than before the changes were co-established with the person, family, and community. Leininger (2002a) asserts in her theory that these three predicted modes of action serve to guide judgments, decisions, and actions, and ultimately culminate in the delivery of culturally congruent care.

Leininger (2002a) describes culturally congruent care as beneficial, satisfying, and meaningful to the individuals, families, and communities served by nurses. In contrast, cultural imposition occurs when nurses and other healthcare professionals impose their own beliefs, practices, and values upon another culture because they believe their ideas are superior to those of the other person or group (Leininger, 2002a). Leininger uses the concepts of cultural congruence and cultural imposition to focus on acceptable (caring) and unacceptable (noncaring) behavior by nurses in the practice, education, and research arena.

UTILITY OF THE THEORY IN NURSING RESEARCH AND PRACTICE

In addition to the development of the theory of cultural care, Leininger (1991a) has developed a research method that is very useful in understanding the phenomenon of culturally based care for vulnerable populations. As described earlier, vulnerability includes culture differences. Leininger's qualitative ethnonursing research method was created to work in conjunction with the theory (and the sunrise model) as a guide for research. The ethnonursing research method according to Leininger and McFarland (2006) is described as "a qualitative nursing research method focused on naturalistic, open discovery and largely inductive (emic) modes to document, describe, explain and interpret informants' worldview, meaning and symbols and life experiences as they bear on actual or potential nursing care phenomena" (p. 21). Leininger (2002a) suggests that this method can be used in conjunction with research enablers such as (1) Leininger's Observation–Participation–Reflection Enabler, (2) Leininger's Stranger to Trusted Friend Enabler, (3) the Sunrise Model Enabler, (4) the Specific Domain of Inquiry Enabler, and (5) Leininger's Acculturation Enabler.

These enabler guides can also be used in the clinical setting in an attempt to move from stranger to trusted friend in the new relationship between the nurse and client. The notion of being viewed as a friend can promote culturally congruent care in many cultures (Zoucha & Reeves, 1999). Such a friend-like or personal relationship between the nurse and the client/patient can decrease the cultural difference vulnerability of the person, as it permits the cultural care needs of the client to become known to the nurse. The nurse is then able to promote care that is congruent with the person's culture and, essentially, to promote the health and well-being needs of the person, family, and community.

The connection between theory, research, and practice is addressed by using the identified enablers to promote a deeper understanding of the cultural phenomenon of interest, regardless of the context (research or clinical practice). This allows for a holistic and comprehensive view of the domain of inquiry and the particular culture being studied. As transcultural nurse researchers and clinicians seek to understand the phenomena of interest for vulnerable populations, it becomes possible to decrease the aspect of vulnerability described as cultural differences. If transcultural nurses do utilize the findings from relevant studies in their actual clinical practice, then each nurse's understanding of the person, family, and community can be viewed from a cultural care perspective, thereby not only increasing the understanding of the cultural care needs but also exposing the vulnerability related to being culturally different.

The concern with personal, family, and community vulnerability regarding cultural differences is that if nurses pursue an understanding of culture in relation to health and well-being, then they have an ethical motivation to promote care that is culturally congruent. This motivation might potentially decrease the vulnerability of the individual, family, and community. Zoucha and Husted (2000) contend that cultural caring should consider the person, family, and community in the context of their culture, with this perspective resulting in the promotion of ethical and culturally congruent care. In agreement with Leininger's theory, Zoucha and Husted (2000) believe that it is the ethical responsibility and duty of the nurse to promote, provide, and encourage care that is culturally based and congruent with the values, beliefs, and traditions of the individual, family, and community.

Leininger's theory provides a holistic and emic view of those factors that describe culture and those cultural values and beliefs that are meaningful to individuals, families, and communities. However, the theory does not explicitly state, in the context of either the sunrise model or the theory, the related factors of racism, poverty, and history of oppression that are commonly encountered among people from other than the dominant culture in the United States. Leininger does consider these issues in her writing and presentations but does not make them clear in the explication of the theory and sunrise model in relationship to research and clinical practice. Adding the factors of racism, poverty, and history of oppression to the sunrise model as part of the experience for people of different cultures (other than the dominant culture) may assist nurses and other healthcare professionals in better understanding the meaning of vulnerability. Through the use of such theory, nurses and other healthcare professionals can promote health and well-being while decreasing the experience of being vulnerable.

In summary, individuals, families, and communities that are identified as vulnerable due to cultural differences can be understood in a manner that seeks to expose the source of that vulnerability and focus on the cultural care needs. Leininger's theory of culture care diversity and universality promotes a deep and clear understanding of the individual, family, and community from a unique cultural perspective. Using this theory and the identified enablers for research and clinical practice allow the nurse to view the individual, family, and community from the perspective of the seven cultural factors identified in the sunrise model (religion, kinship, technology, education, economic, political and legal, and cultural lifeways). By adopting this viewpoint, nurses and other healthcare professionals can decrease the vulnerability of the individual, family, and community by uncovering the concerns deriving from cultural difference and promoting ethical practice that is congruent with the cultural beliefs of those in the caring relationship with nurses and other healthcare professionals.

For a full suite of assignments and additional learning activities, use the access code located in the front of your book to visit this exclusive website: http://go.jblearning.com/dechesnay. If you do not have an access code, you can obtain one at the site.

REFERENCES

Andrews, M. M., & Boyle, J. S. (1999). *Transcultural concepts in nursing care* (3rd ed.) Philadelphia: Lippincott.

Andrews, M. M., & Boyle, J. S. (Eds.). (2008). *Transcultural concepts in nursing care* (5th ed.). Philadelphia: Wolters Kluwer Health.

Campos-Outcalt, D., Fernandez, R., Hollow, W., Lundeen, S., Nelson, K., & Schuster, B. (1994). Providing quality health care to vulnerable populations. Retrieved from http://www.primarycaresociety.org/1994d.htm

Clarke, P. N., McFarland, M. R., Andrews, M. M., & Leininger, M. (2009). Caring: Some reflections on the impact of the culture care theory by McFarland & Andrews and a conversation with Leininger. *Nursing Science Quarterly, 22*(3), 233–239.

Frohlich, K. L., & Potvin, L. (2008). Transcending the known in public health practice: The inequality paradox: The population approach and vulnerable populations. *American Journal of Public Health, 98*(2), 216–221.

Leininger, M. M. (1991a). Ethnonursing: A research method with enablers to study the theory of culture care. *NLN Publishing, 15*(2402), 73–117.

Leininger, M. M. (1991b). The theory of culture care diversity and universality. *NLN Publishing, 15*(2402), 5–68.

Leininger, M. (1996a). Culture care theory, research, and practice. *Nursing Science Quarterly, 9*(2), 71–78.

Leininger, M. (1996b). Response to Swendson and Windsor: Rethinking cultural sensitivity. *Nursing Inquiry, 3*(4), 238–241.

Leininger, M. (2002a). Culture care theory: A major contribution to advance transcultural nursing knowledge and practices. *Journal of Transcultural Nursing, 13*(3), 189–192.

Leininger, M. (2002b). Madeleine Leininger on transcultural nursing and culturally competent care. Interview by Mary Agnes Seisser. *Journal of Healthcare Quality, 24*(2), 18–21.

Leininger, M., & McFarland, M. (2002). *Transcultural nursing: concepts, theories, research and practice.* New York: McGraw Hill.

Leininger, M., & McFarland, M. (2006). *Culture care diversity and universality: A worldwide nursing theory* (2nd ed.). Sudbury, MA: Jones and Bartlett.

Locke, D. (1998). *Increasing multicultural understanding: A comprehensive model* (2nd ed.). Newbury Park, CA: Sage.

Reynolds, C. L., & Leininger, M. M. (1993). *Madeline Leininger, culture care diversity and universality theory.* Newbury Park, CA: Sage.

Shi, L., & Stevens, G. (2005). *Vulnerable populations in the United States.* San Francisco: Jossey-Bass.

Zoucha, R. (2006). Considering culture in understanding interpersonal violence. *Journal of Forensic Nursing, 2*(4), 195–196.

Zoucha, R., & Husted, G. L. (2000). The ethical dimensions of delivering culturally congruent nursing and health care. *Issues in Mental Health Nursing, 21*(3), 325–340.

Zoucha, R., & Husted, G. L. (2002). The ethical dimensions of delivering culturally congruent nursing and health care. *Review Series Psychiatry, 3*, 10–11.

Zoucha, R. D., & Reeves, J. (1999). A view of professional caring as personal for Mexican Americans. *International journal for Human Caring, 3*(3), 14–20.

CHAPTER 12

Positive Skills, Positive Strategies: Solution-Focused Nursing

Margaret McAllister

Objectives

At the end of this chapter, the reader will be able to

1. Describe the concepts of solution-focuses nursing.
2. Explain how solution-focused nursing expands the nurse's ability to work with vulnerable populations.
3. Distinguish solution-focused nursing from problem solving.

WWW

Nurses I teach frequently make me aware of the frustration and powerlessness they and others feel when working with clients who self-harm. How can you be recovery oriented, be empowering, and retain optimism for change when such clients appear to be deliberately hurting themselves, delaying recovery, and sabotaging efforts to help them?

This chapter outlines a practical philosophy for being strategic, forward-looking, and positive with clients. Called solution-focused nursing (SFN), it is derived from critical social theory and positive psychology ideas. The chapter begins with a client's experience of emergency health care. The narrative is analyzed and key lessons are drawn from it, before moving on to introduce a philosophical framework for nursing that helps clinicians be solution focused and strategic, rather than reactive and overwhelmed.

WWW ZARA'S EXPERIENCE

Zara tells her story:

> A while ago I had an experience that I don't ever want to repeat. I had developed a headache that just wouldn't go away. The pain had become so bad that I

was throwing up and beginning to have panic attacks. I'd had headaches before, but never this bad. I'd also had long-standing anxiety, treated with medications, which developed as a consequence of childhood abuse issues that I considered pretty much resolved, after quite a few years of therapy.

After about 6 hours of trying to relieve the headache with paracetamol, cold compresses, and resting, the pain was just not easing. When I began vomiting, I knew I needed help. I called an ambulance and was taken to the public emergency department.

I was placed on a gurney and wheeled into a room away from the nurses' station. No one told me what was happening, whether I'd be okay, or even if they'd be watching me. Sometime later, a nurse came to take my temperature and blood pressure. He also asked me to rate the severity of my pain.

Then, a doctor came in. She seemed kind and sympathetic at first—holding my hand, gently asking me questions, and reassuring me that the pain would subside with IV medications. She said she wanted me to stay overnight, but I told her that I felt panicky in hospitals and if the pain subsided, I'd be better off at home.

The nurse asked me why I felt panicky and I told them both that I had a lot of experience with hospitals—the last being a year ago when I was in the psychiatric unit. The doctor asked me about the reason for this stay and I told her that it was to prevent any risks of problems that might arise following gynecological surgery. My psychiatrist had been concerned that the surgery could be a triggering event, because I had a history with dissociation disorder.

Revealing this information seemed to cause a sudden change in the doctor's attitude. She stopped asking me questions and just pushed up my shirt to examine my body. She saw some old scars and asked me how they were caused. Again I was honest and told her I used to self-harm. That's when she pulled away immediately. It seemed like she was disgusted and I felt terribly ashamed.

Without a word of explanation, the doctor left the room. At this point I had not been given anything for my headache and was still feeling panicky and nauseous. I looked toward the nurse. In that moment, I really needed him.

Reflective Activity

Imagine you were that nurse whose client was in pain and distress. Your colleague has acted in a way that led the person to feel ashamed. Now you must provide for the client's physical and psychological safety, and minimize risks of mounting anxiety and panic. And what about the longer term? Two issues of concern come to mind: the client's future well-being and health service utilization and the promotion of more effective clinician–client interactions.

Analysis of the Narrative

In generating a satisfactory, complete response to these questions and in suggesting an effective care pathway for this nurse, it is helpful to reflect on what some of the significant elements within this story might mean for practice. First, the experience of ill health can be fundamentally disempowering. Second, people who come to health services are vulnerable and need nursing support. Finally, nursing work frequently involves change-oriented work not only with clients, but also with the healthcare culture itself.

The Experience of Ill Health: Must It Always Be Fundamentally Disempowering?

The experience of illness is not comfortable or pleasant at the best of times, but when a client presents to a health service expecting timely, quality care and is not helped to feel safe and secure—and, indeed, is made to feel worse—the experience can be traumatizing (Kendall-Tackett, 2003).

In Australia, for example, clients who have mental health histories continue to complain of substandard care (Hickie, Groom, McGorry, Davenport, & Luscombe, 2005). Despite the goal of a mainstreaming policy to equalize access to health care, fewer than 40% of people with mental disorders receive any mental health care in a 12-month period, and as many as 15% of clients who do present to emergency centers do not have adequate psychosocial assessments completed, leave before being seen, and are lost to follow-up (Brand, Kennedy, MacBean, Sundararajan, & Taylor, 2005). Additionally, when they have preexisting mental health problems, they commonly feel labeled, judged, objectified, and ashamed (Cook, Clancy, & Sanderson, 2004).

This kind of profoundly disempowering experience can have long-term negative health and social consequences. Such clients may be unwilling to want to use the health service again, they may later act out their negative feelings by directing them toward others with hostility or violence, or they may turn inward and allow shame and guilty feelings to spill into a vicious cycle, such as the cycle of self-harm (Link & Phelan, 2006; Sutton, 2007). (See **Figure 12–1**.)

Similarly, nurses who work in these busy environments, without mental health training to correct their stigmatizing and inaccurate perceptions and without backup or referral sources, frequently find that they are themselves disempowered, out of their depth, and unable to confidently or effectively provide care (McCann, Clark, McConnachie, & Harvey, 2006; Urquhart Law, Rostill-Brookes, & Goodman, 2009). Without adequate strategies to effectively intervene in such situations, nurses become disillusioned, disaffected, and demoralized.

In a study examining everyday conversations of nurses working with clients who self-injure (Estefan, McAllister, & Rowe, 2004), researchers found that only the outward acts of injury tended to be the focus of care by nurses. Most did not focus on events that might trigger the urge to self-harm, did not discuss the need to empathize with the individual's specific and present concerns, and did not reveal a concern for helping clients address issues of self-injury or work with them to find safer ways to express distress and communicate their needs. The study also revealed that nurses frequently felt unprepared, lacked clear frameworks for practice, and were

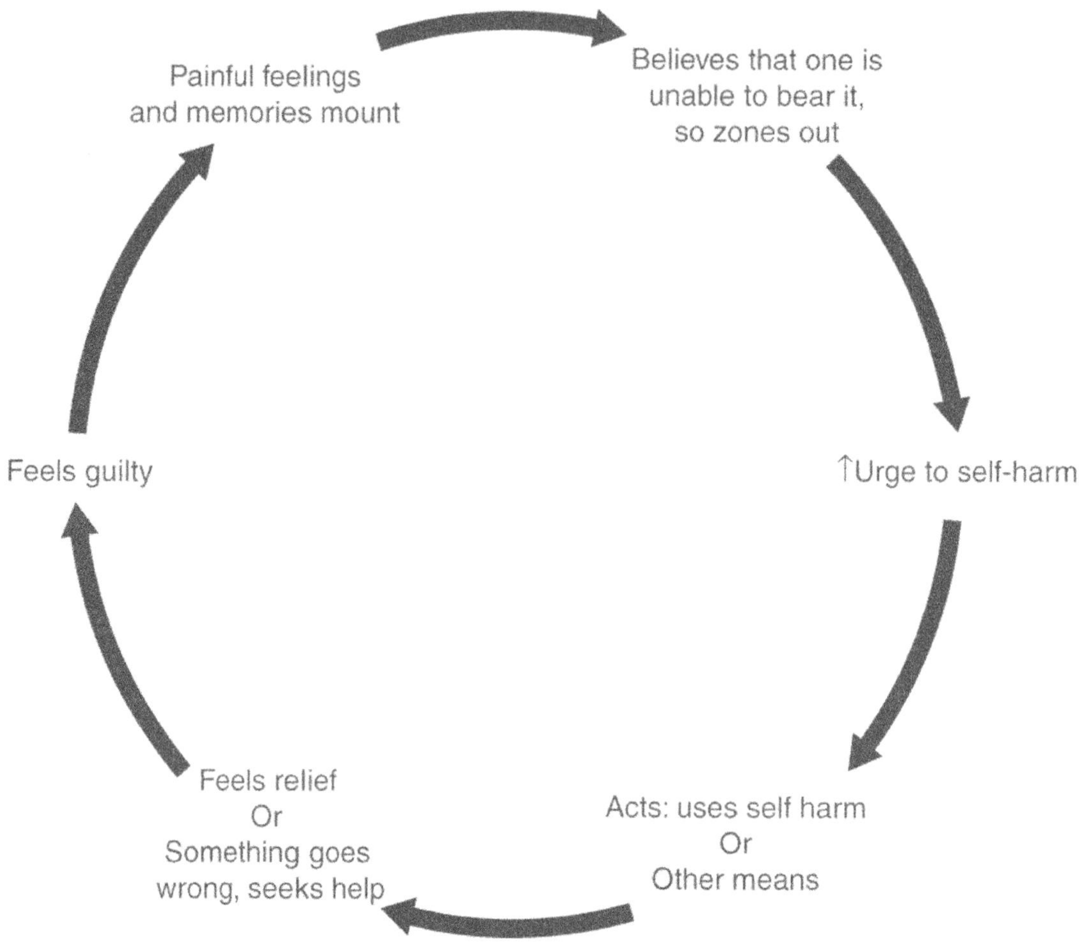

Figure 12–1 The cycle of self harm.

vulnerable to subtle tensions in practice that led to (1) managing before caring, (2) valuing diagnosis before understanding, and (3) focusing on behaviors rather than personal meanings and client The implication for patients and for care is that alienating, unhelpful diagnostic and socially loaded labels are attributed to people. For example, in the narrative that opened this chapter, the fact that the client had been a past psychiatric patient led to substandard health care and a negative experience. The patient was passive and alienated. The caregiving experience was also burdensome for the doctor.

As many have argued, a model of care that is problem centered is unlikely to offer inspiring or sustainable positive outcomes for clinicians or patients, yet it remains dominant across health care (Hall, 1996; Lopez & Gallagher, 2009; Seligman, 2002). As Johnson (2005, p. 48) has argued:

> Solutions to social problems are often relegated to the brief end of chapters and end of classes where they are given little attention or academic rigor. Without adequate coverage of structural solutions many students are left feeling that the world is a terribly unjust place—full of powerful people who use their advantage to exploit others and retain their power—and that it cannot be realistically changed for the better.

A problem orientation may be useful in helping isolate problems, target areas of change, and apply interventions dispassionately and rationally, but these actions are not always appropriate. Constantly searching for problems may prevent appreciating those things that are going right for a person. Perhaps some problems may never be resolved completely, so that a focus on the negative is inherently pessimistic. With a problem-centered focus, problems and difficulties become individuals' main concern, rather than feats and achievements. Problems are seen as something to be overcome rather than tolerated and perhaps integrated into the larger picture.

When this perspective is employed, positive and protective client outcomes are unlikely to be developed and achieved. Indeed, the focus on the problem in relation to self-harm is readily apparent in the abundance of research focusing on the nature of the dysfunction, and the dearth of evidence for effective interventions (Crawford & Kumar, 2009).

What are needed are strategies to help clients manage distress, delay their urges to self-harm, and develop health-seeking behavior, optimism, and self-belief (Barnes, Mitic, Leadbeater, & Dhami, 2009). Without them, nurses continue to be at risk of experiencing vicarious trauma (Urquhart Law et al., 2009), anxiety, frustration, and the need to use defense mechanisms, such as emotional distancing and displacement, that can harm the very person whom nurses are there to help (McAllister, 2001).

In contrast, clinicians who respond with empathy, assume a nonjudgmental stance, facilitate connection and limit setting and provide supportive counselling skills have a positive effect on outcomes for clients (Kool, van Meijel, & Bosman, 2009). Clients report feeling less distressed and are more likely to stay for treatment, to use the health service again rather than attempt to inadequately self-manage, and to accept organized follow-up care under such circumstances (Shaw, 2002; Sinclair & Green, 2005). This relationship suggests that nurses can do a great deal to instill hope, facilitate effective meaning making, and, importantly, provide supportive connections for these clients.

It is not sufficient to prepare nurses to be proficient in technical procedures in this kind of situation. Rather, what they need is a collaborative way of working with both clients and colleagues, one that is actively peace building, so that the negative emotions generated in such an encounter are prevented or contained. It is crucial that nurses be part of the solution, as this adaptation of bell hooks' words (1994) reflects:

> When those who know oppress and dominate others and continue to discriminate and attempt to disempower, then they become part of the problem.

Toward a Power-Building Practice

At some level, nurses who are complicit in allowing a disempowering environment to persist are likely unhappy and unfulfilled; this factor may account for why so many become disenchanted with their work and leave the profession. It is crucial that nurses find a way to circumvent this situation, by inventing a way of working that gives nurses responsibility for engendering a supportive environment. In this framework of care, it is not just technical skills that are important; rather, the psychosocial health and well-being of all players must be a paramount concern.

Solution-focused nursing is a philosophy of care that I developed after years of being confronted with the reality that nurses do tend to take a reactive approach with patients (McAllister, 2007). Nurses have a tendency to be concerned with problems, and problem resolution, rather than to employ an approach that is preventive, strategic, and proactive. Perhaps this tendency explains why the nurse in Zara's story was very efficient at responding to his client's pain. He has assessed the person's physiological status and gathered some baseline data on the severity and nature of the discomfort. Unfortunately, he has not been equally adept at engendering a comfortable, comforting environment for the person. A clinical colleague has acted tactlessly, even damagingly, but the nurse has not felt in a position to act—either in reaction to the clinician's thoughtlessness or preemptively.

This failure to act is not surprising. In most health service cultures, the dominant philosophy is one that favors a problem orientation and a medical model. In this worldview, it is the person's presenting problems or illnesses that take priority, and the concern is to stabilize the body, whether the issue at hand be the physical or psychological parts of that body. Further, in this model, the nurse's role is primarily that of assistant to medical practitioners, with the goal to ameliorate suffering and promote restoration of health and well-being.

Consider this quotation discussing why clinicians negatively label and ostracize clients such as these:

> When time and resources are limited and no one really knows how best to help, it's easier to make judgments and use labels than to spend time looking for possible causes of distress. (Harrison, 1994, p. 4)

Yet health services will always have limited resources, and clients who present for emergency care will always have more concerns than just their physical ailment. As human service workers, it is a health professional's responsibility to know how to act in compassionate, yet effective ways.

Moving Toward Empowerment

The approach presented here is drawn from critical social theory and the positive psychology movement, with the goal of seeing which other possibilities emerge for nursing practice. Critical social theory alerts us to the reality that people in society who are in submissive or marginalized positions—in this situation, patients—are likely to have power removed from them, to not be free to speak their minds, and to experience further effects of being oppressed and alienated. These effects typically include both self-directed hostility and violence, anger, and avoidance directed toward others (Roberts, DeMarco, & Griffin, 2009). Critical social theory suggests that power needs to be shifted so that it is shared between the people in positions of authority and those who are subordinate (Brookfield, 2005). In health services, there is a desire to encourage clients to take a more active role in their own health care and to be more responsible service users; thus such an approach makes perfect sense in this setting. Clinicians who share power with clients, and who are explanatory, consultative, and collaborative, are more likely to achieve their service goals. Adopting this approach, by its nature, ensures a proactive role for clinicians such as nurses.

Positive psychology says that people are more likely to become healthy when their strengths and capacities are being tapped. In contrast, when there is over-focus on the person's vulnerabilities and deficiencies, the client and the caregiver can begin to lose hope, become helpless, and give up (Seligman, 2002). In such cases, chronicity, depression. and a self-fulfilling prophecy of doom and gloom can set in (Johnson, 2005).

Models of care are subtle and can become so deeply embedded in clinicians' daily working life that they are reproduced unconsciously, without thought. When they are subjected to critical reflection, however, they can be challenged and replaced. Many nurses probably feel uncomfortable with the degree of influence the medical model has over their professional practice. Yet, because the medical model is the most familiar worldview in health services, it is also the perspective that people will tend to resort to when they lack an alternative. Critical social theory would urge that alternative worldviews be brought in from the margins and consciously used so that the new perspectives begin to compete with the taken-for-granted medical model.

One effective way that nurses can challenge themselves to not unconsciously reproduce the medical model in their day-to-day interactions with clients is to exercise their abstract, creative brain, thereby rethinking practice—a process known as conscientization (Freire, 1972; Martin & Younger, 2000). Harden (1996) argues that such a process is crucial for all groups seeking emancipation. She states that only when oppression in nursing has been recognized, and a critical consciousness achieved, can true humanistic care be given. Try the consciousness-raising activity shown here to see how the conscientization process works.

Box 12–1 See with New Eyes

Go to a collection of paintings by Frida Kahlo (e.g., in Herrera, 1991), and find the picture entitled *The Little Deer.* Complete a surface-level reading of this picture, by writing down all of the elements you see within the frame.

Now try to look more deeply and make an attempt to answer these questions:

- Imagine this "person" is the client in the story just recounted. How might she be feeling? Which factors are contributing to this feeling state?
- Where is the light coming from in this painting? What might it signify?
- If the role of the nurse is to take the person from a position of darkness and fear to a position of light and comfort, what could a nurse do if he or she was painted into this frame?

Frida Kahlo, the Mexican artist, has created many vivid, evocative expressions (many of them autobiographical) of the experience of pain and vulnerability. In this and other paintings of hers, one gets a sense of here strength, endurance, and resilience. Through all this pain and loneliness, her spirit retains its power.

At a conference on nursing practice development, I showed this image to attendees to promote thought on reframing care by thinking about the lived experience of being a patient and being in pain. I asked participants to tell me what they saw in this image, what it meant to them. The insights drawn from the audience remain with me, and perhaps they resonate for other nurses as well: that people can be wounded, in pain, dehumanized, lost, vulnerable, and at risk, but that good nursing care—good health care—comes when clinicians are able to be with clients, and perhaps reorient them. Just by turning around and facing a new direction, we can help to show clients ways out of their dilemmas. In short, good health care is about finding ways to turn crises into turning points.

Thinking about this image and the role of nursing whenever nurses find themselves in a difficult position with clients or colleagues is illuminating. It suggests a way forward, emphasizes shared humanity, and encourages nurses to notice people's inherent strengths that can be enduring even within hardships and challenges.

SOLUTION-FOCUSED NURSING

Many nursing scholars argue for a model of practice that is anti-oppressive, but do not clearly show how such a model may be created (Hopton, 1997; Martin & Younger, 2000). Solution-focused nursing attempts to fill this gap by stating a simple philosophy and clarifying practices that nurses can use in a range of healthcare situations. SFN comprises six principles, as outlined in **Table 12–1**.

Table 12–1 The Principles of Solution-Focused Nursing

1. The person, not the problem, is at the center of inquiry.
2. Problems and strengths may be present at all times. Looking for and then developing inner strengths and resources will be affirming and assist in coping and adaptation. By working with what is going right with a client, the nurse can enhance the client's hope, optimism, and self-belief, thereby maximizing his or her health capacity.
3. Resilience is as important as vulnerability.
4. The nurse's role moves beyond illness care toward adaptation and recovery.
5. The goal is to create change at three levels: in the client, nursing, and society.
6. The way of being with clients is proactive, rather than reactive.

This model of care is very much focused on achieving empowerment for clients and emancipation for nursing. Whereas clients may have been overlooked, patronized, and marginalized in the healthcare relationship, nurses may have similarly had their power constrained and their potential reduced.

In addition to principles and phases of the working relationship, several concepts inherent to empowerment need close analysis and perhaps reframing. These are power, skill, awareness, and language (**Table 12–2**).

Table 12–2 Elements of Empowerment

Power	Rather than avoid power, nurses can see power as having positive influence, as being a resource to be shared, and as something that can be used "softly."
Nursing skill	The skill of nursing is not just about technical proficiency, nor is it something that remains within the individual nurse's sphere of ownership. Skill also refers to being able to be with a patient supportively—that is, knowing what not to say as well as how best to communicate. Skill is something to be shared, both with clients and with colleagues. It is in the sharing where sustainable development occurs and advancements are to be made.
Awareness	Awareness is a state of being as well as a goal within the nurse–client relationship. Being aware means not being unconscious to the practices that keep groups disempowered. Achieving awareness as a goal refers to the sharing of knowledge, skills, and understanding.
Language	Language provides the codes through which we talk about and understand the world we live in. Language transmits powerful messages. Unconscious use of language can lead to oppression and ongoing marginalization. Conscious usage can be the tool by which nurses move toward an alternative to dominating practices.

It is not uncommon for clinicians working in a deficit model to feel disempowered, out of their depth, and directionless. For example, in their study, Bowles, Mackintosh, and Torn (2001) identified that expressions like this were commonly uttered by nurses: "I really didn't feel like I was offering anything in terms of solutions." Nurses also felt as if they had no direction with patients. One nurse said, "[There was] lots of waffling going on; I let people waffle . . . I was a good listener—I can listen for weeks with no solution in sight."

Educational interventions that provide communication training (Bowles et al., 2001; Polaschek & Polaschek, 2007) do have positive effects. In my own study, I was able to demonstrate that not only did the nurse participants report more understanding and tolerance for the patients' concerns following receipt of such an intervention, but they also developed new response skills, such as the ability to ask more focused uqestions and to communicate in more supportive and motivating ways (McAllister, Moyle, Billett, & Zimmer-Gembeck, 2009).

After training in SFN, participants said things like this:

- "I definitely feel more confident with the communication side of it. It doesn't actually take that much time. You can say, 'Hi, this is my name, I'm really glad you came in and I'm here to help you."

- "I am more tolerant now. If I feel frustrated, I step back away from it and leave it to the [mental health] professionals but without producing a negative effect by putting attitude into it—you know, do no harm."
- "I can recommend to patients that there are ways to break the cycle and take some proactive ways to deal with their lives. Knowing that you don't have to fix everybody's problems takes away the pressure of feeling that you're not doing anything for the person."
- "I can actually—if they're willing to—talk to them about why they did it, that they are not alone and that they should be here, this is where they are supposed to be. There was one person; I said to her, 'It's okay—you need to be here, you're not wasting a bed, and we want you here,' and she felt a lot better in herself."

The SFN Difference

Instead of looking only for causes of problems, clinicians trained in solution-focused nursing began to rely less on expert-centered interventions and more on strategies to help clients construct their own solutions to their present difficulties. This requires not just verbal skills but also therapeutic engagement, the ability to gently probe and challenge, the ability to facilitate goal setting, and the capacity to motivate change (McKergow & Clarke, 2007).

In addition, instead of being focused only on the present—for example, the fact that the client has once again returned to the service for the exact same problem—SFN shifts the orientation toward the future, where the clinician is attempting to facilitate transitions for clients, and transforming the present crisis into a turning point. From this standpoint, the clinician is not just interested in treating problems, but in promoting future health and well-being. Thinking about the future is an important change for nurses—it means that they do not become preoccupied with just what is happening in the present. This subtle shift can be liberating for both clients and nurses. In mental health, this perspective seems particularly important. Consider, for example, the person who feels depressed. Present feelings of sadness, hopelessness, and pain are important for the empathic nurse to acknowledge and even to explore, but equally important are attempts to de-emphasize, shift, and de-center the negative emotions so that the person can notice small changes and develop hope for the future.

SFN Goals: Targeted at Three Levels

Unlike most other nursing theories, SFN targets three areas for change: the client, the nurses themselves, and society. That is, a nurse's focus may be at the interpersonal level between client and nurse, at the social level between colleagues, and at the cultural level with groups. This multiple-level approach acknowledges two key truths: Not only do challenges arise in all three of these areas, but solutions to challenges affecting clients may sometimes be found by effecting changes in the world *around* them, rather than directly through them. For example, when a client requires a predictable, safe, and reliable environment, nurses need to behave cohesively as a single unit. When the nurse aims to create change at the social level and encourages team solidarity, the client may benefit.

Three Phases of Care

The SFN approach involves three phases: joining, building, and extending.

Joining

In the joining phase, effort is made to get to know who the person is, what his or her strengths and vulnerabilities are, and what the nature of the client's condition is, both physically and psychosocially. It is important to notice and develop areas in the person that are healthy and adaptive, as this reinforcement leads to appropriate behavior.

In Zara's case, the nurse could have used the time when he was measuring her vital signs to spend just a few moments engaging the client. This requires a conscious stance wherein you move away from the position of detached, dispassionate expert and become someone who is—to put it simply—human. In this way, a connection is made based on what is shared between a client and a clinician, rather than what keeps them separate. In the scenario with the Zara, the nurse might say:

> Zara, my name is Paul. I'm your nurse. You must be feeling awful [wait and listen]—being in pain, being here alone. You have made a good decision in getting help now. I need to tell you that there will be a wait ahead because the team is really busy here.
>
> By trying to relax, you may help to contain the pain. Have you found, in the past, effective ways to be calm? How would you feel about using those strategies or some that I could suggest?

Even if answers from the client are not forthcoming, the nurse has made an effort to show his concern and opened up a pathway to collaboration. Such an introduction sets a respectful tone, and invites the person to become active in his or her own health care.

Building

In the building phase, the aim is to be educative and supportive. Empowerment is all about giving the skills to clients so that they can better understand health and well-being and better self-manage. It aims to develop in the client a sense of capability and inner strength, and to provide motivation to get through the present health challenge.

Solution-focused nursing is not about a forced optimism. It is also not about being solution forced, because it involves appreciation for the fact that people have vulnerabilities as well as strengths. Thus, in a respectful, empowering relationship, the person feels both supported and motivated. Skill deficits (such as ways to relax and relieve head tension) and excesses (such as the mechanism of self-injury, which can be very effective in managing pent-up distress) can be discussed as part of the building phase.

In emergency health care, such as in Zara's case, the building phase may be brief, perhaps taking only a few minutes, but it is nonetheless at the heart of the nurse–client relationship. Without the building phase, nursing work has no purpose. This step may be as simple as conveying the value of optimism in change or as complex as showing a client ways to self-manage a chronic, debilitating disease. Once the nurse knows the source of Zara's headache, for example, he might say this:

> Zara, this kind of headache is something that, with effort, you could minimize and even prevent. Would you like to learn more about factors that influence headaches?

Together, the nurse and the client might work on building a repertoire of coping skills to help with the immediate situation, talking through issues such as relationships, tension management, and being both capable and strong while simultaneously feeling vulnerable and emotional. This discussion may help to build up in the client feelings of optimism, so that the client can adapt, recover, and get stronger in the longer term.

In this phase, the work may not be exclusively focused on the nurse–client relationship. Indeed, nurses may find that the necessary change exists within their own workplace culture and not within the client. Solution-focused nursing sees that the possibilities for change rest equally within the cultural and social sphere and within the client relationship. This notion is quite a departure from the medical model, and even from other nursing models that emphasize and centralize concern for the individual client (Gordon, 1994; Roper, Logan, & Tierney, 1980). The implication of these models is that the profession of nursing plays no part in creating and sustaining ill health, when, all too often, it patently does.

Zara's experience clearly demonstrates the importance of recognizing the nurse's role in engendering ill health. The nurse in her story, by failing to intervene tactfully and assertively with the doctor, is being complicit in harmful care. Conversely, in being ethical and empowering, nurses have a duty and a moral obligation to protect the person's dignity. But how does one act in a delicate situation such as this scenario? Again, the answers rest in simply being human—in thinking of a way to be empathic and respectful, yet advocating for better care for clients. You could say to the doctor at an appropriate time:

> Sue, got a few minutes? I noticed back there with Zara that you looked uncomfortable and you didn't speak much to her. [Waits and listens] . . . It's a challenge sometimes to be nonjudgmental, yet it's so important. Want to talk some more about this?

Thus the SFN model values moving beyond individual-focused care, to valuing the role of social and cultural care. It involves noticing discourses, practices, actions, and inactions that constrain, obscure, or mislead nurses' aim to be empowering and enabling, and it requires nurses to suggest more enabling ways of thinking about and practicing nursing and health care.

Extending

In the extending phase, the emphasis is on encouraging the person to transfer the skills learned in the nurse–client relationship so they can be used in other contexts, such as when the individual is faced with upsetting social situations. It also involves ensuring that the client has social supports that can be used in place of the clinician–client relationship and, therefore, will be more enduring and sustainable.

In Zara's case, this phase would be brief—perhaps a matter of seconds. Time and duration are not important. Rather, the key issue is conveying the belief that change has been made, and that the way ahead is positive are. You could say:

> If you need help again, Zara, you know what to do and you know more about ways to self-manage, yeah? [Waits for confirmation]

Note that all of these examples of being solution focused are not unidirectional, which is often the case in expert-care models, but rather that the model emphasizes working alongside the client and negotiating care with that individual. The nurse relies on the client giving feedback that the message has been received. The nurse makes an effort to engage in conversation and real dialogue. The belief is that in a partnership model, the person is more likely to feel understood, cared for, and motivated to resume self-caring work.

CONCLUSION

Positive nursing strategies are about taking action, in the knowledge that small steps in the right direction can have a huge impact. They focus on nurturing the things you want to grow—in clients, in the relationship, and in the health service culture. They encourage innovation, creativity, and bright ideas. Solution-focused nursing is about moving beyond the routine and mechanical, in the knowledge that technical competence is only half of the story with nursing practice. It means making a commitment to collaborate, to question, to practice humanism in the everyday, and to have the courage to do things differently.

For a full suite of assignments and additional learning activities, use the access code located in the front of your book to visit this exclusive website: http://go.jblearning.com/dechesnay. If you do not have an access code, you can obtain one at the site.

REFERENCES

Barnes, G., Mitic, W., Leadbeater, B., & Dhami, M. (2009). Risk and protective factors for adolescent substance use and mental health symptoms. *Canadian Journal of Community Mental Health*, *28*(1), 1–15.

Bowles, N., Mackintosh, C., & Torn, A. (2001). Nurses' communication skills: An evaluation of the impact of solution-focused communication training. *Journal of Advanced Nursing*, *36*(3), 347–354.

Brand, C., Kennedy, M., MacBean, C., Sundararajan ,V., & Taylor, D. (2005). *Patients who "leave without being seen" (LWBS) from an emergency department.* Literature review commissioned by the Department of Human Services Victoria. Melbourne, Australia.

Brookfield, S., (2005). *The power of critical theory: Liberating adult learning and teaching.* San Francisco: Teachers College Record.

Cook, S., Clancy, C., & Sanderson, S. (2004). Self-harm and suicide: Care, interventions and policy. *Nursing Standard, 18*(43), 43–55.

Crawford, M., & Kumar, P. (2007). Intervention following deliberate self-harm: Enough evidence to act? *Evidence Based Mental Health, 10*, 37–39 doi: 10.1136/ebmh.10.2.37

Estefan, A., McAllister, M., & Rowe, J. (2004). Difference, dialogue and dialectics: A study of caring and self-harm. In K. Kavanagh & V. Knowlden (Eds.), *Interpretive studies in healthcare and the human sciences. Volume III: Many voices: Toward caring culture in healthcare and healing* (pp. 21–61). Madison, WI: University of Wisconsin Press.

Freire, P. (1972). *Pedagogy of the oppressed.* Harmondsworth: Penguin.

Gordon, M. (1994). *Nursing diagnosis: Process and application* (3rd ed.). St. Louis, MO: Mosby.

Hall, B. (1996). The psychiatric model: A critical analysis of its undermining effects on nursing in chronic mental illness. *Advanced Nursing Science, 18*(3), 16–26.

Harden, J. (1996). Enlightenment, empowerment and emancipation: The case for critical pedagogy in nurse education. *Nurse Education Today, 16*(1), 32–37.

Harrison, D. (1994). *Understanding self-harm.* London: Mind Publications.

Herrera, H. (1991). *The little deer.* In *Frida Kahlo: The paintings.* (p. 189). London: Bloomsbury.

Hickie, I., Groom, G., McGorry, P., Davenport.T., & Luscombe,G., (2005). Australian mental health reform: time for real outcomes. *Medical Journal of Australia, 182*(8), 401–406.

Hooks, B. (1994). *Teaching to transgress: Education as the practice of freedom.* New York: Routledge.

Hopton, J. (1997). Towards anti-oppressive practice in mental health nursing. *British Journal of Nursing, 6*(15), 874–878.

Johnson, B. (2005). Overcoming "doom and gloom": Empowering students in courses on social problems, injustice and inequality. *Teaching Sociology, 33*(1), 44–58.

Kendall-Tackett, K. (2003). *Treating the long-term health effects of childhood abuse: A guide for medical, mental health, and social service professionals.* Kingston, NJ: Civic Research Institute.

Kool, N., van Meijel, B., & Bosman, M. (2009). Behavioral change in patients with severe self-injurious behavior: A patient's perspective. *Archives of Psychiatric Nursing, 23*(1), 25–31.

Link, B., & Phelan, J. (2006). Stigma and its public health implications. *Lancet, 367*, 528–529.

Lopez, S., & Gallagher, M. (2009). A case for positive psychology. In C. Snyder & S. Lopez (Eds.), *Oxford handbook of positive psychology* (2nd ed., pp. 3–6). New York: Oxford University Press.

Martin, G., & Younger, D. (2000). Anti oppressive practice: A route to the empowerment of people with dementia through communication and choice. *Journal of Psychiatric & Mental Health Nursing, 7*(1), 59–67.

McAllister, M. (2001). In harm's way: Hidden aspects of deliberate self harm. *Journal of Psychiatric and Mental Health Nursing, 8*(5), 391–398.

McAllister, M. (Ed.). (2007). *Solution focused nursing: Rethinking practice.* London: Macmillan-Palgrave.

McAllister, M., Moyle, W., Billett, S., & Zimmer-Gembeck, M. (2009). "I can actually talk to them now": Qualitative results of an educational intervention for emergency nurses caring for clients who self-harm. *Journal of Clinical Nursing, 18*(20), 2838–2845.

McCann, T., Clark, E., McConnachie, S., & Harvey, I. (2006). Accident and emergency nurses' attitudes towards patients who self-harm. *Accident and Emergency Nursing, 14*(1), 4–10.

McKergow, M., & Clarke, J. (2007). *Solutions focus working: 80 real life lessons for successful organisational change.* London: Solutions Books.

Polaschek, L., & Polaschek, N. (2007). Solution-focused conversations: A new therapeutic strategy in well child health nursing telephone consultations. *Journal of Advanced Nursing, 59*(2), 111–119.

Roberts, S., DeMarco, R., & Griffin, M. (2009). The effect of oppressed group behaviours on the culture of the nursing workplace: A review of the evidence and interventions for change. *Journal of Nursing Management, 17*(3), 288–293.

Roper, N., Logan, W., & Tierney, A. (1980). *The elements of nursing.* Edinburgh: Churchill Livingstone.

Seligman, M. (2002). Positive psychology, positive prevention and positive therapy. In C. Snyder & S. Lopez (Eds.), *Handbook of positive psychology* (pp. 3–6). Oxford, UK: Oxford University Press.

Shaw, N. (2002). Shifting conversations on girls' and women's self-injury: An analysis of the clinical literature in historical context. *Feminism and Psychology, 12*(2), 191–219.

Sinclair, J., & Green, J. (2005). Understanding resolution of deliberate self harm: Qualitative interview study of patients' experiences. *British Medical Journal, 14*(7500), 111.

Sutton, J. (2007). *Healing the hurt within: Understand self-injury and self-harm, and heal the emotional wounds* (3rd ed.). Oxford, UK: How to Books.

Urquhart Law, G., Rostill-Brookes, H., & Goodman, D. (2009). Public stigma in health and non-healthcare students: Attributions, emotions and willingness to help with adolescent self-harm. *International Journal of Nursing Studies, 46*, 108–119.

CHAPTER 13

Using Self-efficacy Theory to Help Vulnerable Women Breastfeed

Janet L. Engstrom and Paula P. Meier

Objectives

At the end of this chapter, the reader will be able to

1. Review the beneficial effects of breastfeeding.
2. Discuss Bandura's Self-Efficacy Theory as a framework for helping vulnerable women breastfeed.
3. Describe a model that incorporates teaching mothers to breastfeed as an outcome of evidence-based research.

The beneficial health and economic outcomes of breastfeeding are well documented for infants and mothers in both developed and developing countries (Bartick & Reinhold, 2010; Horta, Bahl, Martines, & Victora, 2007; Ip et al., 2007). The nutritional, bioactive, and epigenetic components of human milk ensure better lifetime health for infants, and the lactation process protects mothers from certain cancers and other chronic illnesses long after breastfeeding ceases (Horta et al., 2007; Ip et al., 2007). These better health outcomes translate into health care and societal cost savings equal to billions of dollars annually in the United States alone (Ball & Wright, 1999; Bartick & Reinhold, 2010; Weimer, 2001). These findings form the basis for national health objectives and statements from professional health organizations that prioritize the initiation, continuation, and exclusivity of breastfeeding.

Unfortunately, despite the known health and economic advantages of breastfeeding for the family and society, many women in the United States do not initiate breastfeeding or continue to breastfeed exclusively for the recommended length of time (Centers for Disease Control and Prevention [CDC], 2010a). Breastfeeding rates for initiation, continuation, and exclusivity are lowest among the most vulnerable women and infants, particularly among low-income, adolescent, African American, and rural mothers and infants (CDC, 2010a, 2010d).

This chapter uses self-efficacy theory (Bandura, 1977, 1982, 1994, 1997) as a framework for helping vulnerable women breastfeed their infants. It begins with a review of the beneficial health and economic outcomes of breastfeeding, including a brief overview of the mechanisms by which human milk and the processes of lactation protect the infant and the mother. Also included are official recommendations for the initiation, continuation, and exclusivity of breastfeeding, which are compared with current breastfeeding rates in the United States. Self-efficacy theory is reviewed and applied to breastfeeding scenarios using evidence-based examples of effective breastfeeding interventions. The chapter concludes with an example of a breastfeeding program that applies self-efficacy theory to help vulnerable women breastfeed and/or provide their own milk for their infants.

HEALTH AND ECONOMIC BENEFITS OF BREASTFEEDING

The specific beneficial health outcomes of human milk are numerous, and include optimal growth and protection from specific illnesses during infancy and throughout the life span (American Academy of Pediatrics [AAP], 2005; Horta et al., 2007; Ip et al., 2007). Breastfed infants are significantly less likely than formula-fed infants to develop gastrointestinal illness, acute otitis media, lower respiratory infections, childhood asthma, atopic dermatitis, obesity, types 1 and 2 diabetes, cardiovascular disease, childhood leukemia, sudden infant death syndrome, and other causes of infant death (AAP, 2005; Horta et al., 2007; Ip et al., 2007). Breastfed infants also have higher scores on intelligence tests and better school performance than their formula-fed counterparts (AAP, 2005; Horta et al., 2007; Oddy, Li, Whitehouse, Zubrick, & Malacova, 2011). Premature infants who are fed their mothers' human milk rather than formula have a lower risk of prematurity-specific diseases such as late-onset sepsis, necrotizing enterocolitis, chronic lung disease, retinopathy of prematurity, adverse neurodevelopmental outcome, and rehospitalization after discharge from the neonatal intensive care unit (NICU) (AAP, 2005; Meier, Engstrom, Patel, Jegier, & Bruns, 2010; Patel, Meier, & Engstrom, 2007).

The mechanisms by which breastfeeding affects short- and long-term health outcomes in recipient infants are complex, and are based on the fact that human milk modulates and programs many structural and functional processes during a critical period of human development (Meier et al., 2010). For example, the various components in human milk function synergistically to catalyze tissue growth in the gastrointestinal tract, modulate the immune response, activate enzymes, and "turn on" genetic pathways in the young infant (Meier et al., 2010). These processes occur during a critical window of development in the early post-birth period and have lifelong effects (Meier et al., 2010).

From a nutritional perspective, human milk contains unique types and numbers of species-specific proteins, lipids, and oligosaccharides that are not present in the same form or number in other mammals' milks, and cannot be replicated in commercial infant formulas (AAP, 2005). This unique mixture serves as a nutraceutical, meaning that human milk contains health-promoting nutrients (Baldi & Pinotti, 2008). Indeed, scientists classify human milk as a "medicinal food" or an "edible immunoprotectant."

Human milk also contains an extensive number of bioactive components with immunomodulatory, anti-infective, anti-inflammatory, antioxidant, growth-promoting, and epigenetic actions (Meier et al., 2010; Patel et al., 2007). These substances facilitate the initial colonization of the intestinal tract with commensal bacteria, which serve to downregulate inflammatory processes that are precursors to later health problems such as inflammatory bowel disease, diabetes, and allergic disease (Meier et al., 2010; Patel et al., 2007). Many of these components have a programming or epigenetic role in the immature intestine, such that they change the structure, function, or genetic expression of cells and organs, which has implications for health through the life span (Meier et al., 2010; Patel et al., 2007). Additionally, human milk contains large numbers of undifferentiated stem cells, which have the potential to evolve into a variety of structures over time (Meier et al., 2010; Patel et al., 2007).

Mothers also benefit from the process of lactation. Women who breastfeed their infants have a lower risk of breast and ovarian cancer, type 2 diabetes, hypertension, hyperlipidemia, and cardiovascular disease (Ip et al., 2007; Schwarz, Ray, Stuebe, Allison, Ness, Freiberg, & Cauley, 2009; Stuebe, Rich-Edwards, Willett, Manson, & Michels, 2005). Breastfeeding also confers substantial financial benefits to families. Families save approximately $1200 to $1500 per year by not purchasing infant formula (United States Breastfeeding Committee [USBC], 2002). Families whose infants are breastfeed also save money in healthcare expenses and time lost from work (Weimer, 2001). In the United States, the infant health benefits conferred by breastfeeding translate into billions of dollars of saved healthcare costs (Bartick & Reinhold, 2010; Weimer, 2001).

RECOMMENDATIONS FOR BREASTFEEDING

The beneficial health outcomes of breastfeeding are so well established that health organizations and professional societies uniformly recommend breastfeeding as the optimal method of infant feeding for almost all mothers and infants (AAP, 2005; USBC, 2001; World Health Organization [WHO], 2011). WHO and AAP recommend that human milk (also known as breast milk or mother's milk) be the *only* food given to infants until complementary foods are introduced at approximately 6 months of age. Breastfeeding should continue along with the feeding of complementary foods at least until the child reaches one (AAP) to two years of age (WHO).

CURRENT BREASTFEEDING STATISTICS

Breastfeeding rates are assessed by three measures: initiation, continuation, and exclusivity. Initiation is defined as any breastfeeding such that the infant received any of the mother's milk for any length of time (CDC, 2010c). Recent data indicate that the percentage of women who initiate breastfeeding after birth has recently reached the *Healthy People 2010* goal of 75% (CDC, 2010a, 2010b). Even so, this rate falls far below the levels achieved in other developed countries; in the Scandinavian countries, for example, breastfeeding initiation rates approach 100% (Callen & Pinelli, 2004). Additionally, there are noticeable differences in terms of which women initiate breastfeeding. The women most likely to initiate breastfeeding are white, married, well educated, more affluent, and older (CDC, 2010a, 2010d). In contrast, only 59.7% of

African American women initiate breastfeeding, and lower rates of initiation are also observed in other vulnerable populations such as adolescents (59.7%), low-income women (67%), and rural women (66.4%) (CDC, 2010a).

Continuation, or duration, of breastfeeding is a measure of how long a mother continues to breastfeed her infant. Although the number of women who initiate breastfeeding may have reached the national target, continuation rates in the United States are below the recommendations set in the *Healthy People 2010* and *Healthy People 2020* goals (CDC, 2010b, 2011). The *Healthy People 2010* national targets were 50% for continuation of breastfeeding at 6 months after birth, and 25% for continuation of breastfeeding at 12 months (CDC, 2010b). The *Healthy People 2020* targets are 60.5% for continuation of breastfeeding at 6 months after birth, and 34.1% for continuation of breastfeeding at 12 months (CDC, 2011). Recent data indicate that breastfeeding continuation rates decline precipitously in the first days and weeks after birth. By 6 months after birth, only 43% of women are still breastfeeding, and only 22.4% of women breastfeed for the recommended year (CDC, 2010a). These numbers are even lower in vulnerable mothers, with only 27.9% of African American women breastfeeding for 6 months and just 12.9% continuing breastfeeding for the recommended minimum of 12 months (CDC, 2010a). Similarly, only 22.2% of adolescent women continue breastfeeding for 6 months and only 10.7% for 12 months (CDC, 2010a).

Exclusivity of breastfeeding is defined as giving no food to the infant other than human milk. Although human milk is recommended as the only food for the first 6 months of life, many women supplement their breastfeeding with commercial infant formula or other fluids and foods; this supplementation often begins early in the breastfeeding process. Recent data demonstrate that within the first 2 days after birth, 25.4% of women supplement their breastfeeding with infant formula (CDC, 2010a). By the time children reach 3 months of age, only 33% of women are still breastfeeding exclusively; only 13.3% breastfeed exclusively for the recommended 6 months (CDC, 2010a). These health statistics demonstrate the need for effective interventions to increase the number of women—particularly vulnerable women—who initiate and continue exclusive breastfeeding.

SELF-EFFICACY THEORY AND BREASTFEEDING

Self-efficacy theory can be used as a framework for designing and implementing interventions to help vulnerable women initiate and continue breastfeeding (Dennis, 1999). Self-efficacy is defined as a person's belief or perception about whether he or she can accomplish a task or achieve a goal (Bandura, 1994). Developed by Bandura (1977), this theory proposes that a person's sense of confidence or "self-efficacy" influences whether that individual will attempt and be successful at the activity. Self-efficacy theory has been used extensively in healthcare research, and a large body of research demonstrates that interventions that help people develop self-efficacy are effective methods of changing health behavior (Bandura, 1997). Self-efficacy theory is especially relevant for helping women breastfeed because research demonstrates that a woman's confidence in her ability to breastfeed is an important predictor of whether she will initiate and continue breastfeeding (Dunn, Davies, McCleary, Edwards, & Gaboury, 2005; Mossman, Heaman, Dennis, & Morris, 2008; Thulier & Mercer, 2009). Thus, interventions that target self-efficacy should positively affect the initiation, continuation, and exclusivity of breastfeeding.

The impact of developing a sense of self-efficacy is far greater than the success of achieving one goal or mastering a single activity, even a complex activity with long term health consequences such as breastfeeding. Being successful at an activity enhances a personal sense of self-efficacy and this sense of self-efficacy transfers to other activities (Bandura, 1994). People who have a well-developed sense of self-efficacy feel good about themselves. Self-efficacy reduces the amount of stress perceived by the person and reduces the risk of depression and anxiety (Bandura, 1982). Thus, there are tremendous social and health benefits to developing self-efficacy, and self-efficacy can lead to a change in behavior and, ultimately, social change (Bandura, 1994, 1997).

FACTORS THAT INFLUENCE THE DEVELOPMENT OF SELF-EFFICACY

Four factors influence the development of self-efficacy: mastery experiences, vicarious experience, social persuasion, and a person's perception of his or her physical and psychological state (Bandura, 1977, 1994). These factors can be used to design and implement interventions to develop breastfeeding self-efficacy, especially in vulnerable populations. The development of interventions to increase self-efficacy is important because many of the other factors associated with low breastfeeding rates are demographic (e.g., income, education, race) (CDC, 2010a), and cannot be influenced by healthcare professionals (Dennis, 1999).

Building Mastery Experiences for Breastfeeding

Experiences of mastery are the most important factor in building self-efficacy (Bandura, 1994). Experiences perceived as successes build self-efficacy, whereas experiences perceived as failures impede the development of self-efficacy (Bandura, 1994). Breastfeeding presents unique challenges to the development of mastery because mothers do not have the opportunity to practice or acquire skill in breastfeeding until they are faced with a newborn infant who needs to be fed. Mothers are particularly vulnerable during this time, so that the threat of "failure" may seem overwhelming to them. New mothers know that they are directly responsible for their infants' growth and well-being, and they fear the consequences if breastfeeding is not successful. Further, the initiation of breastfeeding during the immediate post-birth period is often characterized by a complex interaction between an inexperienced mother whose milk supply is not yet established and a newly born infant who must be able to suck effectively to obtain milk and trigger the lactation hormones that are necessary to establish the mother's milk supply.

The challenges to establishing breastfeeding in the early post-birth period make breastfeeding support essential. Numerous studies have demonstrated the importance of support in breastfeeding continuation (Britton, McCormick, Renfrew, Wade, & King, 2007; Shealy, Li, Benton-Davis, & Grummer-Strawn, 2005). Breastfeeding support includes many components.

Women need emotional support and encouragement as well as access to specific breastfeeding knowledge and skills. Breastfeeding support is especially important for vulnerable women who may experience cultural and economic barriers to establishing breastfeeding in addition to the challenges typically experienced by most breastfeeding mothers. During the first two weeks after birth, mothers are most likely to experience the problems that typically result in early discontinuation of breastfeeding, such as perceived inadequate milk supply and sore nipples (Chapman & Perez-Escamilla, 2000). Timely access to a knowledgeable and skilled lactation care is essential during this critical period, especially for vulnerable mothers who may be pressured by friends and family members to "just use formula" to ensure the baby's well-being.

Mastery experiences should be structured to build self-efficacy (Bandura, 1994). For breastfeeding, this means supporting the mother and anticipating her concerns as she begins breastfeeding, rather than waiting until she encounters difficulties to offer help. Bandura (1994) recommends using aids to mastery such as modeling the activity, breaking the activity down into easily managed smaller steps, and performing the activities with an experienced guide. Thus, breastfeeding support should be provided by someone who can guide the mother through the process and who has the skills needed to assist the mother with the most basic of breastfeeding practices, such as assistance with positioning and latch as well as common problems such as sore nipples and perceived inadequate milk supply.

Other interventions may also help women develop mastery. For a mother who is worried about whether her infant is "getting enough" during breastfeeding, milk intake can be measured easily and quickly by weighing the baby before and after a feeding, a procedure known as test-weighing. When an appropriate scale is used, this procedure accurately estimates the volume of intake even for the smallest feedings in premature infants (Meier, Engstrom, Crichton, Clark, Williams, & Mangurten, 1994). Research has demonstrated that this procedure is very reassuring to mothers (Hurst, Meier, Engstrom, & Myatt, 2004), and it can be used to help a mother have confidence that her infant is "getting enough" during breastfeeding. Seeing her infant gain weight during a feeding can help a woman develop a sense of breastfeeding mastery and confidence in her ability to adequately nourish her baby.

Similarly, for a mother who worries that her milk is "not rich enough," a creamatocrit test can be performed using her milk. This procedure, which provides an accurate estimate of the lipid and caloric content of the milk, is quick and can easily be performed by mothers (Griffin, Meier, Bradford, Bigger, & Engstrom, 2000; Meier et al., 2006). Research has demonstrated that mothers are reassured by learning that their milk is "rich enough" to help their baby grow (Griffin et al., 2000).

Providing Vicarious Experiences for Breastfeeding

The second method of developing self-efficacy is by "vicarious" experience obtained through social role models (Bandura, 1994). Vicarious experience involves observing someone who is perceived as being similar to oneself successfully perform an activity, with the implication that the observer will also be able to complete the activity (Bandura, 1994). In addition to providing confidence, vicarious experience provides the opportunity to learn how to perform a task by observing a role model perform the same task (Dennis, 1999).

Historically, vicarious experience has played an important role in breastfeeding. Until the last century, women typically learned about breastfeeding by watching other women breastfeed. Many contemporary women have not had the opportunity to observe breastfeeding, however, and some women do not know anyone who has breastfed. Thus, role models must be obtained from other sources.

Breastfeeding peer counselors (BPCs) and La Leche League members can be powerful role models for breastfeeding women (Rossman, 2007; Rossman, Engstrom, Meier, Vonderheid, Norr, & Hill, 2011). Several recent studies have documented the benefits of having BPCs work with breastfeeding mothers of term and preterm infants (Rossman, 2007; Rossman et al., 2011). These women both model the behavior and possess the knowledge and skills needed to help the mother breastfeed.

A recent study (Reossman et al., 2011) of mothers of premature infants who received care from BPCs in the NICU documented the profound influence of the BPCs on the mothers' ability to provide milk for their infants. Many women revealed that the BPC's story of her own preterm birth and experience of providing her milk for her infant influenced their decision to provide milk for their own infants. Mothers also reported that the BPCs provided four types of support: informational, instrumental, appraisal, and emotional. Informational support included activities such as teaching a woman how to operate a breast pump and safely collect and store her milk. Instrumental support included activities such as helping mothers obtain a breast pump for home use. Appraisal support helped mothers assess their decision to continue pumping. Finally, emotional support was described as "mothering the mother." An important finding of the study was that the BPCs made the mothers feel empowered. Thus, BPCs can be a powerful source of social persuasion and effective role models.

Role models are most effective when they are perceived as having similar characteristics to the learner. In other words, women must be able to "see themselves" in the model. Thus, messages about breastfeeding should be presented by women from diverse ethnic, racial, economic, and geographic backgrounds, and role models should not be overly glamorized. Fortunately, a number of excellent sources of culturally relevant materials are available. For example, the Women, Infants, and Children's (WIC) "Loving Support Makes Breastfeeding Work" campaign provides free, downloadable, copyright-free materials in English and Spanish. The posters and pamphlets depict multicultural women (U.S. Department of Agriculture, 2011). Culturally relevant materials are also available from the Office of Women's Health (2010), which produces a copyright-free booklet entitled "Your Guide to Breastfeeding." This booklet is available online, and editions of the booklet are tailored to African American, American Indian, and Alaskan Native women. The booklet is also available in Spanish and Chinese. Many other culturally relevant resources available in the form of websites and printed materials.

The impact of negative role models on breastfeeding must also be acknowledged. Negative role models are a powerful influence on any person attempting a new activity; indeed, Bandura (1994) suggests that negative role models can be more powerful than positive role models. Negative role models can have a profound impact on a woman's decision to initiate and continue breastfeeding. Many women know other friends or family members who have had negative experiences with breastfeeding, and the problems experienced by these women may make the new mother question her own ability to breastfeed successfully. Given this possibility, it is important to offset these negative examples with positive role models and to provide assurance that the mother will have the lactation support services needed to be able to breastfeed her infant.

Using Social Persuasion to Promote Breastfeeding

Social persuasion can be a particularly powerful method of influencing breastfeeding. Social persuasion entails convincing the person that he or she has the ability to be successful at an activity (Bandura, 1994). Although infant feeding decisions are complex and are affected by a multitude of personal, social, and cultural influences, several studies have demonstrated that a woman's decision can be positively influenced by a healthcare professional's recommendation (Dyson, McCormick, & Renfrew, 2005; Miracle & Fredland, 2007; Miracle, Meier, & Bennett, 2004).

A recent review of the ethics of breastfeeding promotion determined that it was unethical not to inform parents of the beneficial health outcomes of breastfeeding and recommend breastfeeding (Miracle & Fredland, 2007). Although healthcare professionals are often concerned that promoting breastfeeding will make mothers feel guilty or coerce mothers into breastfeeding, recent research demonstrates that mothers do not feel coerced in changing their decision to breastfeed once they learn about the health benefits of human milk (Miracle et al., 2004). Indeed, a study of predominately low-income, African American and Hispanic mothers of premature infants in the NICU found that women were upset that their previous healthcare professionals had not explained the health benefits of human milk and encouraged them to provide their milk for their babies (Miracle et al., 2004).

Social persuasion also entails reassuring the woman that she is performing breastfeeding-related activities correctly (Dennis, 1999). Such reassurance is particularly important for new mothers, especially those from vulnerable populations, because they often have limited or no direct or indirect experience with breastfeeding. Comments such as "You are positioning your baby just right" or "You seem very comfortable with knowing when your baby has finished eating" build the mother's confidence, and are a very important part of social persuasion as practiced by healthcare professionals.

Negative social persuasion, in contrast, can have a deleterious effect on a woman's intent to breastfeed. These powerful influences can take the form of subtle messages that undermine a woman's confidence, such as routine supplemental feedings of formula in the maternity unit, use of complimentary formula gift packs in the hospital, or shipping of free formula to the home after a woman gives birth.

Reducing Perceptions of Physical and Psychological Discomfort

The fourth method of increasing self-efficacy is to reduce the person's perception of physical discomforts and negative emotional states such as stress and anxiety (Bandura, 1994). These issues can be challenging in a woman who has recently given birth, particularly if she has physical discomforts related to birth and the initiation of lactation. Among the most commonly reported types of physical discomfort with breastfeeding in the early post-birth period are engorgement and sore nipples, both of which can lead to early discontinuation of breastfeeding (Chapman & Perez-Escamilla, 2000). Expert lactation care, including correct infant latch and positioning, can prevent or minimize these problems.

Similarly, many new mothers can benefit from knowing how to enlist the help of friends and family members in the home so that the women can rest and breastfeeding frequently. Helpful activities are those that support—rather than replace—breastfeeding (e.g., giving the baby a bottle so the mother can sleep at night is not helpful in establishing breastfeeding). Helpful activities include tasks such as meal preparation, child care for siblings, and household chores.

THE RUSH MOTHERS' MILK CLUB: AN EXAMPLE OF BUILDING BREASTFEEDING SELF-EFFICACY

The Rush Mothers' Milk Club is the name of the lactation program in the 57-bed, tertiary neonatal intensive care unit (NICU) at Rush University Medical Center in Chicago. Founded in 1996, the program provides services to approximately 1000 mothers and their NICU infants annually.

Because of the institution's geographic location and its responsibilities as a state-designated perinatal center, the population of mothers and infants served by this facility is especially vulnerable in many ways. First, all of these infants are either born prematurely or require hospitalization in the NICU, thereby necessitating that mothers use a breast pump to initiate and continue lactation. Second, the population has many demographic characteristics associated with lower breastfeeding rates. For example, 40% of the women are African American and 60% come from low-income households, defined as being eligible for WIC benefits. Although prematurely born African American infants are significantly less likely to receive their mothers' milk than white infants, especially when those infants are born to low-income mothers, 95% of mothers whose infants are admitted to the Rush NICU provide their milk for their infants.

The Rush Mothers' Milk Club incorporates all four factors of self-efficacy in helping mothers provide their milk for NICU infants. First, all NICU care providers use social persuasion by sharing the science of human milk with families, with one consistent message: "Your milk is a medicine, and we need your milk to help prevent complications in your baby during the NICU hospitalization." The neonatologists emphasize the importance of human milk as a central part of the therapeutic management plan, enlisting the parents as partners in their infants' care. Program data reveal that of the 95% of women who initiate lactation, nearly half had intended to formula feed their infants until the physician spoke to them about the unique beneficial outcomes of human milk for NICU infants (Miracle et al., 2004). Of the women who planned to formula feed, 76% were African American and 62% were low income, yet they changed the decision to provide milk for their infants. This study underscores the effectiveness of NICU healthcare professionals' use of social persuasion to influence vulnerable families' decisions to provide milk for their infants.

Second, the program incorporates vicarious experiences to model breastfeeding by employing BPCs as the primary lactation care providers for NICU families. All Rush Mothers' Milk Club BPCs are parents of infants who received care in the Rush NICU, so they share a critical common experience with new families. The Rush BPCs are diverse with respect to race, income, initial intent to breastfeed at the time of their infants' birth, and even gender (there is one male BPC), so parents are able to "see themselves" in the BPC model. Because the BPCs also provide specialist NICU lactation care, the message delivered to families is very clear: "This person was like me when her baby was born. Now she is an expert, and she is helping me. If she was able to be successful with this, and she is here to help me, I can do it, too."

Third, mastery experiences are central to the Rush Mothers' Milk Club program. All mothers begin breast pump use within the first 24 hours after birth, and a BPC is physically available to guide the mother step-by-step through the processes of expressing, collecting, storing, and transporting milk to the NICU for infant feeding. The Rush NICU nurses and physicians relate positive infant outcomes to mothers' milk with comments such as "Look at how much weight your baby has gained on your milk!" or "We're able to increase the amount of milk your baby is fed because he is tolerating your milk so well." Mothers become empowered with these mastery experiences, and they can then use them to overcome negative influences that might arise from other sources.

Fourth, the Rush Mothers' Milk Club's focus on "mothering the mother" achieves the principles of reducing perceptions of physical and emotional discomfort through a variety of mechanisms. Physical discomfort is minimized by ensuring that mothers are custom-fitted with correctly sized breast shields and that they are using state-of-the-art breast pumps that have been evaluated for comfort, effectiveness, efficiency, and convenience (Meier et al., 2008). Mothers are contacted daily by the BPCs during the critical first two weeks post birth to ensure that milk expression is progressing without discomfort or other complications. The NICU nurses encourage mothers to sit in comfortable reclining chairs and use the breast pump at their infant's bedside so that the mothers can relax while expressing their milk, and so that any technique-related problems can be detected by the nurse. Nurses routinely offer to have the postpartum nurse bring analgesics to the NICU so that mothers can receive pain relief while remaining with their infants. These interventions may seem minor, but they convey the message to the mother that she is cared for, and that her lactation is a priority.

The Rush Mothers' Milk Club hosts weekly luncheon meetings that address all of the components of self-efficacy, but are especially helpful in reducing the emotional difficulty that surrounds the birth of an NICU infant and breast pump dependency. The meetings, which are facilitated by the lactation program director, BPCs, and NICU nurses, feature a complimentary, healthy lunch and scientific discussion of mothers' lactation concerns. The focus of the group is on parents sharing experiences, and using one another's experiences to solve their own problems and gain support. During the time that infants are hospitalized in the NICU, parents move from being the novice recipients of lactation support to becoming the experts who help new parents. For example, a common concern among new breast-pump-dependent mothers is that they often experience delayed lactogenesis, or the milk "coming in" later than it would for a mother with a healthy infant (Hurst, 2007). It is easy for these new mothers to feel inadequate, but when they hear from more experienced mothers that they, too, went through this transition prior to establishing a full milk supply, both mothers benefit: The new mother has a role model, and the experienced mother is empowered by her ability to have mastered a task sufficiently to help someone else.

In addition to helping all families with NICU infants provide milk, the Rush Mothers' Milk Club has supports in place to help vulnerable low-income families overcome cost-related barriers to successful lactation. The program features a sliding-scale breast pump rental program so that state-of-the-art breast pumps can be obtained for use in the home. Adequate milk storage space is available in industrial freezers, and one freezer is dedicated to milk storage for families after infants are discharged from the NICU. Thus, no family must discard milk or store it in unsafe conditions because of lack of freezer space in the home. For families with transportation barriers, a complimentary door-to-door taxi service allows them to attend the weekly Milk Club luncheons. BPCs are available to make post-NICU discharge lactation home visits, and for families who require complex lactation care in the home, the program pays for an in-home lactation care visit by a NICU nurse lactation consultant.

SUMMARY

The beneficial outcomes of breastfeeding include better infant health, a reduction in the risk of maternal chronic conditions, and lower costs for society. These beneficial outcomes form the basis for national health objectives and policy statements from professional organizations that prioritize the initiation, continuation, and exclusivity of breastfeeding. Self-efficacy theory is clearly applicable in the development of interventions that target these breastfeeding objectives, especially for vulnerable populations. The healthcare provider can use mastery experiences, vicarious experiences, social persuasion, and interventions to reduce perceptions of discomfort and stress to help mothers breastfeed. The Rush Mothers' Milk Club program applies all of these factors of self-efficacy in an effort to help vulnerable families ensure that their infants receive the mother's milk.

ACKNOWLEDGMENT

Preparation of this chapter was supported by NIH Grant NR 010009.

For a full suite of assignments and additional learning activities, use the access code located in the front of your book to visit this exclusive website: http://go.jblearning.com/dechesnay. If you do not have an access code, you can obtain one at the site.

REFERENCES

American Academy of Pediatrics (AAP). (2005). Breastfeeding and the use of human milk. *Pediatrics, 115*, 496–506.

Baldi, A., & Pinotti, L. (2008). Lipophilic microconstituents of milk. In Z. Bosze (Ed.), *Bioactive components of milk* (pp. 109–125). New York: Springer.

Ball, T. M., & Wright, A. L. (1999). Health care costs of formula-feeding in the first year of life. *Pediatrics, 103*, 870–876.

Bandura, A. (1977). Self-efficacy: Toward a unifying theory of behavioral change. *Psychological Review, 84*, 191–215.

Bandura, A. (1982). Self-efficacy mechanism in human agency. *American Psychologist, 37,* 122–147.

Bandura, A. (1994). Self-efficacy. In V. S. Ramachaudran (Ed.), *Encyclopedia of human behavior* (Vol. 4, pp. 71–81). New York: Academic Press.

Bandura, A. (1997). *Self-efficacy: The exercise of control.* New York: Worth Publishers.

Bartick, M., & Reinhold, A. (2010). The burden of suboptimal breastfeeding in the United States: A pediatric cost analysis. *Pediatrics, 125,* e1048–1056.

Britton, C., McCormick, F. M., Renfrew, M. J., Wade, A., & King, S. E. (2007). Support for breastfeeding mothers. *Cochrane Database of Systematic Reviews 2007, 1,* CD001141.

Callen, J., & Pinelli, J. (2004). Incidence and duration of breastfeeding for term infants in Canada, United States, Europe, and Australia: A literature review. *Birth, 31,* 285–292.

Centers for Disease Control and Prevention (CDC). (2010a). Breastfeeding among U.S. children born 1999–2007: CDC national Iimmunization survey. Retrieved from http://www.cdc.gov/breastfeeding/data/NIS_data/index.htm

Centers for Disease Control and Prevention (CDC). (2010b). Healthy people 2010. Retrieved from http://www.healthypeople.gov/2010/Document/HTML/Volume2/16MICH.htm#_Toc494699668

Centers for Disease Control and Prevention (CDC). (2010c). NIS survey methods. Retrieved from http://www.cdc.gov/breastfeeding/data/NIS_data/survey_methods.htm

Centers for Disease Control and Prevention (CDC). (2010d). Racial and ethnic differences in breastfeeding initiation and duration, by state – National immunization survey, United States, 2004–2008, *Morbidity and Mortality Weekly Report, 59,* 327–334.

Centers for Disease Control and Prevention (CDC). (2011). Healthy people 2020. Retrieved from http://www.healthypeople.gov/2020/topicsobjectives2020/objectiveslist.aspx?topicid=26

Chapman, D. J., & Perez-Escamilla, R. (2000). Lactogenesis stage II: Hormonal regulation, determinants and public health consequences. *Recent Research in Developmental Nutrition, 3,* 43–63.

Dennis, C. L. (1999). Theoretical underpinnings of breastfeeding confidence: a self-efficacy framework. *Journal of Human Lactation, 15,* 195–201.

Dunn, S., Davies, B., McCleary, L., Edwards, N., & Gaboury, I. (2006). The relationship between vulnerability factors and breastfeeding outcome. *Journal of Obstetric, Gynecologic and Neonatal Nursing, 35,* 87–97.

Dyson, L., McCormick, F. M., & Renfrew, M. J. (2005). Interventions for promoting the initiation of breastfeeding. *Cochrane Database of Systematic Reviews 2005, 2,* CD001688.

Griffin, T. L., Meier, P. P., Bradford, L. P., Bigger, H. R., & Engstrom, J. L. (2000). Mothers performing creamatocrit measures in the NICU: Accuracy, reactions, and cost. *Journal of Obstetric, Gynecologic and Neonatal Nursing, 29,* 249–257.

Horta, B. L., Bahl, R., Martines, J. C., & Victora, C. G. (2007). *Evidence on the long-term effects of breastfeeding: Systematic review and meta-analyses.* Geneva, Switzerland: World Health Organization.

Hurst, N. M. (2007). Recognizing and treating delayed or failed lactogenesis II. *Journal of Midwifery & Women's Health, 52,* 588–594

Hurst, N. M., Meier, P. P., Engstrom, J. L., & Myatt, A. (2004). Mothers performing in-home measurement of milk intake during breastfeeding of their preterm infants: Maternal reactions and feeding outcomes. *Journal of Human Lactation, 20,* 178–187.

Ip, S., Chung, M., Raman, G., Chew, P., Magula, N., DeVine, D., … Tau, J. (2007). *Breastfeeding and maternal and infant health outcomes in developed countries.* Evidence Report/Technology Assessment No. 153. ARHQ Publication No. 07-E007. Rockville, MD: Agency for Healthcare Research and Quality.

Meier, P. P., Engstrom, J. L., Crichton, C. L., Clark, D. R., Williams, M. M., & Mangurten, H. H. (1994). A new scale for in-home test-weighing for mothers of preterm and high risk infants. *Journal of Human Lactation, 10,* 163–168.

Meier, P. P., Engstrom, J. L., Hurst, N. M., Ackerman, B., Allen, M., Motykowski, J. E., … Jeiger, B. J. (2008). A comparison of the efficacy, effectiveness, comfort and convenience of two hospital-grade electric breast pumps for mother of very low birthweight infants. *Breastfeeding Medicine, 3,* 141–150.

Meier, P. P., Engstrom, J. L., Patel, A. L., Jegier, B. J., & Bruns, N. E. (2010). Improving the use of human milk during and after the NICU stay. *Clinics in Perinatology, 37,* 217–245.

Meier, P. P., Engstrom, J. L., Zuleger, J. L., Motykowski, J. E., Vasan, U., Meier, W. A., ... Williams, T. M. (2006). Accuracy of a user-friendly centrifuge for measuring creamatocrits on mothers' milk in the clinical setting. *Breastfeeding Medicine, 1,* 79–87.

Miracle, D. J., & Fredland, V. (2007). Provider encouragement of breastfeeding: efficacy and ethics. *Journal of Midwifery & Women's Health, 52,* 545–548.

Miracle, D. J., Meier, P. P., & Bennett, P. A. (2004). Mothers' decisions to change from formula to mothers' milk for very-low-birth-weight infants. *Journal of Obstetric, Gynecologic & Neonatal Nursing, 33,* 692–703.

Mossman, M., Heaman, M., Dennis, C. L., & Morris, M. (2008). The influence of adolescent mothers' breastfeeding confidence and attitudes on breastfeeding initiation and duration. *Journal of Human Lactation, 24,* 268–277.

Oddy, W. H., Li, J., Whitehouse, A. J. O., Zubrick, S. R., & Malacova, E. (2011). Breastfeeding duration and academic achievement at 10 years. *Pediatrics, 127,* e137–e145.

Office of Women's Health. (2010). *Your guide to breastfeeding.* Retrieved from http://www.womenshealth.gov/pub/bf.cfm

Patel, A. L., Meier, P. P., & Engstrom, J. L. (2007). The evidence for use of human milk in very low-birthweight preterm infants. *NeoReviews, 8,* e459–e466.

Rossman, B. (2007). Breastfeeding peer counselors in the United States: helping build a culture and tradition of breastfeeding. *Journal of Midwifery & Women's Health, 52,* 631–637.

Rossman, B., Engstrom, J. L., Meier, P. P., Vonderheid, S. C., Norr, K. F., & Hill, P. D. (2011). "They've walked in my shoes": Mothers of very low birth weight infants and their experiences with breastfeeding peer counselors in the neonatal intensive care unit. *Journal of Human Lactation, 27,* 14–24.

Schwarz, E. B., Ray, R. M., Stuebe, A. M., Allison, M. A., Ness, R. B., Freiberg, M. S., & Cauley, J. A. (2009). Duration of lactation and risk factors for maternal cardiovascular disease. *Obstetrics & Gynecology, 113,* 974–982.

Shealy, K. R., Li, R., Benton-Davis, S., & Grummer-Strawn, L. M. (2005). *The CDC guide to breastfeeding interventions.* Atlanta, GA: U.S. Department of Health and Human Services, Centers for Disease Control and Prevention.

Stuebe, A. M., Rich-Edwards, J. W., Willett, W. C., Manson, J. F. & Michels, K. B. (2005). Duration of lactation and incidence of type 2 diabetes. *Journal of the American Medical Association, 294,* 2601–2610.

Thulier, D., & Mercer, J. (2009). Variables associated with breastfeeding duration. *Journal of Obstetric, Gynecologic and Neonatal Nursing, 38,* 259–268.

United States Breastfeeding Committee (USBC). (2001). Breastfeeding in the United States: A national agenda. Retrieved from http://www.usbreastfeeding.org/LinkClick.aspx?link=Publications%2fNational-Agenda-2001-USBC.pdf&tabid=70&mid=388

United States Breastfeeding Committee (USBC). (2002). Economic benefits of breastfeeding. Retrieved from http://www.usbreastfeeding.org/LinkClick.aspx?link=Publications%2fEconomic-Benefits-2002-USBC.pdf&tabid=70&mid=388

United States Department of Agriculture, Food and Nutrition Service, Women, Infants and Children's Program. (2011). Loving support makes breastfeeding work. Retrieved from http://www.nal.usda.gov/wicworks/Learning_Center/loving_support.html

Weimer, J. (2001). *The economic benefits of breastfeeding: A review and analysis.* Food Assistance and Nutrition Research Report No. 13. Washington DC: Food and Rural Economics Division, Economic Research Service, U. S. Department of Agriculture.

World Health Organization (WHO). (2011). Breastfeeding. Retrieved from http://who.int/topics/breastfeeding/en

UNIT III

Research

Research is the process of going up alleys to see if they are blind.

—Marston Bates

www.quotegarden.com

CHAPTER 14

Research with Vulnerable Populations

Mary de Chesnay, Patrick J. M. Murphy, Lynda Law Wilson, and Maile Taualii

Objectives

At the end of this chapter, the reader will be able to

1. Compare and contrast key issues in research with vulnerable populations.
2. Describe an outline for research proposals that incorporates material on research with vulnerable populations.
3. Describe the Institutional Research Board guidelines for research with vulnerable populations.

INTRODUCTION

The purpose of the research unit is to explore ways to study phenomena of interest to nurses who work with vulnerable populations. Particular attention is given to differences and similarities between qualitative and quantitative designs, methods of data collection, analysis strategies, issues of informed consent, and use of data. Following Chapter 14, which presents an overview of research with vulnerable populations, are several chapters that report on specific studies involving participants who might be considered vulnerable.

One of the issues in studying vulnerable populations is the lack of a consistent definition of "vulnerability," which often leads to problems when specifying exactly how vulnerable populations should be protected (Coleman, 2009). For example, many potential research participants might be members of traditionally defined "vulnerable populations," yet the individuals themselves might be perfectly capable of making their own decisions and giving informed consent. An example might be when pregnant women are studied. In the early days of institutional review boards (IRBs), pregnant women were mandated to be protected from medical research that involved invasive procedures or drug trials in which the medications might have unknown effects on fetuses. However, it is peculiar to think of pregnant women as being any more vulnerable than nonpregnant women in situations in which they are simply asked to respond to questionnaires.

DEVELOPING THE PROPOSAL

The following guidelines describe one way of developing a thesis or dissertation research proposal and can be adapted for other purposes. In terms of writing a proposal for funding, the guidelines specified by the sponsor must be followed, but the outline presented here covers all the aspects that would generally be found in a funding proposal (although the formats may vary). These guidelines are offered with the expectation that readers will adapt the outline for their own preferences and institutional requirements. Much of the work of developing a research proposal is universal and appropriate to all types of research with all kinds of populations, but our focus in this chapter is research issues with vulnerable populations. Although some proposals have fewer or more chapters or headings, the content covered here is generally appropriate for most research proposals.

At the heart of all good research proposals is a meaningful question that the researcher, and subsequently the proposal reviewer, feels a compelling need to answer. While one can quite literally investigate anything under the sun, research involving vulnerable populations should take care to identify questions that will likely have a beneficial impact on the populations being studied. It is becoming increasingly common for IRBs that are charged with protecting human subjects to decline research proposals based on the writer's failure to demonstrate the significance of the proposed study (Olsen & Mahrenholz, 2000). Considering the significance of a proposed research question early in the process will help ensure that the best question is addressed and the most meaningful proposal is written.

It might be helpful to think of the process of preparing a research proposal as having two main phases: (1) the *conceptualization phase*, in which the researcher thinks through the basic problem and reviews the literature, and (2) the *design phase*, in which the researcher describes the detailed plan for conducting the study. After the work has been completed, the investigator enters the *dissemination phase*, in which the study's findings are reported to the scientific community. In most disciplines, research reports in peer-reviewed journals are the gold standard, but presentations at professional meetings are also appropriate and are particularly helpful for obtaining feedback prior to publishing the research. In nursing, it may be useful to the general public to present results in nonscientific literature when the work has important clinical implications. Nurses can be particularly effective in writing columns and addressing health issues on radio and television programs because they have high credibility with the general public.

Although one might be tempted to view proceeding from the conceptualization phase to the design phase as the shortest possible distance from point A to point B, preparing a scientifically rigorous research proposal is rarely a linear process. Indeed, the question that the researcher initially intends to ask may not be the one ultimately pursued. At each step in the proposal preparation process, the writer becomes more knowledgeable about the subject matter. This solid foundation permits a greater understanding of the population being studied as well as more in-depth analysis of the literature on the topic. If the researcher is willing to be reflective during this process, modifications (or quite possibly an entirely new research question) may arise as a result of considering the information uncovered at this stage in the proposal process. Although this step makes for a more cyclical path, it is an important mechanism to ensure the researcher is investigating a significant question.

CONCEPTUALIZATION PHASE

During the conceptualization phase of developing a proposal, the researcher commits to a problem to study, finds a way to ask the question so that the problem can be studied, and describes the theoretical underpinnings of the study. So many people are affected by disparities in health care at so many levels that researchers should have no difficulty identifying researchable problems. The challenge is to design studies that will benefit vulnerable populations and reduce health disparities. Even seemingly small proposals have the potential to provide enormous benefits for and have long-lasting effects on a local community.

Usually the conceptualization phase starts with the basic idea or problem. Some researchers refer to the idea as an "itch" that grabs their attention from some observation in the real world. For example, a nurse might question a practice or policy that the institution maintains out of habit. One might think of these practices as "cherished delusions" because they are rooted in institutional folklore rather than in science; even so, people in authority in institutions in which they have a long vested interest in the status quo tend to hold onto them.

For example, in the 1960s, although the concept of vulnerable populations had not yet been articulated, obstetrical units were quite protective of newborns as vulnerable to infection. Rightly so—but the best practice at the time focused on minimizing contact with newborns. Nursing students of this generation were taught not to let new fathers hold their newborn infants because of the risk of infection. Even though aseptic techniques were known and could have been applied just as well to new fathers as to the newborn nursery staff, it was a sacred belief among the nursery staff that fathers would contaminate their infants. Hence policies called for not letting newborns leave the nursery except for brief and reluctantly granted visits to mothers. Fortunately, after a large body of research was generated on family-centered care, this particular policy was relegated to the history books.

Ideally, many other nursing processes based on folklore, "rules of thumb," and tradition would follow suit and become historical relics. In fact, there is reason for encouragement on this front. Evidence-based medicine and evidence-based nursing practice have increasingly become the standard of care in the United States and many other countries. Evidence-based nursing practice requires scientific justification for clinical decisions and follows the same general principles as a well-conducted research proposal, requiring that decisions are grounded in empirical observations that are based on reproducible data (McAlister, Straus, Guyatt, & Haynes, 2000). To ensure the best research outcome, the researcher must develop a hypothesis that predicts what the answer to the studied research question will be. The more commonplace evidence-based practice and hypothesis-directed research become as part of providing care to vulnerable population, the less need there will be for cherished delusions.

The act of articulating a research question as a problem that can be studied is no small task. Fortunately, it is possible to develop a research proposal that builds on the work of others. Nursing science and vulnerable populations research can be viewed as an ongoing dialogue conducted through thousands of peer-reviewed research articles in dozens (if not hundreds) of reputable journals. This wealth of information is one reason why conducting a thorough literature review is essential for developing the best proposal possible.

Numerous approaches may be employed for successfully undertaking a comprehensive literature review (Oxman & Guyatt, 1993). As the researcher begins reading through published articles related to the vulnerable population and research question of interest, it is advisable to take note of which questions appear to have been asked, which approaches were used to answer those questions, and which questions remain unanswered. Conducting a thorough literature review will help hone a research question and assist in developing the best methodology for the proposed study.

Special Considerations with Vulnerable Populations: The Significance of the Study

As a clinical discipline, nursing should describe the significance of research to the population. This section provides an example of ethical issues related to research with indigenous populations as well as the need for studies that can actually be useful to the population. Indigenous people are particularly vulnerable populations (Liao, 2004). Because they experience the worst health disparities in the country, the first inhabitants of the United States are often targeted for research projects (Norton & Manson, 1996). Research in American Indian, Alaska Native, and Native Hawaiian communities must be conducted with respect and sensitivity. In the past, indigenous people have been subjected to immoral treatment by researchers (Udall, Brugge, Benally, & Yazzie-Lewis, 2006). This historical mistreatment by the scientific community has contributed to the distrust of researchers, such that an increased sensitivity must be implemented when working with indigenous communities (Wolf, 1989).

This chapter thoughtfully outlines the importance of designing a meaningful research proposal that both contributes to the scientific knowledge and is beneficial to the community in which the research is conducted. This issue is especially critical when research in indigenous communities is considered, and there are a number of reasons why designing a meaningful research proposal is, in fact, imperative.

The first is related to the severity of health disparities among indigenous populations. Indigenous communities are facing epidemics of disease and cannot afford to focus on issues that will not provide a genuine benefit to their communities.

Second, indigenous communities are under constant political threat. Examples of these threats include the 1954 termination bills that eliminated the existence of six tribes, the 2007 and 2008 federal budget proposals that called for eliminating health programs for the 61% of American Indians and Alaska Natives who happen to reside in cities, and the denial of federal recognition to Native Hawaiians. Producing meaningful research for indigenous communities will assist these groups in describing the burden of disease and advocating for continued efforts to reduce that burden.

Third, conducting meaningful research in indigenous communities contributes to scientific knowledge. Effective and meaningful research can assist in identifying the true rate of disease and correct the inaccuracies reported in health statistics.

Finally, conducting meaningful research in indigenous communities helps to restore trust, by helping to heal some of the pain and suffering caused by past criminal research studies. By "criminal research," we mean unethical treatment of research subjects and lack of respect for the rights of communities.

METHODOLOGICAL PHASE

In the methodological phase of developing a research proposal, it is important to make all the decisions related to designing the study, recruiting the sample, collecting data, and analyzing data. The methodological phase is a natural extension of the groundwork laid during the conceptual development. Deciding the details of the study enables the researcher to organize the concepts and ideas that have been swirling around into a plan of action that can answer the central research question and test the proposed hypothesis.

Special Methodological Considerations with Vulnerable Populations

Appropriate Designs

Scholars may debate the relative merits of qualitative and quantitative designs, but the question of which is better is a form of misdirection. The point of research is to answer questions. Some questions lend themselves to generating emic (from the participant's point of view) data. Usually qualitative designs are best for this purpose, as they generate rich data that may or may not be generalizable. At some point, in a discipline such as nursing, it becomes useful to generate data that provide the basis for predicting and controlling outcomes. These quantitative data are usually etic (from the researcher's point of view) and form the basis for evidence-based practice. Both types of designs are useful for different purposes.

Qualitative designs lend themselves to research with vulnerable populations because these designs, by nature, are implemented with great attention to respecting the autonomy of those who participate in the study. Indeed, the terms "participant," "co-researcher," "respondent," and "cultural informant" may be used in place of the term "subject." Quantitative designs can be implemented effectively as well, provided there is particular attention paid to the rights of subjects.

Protecting the Rights of the Population

It is the job of the IRB to ensure that the rights of all human subjects are protected, and federal guidelines mandate that full reviews be completed for those persons considered vulnerable before they may participate in research. For example, when subjects are children, pregnant women, prisoners, mentally disabled, and frail elderly people, full IRB reviews are required. IRBs have great latitude in interpreting the federal guidelines, however, and some might designate other groups as vulnerable. The ethical treatment of participants is assured through extensive review by such bodies as the IRB (Sutton, et. al., 2003.)

Olshansky's example in this book represents the advantages of participatory action research (PAR), which is a way of involving the community in decision making about the research. Olshanky's detailed account of the processes involved in PAR is applicable to both qualitative and quantitative research. Examples of PAR studies can be found in the first edition of this book as well as in the nursing and social studies literatures (Colvin, de Chesnay, Mercado, & Benavides, 2005; Crandall, Senturia, Sullivan, & Shiu-Thornton, 2005; Evans, Butler, Etowa, Crawley, Rayson, & Bell, 2005; Kelly, 2005; McAllister, 2005; Sullivan, et al 2005; Young, 2006).

Another technique for protecting the rights of vulnerable populations in research is to name an advisory board that includes members of the target population. These individuals not only are helpful in speaking on behalf of the population, but also can be valuable consultants on a variety of cultural and language problems that might arise in the course of conducting research. One area where advisory board members from the target population can be of assistance is in resolving the issue of intellectual property rights. Increasingly, communities are insisting on their rights to own the data generated from their participation in a study.

Incentives

Whether to offer incentives is a controversial point. Some researchers believe that offering any incentive to poor subjects represents undue coercion (Hutz & Koller, 1999). Most authors, however, believe that incentives are acceptable if they are balanced against the degree of deprivation of subjects. For example, small food gifts, telephone calling cards, small amounts of cash, and bus passes are minor gifts that would usually not be seen as coercive (Ensign, 2003).

A more insidious form of coercion concerns research on prisoners. In the mid-twentieth century, abuses of prisoners were rampant. They were unknowing and ill-informed participants in many clinical trials for drugs and cosmetics. Today, prisoners often enroll in clinical trials out of desperation to obtain medical care at crowded, understaffed prisons (Gostin, Vanchieri & Pope, 2007).

Informed Consent

With the increase in regulations focused on research with human subjects, special attention is being given to informed consent—a sticky issue when people cannot speak for themselves, which is resolved by having someone else speak for them. Over-protectiveness may sometimes lead to denial of consent on behalf of vulnerable persons, placing them in the position of not benefiting from the research. For example, research with developmentally disabled persons requires consent by a legal guardian, and there must be provision for the disabled person to participate to his or her capacity (Slayter, 2010). If the guardian does not consent, the person does not receive the benefit of the study.

Cultural issues can also affect informed consent. Rashad, Phipps, and Haith-Cooper (2004) discuss the difficulties of obtaining informed consent from Egyptian women. Although poor

Egyptian women are often research subjects, their low literacy level prevents their full understanding of the study if British or American consent forms are used. Although personal autonomy and accountability to God are key concepts of Islam, Egyptian women tend to defer to the male authority figures in their families (a cultural issue). Signing a consent form is a major commitment in many cultures, and obtaining signed consents (preferred in Western research) is often difficult or impossible (Davison, Brown & Moffitt, 2006).

OUTLINE OF A RESEARCH PROPOSAL

The following outline is offered to assist nurses who are developing research proposals in thinking through the decisions involved in research, particularly with regard for vulnerable populations. For novice researchers, it might be helpful to write the first draft in the first person—a technique that is *not* acceptable in final drafts and most scientific writing. Writing in the first person helps the novice to "own" the study by picturing each step in a logical order.

Chapter I: Overview of the Study (Preview of Coming Attractions)

- What you are going to investigate (purpose or statement of the problem and research questions or hypotheses, including null hypotheses)

  Qualitative Example: What is the lived experience of currently pregnant women whose pregnancy is a result of rape.

  Quantitative Example: Are there significant differences between men and women on a stress scale that measures reaction to the diagnosis of cancer.

  Null Hypothesis: (1) There is no significant difference or (2) the mean of the male group equals the mean of the female group.

  Research Hypothesis: (1) The female group will score significantly higher than the male group or (2) the means will not be equal.

- What theoretical support the idea has (conceptual framework or theoretical support)

  Qualitative Example: Often, qualitative researchers do not specify a theoretical framework prior to conducting the study. The rationale is that the researcher might become biased and not be able to view the data with adequate scientific objectivity.

  Quantitative Example: In quantitative research, it is customary to consider the research to be testing a theory, even if the investigator is conducting descriptive research as a "fishing expedition" to see whether any interesting relationships appear. The researcher often uses theory to support the logic of the study, if not to test a particular theory.

- Which assumptions underlie the problem. It is useful to think of this section as statements that you must accept as true to do the work. For qualitative interviews (and quantitative surveys,) you must be able to trust what people tell you.

Qualitative Example: Participants will tell the truth as they see it.

Quantitative Example: The sphygmomanometer is calibrated accurately for the purposes of the study.

- Which definitions of terms are important to state. Typically these definitions in quantitative research are called *operational definitions* because they describe how you will know the item when you see it. (An operational definition usually starts with the phrase like this: "a score of [number] or higher on the [name of instrument]." You may also want to include a conceptual definition, which is the usual meaning of the concept of interest or a definition according to a specific author. In contrast, qualitative research usually does not include measurements, so operational definitions are not appropriate, although it may be important to state conceptual definitions.

  Qualitative Example: Bereavement is defined as the process of grieving the loss of a loved one that occurs through the death of the loved one.

  Quantitative Example: In a study involving adolescent pregnancy, *adolescents* are defined as males and females between the ages of 13 and 18.

- Any expected limitations to the study design (not delimitations, which are intentional decisions about how to narrow the scope of the population or focus).

  Qualitative Example: For the interview with the third participant, there were distractions present at the setting (children running around the room).

  Quantitative Example: Sample size may not have been sufficient to capture meaningful differences between groups.

- How important the study (significance) is to nursing. In vulnerable populations research, will the study contribute to reducing health disparities?

For both qualitative and quantitative designs, it is critical to discuss the importance of conducting the study in specific terms. It is not enough to make a sweeping pronouncement that the study is significant; rather, the investigator must state *how* it is significant. How will it benefit the population, if not the subjects in the study? How will the study enable nurses in the clinical setting to provide better care? How will the study increase knowledge about a little-known or understudied phenomenon? How can the results help to reduce health disparities? How can the study results be applied to benefit the community being studied?

Special Considerations for Vulnerable Populations in Stating the Problem

The statement of the problem is critical in defining the researcher's approach to the problem. Have the research questions or hypotheses been stated in ways that are appropriate to the design? Will the research question advance understanding of health disparities or interventions with vulnerable populations? Although not all research must address the needs of vulnerable populations, it does seem appropriate that nurse researchers pay more attention to conducting studies that are likely to lead to improved nursing interventions. Both quantitative and qualitative designs are needed and should be logically related to the statement of the problem.

The assumptions of the study are particularly relevant to research with vulnerable populations and worthy of special mention. While researchers attempt to control bias in quantitative research and acknowledge bias in qualitative research, a particular type of bias occurs when the researcher is not a member of the same population as the subjects or participants. *Ethnocentric bias* is an anthropological concept that means the researcher might assume things about the study population or about the way that the conceptual framework of the study works for the population based on ideas derived from his or her own culture. This kind of bias may also be a limiting factor in studies of populations within one's own culture. There could be a tendency for the investigator to accept as true for all people those ideas held to be true within his or her own narrow circle of family and friends and to disregard ideas that conflict with those of his or her own circles.

Ethnocentric bias is not necessarily malicious, as when individuals express racial prejudices, but it does affect the investigator's ability to interpret data from the emic (participant's) point of view, because it relies on preconceived ideas about how people "ought" to behave or think. For example, one of the critical assumptions in qualitative research is that the participants will tell the truth as they see it. If they feel antagonized by comments that reflect ethnocentric bias on the part of the researcher, they may be inclined either to mislead the investigator or to simply not answer questions. This reaction is similar to the dynamic in which subjects try to please the researcher by responding as they think the researcher wishes them to respond.

From the researcher's perspective, the danger lies in misinterpreting data. If the investigator cannot bracket his or her biases, then it becomes highly likely that he or she will miss the point of what participants were trying to say. One way of minimizing ethnocentric bias in a study is to consult a cultural informant to review the study proposal and to assist in monitoring the data. This person can also be useful in explaining the norms of the culture to the researcher (Beattie & VandenBosch, 2007).

Chapter II: The Review of Research Literature (Why You Are Not Reinventing the Wheel)

During the conceptual phase of preparing a research proposal, the researcher first surveys the literature for a general sense of what has been previously done and which questions have already been asked. This search is then followed by a more detailed examination of the literature, focusing on how specific research questions have been articulated and which methods have been employed to investigate the issues. Once the researcher makes any necessary revisions to the proposed research question, it is then possible to thoroughly scour the literature for the most crucial articles relating to the anticipated research. The literature describing vulnerable populations is large and complicated. The explosion of vulnerable-population studies and research publications, although clearly events to celebrate, make sorting through an exponentially growing body of knowledge a bit of challenge (Dixon-Woods et al., 2006). For this reason, a variety of search strategies may need to be employed.

Literature searching contains elements of both science and art. Like the development and redevelopment of the research question itself, a successful literature search often requires multiple iterations as the researcher crafts a specific hypothesis and devises a research plan. As the number of articles in the researcher's possession grows, it is particularly worthwhile to identify apparent gaps in the literature. This step can be useful for helping revise a literature search strategy as well as for potentially identifying an unexplored area of research within the field. The next challenge for the researcher is to selectively and succinctly summarize the current state of the literature in the literature review section of the research proposal.

In this section of the proposal (Chapter II), the researcher frames the problem within the context of knowledge in the discipline. For quantitative studies, the main literature review is conducted before the study. In contrast, for qualitative studies, the major part of the literature review might be done after the study and would be based on the concepts that emerged from the data.

Organize this chapter according to the concepts in your conceptual framework in Chapter I and describe the studies in the literature review first, followed by discussion of the state-of-the-art literature and the manner in which the study fills gaps in the existing literature.

- Concept 1: Brief description of each study reviewed that supports concept 1 within the conceptual framework. The brief description should include the highlights of the study such as the sample size and type, design, key findings, and anything relevant to the point you are trying to make.
- Repeat this step for as many concepts as are included in conceptual framework.
- Areas of agreement in literature: A paragraph or two that summarizes the main points on which authors agree.
- Areas of disagreement: Summary of where authors disagree.
- State of the art on the topic: A few paragraphs that clearly articulate where the literature is strong and where the gaps are.
- A brief statement of how your study fills the gaps or why your study needs to be done to replicate what someone else has done.

Research Examples Illustrating Special Considerations for Vulnerable Populations

In this section, examples of special considerations in conceptualizing and planning research with vulnerable populations are presented from two separate studies: one study that focused on the effects of a gentle touch intervention for preterm infants in the neonatal intensive care unit (Harrison, Williams, Berbaum, Stem, & Leeper, 2000) and a second study that involved focus groups with Latino immigrant parents to identify parents' perceptions of their children's health needs (Harrison & Scarinci, 2007). Preterm infants are considered vulnerable because of their physiologic fragility, and Latino immigrant parents are considered vulnerable both because of their status as ethnic minorities and because of the economic, cultural, and language barriers to obtaining healthcare services that they face.

Given the physical vulnerability of preterm infants, it was essential for the investigators to carefully review previous research during the conceptualization phase to ensure that there were no reports of risks that might arise from the proposed tactile intervention, and that the significance of the proposed study justified any potential risks that might ensue during the study. It was also critical to identify a conceptual framework that supported the proposed intervention and to identify potential extraneous variables that should be considered to minimize any unnecessary risks to the infants who were assigned to the intervention group. Harrison et al. (2000) developed a conceptual framework based on a thorough review of previous research and discussions with other researchers who had conducted studies evaluating preterm infants' responses to touch and massage, and briefly summarized the framework in one of the publications that presented the findings from this study:

> The conceptual framework for this study was based on the premise that Gentle Human Touch (GHT) would stimulate tactile and pressure receptors promoting infant comfort and reducing stress, resulting in positive immediate and longer-term outcomes. Immediate outcomes would be reflected in physiologic indicators of reduced stress and of maintenance of comfort during the GHT intervention, including maintenance of heart rate and levels of oxygen saturation (O_2 sat) within normal ranges. Immediate outcomes would also be reflected by reduced levels of stress during the GHT intervention as evidenced by decreased levels of behavioral distress cues. Immediate outcomes would also be reflected by decreased energy expenditure as evidenced by decreased levels of motor activity and maintenance of a sleep state as opposed to an active awake or fuss/cry state during and after the GHT intervention. By reducing stress and energy expenditure during the early weeks in the NICU, it was predicted that the GHT intervention would result in longer-term benefits including reduced levels of morbidity and increased weight gain during the infant's hospitalization, and reduced levels of motor activity and increased quiet sleep when the infants were 17–20 days of age. It was also predicted that providing supplemental tactile stimulation would enhance sensory maturation and thereby promote more optimal behavioral organization at the time of hospital discharge among infants in the GHT group as compared to infants in the control group. (Harrison et al., 2000, p. 438)

Because of the vulnerability of preterm infants, any type of supplemental stimulation poses some risk of adverse physiologic and behavioral response. Thus it was also important to outline procedures for identifying and responding to any adverse responses that might arise during the course of the study. To minimize any potential adverse effects of the GHT intervention, the researchers used a "decision tree" protocol throughout their study. This protocol involved establishing criteria that would be considered indicators of adverse physiologic responses to the GHT, and specifying procedures that would be followed if the infants demonstrated any of these indicators:

> The GHT lasted for up to 10 minutes but was discontinued if the infant demonstrated signs of physiological distress (heart rate ≤ 100 or ≥ 200 beats per minute

> [bpm] for 12 seconds or more; or arterial O_2 saturation levels < 90% for longer than 30 seconds). If the touch had to be discontinued early due to changes in either heart rate or oxygen saturation levels, the researcher waited at least 30 minutes before instituting another GHT intervention. The decision to provide the GHT for 10 minutes was based on findings from previous studies of gentle touch and massage in which positive outcomes were noted following supplemental tactile interventions that lasted from 10–15 minutes. (Harrison et al., 2000, p. 440)

In a study that involved focus groups with 82 Latino immigrant parents, there were also special issues to consider when conceptualizing and planning the study (Harrison & Scarinci, 2007). Of particular importance in this study was the need to identify and minimize potential sources of ethnocentric bias both in planning the study and in collecting and analyzing the data. One strategy that was used was to involve members of the community where the research was conducted in planning the study, including plans for recruitment of focus group participants as well as the format of the questions that would guide the focus groups. Native Spanish speakers led the focus groups and participated in training to help them learn to maintain objectivity during the sessions and respond to themes and concerns that arose during the groups. Each focus group was tape recorded, and following each session, the principal investigator met with the group leaders to review the sessions and share concerns and perceptions about the sessions. These "debriefing" sessions provided important guidance and learning opportunities for both the focus group facilitators and the principal investigator (PI), and they helped to minimize problems with bias.

During the focus groups, there were many instances in which it appeared that group participants were trying to please the researcher by responding as they thought the researcher wanted them to respond; thus it was important for the investigators to help the group facilitators learn to identify these situations and appropriate responses to them. For example, in one of the groups, mothers were sharing diverse opinions about whether it was appropriate to spank their children. After several mothers had expressed differing opinions on this topic, one asked the group leader what she thought, as though seeking reinforcement for her own opinion. The leader stated that her role was to listen and facilitate discussion, not to provide her own view or opinion.

Another consideration in planning this study was planning procedures for obtaining informed consent. All consent forms were translated and available in Spanish, although the researchers recognized that there were some Guatemalan immigrants in the study community who did not speak Spanish and were not able to read their Mayan language. Special approval was obtained from the IRB to have the consent forms read to these participants in their native language (Canjobal) by a bilingual translator.

DESIGN PHASE

During the design phase of developing a proposal, the researcher presents the detailed plan of the activities in the study along with a rationale for each methodological decision and the approach to be used for data collection and analysis. It is also helpful to the reader of the proposal for the investigator to not only state what is planned, but also explain why alternative decisions might be less desirable. For example, certain design decisions might be particularly appropriate in research with vulnerable populations.

Chapter III: Methodology (Plan for the Study)

The outline for Chapter III presented here constitutes a proposal for a thesis or dissertation. For grants, the same decisions have to be made, but the format varies based on the sponsor's requirements.

Design

Name and describe the design—for example, ethnographic, experimental, survey, cross-sectional, phenomenological. One of the fundamental decisions that the researcher needs to make at this stage of the proposal development is whether to collect quantitative data, qualitative data, or a combination of the two. All three approaches have been successfully used in conducting nursing research focusing on vulnerable populations (Carr, 1994), but each has distinct advantages and drawbacks that should be considered. *Qualitative research* aims to provide a robust description of the data that cannot be readily reduced to a numerical format. *Quantitative research* involves the examination of numerical data and the construction of mathematical models to describe the events that are observed.

Qualitative data are collected directly by the researcher and may include quoted words, pictures, or objects. Quantitative data are collected by using a research instrument that translates the researcher's observations into numerical data. Although qualitative data may be regarded as more robust and paint a more contextualized picture of the researcher's observations, quantitative data may be regarded as substantially more efficient for analyzing large data sets and enable the researcher to be further removed from data collection and interpretation (Corner, 1991).

One notable trend in vulnerable populations research is the practice of conducting studies that include both quantitative and qualitative research components, referred to as "triangulation" by Halcomb and Andrew (2005). One major benefit to collecting both quantitative and qualitative data for the same sample set is that this approach may increase the researcher's confidence in the collected data and provide for a more complete data analysis and interpretation.

Although the collection of qualitative and quantitative may be an added encumbrance for the researcher, it may be the approach that enables a researcher to produce the most inclusive results on a complex and multifaceted population.

Sample

Describe the number of people who will serve as the sample and the sampling method—that is, where and how the sample will be recruited. State the sample inclusion and exclusion criteria (delimitations). Provide a rationale for selection of the sample, including statements about inclusion of women and minorities. Include the IRB statement and explain how the rights of subjects or participants will be protected, including how you will obtain informed consent, code the data, and store the data. The IRB statement is usually a sentence that simply states that approval will be sought from the institution's IRB before the study is initiated.

Setting

Where will data collection take place? How will any potential distractions be controlled?

Incentives

Discuss whether incentives will be offered (e.g., bus fare to site of data collection, reimbursement, free lab tests). Incentives should not be so great that people feel coerced to join the study—that they cannot pass up the incentive.

Tools

This section covers instruments and data analysis. How will the variables of interest be measured? How will you make sense of the data—that is, analyze the data?

Validity and Reliability

How will you know if you have good data? (In qualitative research, the corresponding terms are "accuracy" and "replicability.")

Procedures

Which procedures for data collection and analysis will be followed? Outline a 1-2-3, step-by-step plan of action.

Timeline

Provide a chart that lists the activities in the research plan on a month-by-month schedule.

Chapter IV: Results (What Happened? Presentation of the Raw Data)

The results section of a thesis or dissertation can be summarized by recalling the intentional dryness of a 1950s TV police officer who has only one thing on his mind: "Just the facts, ma'am." While Chapters I through III walk the reader through the development of the research question and act as a scholarly tour guide of the literature, the results section should be written in a way that allows the readers to interpret the data directly. Graphs, figures, and tables may aid in the visual presentation and organization of the data, but the researcher's own interpretation of what the data mean are intentionally and conspicuously absent. By this point in the proposal, the reviewers should be aware of the researcher's question, hypothesis, and methodology for attempting to answer the problem. One can consider this lack of commentary in the results section to be an academic courtesy to the reviewers, allowing them to arrive at their own conclusions as to what the researcher's data are saying.

Some researchers like to describe the sample in this section as a way to lead off the discussion of findings. A simple chart that shows the demographics of the sample can help the reader frame the results for the population.

Following the order in which the various hypotheses or research questions were presented, describe the data that addressed each question. Use raw data only, do not draw any conclusions from the data, and make no interpretations.

Chapter V: Discussion (What Sense Do You Make of What You Learned and What Are You Going to Do for an Encore?)

Conclusions

Provide a concise statement of the answer to each research question or hypothesis. Some researchers like to add interpretation here—that is, say how confident the investigator is in each conclusion. The thorough discussion that follows each conclusion incorporates the investigator's interpretation of data and should tie the data back to the literature. If the study has extended over a long time period, it is advisable to conduct a new literature search to capture any recent studies.

Implications

How can each conclusion be used to help address the needs of vulnerable populations or nursing practice, education, administration, or health policy.

Recommendations

These statements indicate which kind of research should be conducted or which directions should be followed based on the findings.

SUMMARY

This chapter provided a framework for developing research proposals. Potential sponsors may have different guidelines, but the outline provided here includes the most important considerations of designing research involving vulnerable populations. Some sample proposals appear in subsequent chapters that illustrate some of the key points made in this chapter.

For a full suite of assignments and additional learning activities, use the access code located in the front of your book to visit this exclusive website: http://go.jblearning.com/dechesnay. If you do not have an access code, you can obtain one at the site.

REFERENCES

Beattie, E., & VandenBosch, T. (2007). The concept of vulnerability and the protection of human subjects. *Research and Theory for Nursing Practice: An International Journal, 21*(3), 156–173.

Carr, L. T. (1994). The strengths and weaknesses of quantitative and qualitative research: What method for nursing? *Journal of Advanced Nursing, 20*(4), 716–721.

Coleman, C. (2009). Vulnerability as a regulatory category in human subject research. *Journal of Law, Medicine and Ethics, 37*(1), 12–18. Doi: 10.1111/j.1748-720x.2009.00346.x

Colvin, S., de Chesnay, M., Mercado, T., & Benavides, C. (2005). Child health in a barrio of Managua. In M. De Chesnay (Ed.), *Caring for the vulnerable: Perspectives in nursing theory, practice and research* (pp. 161–170). Sudbury, MA: Jones and Bartlett.

Corner, J. (1991). In search of more complete answers to research questions: Quantitative versus qualitative research methods: Is there a way forward? *Journal of Advanced Nursing, 16*(6), 718–727.

Crandall, M., Senturia, K., Sullivan, M., & Shiu-Thornton, S. (2005). Latina survivors of domestic violence: Understanding through qualitative analysis. *Hispanic Health Care International, 3*(3), 179–187.

Davison, C., Brown, M., & Moffitt, P. (2006). Student researchers negotiating consent in northern aboriginal communities. *International Journal of Qualitative Methods, 5*(2), 1–10.

Dixon-Woods, M., Cavers, D., Agarwal, S., Annandale, E., Arthur, A., Harvey, J., . . . Sutton, A. J. (2006). Conducting a critical interpretive synthesis of the literature on access to healthcare by vulnerable groups. *BMC Medical Research Methodology, 26*(6), 35.

Ensign, J. (2003). Ethical issues in qualitative health research with homeless youths. *Journal of Advanced Nursing, 43*(1), 43–50.

Evans, J., Butler, L., Etowa, J., Crawley, I., Rayson, D., & Bell, D. (2005). Gendered and cultural relations: Exploring African Nova Scotians' perceptions of breast and prostate cancer. *Research and Theory for Nursing Practice, 19*(3), 257–273.

Gostin, L., Vanchieri, C. & Pope, A. (2007). *Ethical Considerations for Research Involving Prisoners*. Washington, D.C.: Institute of Medicine.

Halcomb, E., & Andrew, S. (2005). Triangulation as a method for contemporary nursing research. *Nurse Researcher, 13*(2), 71–82.

Harrison, L., & Scarinci, I. (2007). Child health needs of rural Alabama Latino families. *Journal of Community Health Nursing. 24*(1), 31–47.

Harrison, L. L., Williams, A., K., Berbaum, M. L., Stem, J. T., & Leeper, J. (2000). Physiologic and behavioral effects of gentle human touch on preterm infants. *Research in Nursing & Health, 23*, 435–446.

Hutz, C. & Koller, S. (1999). Methodological and ethical issues in research with street children. *New Directions in Child and Adolescent Development, 85*(1), 55–70.

Kelly, P. (2005). Practical suggestions for community interventions using participatory action research. *Public Health Nursing, 22*(1), 65–73.

Liao, Y. (2004). REACH 2010 Surveillance for health status in minority communities—United States, 2001–2002. *MMWR Surveillance Summary, 53*, 1–36.

McAlister, F. A., Straus, S. E., Guyatt, G. H., & Haynes, R. B. (2000). Users' guides to the medical literature: XX: Integrating research evidence with the care of the individual patient. Evidence-Based Medicine Working Group. *Journal of the American Medical Association, 283*(21), 2829–2836.

McAllister, M. (2005). Women with dissociative identity disorder: Solution-focused nursing. In M. de Chesnay (Ed.) Caring for the vulnerable: Perspectives in nursing theory, practice and research (pp. 181-188). Sudbury, MA: Jones and Bartlett.

Norton, I. M., & Manson, S. M. (1996). Research in American Indian and Alaska Native communities: Navigating the cultural universe of values and process. *Journal of Consulting Clinical Psychology, 64*(5), 856–860.

Olsen, D. P., & Mahrenholz, D. (2000). IRB-identified ethical issues in nursing research. *Journal of Professional Nursing, 16*(3), 140–148.

Oxman, A. D., & Guyatt, G. H. (1993). The science of reviewing research. *Annals of the New York Academy of Science, 31*(703), 125–133.

Rashad, A., Phipps, F. M., & Haith-Cooper, M. (2004). Obtaining informed consent in an Egyptian research study. *Nursing Ethics, 11*(4), 394–399.

Slayter, E. (2010). Clinical and demographic characteristics of adults with intellectual disabilities in a Medicaid population. *Intellectual/Developmental Disabilities. 48*(6), 417–431.

Sullivan, M., Buyan, R., Senturia, K., Shiu-Thornton, S., & Ciske, S. (2005). Participatory action research in practice: A case study in addressing dometic violence in nine cultural communities. Journal of Interpersonal Violence, 20(8), 977–995.

Sutton, L. B., Erlen, J. A. Glad, J. M., & Siminoff, L. A. (2003). Recruiting vulnerable populations for research: Revisiting the ethical issues. *Journal of Professional Nursing, 19*(2), 106–112.

Udall, S., Brugge, D., Benally, T., & Yazzie-Lewis, E. (2006). *The Navajo people and uranium mining.* Albuquerque, NM: University of New Mexico Press.

Wolf, A. S. (1989). The Barrow studies: An Alaskan's perspective. *American Indian and Alaska Native Mental Health Research, 2,* 35–40.

Young, L. (2006) Participatory action research: A research strategy for nursing? *Western Journal of Nursing Research, 28*(5), 499–504.

CHAPTER 15

Sample Qualitative Research Proposal: Childhood Obesity in Latino Families

Nicole Mareno

Objectives

At the end of this chapter, the reader will be able to

1. Using the outline from Chapter 14, propose a qualitative study that can be conducted with vulnerable populations.
2. Describe the special ethical implications of conducting qualitative research with Latino parents of overweight children.

The following is a shortened version of a sample research proposal for qualitative designs. The study has not been conducted.

CHAPTER 1: STUDY OVERVIEW

Research Question

What are the perceptions of family dietary and physical activity patterns for Latino parents of overweight 6- to 12-year-old children in northern Georgia?

Theoretical Support

The prevalence of overweight (OW) and obesity (OB) among U.S. children and adolescents has reached epidemic proportions. According to the most current data, 31.7% of 2- to 19-year-old children and adolescents exceed the 85th percentile for body mass index (BMI) for age, with 11.9% of the group exceeding the 95th percentile (Odgen, Carroll, Curtin, Lamb, & Flegal, 2010). Among children aged 10 to 17, the prevalence of OW and OB has increased from 30.6% to 31.6% from 2003 to 2007 (Bethell, Simpson, Strumbo, Carle, & Gombojav, 2010).

Childhood OW and OB can track into adulthood, increasing the risk of chronic diseases and premature death (Franks, Hanson, Knowler, Sievers, Bennett, & Looker, 2010; Raghuveer, 2010). OB contributes to all major chronic diseases, including cardiovascular diseases, diabetes, cancer, asthma, liver disease, and joint disorders (Barlow, 2007; Fennoy, 2010; Raghuveer, 2010). In addition, obesity may contribute to mental health issues, including self-esteem problems and decreased quality of life (Barlow, 2007).

The causes and risk factors for OW and OB have been fiercely debated in the scientific community. A complex web of genetic, familial, environmental, societal, social, and cultural factors is believed to lead to these conditions (Barlow, 2007; Birch & Ventura, 2009; Golan & Crow, 2004). Modifiable lifestyle behaviors, including a caloric-dense diet and inadequate physical activity, have contributed to increased rates of OW and OB (Barlow, 2007; Collins, Warren, Neve, McCoy, & Stokes, 2007; Golan & Crow, 2004).

Education on modifiable lifestyle behaviors, including dietary intake and physical activity, have become the primary approaches to prevention and treatment of OW and OB. Parents serve as children's primary role models for eating and physical activity and are the key change agents within the family system. Health behaviors are learned in the home environment, and children begin to emulate parental dietary and physical activity patterns from an early age (Golan & Crow, 2004). Thus OW and OB issues affect the entire family unit. Likewise, prevention and treatment start with the family— and particularly with the parents.

Conceptual Framework

The proposed qualitative study consists of generating emic data. The literature review is to be conducted on key themes that emerge after data analysis so as to increase the likelihood of interpreting the data correctly.

Assumptions

The primary assumption in this study is that people will tell the truth as they see it within their sociocultural context.

Definitions

BMI—an indirect measure of body fat—is the primary accepted screening measure for childhood OW and OB. BMI is a measure of weight adjusted for height and is defined as the weight in kilograms divided by the square of the height in meters (kg/m^2). For children and adolescents aged 2 to 19 years, BMI is plotted on a gender-appropriate growth chart to obtain a percentile ranking. This ranking is referred to as BMI for age (Centers for Disease Control and Prevention, 2009)

The current recommendations for categorizing body weight are as follows: (1) children and adolescents under the 5th percentile for BMI are categorized as "underweight"; (2) children and adolescents between the 5th and 85th percentiles for BMI are categorized as "healthy weight"; (3) children and adolescents with a BMI greater than or equal to the 85th percentile but less than the 95th percentile (or BMI less than 30 kg/m^2, whichever is smaller) are categorized as "overweight"; and (4) children and adolescents whose BMI is greater than or equal to the 95th percentile or whose BMI is greater than or equal to 30 kg/m_2 (whichever is smaller) are categorized as "obese" (Barlow, 2007; Krebs, Himes, Jacobson, Nicklas, Guilday, & Styne, 2007).

Limitations

The study is designed to amass rich data from each participant's unique perspective. Generalizability of the findings, therefore, is neither an expectation nor a concern.

Ethnocentric bias is a concern in conducting qualitative research with vulnerable populations. To eliminate ethnocentric bias in the research, the researcher will bracket any preconceived notions or assumptions to prevent misinterpretation of the data.

Significance of Findings to Nurses Working with Vulnerable Populations

Health promotion and disease prevention are vital nursing roles. The high rates of OW and OB among children and adolescents are a public health threat and one of the primary target areas of governmental programs, including *Healthy People 2020* and Let's Move! Access to early preventive health care and education is a fundamental strategy to lower the rates of OW and OB in the United States.

Racial, ethnic, and socioeconomic disparities in the rates of childhood OW and OB have been widely publicized. Among 2- to 19-year-old children and adolescents, the prevalence of OW or OB is higher in Latino (41% to 42.6%) and African American (37.6% to 41.1%) children than among Caucasian children (26.8% to 34.5%) (Bethell et al., 2010; Odgen et al., 2010). Notably, the rate of childhood OW and OB increases when family income falls below the poverty level (Bethell et al., 2010). Rates of OB are higher among Latino preschool-aged children from low-income families (18.5%) than among Caucasian (12.6%) and Asian (12.3%) children from low-income families (Sharma et al., 2009).

Individuals from economically disadvantaged backgrounds and ethnically diverse families often face barriers to preventive health care, including lack of access, lack of insurance, lack of transportation, discrimination, and difficulty navigating the healthcare system (Richardson & Norris, 2010). Barriers at the familial, community, provider, and systemic levels often make it difficult for families to be recruited and retained in preventive weight management programs. There is a lack of research on culturally sensitive weight management strategies for ethnically diverse families, especially Latino families. It is imperative to understand modifiable lifestyle factors, including dietary and physical activity patterns, from the perspective of Latino parents so as to develop culturally sensitive weight management interventions for families.

CHAPTER II: REVIEW OF THE RESEARCH LITERATURE

The literature review provides a foundation for the proposed study. A comprehensive literature review will be completed after themes emerge from the data.

Prevalence

OW and OB are a concern both in the United States and abroad. In the United States, there has been a threefold increase in the rate of OB since 1980 (Odgen et al., 2010; Odgen, Carroll, Curtin,

McDowell, Tabak, & Flegal, 2006). According to recent data from the World Health Organization (WHO, 2010), OB is now the fifth leading mortality risk worldwide. The estimated worldwide prevalence of OW and OB among children aged 5 years and younger is 43 million. According to WHO (2010), the prevalence is higher among children living in developing countries (35 million) than among children living in developed countries (8 million).

OB costs the United States an estimated $147 billion per year. The increased prevalence of OB in this country has accounted for a $40 million increase in healthcare spending since 2006 (Finkelstein, Trogden, Cohen, & Dietz, 2009). These costs are based on estimates from Medicare, Medicaid, and private insurance companies (Finkelstein et al, 2009.) and do not account for indirect costs of disease burden including, but not limited to, individual out-of-pocket expenditures, comorbid health conditions, disability, and job absenteeism (Cawley, 2010).

Genetic, environmental, cultural, social, familial, socioeconomic, and lifestyle factors have all contributed to the current obesity epidemic in the United States. Cawley (2010) reviewed economic, environmental, and social trends implicated as contributors to the increased rates of childhood OW and OB. This author asserts that factors including food prices, subsidization of corn products, low family income, increased maternal work hours outside of the home, and increased use of technology have been linked to increased rates of childhood OW and OB. Family cultural beliefs regarding feeding practices, physical activity, and body weight can be either supportive or detrimental to family weight management.

Researchers have uncovered evidence indicating that the rates of OW and OB are higher among children who watch more television, consume higher amounts of sugar-sweetened beverages, eat increased amounts of fast food, and have parents with higher BMIs (Starling Washington, Reifsnider, Bishop, Domingeaux Ethington, & Ruffin, 2010; Taveras, Gillman, Kleinman, Rich-Edwards, & Rifas-Shiman, 2010). There are also strong correlations between high maternal BMI and high child BMI, especially among Latino families (Elder et al., 2010; Fuentes-Afflick & Hessol, 2008). In one study, in households where children had limited television or computer screen time, had adequate sleep, and consumed dinner as a family, the prevalence of OB was 40% lower than that in households that did not participate in these routines (Anderson & Whitaker, 2010).

Ethnic Disparities

The rates of OW and OB are higher among Latino children (Hispanic and Mexican American) than among non-Hispanic Caucasian children. When Bethell et al. (2010) examined the 2007 data from the National Survey of Children's Health ($n = 44{,}101$), these researchers found that the prevalence of OW and OB among Latino children from Spanish-speaking households was 45%, which is 18.2% higher than the prevalence among non-Hispanic Caucasian children. The same researchers also found a slight decrease in the prevalence of OW and OB among Latino children from English-speaking households (37.9%), although this rate was still 11.1% higher than the rates among non-Hispanic Caucasian children. Bethell et al. (2010) also reported that the likelihood of OW and OB increased among children from low-income households, children of Hispanic ethnicity, and families participating in public insurance programs.

Odgen et al. (2010) also found a higher prevalence of OW and OB among 2- to 19-year-old Latino children (38.2%) in comparison to non-Hispanic Caucasian children (29.2%). In addition, these researchers reported that Latino boys had higher odds of developing OW and OB in comparison to other racial/ethnic groups.

Studies of parental perceptions of child OW and OB indicate trends in parental inability to recognize children as overweight or obese. Mothers—especially those with higher BMIs—are less likely to recognize OW or OB in their children and may not be concerned about the risks of OW (Doolen, Alpert, & Miller, 2009; Towns & D'Auria, 2009). In two separate studies, researchers found that more than half of parents did not recognize their child as OW and determined that parents of younger children were more likely to underestimate their child's weight than parents of adolescents (Hackie & Bowles, 2007; West, Raczynski, Phillips, Bursac, Health Gauss, & Montgomery, 2008). Eckstein and colleagues (2006) found that few parents of OW or at risk for overweight (AROW) children felt that their child was OW; they were more likely to identify their child as OW if they recalled a doctor bringing the topic up at a visit. Carnell, Edwards, Croker, Boniface, and Wardle (2005) found similar results: Only 1.9% of parents of OW children and 17.1% of parents of OB children in their study described their child as OW.

Compounding frequent misperceptions are cultural beliefs about body weight. Many cultural groups value increased body weight as a sign of good health. Garcia (2004) asserts that this is especially true among Latino families, who value baby fat and have difficulty recognizing OW and OB in their children. Goodell, Pierce, Bravo, and Ferris (2008) and Sussner, Lindsay, Greaney, and Peterson (2008) obtained conflicting results when interviewing Latina mothers, however. Both of these research teams reported that longer residence in the United States changed maternal perceptions of weight, leading to less concern with thinness as a sign of poor health.

Understanding cultural beliefs and values about weight, dietary patterns, and physical activity is important prior to planning culturally sensitive weight management interventions. Ward (2008) conducted an integrative review of the literature and identified four significant themes related to childhood OW in the Latino community: parental perceptions of child weight, parenting practices and child feeding, food availability, and acculturation status. As mentioned previously, exploring parents' belief systems about child weight status is an important foundational step in intervention planning.

Moreover, understanding cultural variations in parenting practices is essential. Sussner and colleagues (2008) reported that Latina mothers value child feeding practices that include large quantities of food and encouragement to clean one's plate. Limit setting, monitoring, and positive reinforcement have all been positively associated with healthy eating behaviors, whereas pressuring children to eat and controlling access to foods have been found to correlate with higher levels of unhealthy eating practices (Arredondo, Elder, Ayala, Campbell, Baquero, & Duerksen, 2006; Elder et al., 2010; Matheson, Robinson, Varady, & Killen, 2006).

In addition, food availability may affect child weight status. Sussner and colleagues (2008) reported that Latina mothers perceived less healthy food choices to be available in the United States and that they consumed more natural foods in their native countries. Food insecurity has been found to limit food choices and impact parental feeding practices in Latino families (Matheson et al., 2006).

Finally, acculturation status may have an association with child weight status. Recent research findings have suggested that a lower acculturation status has been significantly associated with higher levels of child OW in the Latino population (Elder et al., 2010; Fuentes-Afflick & Hessol, 2008).

State of the Art

Effective approaches to preventing or treating childhood OW or OB vary depending on the age of the child, the level of involvement of the parents, the education provided, and the methods used to measure success. The evaluation of meta-analyses on the topic of effective approaches to treating childhood OW and OB revealed four common recommendations: (1) child exposure to healthy foods before entry into primary school; (2) proper portion sizes and limit setting on unhealthy foods; (3) multimodal behavioral change treatment that includes non-dieting approaches to healthy eating, increased physical activity, and the reduction of sedentary behaviors; and (4) parent-focused interventions that encourage role modeling of healthy lifestyle behaviors and prevention of restrictive or coercive parenting practices related to child feeding (Birch & Ventura, 2009; Collins et al., 2007; Latzer et al., 2008). Researchers agree that parent-focused interventions are of utmost importance, given that younger children are amenable to complying with parental instructions (Latzer et al., 2008).

For health professionals working with Latino families, attention to parental perceptions of child weight, cultural values and beliefs, parenting practices, and level of acculturation are important factors to consider prior to initiating an intervention (Ward, 2008). When Gallagher (2009) interviewed Latina mothers about childhood OW and OB prevention, the findings revealed that the mothers valued a balanced diet, disciplined eating practices (i.e., regular meals, moderation of unhealthy foods), child activity, and limiting television as approaches to weight management. The results of past research reinforce the importance of understanding cultural values, beliefs, and practices for nurses planning to conduct research with vulnerable populations.

To understand values, beliefs, and practices, researchers must hear the voices of the participants in their studies. This consideration is especially important when working with vulnerable populations, particularly for tailoring interventions to a specific population. One technique to give individuals a voice is use of the Photovoice method. The primary goals of the Photovoice method are to encourage research participants to document personal and community strengths and concerns through photography. This process enables individuals within a community to engage in dialogue in small groups about personal and community issues as well as to become the impetus for policy changes (Wang, 1999; Wang & Burris, 1997). In past studies, Photovoice has been used to elicit information about supportive or detrimental factors affecting health in a variety of populations: family planning for Midwestern Latino adults (Schwartz, Sable, Dannerbeck, & Campbell, 2007); family, maternal, and child health for adults in Northern California (Wang & Pies, 2004); health concerns of college students in the Northeast (Goodhart,

Hsu, Baek, Coleman, Maresca, & Miller, 2006); perceptions of health for preadolescent Latina girls in the Midwest (Vaughn, Rojas-Guyler, & Howell, 2008); healthy eating for low-income women living in homeless shelters in the Northeast (Valera, Gallin, Schuk, & Davis, 2009); and perceptions of health for young adolescent mothers (Stevens, 2006).

Areas of Agreement and Disagreement

Despite uncertainty regarding the degree of impact that genetic, environmental, social, cultural, and socioeconomic factors have on the development of childhood OW and OB, researchers agree these conditions are pervasive problems and priority public health concerns. While the most effective approaches to prevent and treat childhood OW and OB are still being studied and disseminated, parent-focused approaches are almost unanimously supported. Understanding values, beliefs, and health practices is important prior to intervention with vulnerable populations, necessitating further research using qualitative methodologies.

Gaps in the Literature

Given the large body of literature about childhood OW and OB, why does this study need to be done? The purpose of this study is to hear the voices and perspectives of Latino parents in northern Georgia about their family's dietary and physical activity patterns. To date, the Photovoice method has not been used to study assets and concerns about childhood OW and OB from the parents' perspective. The proposed study will make a unique contribution to the profession of nursing, and the results will be useful in assisting researchers to design culturally sensitive weight management interventions that target specific populations of parents. Understanding the voices of parents helps to provide the foundation for realistic and effective strategies to combat childhood OW and OB.

CHAPTER III: METHODOLOGY

Design

The proposed study will employ a community-based participatory research (CBPR) approach using the Photovoice methodology (Wang & Burris, 1997). CBPR, an action research method, allows for critical discussion between community members and researchers about health disparities and concerns (Colvin, de Chesnay, Mercado, & Benavides, 2005). The Photovoice methodology allows individuals to reflect on and communicate their everyday life experiences through the use of constructed images captured with a camera. This method is rooted in a critical, feminist perspective and the primary goal is to elucidate subjective experiences (Wang, 1999). Images are a powerful mechanism for individuals to document how they perceive themselves and the world around them. Social, cultural, and economic conditions affecting health can be illuminated through the creation of photographic images. The three primary goals of the Photovoice method are to produce images, to receive and attach meaning to the images, and to contextualize the content of the images (Wang, 1999).

Contextual information will be obtained from Latino parents older than the age of 18 who have one or more children in the 6- to 12-year-old age group who meet the definition of OW or

OB based on BMI for age. The participants may be English speaking only, Spanish speaking only, or bilingual. Given that the principal investigator (PI) speaks minimal conversational Spanish, a native Spanish-speaking research assistant will be employed to assist the PI during the research process.

The following steps will be used for the Photovoice methodology (Wang, 1999):

1. Community healthcare providers from a northern Georgia university-affiliated community health clinic will be engaged in a discussion about the importance of the study and the need for culturally sensitive weight management interventions in the community. A recruiting plan will be discussed as well as an agreement for use of the facilities for the focus groups.
2. Participants will be recruited from the community health clinic in northern Georgia.
3. An initial session will be conducted to introduce the participants to the Photovoice method, including education on how to use the cameras, how to take meaningful photographs, and which ethical concerns arise with photography in the community (e.g., not taking someone's picture without that person's permission). Individuals wishing to participate will then sign the research consent form. Demographic information from the participants will be collected, including age, gender, marital status, employment status, income level, and number of children.
4. The participants will meet in one of two assigned focus groups. The intent of the first focus group is to identify initial themes related to the topic of dietary and physical activity patterns. The participants will derive one to three key themes that will guide their photography assignment. Disposable 35-mm cameras will be distributed during this session, and each participant will be assigned a number. Participants will be instructed to take photographs of persons, places, and things related to the key themes. A timeline will be established for when the participants will return their cameras to the PI (participants are usually given two to three weeks to capture images).
5. The PI will develop all of the pictures in the interval between the first and second focus group sessions. Each photograph will be labeled on the back with the participant's assigned number.
6. The participants will then meet in their groups for the second set of focus groups. Each participant will select two or three photographs to share with the group. To contextualize and tell stories about the pictures, the acronym "SHOWeD" (Wang & Burris, 1997) will be used to guide the participants:

    - What do you **S**ee here?
    - What is really **H**appening here?
    - How does this relate to **O**ur lives?
    - **W**hy does this situation, concern, or strength exist?
    - What can we **D**o about it?

    Coding of key themes and issues will be completed once all participants have shared their photographs and stories.

7. Plans to share the key themes and photographs with community healthcare providers and community members at the clinic will be made.

Sample

Two groups consisting of 7 to 10 parents each will participate in the proposed study, for a total of 14 to 20 parents. Participants will be identified through the PI's connections at a northern Georgia university-affiliated community health clinic where a large number of Latino families are served. Potential participants must be older than the age of 18 and have one or more children in the 6- to 12-year-age group that meet the definition of OW or OB based on BMI for age. The child's or children's BMI will be determined based on a height and weight reported by the parent.

Setting

The focus groups will take place in a community clinic meeting room in northern Georgia at a date and time mutually agreed upon by the research team and participants. The goal for the setting is to ensure privacy and to be a convenient, familiar location for the participants. During the focus group sessions, a tape recorder will be used to capture participant responses. The PI and native Spanish-speaking research assistant will lead the focus group sessions. In addition to tape recording the session, the PI will take field notes.

Institutional Review Board Statement

The proposed study will be submitted to the university institutional review board (IRB) for approval prior to data collection. Potential participants who express interest in the study will be given a research consent form that will include information about the purpose of the study, procedures, time required to participate, confidentiality, risks, benefits, and voluntary nature of the study. Individuals who wish to participate will sign the consent form and be given a copy of the form. The contact information of both the PI and the university IRB will be given to the participants in the event that questions or concerns arise during the study. All research consent forms, tapes, transcripts, and field notes will be kept in a locked drawer in the PI's university office. All electronic files have three levels of protection: no personal identifiers, password protection, and a firewall-protected computer.

Data Analysis

Data will be analyzed using Diekelman, Allen, and Tanner's (1989) procedural steps. First, all transcripts in Spanish with be translated into English by a translator. Second, the interview transcripts and field notes will then be read in their entirety to gain an overall impression. Third, the PI will summarize key findings and search for overall themes. Fourth, the PI and the research assistant will review the transcripts together. Fifth, the PI and the research assistant will follow up with the participants as needed to clarify concepts. Sixth, the PI will identify emerging patterns among the themes. Seventh, the PI and the research assistant will review the final interpretation of the data and plan to meet with community leaders to share the results and photographs. The findings will serve as a basis for a conceptual framework about how Latino parents from northern Georgia perceive dietary and physical activity patterns for their families.

Final Report

A final report of the study will be written once data collection is complete. The final report will include a summary of the study results, a discussion of the results, conclusions, recommendations, and implications for practice.

Procedures

1. The IRB application will be submitted to the university IRB board.
2. Once approval is obtained, data collection equipment will be purchased.
3. Data entry files will be created for participant lists, demographic information, and transcripts.
4. Potential study participants will be identified at the community health center.
5. An initial session will be conducted to introduce the participants to the study as well as to the Photovoice method. The purpose of the study as well as participant rights and responsibilities will be explained, informed consent will be given, and the research consent forms will be signed. The participants will be assigned to one of two focus groups. The scheduling of focus groups will be made during the introductory session.
6. The first focus group will be conducted, followed by a two-week period during which the participants will take photographs.
7. The PI will develop the photographs.
8. The second focus group will be conducted.
9. The tapes from the focus groups will be transcribed into Microsoft Word.
10. The transcripts will be translated into English by a translator.
11. The data will be analyzed using the procedural steps outlined by Diekelman et al. (1989).
12. The final report will be reviewed and the research findings disseminated orally and in print.

Timeline

It is expected that the study will take between nine months and one year to complete from start to finish. This timeline may be adjusted depending on the availability of space to conduct the focus groups, the participant's availability, and the time it takes to transcribe and translate the research data. Please refer to Appendix A for a detailed timeline.

Budget

Refer to Appendix B for a summary of the proposed budget with justifications.

WWW

For a full suite of assignments and additional learning activities, use the access code located in the front of your book to visit this exclusive website: http://go.jblearning.com/dechesnay. If you do not have an access code, you can obtain one at the site.

REFERENCES

Anderson, S. E., & Whitaker, R. C. (2010). Household routines and obesity in U.S. preschool- aged children. *Pediatrics, 125*, 420–428. Doi:10.1542/peds.2009-0417

Arredondo, E. M., Elder, J. P., Ayala, G. X., Campbell, N., Baquero, B., & Duerksen, S. (2006). Is parenting style related to children's healthy eating and physical activity in Latino families? *Health Education Research, 216*, 862–871. Doi: 10.1093/her/cyll.10

Barlow, S. E. (2007). Expert committee recommendations regarding the prevention, assessment, and treatment of child and adolescent overweight and obesity: Summary report. *Pediatrics, 120*, S164–S192. Doi: 10.1542/peds.2007-2393C

Bethell, C., Simpson, L., Strumbo, S., Carle, A. C., & Gombojav, N. (2010). National, state, and local disparities in childhood obesity. *Health Affairs, 29*, 347–356. Doi: 10.1377/hlthaff.2009.0762

Birch, L. L., & Ventura, A. K. (2009). Preventing childhood obesity: What works? *International Journal of Obesity, 33*, S74–S81.

Carnell, S., Edwards, C., Croker, H., Boniface, D., & Wardle, J. (2005). Parental perceptions of overweight 3–5 yr olds. *International Journal of Obesity, 29*, 353–355.

Cawley, J. (2010). The economics of childhood obesity. *Health Affairs, 29*, 347–356. Doi: 10.1377/hlthaff.2009.0721

Centers for Disease Control and Prevention. (2009). About BMI for children and teens. Retrieved from www.cdc.gov/healthywt/assessing/bmi/childrens_bmi/aboutchildrens_bmi.html

Collins, C. E., Warren, J. M., Neve, M., McCoy, P., & Stokes, B. (2007). Systematic review of interventions in the management of overweight and obese children, which include a dietary component. *International Journal of Evidence Based Healthcare, 5*, 2–53. Doi: 10.1111/j.1479-6988.2007.00061.x

Colvin, S., de Chesnay, M., Mercado, T., & Benavides, C. (2005). Child health in a barrio of Managua. In M. de Chesnay (Ed.), *Caring for the vulnerable: Perspectives in nursing theory, practice and research* (pp. 161–170). Sudbury, MA: Jones and Bartlett.

Diekelman, N. L., Allen, D., & Tanner, C. (1989). *The NLN criteria for appraisal of baccalaureate programs: Critical hermeneutic analysis*. New York: National League for Nursing.

Doolen, J., Alpert, P. T., & Miller, S. K. (2009). Parental disconnect between perceived and actual weight status of children: A metasynthesis of current research. *Journal of the American Academy of Nurse Practitioners, 21*, 160–166. Doi:10.1111/j.1745-7599.2008.00382.x

Eckstein, K. C., Mikhail, L. M., Ariza, A. J., Thomson, S., Millard, S. C., & Binns, H. J. (2006). Parents' perceptions of their child's weight and health. *Pediatrics, 117*, 681–690. Doi: 10.1542/peds.2005-0910

Elder, J. P., Arredondo, E. M., Campbell, N., Baquero, B., Ayala, G., Crespo, N.C., . . . McKenzie, T. (2010). Individual, family, and community environmental correlates of obesity in Latino elementary school children. *Journal of School Health, 80*, 20–30.

Fennoy, I. (2010). Metabolic and respiratory comorbidities of childhood obesity. *Pediatric Annals, 39*, 140–146.

Finkelstein, E. A., Trogdon, J. G., Cohen, J. W., & Dietz, W. (2009). Annual medical spending attributable to obesity: Payer and service specific estimates. *Health Affairs, 28*, W872– W831.

Franks, P. W., Hanson, R. L., Knowler, W. C., Sievers, M. L., Bennett, P. H., & Looker, H. C. (2010). Childhood obesity, other cardiovascular risk factors, and premature death. *New England Journal of Medicine, 362*, 485–493.

Fuentes-Afflick, E., & Hessol, N. A. (2008). Overweight in young Latino children. *Archives of Medical Research, 39*, 511–518.

Gallagher, M. R. (2009). Maternal perspectives on lifestyle habits that put children of Mexican descent at risk for obesity. *Journal for Specialists in Pediatric Nursing, 15*(1), 16–25. Doi: 10.1111/j.1744-6155.2009.00213.x

Garcia, R. S. (2004). No come nada. *Health Affairs, 23*, 215–219. Doi: 10.1377/hlthaff.23.2.215

Golan, M., & Crow, S. (2004). Parents are key players in the prevention and treatment of weight-related problems. *Nutrition Reviews, 82*, 39–50.

Goodell, L. S., Pierce, M. B., Bravo, C. M., & Ferris, A. M. (2008). Parental perception of overweight during early childhood. *Qualitative Health Research, 11*, 1548–1555.

Goodhart, F. W., Hsu, J., Baek, J. H., Coleman, A. L., Maresca, F. M., & Miller, M. B. (2006). A view through a different lens: Photovoice as a tool for student advocacy. *Journal of American College Health, 55*, 53–56.

Hackie, M., & Bowles, C. L. (2007). Maternal perception of their overweight children. *Public Health Nursing, 6*, 538–546. Doi: 0.1111/j.1525-1446.2007.00666.x

Krebs, N. F., Himes, J. H., Jacobson, D., Nicklas, T. A., Guilday, P., & Styne, D. (2007). Assessment of child and adolescent overweight and obesity. *Pediatrics, 120*, S193–S228. Doi: 10.1542/peds.2007-2329D

Latzer, Y., Edmunds, L., Fenig, S., Golan, M., Gur, E., Hochberg, Z., . . . Stein, D. (2008). Managing childhood overweight: Behavior, family, pharmacology, and bariatric surgery interventions. *Obesity, 17*, 411–423. Doi:10.1038/oby.2008.553

Matheson, D. M., Robinson, T. N., Varady, A., & Killen, J.D. (2006). Do Mexican American mothers' food-related parenting practices influence their children's weight and dietary intake? *Journal of the American Dietetic Association, 106*, 1861–1865.

Odgen, C. L., Carroll, M. D., Curtin, L. R., Lamb, M. M., & Flegal, K. M. (2010). Prevalence of high body mass index in US children and adolescents, 2007–2008. *Journal of the American Medical Association, 303*, 242–249.

Odgen, C. L., Carroll, M. D., Curtin, L. R., McDowell, M. A., Tabak, C. J., & Flegal, K. M. (2006). Prevalence of overweight and obesity in the United States, 1999–2004. *Journal of the American Medical Association, 295*, 1549–1555.

Raghuveer, G. (2010). Lifetime cardiovascular risk of childhood obesity. *American Journal of Clinical Nutrition, 91*, 1514S–1519S. Doi: 10.3945/ajcn.2010.28701D

Richardson, L. D., & Norris, M. (2010). Access to health and health care: How race and ethnicity matter. *Mount Sinai Journal of Medicine, 77*, 166–177.

Schwartz, L., Sable, M., Dannerbeck, A., & Campbell, J. (2007). Using Photovoice to improve family planning for immigrant Hispanics. *Journal for Health Care of the Poor and Underserved, 18*, 757–766.

Sharma, A. J., Grummer-Strawn, L. M., Dalenius, K., Galuska, D., Anandappa, M., & Borland, E. (2009). Obesity prevalence among low income preschool aged children in the US 1998–2008. *Morbidity and Mortality Weekly Report, 58*, 769–773.

Starling Washington, P., Reifsnider, E., Bishop, S., Domingeaux Ethington, M. E., & Ruffin, R. (2010). Changes in family variables among normal and overweight preschoolers. *Issues in Comprehensive Pediatric Nursing, 33*, 20–38.

Stevens, C. A. (2006). Being healthy: Voices of adolescent women who are parenting. *Journal for Specialists in Pediatric Nursing, 11*, 28–40.

Sussner, K. M., Lindsay, A. C., Greaney, M. L., & Peterson, K. E. (2008). The influence of immigrant status and acculturation on the development of overweight in Latino families: A qualitative study. *Journal of Immigrant and Minority Health, 10*, 497–505. Doi: 10.1007/s10903-008-9137-3

Taveras, E. M., Gillman, M. W., Kleinman, K., Rich-Edwards, J. W., & Rifas-Shiman, S. L. (2010). Racial/ethnic differences in early-life risk factors for childhood obesity. *Pediatrics, 125*, 686–695. Doi:10.1542/peds.2009-2100

Towns, N., & D'Auria, J. (2009). Parental perceptions of their child's overweight: An integrative review of the literature. *Journal of Pediatric Nursing, 24*, 115–130. Doi: 10.1016/j.pedn.2008.02.032

Valera, P., Gallin, J., Schuk, D., & Davis, N. (2009). "Trying to eat healthy": A Photovoice study about women's access to healthy food in New York City. *Affila: Journal of Women and Social Work, 24*, 300–314.

Vaughn, L., Rojas-Guyler, L., & Howell, B. (2008). "Picturing" health: A Photovoice pilot of Latina girls' perceptions of health. *Family and Community Health, 31*, 305–316. Doi: 10.1097/01.FCH.0000336093.39066.e9

Wang, C. C. (1999). Photovoice: A participatory action research strategy applied to women's health. *Journal of Women's Health, 8*, 185–192.

Wang, C., & Burris, M. (1997). Photovoice: Concept, methodology, and use for participatory needs assessment. *Health Education & Behavior, 24*, 369–378.

Wang, C. C., & Pies, C. M. (2004). Family, maternal, and child health through Photovoice. *Maternal and Child Health Journal, 8*, 95–102.

Ward, C. L. (2008). Parental perceptions of childhood overweight in the Mexican-American population: An integrative review. *Journal of School Nursing, 24*, 407–416.

West, D. S., Raczynski, J. M., Phillips, M. M., Bursac, Z., Health Gauss, C., & Montgomery, B. E. (2008). Parental recognition of overweight in school-aged children. *Obesity, 16*, 630–636.

World Health Organization (WHO). (2010). Population-based strategies for childhood obesity. Retrieved from http://www.who.int/dietphysicalactivity/childhood/report/en

APPENDIX A

Detailed Timeline

Specific Activities or Steps	Month of Activity or Step											
	1	2	3	4	5	6	7	8	9	10	11	12
Prepare and submit IRB application	X											
Recruit co-PI, co-investigators, and clerical personnel	X											
Orient project team to roles		X										
Duplicate IRB consent forms		X										
Advertise study			X									
Recruit participants			X									
Conduct first focus group				X								
Transcribe first focus group session				X								
Develop photographs					X							
Conduct second focus group						X						
Transcribe second focus group session						X						
Analyze data							X	X	X			
Prepare final report									X			
Prepare manuscripts										X	X	
Disseminate results through publications and presentations											X	X→

APPENDIX B

Proposed Budget

A.	**Personnel**		**$81,570**
	1. Principal investigator: Dr. Nicole Mareno		
	Academic year salary (sample salary = 50,000)		
	Stipend requested (40% effort = 50,000) =	20,000	
	Fringe benefits (30% of salary × 50,000) =	15,000	
	Summer stipend (30% of 9 months' salary × 50,000) =	15,000	
	Summer fringe benefits (30% × 15,000) =	4,500	
	2. Co-principal investigator: Dr. Mary de Chesnay (donated time)	0	
	3. Co-investigator: Ms. Donna Chambers (donated time)	0	
	4. Clerical support		
	a. Clerical manager ($10/hr × 40 hr/week = 50 weeks ×	20,000	
	Fringe benefits (30% × 20,000 =)	6000	
	b. Interpreter		
	$20/hour for 10 hours total interpretation	200	
	No fringe benefits		
	c. Transcriptionist		
	$15/hour for 30 hours total translation	450	
	No fringe benefits		
	d. Graduate research assistant		
	$14/hour for 30 hours total		
	No fringe benefits	420	
B.	**Project Operating Expenses**		**$3343**
	1. Cameras and developing		
	a. 35-mm, 27-exposure cameras	114	
	b. Developing	129	
	2. Office supplies	100	
	3. Travel	3000	
Total Funding Request			**$84,913**

BUDGET EXPLANATION/JUSTIFICATION

A. Personnel

1. *Principal Investigator:* Dr. Nicole Mareno's role is to train the research team, manage the project, coordinate the data collection, analyze the data, write the final reports, and prepare publications and presentations for dissemination.
2. *Co-principal Investigator:* Dr. Mary de Chesnay, who is experienced in conducting action research, will serve as a methodology consultant on the project. Dr. de Chesnay will assist Dr. Mareno with management of the budget. In her role as Director of the School of Nursing, she is experienced in managing budgets and will also work with Dr. Mareno to ensure adequate course release time to complete the research. No funds are requested, as her time is donated.
3. *Co-investigator:* Ms. Donna Chambers, the FNP clinical coordinator of the clinic, will assist in gaining access to the sample. Her time is donated.
4. *Clerical Support*
   a. *Clerical Manager:* The clerical manager's role is to assist with recruitment of the study participants, schedule appointments, arrange meeting rooms, call participants to remind them of focus group sessions, and assist in writing reports.
   b. *Interpreter:* Because a large proportion of the sample is Spanish speaking, an interpreter will be needed to assist with informed consent, instructions for data collection, and interpretation during the focus group sessions.
   c. *Transcriptionist:* A transcriptionist is needed to transcribe tapes from the interviews.
   d. *Research Assistant:* The research assistant will assist with data collection and report writing. The research assistant will be mentored by Dr. Mareno to conduct spin-off studies for a graduate project or dissertation. If a graduate research assistant cannot be recruited, an attempt will be made to recruit an undergraduate research assistant.

B. Project Operating Expenses

1. *Cameras/Developing:* Costs to cover disposable cameras and developing at a local drugstore. In addition, 6% state sales tax is included. Thirty 35-mm, 27-exposure cameras are needed (three 10-packs at $38.00 apiece). Developing costs include 810 prints × $0.15 plus 6% tax.
2. *Office Supplies:* Legal pads, pens, and other items are needed for taking field notes.
3. *Travel:* Both the research assistant and the interpreter will be traveling to the research data collection sites. Travel costs for the research assistant (four site visits) and the interpreter (three site visits) were calculated by multiplying the number of trips by the state rate of $0.50 per mile for 309 miles. Travel to a conference for the principal investigator will include airfare, hotel, conference fee, and meals.

CHAPTER 16

Sample Quantitative Research Proposal: Effect of Video-Based Education on Knowledge and Perceptions of Risk for Breast Cancer Genes *BRCA1* and *BRCA2* in Urban Latina Populations

Janice B. Flynn and Janice Long

Objectives

At the end of this chapter, the reader will be able to

1. Using the outline from Chapter 14, propose a quantitative study that can be conducted with urban Latinas at risk for breast cancer.
2. Describe the ethical implications of conducting quantitative research with this particular vulnerable population.

WWW

This chapter is a shortened version of a sample outline of a quantitative research proposal. The study has not been conducted.

CHAPTER I: STUDY OVERVIEW

The purpose of this study is to determine the effect of a video-based educational intervention for knowledge and perceptions of risk for *BRCA1* and *BRCA2* (*BRCA1/2*) in an urban Latina population. It is hypothesized that the intervention will increase knowledge about risk for inherited breast cancer (IBC) associated with *BRCA1/2* and increase awareness of the risk of having a mutation in *BRCA1/2*.

Research Questions

1. What is the effect of a video-based educational intervention on knowledge of *BRCA1/2* testing among Latinas?
2. What is the effect of a video-based educational intervention on perception of risk for a gene mutation in *BRCA1/2* for Latinas?

Null Hypothesis

1. There are no significant differences in pre- and post-test scores for knowledge about *BRCA1/2* between intervention and control groups.
2. There are no significant differences in pre- and post-test scores for perception of risk of *BRCA1/2* between intervention and control groups.

Background

Among all breast cancers, 5% to 10% have been linked to genetic mutations in two identified breast cancer genes, *BRCA1/2.* Germline genetic mutations in *BRCA1/2* have been linked to an 85% lifetime risk of developing breast cancer at an average age of 30 to 40 years (King, Marks, & Mandell, 2003; Schwartz et al., 2009). Development of gene sequencing technology led to the commercial availability of deoxyribonucleic acid (DNA) testing for *BRCA1/2.* This kind of DNA testing (also referred to as genetic testing) for *BRCA1/2* is not considered a population screening tool. Instead, individuals with preliminary risks for IBC should be identified and referred for further analysis of risk including detailed pedigree development. Research is needed to identify best practices for teaching women about the risks for IBC related to *BRCA1/2.* Women need to know and understand their own risk for IBC to decrease their anxiety and worry if they are not at high risk of carrying the mutations in *BRCA1/2.* Knowledge of risk can inform decision making related to genetic testing for the abnormal genes.

In the sparse literature related to knowledge and perceptions about genetic testing, some researchers have found that Latinas have low knowledge (Honda, 2003; Kinney, Gammon, Coxworth, Simonsen, & Arce-Laretta, 2010; Ramirez, Aparicio Ting, de Majors, & Miller, 2006) and negative perceptions of genetic testing (Thompson, Valdimarsdottir, Jandorf, & Redd, 2003). In contrast, other researchers have identified positive attitudes in this population, including increased interest in participating in cancer genetics services and testing (Ramirez et al., 2006; Ricker et al., 2007; Ramirez et al. (2006) concluded that high interest in genetic testing may be driven by lack of knowledge of risk factors for IBC. Kinney et al. (2010) concluded there was a need for bilingual media to increase awareness about IBC. Further study is needed to describe knowledge and perceptions of IBC linked to *BRCA1/2* status in Latinas.

Theoretical Framework

The theoretical base for the study is health belief model (HBM), as defined in **Table 16–1**. Using constructs of the HBM, this study will describe the effectiveness of an educational intervention as the modifying factor (knowledge about *BRCA1/2*) and the individual perception of perceived risk of having an altered breast cancer gene. From these variables, the study will explore knowledge and perceptions about *BRCA1/2* in Latinas.

Assumptions

For this study, the following assumptions are identified:

1. Subjects are capable of understanding the instruments.
2. The subjects' responses to the instruments represent their perceptions.

Table 16–1 Organizational Constructs of the Health Belief Model Applied to Genetics

Individual Perceptions	Modifying Factors	Cues to Action	Likelihood of Action
Breast cancer susceptibility	Age, race	Genetic testing awareness	Intent to obtain testing for breast cancer genes
Altered gene susceptibility	Knowledge of *BRCA1/2*		
Breast cancer seriousness	Breast cancer family history		
Genetic testing—benefits, barriers	Personal breast cancer risks		

Sources: Flynn, 2001. Adapted from Champion & Scott, 1997; Lerman et al., 1997; Rosenstock, 1966.

3. Knowledge about *BRCA1/2* and perceptions of risks of inherited breast cancer can be measured in women.
4. Women who have mutations in *BRCA1/2* are at higher risk for developing breast cancer at an earlier age.
5. Acculturation in Latina immigrants to the United States may have an effect on these women's knowledge of *BRCA1/*2 and perceptions of risk for IBC.

Definitions

1. Breast Cancer Genes (*BRCA1/2*)

   Theoretical definition: *BRCA1/2* are tumor suppressor autosomal dominant genes that are carried in paternal and maternal blood lines (Schwartz et al., 2009; Turnpenny & Ellard, 2005). *BRCA1* is located on the long arm of chromosome 17 (q12–21), while *BRCA2* is on the long arm of chromosome 13. *BRCA1* is thought to account for 30% to 40% of breast cancer in families with a high incidence of breast cancer and as much as 90% of combined breast and ovarian cancer (Schwartz et al., 2009; Yarbro, Frogge, & Goodman, 2005). *BRCA2* is considered to be responsible for 35% of early-onset breast cancer, but also has been linked with other cancers such as pancreatic, fallopian tube, and uterine cancers, male breast cancer, and adult leukemia (Turnpenny & Ellard, 2005). Multiple mutations of both genes have been reported. While the two genes are modestly different in molecular characteristics, *BRCA1/2* are commonly grouped together given that their similarities outweigh the differences.

   Operational definition: Risk factors for both genes include the client or a first-degree blood relative with early-onset breast cancer; the client or a first-degree blood relative with ovarian cancer; bilateral breast cancer in the client or a first-degree blood degree relative; both ovarian and breast cancer in the client or a first-degree blood relative; the client or a blood relative known to have a *BRCA1* or *BRCA2* mutation; Ashkenazi Jewish women who have breast or ovarian cancer or a family history of one or both diseases; and breast cancer in a male family member (Narod, 2006; Schwartz et al., 2009; Turnpenny & Ellard, 2005).

2. Knowledge About Inherited Breast Cancer and *BRCA1*

   Theoretical definition: An understanding of inheritance of breast–ovarian cancer susceptibility and genetic testing (Flynn, 2001; Lerman et al., 1996).
   Operational definition: Knowledge about inherited breast cancer and *BRCA1/2* based on the score on the Knowledge About Inherited Breast Cancer and *BRCA1/2* Questionnaire (Lerman, et al., 1996). The 11-item true/false scale measures knowledge of inheritance patterns and risk factors for *BRCA1/2*.

3. Health Beliefs

   Theoretical definition: An individual's feelings of personal vulnerability to a specific health problem and the conviction that the benefits of taking action to protect health outweigh the barriers that will be encountered. Beliefs about personal susceptibility and seriousness of disease combine to produce the degree of threat or negative valence of a particular disease (Rosenstock, 1966).
   Operational definition: Perceived risk of having a *BRCA1/2* mutation is the score on the Perceived Risk of Having a *BRCA1* Mutation Scale (Lerman et al., 1996).
4. Latino Culture: The attitudes and behavior that are characteristic of the Latino population.
5. Promotores de Salud: Hispanic/Latino community health workers who advocate for healthy lifestyles, serve as lay health educators, and act as communicators between health consumers and providers.
6. Faith-Based Settings: A group of individuals united on the basis of religious or spiritual beliefs (Ransdell & Rehling, 1996).

Limitations

1. Caution must be exercised in making inferences from the results of this study to Latinas outside the geographic region or to Latinas from ethnic groups other than those included in the study.
2. Subjects may be reluctant to answer questions related to genetics due to a lack of knowledge or understanding of the meanings of the terms. They may also be fearful or uncertain about the implications for their own family.
3. Data provided by the participants are expected to consist of their own perceptions of their risk for inherited breast cancer and their own knowledge of the condition. Some participants may have experience in the past with *BRCA1/2* and may have communicated with other subjects.

Significance to Latinas

In the United States, breast cancer is the second leading cause of death from cancer in women, and the most frequently diagnosed cancer in women. In general, women have a 10% chance of developing breast cancer in a lifetime, with the average onset between 60 and 70 years of age (American Cancer Society [ACS], 2010). Among Latinas, breast cancer is the most frequently diagnosed cancer and leads to higher mortality in this group. While the breast cancer incidence rate in Latinas is lower than that in non-Hispanic white women, breast cancer among Latinas is more likely to be underdiagnosed (ACS, 2007). For those Latinas who are diagnosed with breast cancer, more are likely to have reached a late-stage breast cancer level compared with non-Latina whites (Shavers, Harlan, & Stevens, 2003; Vanderpool, Kornfeld, Rutten, & Squiers, 2009).

In general, Latinos do not have a significantly higher rate of carrying the *BRCA1/2* genes than other ethnic groups. The one ethnic group that has been identified as having a higher incidence of *BRCA1/2* is Ashkenazi Jews. Early haplotype studies suggest a founder effect between Ashkenazi Jews and individuals of Mexican descent; however, this linkage has not been broadly confirmed in the literature (Weizel et al., 2005). It is important to reach the Latina population early to identify risk and implement education programs on the urgency for early recognition of breast cancer.

Feasibility and Application

Examining the effects of a video educational intervention on knowledge and perception of risk for *BRCA1/2* among Latinas appears to be a feasible, researchable study. It can be measured quantitatively and is easily implemented. Exploring this research question may provide information useful to nurses in diverse settings, ranging from public health and home care to acute care settings. The findings could also prove helpful for nurse practitioners and other healthcare providers who are uniquely positioned to provide education on breast health and cancer prevention for Latinas. If educational videos are effective in increasing the knowledge and awareness of risk for *BRCA1/2*, it is possible that more Latinas will be better informed about their personal risk for *BRCA1/2*.

CHAPTER II: REVIEW OF THE RESEARCH LITERATURE

BRCA1 and BRCA2

Four genetic mutations have been linked to breast cancer: *BRCA1*, *BRCA2*, p53 (associated with Li-Fraumeni syndrome), and *CD1* (associated with Cowden syndrome and possibly ataxia telangiectasia [ATM]). Of these genetic mutations, the *BRCA1/2* set has been implicated in more direct causation of breast and ovarian cancers (Schwartz et al., 2009). *BRCA1* and *BRCA2* were identified with positional cloning in 1994 and 1995, respectively (Futreal et al., 1994; Miki et al., 1994; Wooster et al., 1995). Schwartz and colleagues (2009) also concluded that familial breast cancers in clients who test negative for the *BRCA1/2* genes are presumably due to other, as yet unidentified, high-penetrance genes.

Soon after the cloning of *BRCA1/2*, multiple studies of high-risk families identified risk factors associated with mutation in *BRCA1* and *BRCA2* (Frank et al., 1998; Narod, 2006). Those findings have held up throughout the past 15 years and were reaffirmed by Schwartz and colleagues (2009) at the International Consensus Conference on Breast Cancer Risk, Genetics, and Risk Management. Risks for *BRCA1/2* include the following:

- Client or first-degree blood relative with early-onset breast cancer
- Client or first-degree blood relative with ovarian cancer
- Bilateral breast cancer in client or first-degree blood relative
- Both ovarian and breast cancer in client or first-degree blood relative
- Client or blood relative known to have a *BRCA1* or *BRCA2* mutation
- Ashkenazi Jewish women who have breast or ovarian cancer or a family history of one or both diseases
- Breast cancer in a male family member

Because mutations in *BRCA1/2* are rare, screening for these mutations in the general population is unwarranted. However, in this information age, news of genetic advances is instantly available to the general public through media and the Internet and may increase expectations, anxiety, and worry about genetic testing (Lerman et al., 1996; Wang, Gonzalez, Janz, Milliron, & Merajver, 2007). One of the greatest challenges in the immediate future will be for healthcare providers to assist individuals with the interpretation of genetic advances and applications of these advances in the diagnosis and treatment of genetically linked adult-onset disease.

Most scientists agree that testing for the genetic alterations *BRCA1/2* should include extensive genetic counseling. Contrary to that recommendation, the reality is that biotechnology companies are offering genetic testing for the breast cancer genes to healthcare providers and to the general public (Turnpenny & Ellard, 2005). Studies in the literature of women's knowledge and perceptions about genetic testing for breast cancer are few in number and mostly limited to women in high-risk populations (Lerman et al., 1997; Lerman et al., 1996; Ramirez et al., 2006).

Studies on genetic testing for cancer susceptibility suggest that the motivation for genetic testing may diminish as individuals at low to moderate risks receive education about the limits and risks of testing. Following a study of families with high-risk kindreds, Lerman and colleagues (1997) concluded that standard educational approaches may be equally effective as expanded counseling approaches in enhancing knowledge for decision making about genetic testing. Confirming Lerman et al.'s earlier findings, Ramirez et al. (2006) concluded that culturally sensitive educational materials are needed to inform Hispanics about hereditary risk for breast cancer. Descriptions of the systematic study of what women in the general population know and think about inherited breast cancer and associated genetic testing are extremely limited in the literature, and this topic clearly warrants further study. Reports on the implementation of educational programs for women who may not be at high risk for IBC are absent in the literature. Additionally, further study is needed to determine whether individuals outside identified high-risk kindreds have an inflated view of their personal risk of having a genetic mutation in *BRCA1/2*.

Health Belief Model

The health belief model was originally proposed as a theoretical framework for explaining why some people who are free of disease or illness take actions to avoid illness, whereas others fail to take protective actions (Rosenstock, 1966). The intention of the model was to predict who would or would not use preventive measures to maintain health as well as to recommend interventions that might increase the predisposition of resistant individuals to adopt health-protecting behaviors. HBM is based on the assumption that behavior is determined by the individual's subjective perception of the environment (Rosenstock, 1974). Cues or stimuli to health behavioral action may be internal, such as a symptom, or external, such as interaction with others or the mass media (Maiman & Becker, 1974). Other assumptions of the HBM include the premise that health is a valued goal for most individuals and that people can accept the possibility that they may have a serious illness in the complete absence of symptom.

Based on the social–psychological work of Lewin (1935), HBM reflects health protection as avoidance of negatively valence regions of illness and disease (Davidhizar, 1983). To further explain a negative valence region, Lewin (1935) described the life space in which an individual exists as being composed of regions—some having negative valence, some having positive valance, and others being relatively neutral. Illness is conceived to exist in the region of negative valence, and has the potential to move an individual from neutral or positive valence to negative valence.

Becker (1974) modified the HBM to further define variables that predict the likelihood of taking recommended preventive health actions. Variables proposed as directly affecting predisposition to take action include the perceived threat to personal health and the belief that the benefits of preventive action outweigh the perceived barriers to action.

In analyzing this model's utility for health protective behaviors, Pender (1996, pp. 35–36) summarized it as including the following propositions:

1. Beliefs about personal susceptibility and the seriousness of a specific disease combine to produce the degree of threat or negative valence of a particular disease.
2. Perceived susceptibility reflects individuals' feeling of personal vulnerability to a specific health problem.
3. Perceived seriousness or severity of a given health problem can be judged either by the degree of emotional arousal created by the thought of having the disease or by the medical and clinical or social difficulties (family and work) that individuals believe a given health condition would create for them.
4. Perceived benefits are beliefs about the effectiveness of recommended actions in preventing the health threat.
5. Perceived barriers are perceptions concerning the potential negative aspects of taking action, such as expense, danger, unpleasantness, inconvenience, and time required.
6. Modifying variables such as demographic, sociopsychologic, and structural variables, as well as cues to action, only indirectly affects action tendencies through these variables' relationship with the perception of threat.

After reviewing a 10-year period of HBM research, Janz and Becker (1984) concluded that perceived barriers are the most powerful of the HBM dimensions in explaining or predicting health behavior. These authors also noted the implication that perceived susceptibility is an important variable in understanding protective health behaviors. Pender (1996) credits HBM as being foundational to the development of the health promotion model, in which she defines health protection as "decreasing the probability of experiencing health problems by active protection against pathologic stresses or detection of health problems in the asymptotic stage. Health protection focuses on efforts to move away from or avoid the negatively valenced states of illness" (p. 34).

While not a formal part of the HBM, the concepts of primary, secondary, and tertiary prevention have been used to describe health protection activities. According to Fensler and Miller (1997). the HBM has been used "extensively as a framework for the identification of individuals who engage in behaviors relevant to primary and secondary prevention" (p. 82). Primary prevention is the specific protection against a disease to prevent its occurrence. Examples include mass immunizations to prevent disease, reductions in risk factors, and control of air, water, and noise pollution so as to prevent chronic diseases. Secondary prevention is defined as organized, direct screening efforts or education of the public to promote early case finding of individuals with disease so that treatments can be implemented to halt pathologic process and limit disability. Examples include use of home kits for detection of occult blood in the stool and public education to promote health behaviors such as mammography and breast self-examination. Tertiary prevention is aimed at minimizing residual disability from disease and promoting a productive life, within the limitation of the residual effects. Examples include cardiac rehabilitation and stroke rehabilitation (Pender, 1996).

In cancer research, the HBM has been used extensively as a theoretical framework for identifying behaviors relevant to primary and secondary prevention. Specific to breast cancer, this model has been used to study breast self-examination practices (Champion, 1994, 1995; Rutledge & Davis, 1998; Sensiba, 1995) and mammography screening for breast cancer (Champion, 1994; Fischera & Frank, 1994; Johnson & Meischke, 1994).

The utility of the HBM in cancer research and screening is well established. Health motivation and perceived barriers have been validated as strong predictors of individuals' intentions and behaviors related to cancer prevention and screening (Champion, 1995; Cody & Lee, 1990; Johnson & Meischke, 1994; Kelly, Zyzanski, & Alenagno, 1991; Sensiba & Stewart, 1995; Wyper, 1990).

Use of the HBM in genetic testing for breast cancer has been primarily limited to women in high-risk populations (Lerman et al., 1997; Lerman et al., 1996). In an effort to evaluate health beliefs about *BRCA1/2* in a more general population, Flynn (2001) studied 270 women with no prior diagnosis of breast cancer. The results revealed that perceived susceptibility to breast cancer, intent to obtain genetic testing, and the number of first-degree relatives with ovarian cancer were significant predictors of perceived risk of having an altered breast cancer gene. In 2007, Wang et al. surveyed 205 women prior to their genetic counseling appointments, and then completed a chart audit to determine genetic testing decisions. A significant three-way interaction existed between perceived susceptibility, perceived severity, and worry about being a *BRCA1/2* carrier that affected testing decisions. McGarvey et al. (2003) used the HBM to investigate differences among ethnically diverse, low-income women. This study concluded that barriers and health beliefs differ among ethnic groups and that clients should not be collapsed into general categories, but rather grouped according to country of origin.

Methods of Education for Latinas

No studies were found that provided evidence for effective health education methods for teaching Latinas about genetic testing for *BRCA1/2*. However, a few studies did suggest that Latinos might benefit from video-based education. A study conducted by Gordon and Iribarren (2008), for example, found that participants who were dominant Spanish speakers preferred education in video form or in their homes on television. Another study conducted with Latinos regarding end-of-life decision making supported the concept that videos were a useful teaching strategy but must be culturally sensitive to the ethnic group's beliefs and practices (Volandes, Ariza, Abbo, & Paasche-Orlow, 2008). Murphy et al. (2007) used culturally sensitive video vignettes that were specific to the patient's own ethnic group to teach a variety of health topics. These educational vignettes were found to be effective in communicating health messages compared to the usual brochure.

CHAPTER III: METHODOLOGY

Design

An experimental, comparison design will be used to examine participant knowledge and perception of risk for *BRCA1/2* before and after exposure to a culturally sensitive, Spanish-language video. To control for testing bias, a randomly selected sample of participants will receive the same pre- and post-testing over an identical time frame as the participants who view the video education program. It is anticipated that the intervention group results will demonstrate significantly higher knowledge level and awareness of *BRCA1/2* compared to the control group. The researchers are fluent in the Spanish language, and promotores de salud from the two faith-based settings will be trained as research assistants for each of the on-site groups. This project proposal will be sent to the institutional review board (IRB) for approval prior to implementation of the actual study.

Sample

A convenience sample of approximately 50 Latinas from 18 to 50 years of age will be recruited for participation in the study through a partnership with two local promotores de salud faith-based programs. The two faith-based settings have Latino memberships numbering more than 2000, and each has from six to eight promotores de salud who work with the congregations.

Once candidates demonstrate an interest in participating, they will be invited to a meeting at a designated community setting. All participants will initially gather into one room, where each will receive a copy of the consent form for participation. Consent forms will be written in Spanish and English. The consent form will include the following information: (1) the purpose of the study, (2) description of the intervention, (3) length of time involved, (4) descriptions of the risks and benefits, (5) strategies for maintaining confidentiality, and (6) contact information for the primary researcher and the IRB. A researcher will read the consent form aloud and answer questions. All participants will be asked to complete a demographic questionnaire.

The Knowledge About Inherited Breast Cancer and *BRCA1* Questionnaire and the Perception of Risk for *BRCA1/2* instruments (pre- and post-tests, respectively) will be administered to all participants. Once the consent forms are read and signed, and the pre-tests collected, 25 participants who are randomly assigned to the intervention group will leave the room with one researcher and promotore de salud research assistant. A total of 25 participants will be present in each of the two locations. Participants remaining in the control group setting will not be subjected to the intervention.

Setting

The study will take place at a community meeting site where two rooms are available, one of which can accommodate as many as 50 participants. The two rooms will be isolated from each other to assure that no sound from either can be overheard.

Instrumentation

Two instruments (pre- and post-tests) and a demographic form will be used for the study:

Knowledge About Inherited Breast Cancer and BRCA1 *Questionnaire.* The Knowledge About Inherited Breast Cancer and *BRCA1* Questionnaire is an 11-item true/false scale used to assess knowledge of inherited breast–ovarian cancer susceptibility and genetic testing. It is scored based on the number of correct responses (range = 0–11). Permission is not necessary for use this instrument, which was developed by the National Center for Human Genome Research Cancer Studies Consortium (Lerman et al., 1996) as a part of a set of core instruments. This document is in the public domain.

Perception of Risk for BRCA1 *and* BRCA2. Perception of Risk for *BRCA1* and *BRCA2* is the score on the Perceived Risk of Having a *BRCA1* Mutation Scale. Permission is not necessary for use this instrument, which was developed by the National Center for Human Genome Research Cancer Studies Consortium (Lerman et al., 1996) as a part of a set of core instruments. This document is in the public domain.

Demographic Data (Investigator Developed)

A demographic questionnaire developed by the investigator will be used to gather descriptive data for subjects. Demographic data will include age, marital status, geographical origin of ancestors, ethnic background, education (highest level), occupation, employment status, ethnic background, family income, family background (e.g., adopted), and number of children.

Data Analysis

The data from each demographic, pretest, and posttest will be entered into SPSS for analysis using unique identification codes for each participant. Two researchers will examine the data independently to assure accuracy.

Frequency distributions will be examined for central tendencies and for possible outliers and missing variables. A two-variable analysis of variance (ANOVA) will be conducted to examine differences between participants' pre- and post-test scores on each of the two instruments. Both within-group and between-group analysis will provide a means to determine whether either the control group or the intervention group achieves statistically significant improvement between the predictor variable or pre-test of knowledge and awareness of *BRCA1* and *BRCA2* compared to the post-test awareness and knowledge.

Validity and Reliability

The *Knowledge About Inherited Breast Cancer Questionnaire* has been tested in previous studies and found to be reliable (alpha = .74) and valid (Flynn, 2001; Lerman et al., 1997; Lerman et al., 1996). Reliability and validity cannot be determined for the *Perception of Risk for* BRCA1 because it is a one-item scale.

Procedures

1. Funding to conduct the study will be obtained.
2. Community partners will be identified.
3. The IRB application will be submitted to the university IRB committee.
4. An advisory board will be formed and will include a representative from the university and other community partners, and one promotore de salud from each of the faith-based settings.
5. Once IRB approval is obtained, computer software (SPSS) will be purchased and forms for data collection printed.
6. Flyers will be developed explaining the intent of the study, the date and time, and the location for each setting. Each flyer will be written in both Spanish and English.
7. Promotores de salud at each setting will be trained on the purpose of the study, the methods involved in recruiting, and their role in recruiting participants. Flyers will be given to each promotore de salud to distribute on a designated date to that individual's congregation.
8. With the help of the promotores de salud, two rooms will be reserved at a central location that is convenient for participants from each of the two faith-based settings.
9. A database will be created using the list of participants provided by each promotore de salud from each location.
10. A two-hour meeting will be held at the designated setting. At the start of the meeting, the researchers will introduce the participants to the study and explain and obtain informed consent from all participants. The purpose of the study will be explained as well as participants' right to leave if they do not wish to participate. The participants will be asked to complete three forms: one covering demographics, the *Knowledge About Inherited Breast Cancer Questionnaire*, and the *Perceptions of Risk for* BRCA1 instrument. All participants will hear the same instructions. Once the initial forms are completed, a randomly selected group (Group 1) will be asked to move to a

second room, where they will receive the video education intervention on *BRCA1/2*. All other participants will be designated as Group 2.

11. While Group 1 is viewing the video, Group 2 will view a general health and wellness video. After watching the video, the participants will be asked to complete the post-test.
12. The group randomized to view the video education program will view the video vignette education on *BRCA1/2*. They will then be provided with refreshments and the post-tests will be completed.
13. The participants will be thanked for their participation and the meeting will be dismissed at least two hours from the time it began.
14. The data will be entered by the two researchers into SPSS, and analysis conducted using SPSS. Data will then be presented to the advisory board for discussion and determination of next steps.
15. The research findings will be prepared in a final report to the funder, the advisory committee, and the community partners including the promotores de salud. The findings will then be disseminated through poster and/or oral presentations.

Timeline

After funding is secured, it is expected that the study will take place over six months with the meeting itself occurring in one two-hour time frame (Appendix A). This timeline may be adjusted depending on the availability of promotores de salud to recruit participants and adequate space to conduct the meetings.

Budget

Refer to Appendix B for a summary of the proposed budget with justifications.

WWW

For a full suite of assignments and additional learning activities, use the access code located in the front of your book to visit this exclusive website: http://go.jblearning.com/dechesnay. If you do not have an access code, you can obtain one at the site.

REFERENCES

American Cancer Society (ACS). (2007) *Cancer facts and figures for Hispanic/Latinos 2006–2008*. Atlanta, GA: Author.

American Cancer Society (ACS). (2010). *Facts and figures*. Atlanta, GA: Author.

Becker, M. (Ed.). (1974). *The health belief model and personal health behavior*. Thorofare, NJ: Slack.

Champion, V. (1994). Beliefs about breast cancer and mammography by behavioral stage. *Oncology Nursing Forum*, *21*, 1009–1014.

Champion, V. (1995). Results of a nurse delivered intervention on proficiency and nodule detection with self breast examination. *Oncology Nursing Forum*, *22*, 819–824.

Champion, V., & Scott, C. (1997). Reliability and validity of breast cancer screening beliefs scales in African American women. *Nursing Research, 46,* 331–338.

Cody, R., & Lee, C. (1990). Behaviors, beliefs and intentions in skin cancer prevention. *Journal of Behavioral Medicine, 13,* 373–389.

Davidhizar, R. (1983). Critique of the health belief model. *Journal of Advanced Nursing, 8,* 46–72.

Fensler, J., & Miller, M. (1997). Factors affecting health behavior. In S. Groenwald, M. Frogge, M. Goodman, & C. Yarbro (Eds.), *Cancer nursing: Principles and practices* (4th ed., pp. 77–93). Sudbury, MA: Jones and Bartlett.

Fischera, S. D. & Frank, D. I. (1994). The health belief model as a predictor of mammography screening. *Health Values: The Journal of Health Behavior, Education & Promotion, 18*(4), 3–9.

Flynn, J. B. (2001). *Health beliefs about inherited breast cancer and genetic testing for* BRCA1 *and* BRCA2 *in women who have never been diagnosed with breast cancer and who use mammography services.* Doctoral dissertation. Retrieved from CINAHL (2003135289).

Frank, T., Manley, S., Olopade, O., Cummings, S., Garber, J., Bernhardt, B., . . . Thomas, A. (1998). Sequence analysis of *BRCA1* and *BRCA2*: Correlations of mutations with family history and ovarian cancer risk. *Journal of Clinical Oncology, 17*(7), 2417–2425.

Futreal, P., Liu, Q., Shattuck-Eidens, D., Cochran, C., Harshman, K., Tavigian, S., . . . Miki, Y. (1994). *BRCA1* mutations in primary breast and ovarian carcinomas. *Science, 266,* 120–122.

Gordon, N. P., & Iribarren, C. (2008). Health-related characteristics and preferred methods of receiving health education according to dominant language among Latinos aged 25 to 64 in a large northern California health plan. *BMC Public Health, 8,* 305. Doi: 10.1286/1471-2458-8-305

Honda, K. (2003). Who gets the information about genetic testing for cancer risk? The role of race/ethnicity, immigration status, and primary care clinicians. *Clinical Genetics, 64*(2), 131–136.

Janz, N., & Becker, M. (1984). The health belief model: A decade later. *Health Education Quarterly, 11,* 1–47.

Johnson, J., & Meischke, H. (1994). Factors associated with adoption of mammography screening: Results of a cross-sectional and longitudinal study. *Journal of Women's Health, 3,* 97–105.

Kelly, R., Zyzanski, S., & Alenagno, S. (1991). Prediction of motivation and behavior change following health promotion: Role of health beliefs, social support, and self efficacy. *Social Science Medicine, 32,* 311–320.

King, M., Marks, J., & Mandell, J. (2003). Breast and ovarian cancer risks due to inherited mutations in *BRCA1* and *BRCA2. Science, 302*(5645), 643–646. Retrieved from MEDLINE with Full Text database.

Kinney, A. Y., Gammon, A., Coxworth, J., Simonesen, W. E., & Arce-Laretta, M. (2010). Exploring attitudes, beliefs, and communication preferences of Latino community members regarding *BRCA1/2* mutation testing and preventive strategies. *Journal of Genetics in Medicine, 12*(2), 105–115.

Lerman, C., Biesecker, B., Benkendorf, J., Kerner, J., Gomez-Caminero, A., Hughes, C., & Reed, M. M. (1997). Controlled trial of pretest education approaches to enhance informed decision-making for *BRCA1. Journal of the National Cancer Institute, 89*(2), 148–157.

Lerman, C., Narod, S., Schulman, K., Hughes, C., Gomez-Caminero, A., Bonney, G., . . . Lynch, H. (1996). *BRCA1* testing in families with hereditary breast–ovarian cancer: A prospective study of patient decision making. *Journal of the American Medical Association, 24,* 1885–1892.

Lewin, K. (1935). *A dynamic theory of personality: Selected papers.* New York: McGraw-Hill.

Maiman, L., & Becker, M. (1974). The health belief model: Origins and correlates in psychological theory. In M. Becker (Ed.), *The health belief model and personal health behavior* (pp. 9–26). Thorofare, NJ: Slack.

McGarvey, E., Clavet, G., Johnson, J., Butler, A., Cook, K., & Pennino, B. (2003). Cancer screening practices and attitudes: Comparison of low-income women in three ethnic groups. *Ethnicity and Health, 8*(1), 71–82.

Miki, Y., Swensen, J., Shattuck-Eidens, D., Futreal, P. A., Harshman, K., Tavtigian, S., . . . Ding, W. (1994). A strong candidate for the breast and ovarian cancer susceptibility gene *BRCA1. Science,* 266(5182), 66–71.

Murphy, D., Balka, E., Poureslami, I., Leung, D. E., Nicol, A. M., & Cruz, T. (2007). Communicating health information: The community engagement model for video production. *Canadian Journal of Communication, 32*, 383–400.

Narod, S. (2006). Modifiers of risk of hereditary breast cancer. *Oncogene, 25*(43), 5832–5836. Retrieved from MEDLINE database.

Pender, N. (1996). *Health promotion in nursing practice* (3rd ed.). Stamford, CT: Appleton & Lange.

Ramirez, A. G., Aparicio-Ting, F. E., de Majors, S. S., & Miller, A. R. (2006). Interest, awareness, and perceptions of genetic testing among Hispanic family members of breast cancer survivors. *Ethnicity & Disease, 16*(2), 398–403.

Ransdell, L. B., & Rehling, S. L. (1996). Church-based health promotion: A review of the current literature. *American Journal of Health Behavior, 20*(4), 195–207.

Ricker, C. N., Hiyama, S., Fuentes, S., Feldman, N., Kumar, V., Uman, G. C., . . . Weitzel, J. N. (2007). Beliefs and interest in cancer risk in an underserved Latino cohort. *Preventive Medicine, 44*(3), 241–245.

Rosenstock, I. (1966). Historical origins of the health belief model. In M. Becker (Ed.), *The health belief model and personal health behavior* (pp. 1–8). Thorofare, NJ: Slack.

Rosenstock, I. (1974).Why people use health services. *Milbank Memorial Fund Quarterly, 44*, 94–127.

Rutledge, D., & Davis, G. (1998). Breast self-examination compliance and the health belief model. *Oncology Nursing Forum, 15*, 175–179.

Schwartz, G. F., Hughes, K. S., Lynch, H. T., Fabian, C. J., Fentiman, I. S., Robson, M. E., . . . Untch, M. (2009). Proceedings of the International Consensus Conference on Breast Cancer Risk, Genetics & Risk Management. *Breast Journal, 15*(1), 4–16.

Sensiba, M., & Stewart, D. (1995). Relationship of perceived barriers to breast self-examination in women of varying ages and levels of education. *Oncology Nursing Forum, 22*, 1265–1268.

Shavers, V. L., Harlan, L. C., & Stevens, J. L. (2003). Racial, ethnic variation in clinical presentation, treatment, and survival among breast cancer patients under age 35. *Cancer, 97*(1), 134–147.

Thompson, H. S., Valdimarsdottir, H. B., Jandorf, L., & Redd, W. (2003). Perceived disadvantages and concerns about abuses of genetic testing for cancer risk: Differences across African American, Latina and Caucasian women. *Patient Education & Counseling, 51*(3), 217–227.

Turnpenny, P., & Ellard, S. (2005). *Emery's elements of medical genetics*. London: Elsevier Churchill Livingston.

Vanderpool, R. C., Kornfeld, J., Rutten, L. F., & Squiers, L. (2009). Cancer information-seeking experiences: The implications of Hispanic ethnicity and Spanish language. *Journal of Cancer Education, 24*(2), 141–147.

Volandes, A. E., Ariza, M., Abbo, E. D., & Paasche-Orlow, M. (2008). Overcoming educational barriers for advance care planning in Latinos with video images. *Journal of Palliative Medicine, 11*(5), 700–706. Doi: 10.1089/jpm.2007.0172.
Wang, C., Gonzalez, R., Janz, N. K., Milliron, K. J., & Merajver, S. D. (2007). The role of cognitive appraisal and worry in *BRCA1/2* testing decisions among a clinic population. *Psychology and Health, 22*(6), 719–736.

Weizel, J., Langos, V., Blazer, K., Nelson, R., Ricker, C., Herzog, J., . . . Neuhausen, S. (2005). Prevalence of *BRCA* mutations and founder effect in high-risk Hispanic families. *Cancer Epidemiology, Biomarkers and Prevention, 14*(7), 1666–1671.

Wooster, R., Bignell, G., Lancaster, J., Swift, S., Seal, S., Mangion, J., . . . Micklem, G. (1995). Identification of the breast cancer susceptibility gene *BRCA2. Nature, 378*(6559), 789–792.

Wyper, M. (1990). Breast self-examination and the health belief model: Variations on a theme. *Research in Nursing Health, 13*, 421–428.

Yarbro, C., Frogge, M., & Goodman, M. (2005). *Cancer nursing principles and practice* (6th ed.). Sudbury, MA: Jones and Bartlett.

APPENDIX A

Detailed Timeline

Activities	Months					
	1	2	3	4	5	6
Identify community partner(s) Establish advisory committee	X					
Prepare and submit IRB application	X					
Recruit co-investigator, promotore de salud	X					
Orient project team to roles Train promotores de salud in on-site research assistant role		X				
Develop flyers for recruitment of participants and provide them to promotores de salud		X				
Print forms in Spanish (demographic forms, pre-tests, and post-tests)			X			
Recruit participants			X			
Secure the meeting location			X			
Formally invite participants to the meeting date and time				X		
Prepare random assignment numbers using SPSS				X		
Conduct the meeting				X		
Enter data in SPSS					X	
Analyze data					X	
Discuss findings with advisory committee and determine implications for the population and next steps						
Prepare reports to the advisory committee and other community partners (including promotores de salud)					X	
Prepare manuscripts						X
Disseminate results to providers and nurses through department meetings, publications, and presentations						X

APPENDIX B

Proposed Budget

A.	**Personnel**		**$46,580**
	1. Principal investigator: Dr. Jan Flynn		
	Academic year salary (sample salary = 50,000)		
	Stipend requested (25% effort × 50,000) =	12,500	
	Fringe benefits (30% of salary × 50,000) =	3,750	
	2. Co-principal investigator: Dr. Janice Long		
	Academic year salary (sample salary = 50,000)		
	Stipend requested (25% effort × 50,000) =	12,500	
	Fringe benefits (30% of salary × 50,000) =	3,750	
	3. Promotores de Salud		
	2 positions (@ 50% effort): $10/hr × 20 hr/week		
	× 26 weeks =	10,400	
	Fringe benefits (30% × 20,000) =	3,120	
	4. Graduate research assistant		
	$14/hr for 40 hr total		
	No fringe benefits	560	
B.	**Project Operating Expenses**		**$1600**
	1. Video *BRCA1/2* (Spanish and English versions)	1,250	
	2. Office supplies	200	
	3. Travel	150	
	Total Funding Request		**$48,180**

BUDGET EXPLANATION/JUSTIFICATION

A. Personnel

1. Principal Investigator: Dr. Jan Flynn has expertise in genetic research and testing and in teaching patients about inherited breast cancer risk. Dr. Flynn's role in the study is to oversee the general operations of the study, including the budget and assurance of human subjects' protection. She will lead the research advisory committee.
2. Co-principal Investigator: Dr. Janice Long has expertise in working with the Latino population and has conducted research and oversight of a faith-based promotores de salud program where the study subjects will be recruited. Dr. Long will be responsible for recruiting two promotores de salud to work with the study and for training the two promotores de salud as research assistants in collaboration with Dr. Flynn. Consent forms will be read to participants in Spanish. Drs. Flynn and Long will collaborate on writing the final reports and dissemination of study findings.
3. Promotores de Salud: Two promotores de salud who are experienced in working with the clients in the two faith-based settings will assist the researchers in coordination of activities for recruitment of study participants. They will deliver flyers to the congregants at each of the two settings and will coordinate acquisition of the location and rooms where the study will take place. The promotores de salud will also communicate with the candidates prior to and during the two-hour study session, and each will attend the research advisory committee meetings.
4. Graduate Research Assistant: The research assistant will assist with form preparation for the study (including copying and making packets for each participant), data entry, and report writing. If a graduate research assistant cannot be recruited, an attempt will be made to recruit an undergraduate research assistant.

B. Project Operating Expenses

1. A culturally sensitive video on *BRCA1* testing in Latinos will be purchased for the study. A second copy of the same video in English will also be purchased and made available for researchers to review. The cost of the two videos is expected to be $1250.
2. Office supplies (ink cartridges, paper, folders and binders for each participant as well as materials for duplicating the forms to be used for the study for 50 participants) are expected to cost $4/participant, for a total cost of $200.
3. Both the researchers and promotores de salud will be traveling to the research site, to research advisory committee meetings, and to investigate locations to conduct the study. Travel for the researchers and promotores de salud was calculated based on the total number of trips estimated (20 trips at 15 miles per trip) multiplied by the state rate of $0.50 per mile for 300 miles for a cost of $150.00.

CHAPTER 17

Mobile Clinics as Outreach to the Underserved

Mary de Chesnay and Heather Payne

Objectives

At the end of this chapter, the reader will be able to

1. Describe the utility of mobile clinics in the United States for serving vulnerable populations.
2. Compare and contrast the key differences and similarities among the clinics presented in the chapter.
3. Suggest other ways in which mobile clinics can be used to present health services other than nursing in a team effort that includes nursing.

INTRODUCTION

From remote areas of the isolated regions of the world to inner cities in the United States, mobile clinics bring health care to vulnerable populations as well as convenient health care to those who might not otherwise have the time or resources to seek help. Mobile health clinics range from simple vans to highly sophisticated buses that include examination rooms and laboratories. Their purposes vary from full-scale health assessments to specific interventions or screenings for particular diseases. This chapter outlines a descriptive study on mobile health clinics that was conducted in the United States.

STATEMENT OF THE PROBLEM

The study was conducted for the purpose of documenting the demographic characteristics of selected mobile health clinics. These clinics provide a great service to their communities by assisting vulnerable and medically underserved populations and relieving the burden on the healthcare delivery system. Most of the data collected for the study involve public information obtained from the websites of the clinics and the professional literature about the clinics. In addition, interviews were conducted with key personnel at some clinics to determine common characteristics.

THE LITERATURE

There is a growing body of literature on mobile clinics in terms of describing their services and outcomes of screenings. Much of the literature found concerned mobile clinics in other countries, even though they are widely used in the United States. An Internet search for mobile clinics yielded more than 110,000 entries. An excellent resource on mobile clinics is the organization known as Mobile Clinic Network; its website (www.mobilehealthclinicsnetwork.org) presents a wealth of anecdotal and scientific materials.

Many local news items describe clinics that serve specific communities. For example, in Australia, a project has been described as a means to provide comprehensive screenings to aboriginal communities ("Increase Mobile Nurse Clinics," 2010). Nurses in rural mobile clinics conduct screenings using simple tests for chronic diseases. One such screening in the Australia study found that a woman who had presented with eight urinary tract infections had been using a swimming pool with sodium chloride levels that were three-fourths of the normal level. Another more detailed report has described the effectiveness of mobile clinics used by disaster relief teams from the U.S. military after a tsunami devastated Sri Lanka (Lane, 2006); after the earthquakes in Taiwan (Lee et al., 2010) and California (Weiss, Weiss, Teeter, & Geraci, 1999); and as means to help war victims in Somalia (VanRooyen, VanRooyen, Sloan, & Ward, 1995).

Many countries around the world use mobile clinics to provide both basic and targeted services. For example, patients with early-stage chronic kidney and cardiovascular diseases have been identified through mobile clinics in Mexico (Gutierrez-Padilla et al., 2010). In Thailand, an ambitious project aims to screen all Thai women ages 35 to 60 for cervical cancer (Sriamporn, Khuhaprema, & Parkin, 2006). In Malawi, sex workers attending mobile clinics are screened for sexually transmitted diseases (Zachariah, Spielman, Harries, Nkhoma, Chantulo, & Arendt, 2003). Uganda provides antiretroviral therapy to clients of its mobile clinics, although researchers found that facility-based clinics were more effective in this case (Babigumira, Sethi, Smyth, & Singer, 2009). South Africa uses nurses in mobile clinics to provide alcohol screening and brief interventions (Peltzer, Seoka, Babor, & Okopt, 2006). Irish providers have found an effective way to provide outreach services for aging and dementia through mobile clinics (McCarron & Lawlor, 2003).

In the United Kingdom, mobile breast screening has been found to substantially decrease the automobile emissions from extensive traveling to clinical facilities (Bond et al., 2009). The team investigating this issue found that the costs and emissions from the vans were significantly less than the costs per year of each patient traveling to facilities. In Canada, street youth have been found to be willing to use mobile clinics more than physician clinics, and the services provided through the mobile clinics include both case finding and treatment (Worthington & MacLaurin, 2009).

Many examples of services provided to U.S. communities can be found in the literature. In Baltimore, researchers have found that rapid HIV testing through mobile clinics can identify people who do not access other types of health services (Ellen et al., 2004; Liang et al., 2005). Frothinger (2008) described the potential for a mobile clinic to assist homeless individuals in Seattle. Kilgore (2000) described provision of services to poor communities along the U.S.–Mexico border. An innovative program to manage childhood asthma in southern California (the Breathmobile Program) has been described by Jones et al. (2005). In Iowa, services are provided to people with Down syndrome (Liston, 1994). The Veterans Administration provides services to veterans via mobile clinics in many rural areas ("VA Mobile Health Clinics Reach Rural Populations.", 2008).

The Canadian Health Measures Survey (Tremblay & Gorber, 2007) used mobile clinics to collect data on more than 5000 Canadians, aged 6 to 79 years. The results enabled the team to establish national baseline data on chronic diseases such as obesity, hypertension, and cardiovascular disease as well as nutrition and exposure to environmental hazards.

METHODOLOGY

Design

The design of the present study was qualitative, utilizing phone interviews with personnel in most of the clinics and an in-person interview in one clinic. All staff gave permission for the names of their clinics to be used. Material that they considered sensitive was not included in the chapter.

Sample

The sample consisted of the key staff of 13 clinics, sometimes including the directors and sometimes including other staff. The sample was recruited purposively to provide data from clinics in all the regions of the United States. The institutional review board (IRB) of Kennesaw State University gave approval prior to data collection.

Setting

Staff from one clinic were interviewed in person at their home offices. This was done because the directors were so excited to be included in the study that they readily offered a visit instead of a simple phone interview. Other staff members were interviewed by phone. Interviews lasted from 20 minutes to 1 hour for the in-person interview.

Instrumentation

The instrument consisted of a series of open-ended questions designed to elicit information about the history, funding base, populations served, and challenges encountered by the clinics. These five major questions were supplemented by several sub-questions to follow up for more detailed information.

Procedures

1. After IRB approval was obtained, the co-investigator called staff at a variety of clinics representing each region of the United States to ask if the staff would agree to be interviewed by phone. The study was explained and questions answered.

2. Phone interviews were scheduled at the convenience of the staff. Sometimes they were conducted immediately, but most occurred at a later time.
3. Interviews were summarized onto an instrument that was then content analyzed for themes, and descriptions were written of the interview content.
4. The principal investigator (PI) visited one site to obtain the same data as the phone interviews. This was done because the staff was excited to discuss the clinic and it was convenient for the PI to make a personal visit. Because the study is descriptive and qualitative in nature, it did not create a validity or reliability issue to visit one site and conduct phone interviews with others.
5. The PI and co-PI met during the course of the study to discuss the results and to compare notes on conclusions.
6. Once the final meeting occurred, the study results were written.

Data Analysis

The primary type of data analysis consisted of description of the various topics of interest at each site. Data were content analyzed by extracting themes and concepts from raw data and comparing results across interviews.

RESULTS

The results were quantified to show major categories for each question, but no attempt was made to perform statistical analysis because the sample size was small ($N = 13$) and the study focus was qualitative description. The following figures summarize the key factors in each response.

Appendix A shows the funding sources for these mobile clinics. Most funding comes from foundations, with a second major source being the federal government for those clinics that have federally qualified health center statues (FQHC) or what is referred to as "look-a-like" status. Other funding sources included colleges, hospitals, a fuel company, states, and a line item in a budget for another entity.

Appendix B depicts the populations served by the mobile clinics. In most cases they are simply described as children or adults, but special populations were also identified: homeless persons, migrants, tribes, women, and immigrants.

Appendix C shows the services provided by the mobile clinics. These include mammography, a variety of primary care services, specialized services to women and children, and laboratory tests. The results are skewed in terms of percentage of services because one van provides only mammography.

Nurse practitioners are the major source of staff for mobile clinics, but a variety of other healthcare professionals also staff these clinics, either as primary staff or secondary staff Appendix D. Nursing students support clinics associated with universities as well. These clinics are viewed as wonderful learning opportunities for students.

Not surprisingly, funding was the key challenge for mobile clinics (Appendix E). Virtually all of the clinics had issues with funding because there were few stable funding bases identified on which staff could depend.

NURSING EXAMPLE FROM SOUTH CAROLINA

The Clemson University mobile clinic began in the 1990s primarily to deliver federal Women's, Infants, and Children (WIC) services to the upstate region of South Carolina near the North Carolina and north Georgia state lines. Originally it was thought that the client population would be Spanish-speaking migrant workers, but as it turned out that most of the migrants at that time were African Americans who traveled along the East Coast every summer and fall to pick apples. The current van is the third vehicle used by the program. Funding is dependent on the type of service provided, and comes from a variety of sources. Its partial reliance on Department of Housing and Urban Development (HUD) funding reinforces Clemson's tradition of teaching, research, and service.

The clinic serves a variety of clients, including university employees, but concentrates on the underserved, underinsured, and uninsured. The overwhelming majority of the client base is rural, located in the upstate counties of Pickens, Oconee, Anderson, and Greenville. The services offered are continually shifting to coincide with community need, so the client demographics change accordingly; a current estimate is that one-third of clients are Hispanic and two-thirds are Caucasian. University-affiliated nurse practitioners rotate shifts on the van, and students are heavily involved in providing services. In 2009, more than 300 students provided in excess of 5000 hours of care. Services can include acute care, screening, wellness programming, surveillance, flu shots, community projects, and community counseling. Sometimes specific programs are offered, such as hormone replacement. A unique characteristic of Clemson's mobile clinic is that the services provided are changeable, because the clinic provides services in the community that no one else is offering.

Funding is always a challenge. Funding waxes and wanes with the state of the economy, and the clinic reports that current times are the toughest it has ever navigated. Grants, gifts, contracts, and endowments are some funding sources employed, and staff "try to be creative" in seeking sources. The clinic maximizes its use of resources in every way possible, by reorganizing, moving people, and examining its structure. The clinic's Dr. Paula Watt states that the clinic has the asset of having "a lot of committed people. The college collaborates in every way, and is so supportive."

NON-NURSING EXAMPLE FROM WISCONSIN

Wisconsin's Marshfield Clinic is saving the lives of rural women through its two mobile mammography/bone density units. In its 10 years of existence under the present award-winning director, Myron Gadke, and his current supervisor, Gene Santilli, more than 11,000 individuals have been screened for breast cancer, and 37 women's lives have been saved by early detection and intervention. The clinic's first unit included primary care by a nurse practitioner. Because rural women found it difficult to undergo Pap tests and other physical assessments in the confines of the van, the team eventually switched to offering just mammography and bone density tests. However, the resurgence of primary care as a healthcare priority has inspired the team to reexamine this modality. The clinic is part of a major medical center serving the state of Wisconsin, and funding is obtained from private sources and the medical center.

DUFFY HEALTH CENTER

Duffy Health Center has been an independent, federally qualified health center since 2002. A 2006 Health Resources and Service Administration (HRSA) grant is the major support for the van and partial operations costs. The Irving Oil Company and insurance companies donate money to fund the mobile clinic, and in return they may advertise on the van. The van travels all over Cape Cod, Massachusetts, so donating companies obtain a great deal of exposure. The interviewee, Ms. DeGroot, stated, "You have to get the initial funding, then build on it."

Duffy serves the homeless. Cape Cod has "hidden homelessness," in which individuals move from place to place because of the tourist economy. Duffy serves Barnstable County (which includes Cape Cod), which is mostly suburban or rural. The population of the county is 95% white, and the patient population is 85% white. Approximately 82% of the clients have incomes less than 100% of the federal poverty level. The rest has incomes less than 300% of the federal poverty level. Duffy coordinates its services with other agencies to provide care, such as operation of a food pantry in Falmouth. The van is staffed by one nurse practitioner and one driver. The driver is able to enroll patients into state health insurance. All persons in Massachusetts are eligible for state health insurance, so the first order of business is to make sure a patient has insurance. The van staff can also work with case managers to accomplish this task.

The primary site provides integrated care. The mobile clinic offers primary care, mental health, substance abuse treatment, case management, and housing programs. It works with the Duffy Health Center primary site to get patients the care they need. This coordination is facilitated through use of the van's electronic medical records. Because the county is not urban, finding the target population can be a challenge. Duffy has received a grant for marketing its services, and has also hired an access educator to help meet this challenge. The access educator will visit county agencies, such as police departments and food pantries, to find ways to make access easier. Ms. DeGroot states, "We see our mobile clinic as the beginning of client interaction. We want to connect people to a 'healthcare home.'"

LEWIS & CLARK COMMUNITY COLLEGE

Efforts to start Lewis & Clark Community College's mobile unit program began around 2006, when the college had a stationary clinic on its campus in a somewhat rural area in Illinois. The following year, the college spoke to an aide for then-Senator Barack Obama. Senator Obama met with college representatives, and ultimately secured a $279,000 earmark through the HRSA. In 2008, a $450,000 nursing and dental van was delivered with fuel donated by Conoco Phillips and by Piasa Fuel Company (a local company). The college funds a full-time driver/intake person.

The mobile unit serves roughly 1800 square miles in the Lower Mississippi River Basin, covering all or portions of seven counties. The area is somewhat rural. Approximately 65% of the population served is uninsured. The unit visits churches, schools, senior centers, corporations, and small communities to provide care. The medical/dental unit is run by four nurse practitioners, three of whom have a joint faculty arrangement. The Illinois Nurse Practice Act (under the "Advanced Practice Nurse Staff" provision) does not require a physician to be present for nurse practitioners to treat patients, but the nurses have a physician and a dentist to collaborate with when needed. Two registered nurses, a dental hygienist, one stationary clerical worker, and one mobile clerical worker are also on staff. The full-time driver is under faculty direction. The college's students also assist with patient care—nursing students help with screenings, interviews, glucose checks, and flu shots; dental students help with fluoride treatments and tooth cleanings.

Medical services offered by the mobile clinic include primary care (acute episodic), prevention, screenings, health education, women's health, breast examinations, cholesterol testing, and sometimes blood draws. If a problem is found during a breast examination, the clinic refers the patient for further care. Dental services include sealants and oral health screenings. No surgical or restorative care is provided. The high need for its services poses a challenge for the mobile clinic. As Donna Meyer, the Dean of Health Services and Project Director, states, "The unit could be out seven days a week." This challenge cannot be resolved without the addition of more staff and another mobile unit.

Dean Meyer wanted the investigators to know that Lewis & Clark is the only community college with a mobile unit. The United States is home to more than 2200 community colleges, and they could make a large impact on health care. A mobile unit is a good way for students to get community health experience. Lewis & Clark has created its own clinical site that students "tend to love."

SARA LINCOLN BUSH HEALTH CENTER

The Sara Lincoln Bush Health Center mobile unit is hospital affiliated. In 2000, a Women and Children First grant for the unit was received through the community. The hospital provides an operational account for the van, which pays for gas and maintenance. The area and population served by the mobile care program is both extensive and diverse. The unit has expanded to serve at least nine counties monthly, with each seen at least one time per month. People of more than 35 ethnicities are served in the area; examples include Amish, Hispanic, and Caucasian. The population is primarily rural, and some are working at the time that they visit the van (e.g., farmers or bankers).

The unit has started to provide mammography in some rural areas, and to serve working women who cannot come during the week. The unit provides osteoporosis heel scans and mammography. The mobile unit staff includes one x-ray technician who specializes in mammography and a driver who also maintains the van. The technicians at the hospital read the images. Health department nurses conduct free blood draws for cholesterol, and the unit picks up the samples and takes them to the hospital. Patients must have a doctor to get their report. The unit prefers that clients schedule their visits by appointment, but also accepts walk-ins.

Funding for new equipment and staff is the mobile unit's biggest challenge. Reimbursement is limited. Staff meets this challenge by continuing to ask for help. The hospital foundation helps raise money for the mobile unit, and local banks often donate to support it. Patients who come are very appreciative that the unit is available in their hometowns, because many do not have access to a hospital. The elderly, for example, may not have a ride to far-off health facilities.

THE VISITING NURSE ASSOCIATION'S FLORENCE NIGHTINGALE EXPRESS

The Visiting Nurse Association is a 3½-year-old nonprofit organization that operates in Florida. Its mobile van, which is known as the Florence Nightingale Express, was purchased by the foundation, rather than being tax funded. The foundation organizes fundraisers and other events to pay for the mobile clinic. Patients' prescriptions are filled for free at Publix or for $4 at Wal-mart. The foundation also provides funding in special cases: Once the unit found a lump in the breast of a male migrant worker and asked for extra money from the board for ultrasound testing, which it provided.

The Florence Nightingale Express serves 15 counties in the middle of the state of Florida. The counties are a combination of suburbs and rural areas. The farthest trip the mobile unit makes is 250 miles. Its patient population has evolved as health and financial crises in the United States have developed. Three locations initially served migrant farmworkers. Today, the clinic serves the homeless, the underinsured, and the unemployed. Some patients who are seen are waiting to become eligible for Medicaid. Patients come from diverse cultures, and the unit serves only adults. The unit can be accessed through soup kitchens and food banks.

One nurse practitioner runs the unit, while another person coordinates patients and takes vital signs. The unit provides urgent care as opposed to primary care. Nurse practitioner Sandy Ripper explains, "We want to keep patients out of the ER, not to use it as primary care. This will directly impact the ER." Examples of services include methicillin-resistant *Staphylococcus aureus* (MRSA) wound care, treatment of fungal infections, removal of stitches, sick diagnostics, treatment for bedbugs, and case management. The mobile unit uses paper records to document its care.

Obtaining resources is the greatest challenge the unit faces. Ms. Ripper states, "We're helping patients. To access local resources so they can get ongoing care is a never-ending battle looking up resources. We've tried to get pharmaceuticals donated, but [the pharmaceutical companies] aren't interested."

Ms. Ripper rounded out her comments by noting, "There are aspects that are very rewarding when you see people getting help who would otherwise be disenfranchised, but that is mixed with people who use money to buy alcohol and drugs. They cycle back to us because they didn't get their scrip and now they're worse. The biggest growing problem is people's teeth as a source of infection—people's teeth are coming out. When the economy crashed, people bought food instead of toothpaste. Nobody takes us for granted. There is a sense of getting worse, not better. We are seeing more and more patients."

UNIVERSITY OF TEXAS, TEXAS MEDICAL CENTER

The mobile clinic project of the University of Texas's Texas Medical Center began in 1988. Over its more than 22 years of existence, the project has had three mobile units, and has been working for four years to acquire a new third unit. Funding is through the state via a special line item. Foundation gifts are also a funding source.

Sometimes the unit travels 400 miles from Houston. The terrain is flat with rivers coursing through. When it rains, there is no runoff, and flood conditions result—which in turn makes parasitic infections a problem. One vulnerable population whom the unit serves lives in Mexican American colonias. Colonias are substandard housing developments in which owners buy real property that lacks water or utilities. Migrant farmworkers are another population served by the mobile unit; many have problems with severe dermatitis from pesticides. The unit also visits Cameron City schools. Telemedicine through encrypted communication allows the mobile unit to communicate securely with the schools. Director Dr. Kathleen Becan-McBride states, "We have provided lots of patient services over 22 years that they otherwise wouldn't have had."

The mobile clinic staff consists of one physician assistant, one medical assistant, and four fourth-year medical students per year. These providers offer primary health care. The unit also has the capability to perform lab tests such as lipids, glucose, and hemoglobin. Stress screening is conducted as well. Gastric ulcers are a common result of parasites, and treatment of this condition is a unit specialty.

Hurricanes pose a challenge for the mobile unit staff, because they have to find a safe place to park the mobile clinic and keep it safe. During emergent situations, the staff must also find generator power to maintain refrigerated items such as vaccines and run the quality control apparatus.

CHILDREN'S HEALTH FUND

Children's Health Fund is a national nonprofit organization serving Orleans, Plaquemines, and St. Bernard parishes in Louisiana. Locally, Tulane School of Medicine runs the mobile clinics. The local response began 5 days post–Hurricane Katrina, on September 4, 2005. Although it was initially intended to be a crisis response, a needs assessment showed continued disparity in healthcare services. Today, the mobile clinics' mission is removing barriers to accessing health care. Persons do not have to live in the three parishes mentioned earlier to receive healthcare services from the vans.

A broad range of people are seen, and the ethnic predominance varies with location. A fixed schedule determines which days the mobile vans will be at which sites. On Mondays, the unit serves the Lower Ninth Ward, and the majority of clients are African American. On Tuesdays, the unit serves Mid City, and the majority of clients are Hispanic. On Wednesdays, the vans go to St. Bernard parish, where the medical van staff sees mostly Hispanics and African Americans, and the mental health van staff see mostly Caucasians and African Americans. The vans go to Gentilly on Thursdays, where mostly Hispanic and African American clients are seen. On Fridays, the vans go to Plaquemines parish to see mostly African American clients.

The mobile clinic effort is extensively staffed. University faculty includes three doctors: one pediatrician, one asthma specialist, and one child psychiatrist. In addition to providing care, the physicians oversee medical students on their clinical rotations. Other staff members include one patient care coordinator who answers phones, three licensed clinical social workers, one addiction counselor, two case managers, one RN, one intern caseworker, one health educator with a master's degree in nursing, two doctoral fellows who do research and marketing, and one program manager who concentrates on finances. In addition, three multitasking field specialists drive, scan documents into medical records, log patients in, and perform other tasks. The mobile clinic staff serves as primary care providers following a medical home model, with the case manager assessing compliance with this model. Thus a comprehensive medical history is taken for each client. Mental health services encompass a broad range of services, from large classroom-based education to medication management. Locally, CARE Center is the mental health partner for the program.

On the topic of challenges, the interviewee commented, "We're pretty adaptable folks." Physical challenges stem from operating very large buses in old cities with low-lying trees: The roots and branches of the trees have an unhappy tendency to break things on the buses. Hurricanes also have the potential to damage the buses.

Another challenge is getting the state to recognize the need for funding this service. The mobile clinic program is an extension of the regular Children's Health Fund project, and is planned to continue indefinitely.

In October 2010, Children's Health Fund responded to individuals affected by the immense oil spill in the Gulf of Mexico. Research at that time noted the need for pediatric mental health services in the Gulf states, where problems were present at an alarming rate.

At the time of interview, the van was parked 200 yards from the waters of the Mississippi River, with levies on both sides. When asked what else the study should know about the clinic, the interviewee stated, "We do a great job."

KIDCARE EXPRESS

Kidcare Express began operating its first mobile medical unit in California in 1998; today the program has three units. One was gifted by a local hospital that tried mobile health but found it did not work out for the institution.

Kidcare Express's funding sources are diverse, in part owing to its reimbursement designation is as a federally qualified health center. It can bill the state's Office of Family Planning, for example. The organization receives an enhanced Medicaid reimbursement rate, as well as special population funding for public housing and the homeless. Funding also comes from grants, fundraisers, and private and public corporation donations.

Kidcare Express serves the central and southern portions of San Diego. Approximately 95% of its patients have incomes that are less than 100% of the federal poverty level. In this urban area, the mobile clinics go to schools, homeless shelters, substance abuse treatment facilities, and public housing. Due to the geographic region served, staff members see many Hispanic/Latino clients. In addition, the program serves many low-income, medically uninsured persons. "Kidcare Express" is actually a misnomer, as services are offered to both children and adults. Although a mix of all ages is seen, clients are predominantly adults.

The mobile clinic is staffed by six or seven mid-level providers, who are physician assistants or nurse practitioners. It has one medical assistant. There is also a patient service representative/driver who checks people in. The mobile clinic offers most of the same services that the stationary clinic sites do, including sick visits, physical examinations, immunizations, STD/HIV counseling and testing, sports physicals, x-rays, lab testing, and treatments for asthma, hypertension, and diabetes. The mobile clinic does not offer prenatal care or adult immunizations.

Despite Kidcare Express's diverse sources of support, funding is a major challenge. Coordinator Tom Stubberud states, "They [the mobile units] don't make money for us. We lose money every year." Another issue is that vehicles age and need maintenance. One unit is 12 years old now, and the worry is that it will break down.

When asked what else the investigators should know about Kidcare Express, Mr. Stubberud proclaimed, "We're fabulous!" He remains enthusiastic about the fact that the program is "mission focused." He says, "We really do follow our mission. It's not just words on a page. We provide to the underinsured. That is guiding our decisions at the top. What is the need, where is the need, how can we provide it. . . . With good partnerships and respect, collaboration is easy. . . . We also get to participate in some of the more controversial things, like transgender health and needle exchanges."

ROCKY MOUNTAIN YOUTH CLINICS

The Rocky Mountain Youth Clinic mobile unit was initially a department of a local hospital in Denver. When the program folded in 1996, a local pediatrician developed a sustainable model for the unit. Today the unit is considered a medical home, and is a tax-advantaged site. The clinic receives both foundation and individual donations, and the vans were donated by Ronald McDonald House.

The clinic serves the Denver metro area, whose population totals approximately 2.2 million people. The population served is primarily urban, but the program also tries to "reach out to rural." It includes 3 regular clinics, 12 school-based clinics, and 2 mobile vans. One van is medical; the other is dental. The mobile units see children ranging in age from newborn to 21 years old, and now with expanded coverage they can see patients older than age 21. There is a sliding fee for the underinsured and uninsured, and the unit is able to accept Medicaid reimbursement.

Ms. Taylor, the Director of Community and School-Based Health Programs, notes, "Our facilities are not roomy." Physician assistants or nurse practitioners are paired with a medical assistant, and one dental assistant and a dental hygienist staff the dental van. Each medical and dental staff member has a commercial driver's license, which saves space. Patients may be referred to a primary care provider if needed, or they can come to the stationary clinics if they do not have their own physician.

The mobile units can do everything that is done in a clinic. Medical services include sick and well visits, primary care, WIC assessments, labs, and rapid *Streptococcus* tests. The units also have the capability to take and develop x-rays. Dental services include preventive cleanings, fluoride treatments, and varnishes, but no restorative care is available. Children needing further dental care can receive services through Kids in Need of Dentistry (KIND). Medicaid pays for one cleaning per year, but the providers believe that two are essential; to facilitate clients in receiving two cleanings, the program charges $10 every 6 months. Both the medical and dental units document their care and findings in electronic medical records.

One challenge for the staff is the small area available for delivering services. As Ms. Taylor explains, "[In the van] they have to be in close quarters for extended periods of time. There has to be a good mix of personalities. We have to rotate providers and [medical assistants]." Maintenance for the vans is also costly. Also, "We have a lot of no-shows. We try to curb the no-show rate. We see where we have the most impact and concentrate on those areas."

When asked what else the study should know about the mobile health clinic, Ms. Taylor answered, "The most important thing is that mobile health is an amazing concept, but if you don't have the structure to support it . . . If a child is diagnosed with diabetes and you have nowhere to refer them . . . Mobile health is just an outreach. You need a robust structure to take care of kids who are uninsured and really sick."

ST. VINCENT HEALTHCARE

The St. Vincent Healthcare mobile clinic was launched in Montana in 2010. The foundation that supports this program is philanthropic and expects no profit. Two Native American reservations—one Crow and one Cherokee—are served, along with rural farmers. The unit works with Riverstone Health, which treats breast and cervical health. Local women already cannot afford mammograms, so if problems are found they can sign up for help with further expenses. A technologist and a driver staff the van. Services offered include screening mammograms, diagnostic mammograms, breast magnetic resonance imaging (MRI), and stereostatic ultrasound for biopsy. Approximately 300 women were screened last year, and more than 2000 others were identified who need screening.

Local relations are the biggest challenge the mobile unit currently faces. Patrick Grimsley states, "We're still working through getting locations to take the coach. Some of the other local institutions don't want this. We don't want to jeopardize relationships with area hospitals."

Other comments from Mr. Grimsley reveal his enthusiasm for the program: "We think it's a great service. It's very rewarding. We get more 'thank you's' from this than anything else." Winnette, Montana, is "not the end of the earth but you can see it from here." When a girl in Winnette lost her stepmother to breast cancer, she called the mobile clinic; the clinic then went to Winnette and did about 20 screenings.

UNIVERSITY OF MEDICINE AND DENTISTRY, NEW JERSEY, AND SCHOOL OF NURSING

The mobile clinic operated by the University of Medicine and Dentistry, New Jersey (UMDNJ) began in 2006–2007 with a $2 million grant from the HRSA. The School of Nursing matched $375,000 of the grant, and Schering-Plough donated $250,000. Children's Health Fund donated the vans. The first van cost $450,000; in 2010, a new van with electronic medical records capability cost $250,000.

The unit serves 19 sites in Newark, Elizabeth, and Urvington, New Jersey, and is expanding to New Brunswick. Its clients are children: 70% of the children are African American, and 30% are Hispanic; 80% are uninsured and 20% receive Medicaid.

The mobile clinic is run by four nurse practitioners who are adult health or family health specialists. Students also play active roles in the clinic. Nursing students complete Community

Health class requirements, BSN students complete Primary Care Practice class requirements, and medical students complete Public Health class requirements. Primary care is provided, such as treatment of family illnesses, well visits, immunizations, and flu shots. Women's health is newly provided through in collaboration with the gynecological department at the clinic's affiliated hospital. The primary issues that the clinic encounters are obesity, hypertension, and asthma.

Ariel Almacin cites follow-up as the main challenge the mobile clinic faces. Most patients are transient, and some are undocumented. Patients typically have no transportation. The clinic has site coordinators, some of whom are social workers. Data analysis has identified two sites that see the most number of follow-up visits. The clinic plans to concentrate on these two sites and merge some of the others to maximize follow-up. Finances are also a challenge, as with other mobile clinics. Mr. Almacin states, "The main selling point of our clinic is that it is mostly nurse run, and that we serve vulnerable populations."

Washington on Wheels

In 1999–2000, a community needs assessment in Northern California revealed that many people in the area were uninsured and lacked transportation to healthcare facilities. Recognizing this need, the Washington on Wheel's affiliated hospital decided to use the money it had received from its annual fundraiser to purchase a mobile clinic. The hospital is community based, so its interest is in serving the health of the larger community. A total of $80,000 from the fundraiser was devoted to the purchase of the mobile unit, $50,000 to $60,000 came from grants, and the hospital donated the rest, thereby financing the unit's $180,000 purchase price. The hospital pays for the unit's ongoing operations.

Washington on Wheels serves a large San Francisco Bay metro area, located approximately one hour outside San Francisco. The unit does not go more than 25 miles from its affiliated hospital. The tri-city area covered includes the suburban communities of Freemont, Newark, and Union City. There is some industry in this area, which is close to Silicon Valley. The community includes large populations of Asians, Indians (from India), Afghans, Chinese, and Filipinos. Many new immigrants reside in the area, and there is a large population of Latinos. The unit reaches out to this highly diverse community through other institutions such as churches, schools, and senior centers. Although another local mobile clinic serves the homeless population in this area, Washington on Wheels gets this unit's patient overflow. Both children and adults are seen by program providers.

In California, nurse practitioners need medical oversight, although supervision does not have to be on-site—an arrangement called a "furnishing license." Nurse practitioners can prescribe medications. A nurse practitioner and a medical assistant staff the van most days of the week. A medical director, along with the clinic's own office physician and his partners, are available for consultation. For referrals, the unit has excellent relationships with community resources such as school nurses and social service agencies. Student nurses work with the program to gain community health experience. Baccalaureate-prepared and master's-degree nurses do one- to four-month rotations on the mobile unit.

The unit offers primary care, physical examinations, blood pressure checks, wellness visits, immunizations, some continuing education, and diabetic management (no insulin). It does not conduct surgery. The unit serves children coming from other countries who need immunizations to attend school in the United States. The mobile clinic sees many patients with hypertension, high cholesterol, and diabetes. As interviewee Ruth Traylor stated, "Often we're the first people who diagnose a problem." The unit transitions people into continuous care. Another focus is to find out what aid patients may qualify for. The unit has a low sliding scale for payment, but also provides free services.

One problem that the mobile clinic faces is simply determining who is qualified to receive aid. Ms. Traylor explains, "We have to apply a standard discount across the board, and there's no validation. We had to implement a screening tool to see who qualifies, which scares off a lot of Latinos who are undocumented. We're working with and through schools to solve this problem. Another problem is getting the word out—of where we are, who we are, and what we're doing."

Ms. Traylor states of the mobile clinic, "It is really useful, especially for vulnerable populations." And its benefits are clear: "Our area had a really high rate of diabetes—through the roof. We had the highest incidence of mortality from it. We offered a free glucose screening in June through September that year. We targeted Asians and migrant workers, and screened over 1000 people. We have the lowest rates now. There's no research to show cause and effect, but it's clear."

SUMMARY

Although several staff members in mobile clinics declined to be interviewed due to their extremely busy schedules, the people who did participate were enthusiastic and proud of their achievements and the services they provided to their communities. The rich diversity of the clinics in terms of services offered, funding bases, and efforts of the staff paint a picture of dedication to the needs of the vulnerable populations in the communities served by the clinics. Their efforts bring hope and healing to people who might not otherwise receive care.

WWW

For a full suite of assignments and additional learning activities, use the access code located in the front of your book to visit this exclusive website: http://go.jblearning.com/dechesnay. If you do not have an access code, you can obtain one at the site.

REFERENCES

Babigumira, J., Sethi, A., Smyth, K., & Singer, M. (2009). Cost effectiveness of facility-based care, home-based care and mobile clinics for provision of antiretroviral therapy in Uganda. *Pharmacoeconomics, 27*(11), 963–973.

Bond, A., Jones, A., Haynes, R., Tam, M., Denton, E., Ballantyne, M., & Curtin, J. (2009). Tackling climate change close to home: Mobile breast screening as a model. *Journal of Health Services Research and Policy, 14*(3), 165–167.

Ellen, J., Liang, T., Jacob, C., Erbelding, E., & Christmyer, C. (2004). Post-HIV test counseling of clients of a mobile STD/HIV clinic. *International Journal of STDs and AIDS, 15*, 728–731.

Frothinger, L. (2008). Mobile care clinic: An integrated program for the homeless. In M. de Chesnay & B. Anderson (Eds.), *Caring for the vulnerable* (pp. 443–450). Sudbury, MA: Jones and Bartlett.

Gutierrez-Padilla, J., Mendoza-Garcia, M., Plascencia-Perez, S., Renoirte-Lopez, K., Garcia- Garcia, G., Lloyd, A., & Tonelli, M. (2010). Screening for CKD and cardiovascular disease risk factors using mobile clinics in Jalisco, Mexico. *American Journal of Kidney Diseases, 55*(3), 474–484.

Increase mobile nurse clinics. (2010). *Australian Nursing Journal, 18*(5), 9.

Jones, C., Clement, L., Hanley-Lopez, J., Morphew, T., Kwong, K., Lifson, F., . . . Guterman, J. J. (2005). The Breathmobile Program: Structure, implementation, and evolution of a large-scale urban, pediatric asthma disease management program. *Disease Management, 8*(4), 205–222.

Kilgore, J. (2000). The road show: Mobile clinics provide care to poor communities along the Texas–Mexico border. *Healthweek, 5*(23), 16–17.

Lane, D. (2006). Medical support to Sri Lanka in the wake of tsunamis: Planning considerations and lessons learned. *Military Medicine, 171*(suppl), 19–23.

Lee, I., Chen, C., Yeh, T., Chen, K., Lee, C., & Chen, P. (2010). A community mental health survey and relief program in Taiwan after the great earthquake: Implementation, clinical observation and evaluation. *Stress and Health: Journal of the International Society for Investigation of Stress, 26*(4), 269–279.

Liang, T., Erbelding, E., Jacob, C., Wicker, H., Christmyer, C., Brunson, S., . . . Ellen, J. M. (2005). Rapid HIV testing of clients of a mobile STD/HIV clinic. *AIDS Patient Care and STDs, 19*(4), 253–257.

Liston, J. (1994). Mobile Down's syndrome clinics initiated in Iowa. *NP News, 2*(4), 8–10.

McCarron, M., & Lawlor, B. (2003). Responding to the challenges of aging and dementia in intellectual ability in Ireland. *Aging and Mental Health, 7*(6), 413–417.

Mobile Health Clinics Network. (2011). Retrieved January 4, 2011, from www.mobilehealthclinicsnetwork.org

Peltzer, K., Seoka, P., Babor, T., & Obot, I. (2006). Training primary care nurses to conduct alcohol screening and brief interventions in South Africa. *Curationis, 29*(2), 16–21.

Sriamporn, S., Khuhaprema, T., & Parkin, M. (2006). Cervical cancer screening in Thailand: An overview. *Journal of Medical Screening, 13*(1), 39–42.

Tremblay, M., & Gorber, S. (2007). Canadian health measures survey. *Canadian Journal of Public Health, 98*(6), 453–456.

VA mobile health clinics reach rural populations. (2008, Fall). *Military Medicine*, 4–5.

VanRooyen, M., VanRooyen, J., Sloan, E., & Ward, E. (1990). Mobile medical relief and military assistance in Somalia. *Prehospital and Disaster Medicine, 10*(2), 118–120.

Weiss, T., Weiss, L., Teeter, D., & Geraci, J. (1999). Care provided by VA mobile clinic staff during Northridge earthquake relief. *Prehospital and Disaster Medicine, 14*(3), 191–197.

Worthington, C., & MacLaurin, B. (2009). Level of street involvement and health and health services use of Calgary street youth. *Canadian Journal of Public Health, 100*(5), 384–388.

Zachariah, R., Spielman, M., Harries, A., Nkhoma, W., Chantulo, S., & Arendt, V. (2003). Sexually transmitted infections and sexual behavior among commercial sex workers in a rural district of Malawi. *International Journal of STD and AIDS, 14*, 185–188.

APPENDIX A

Funding Sources

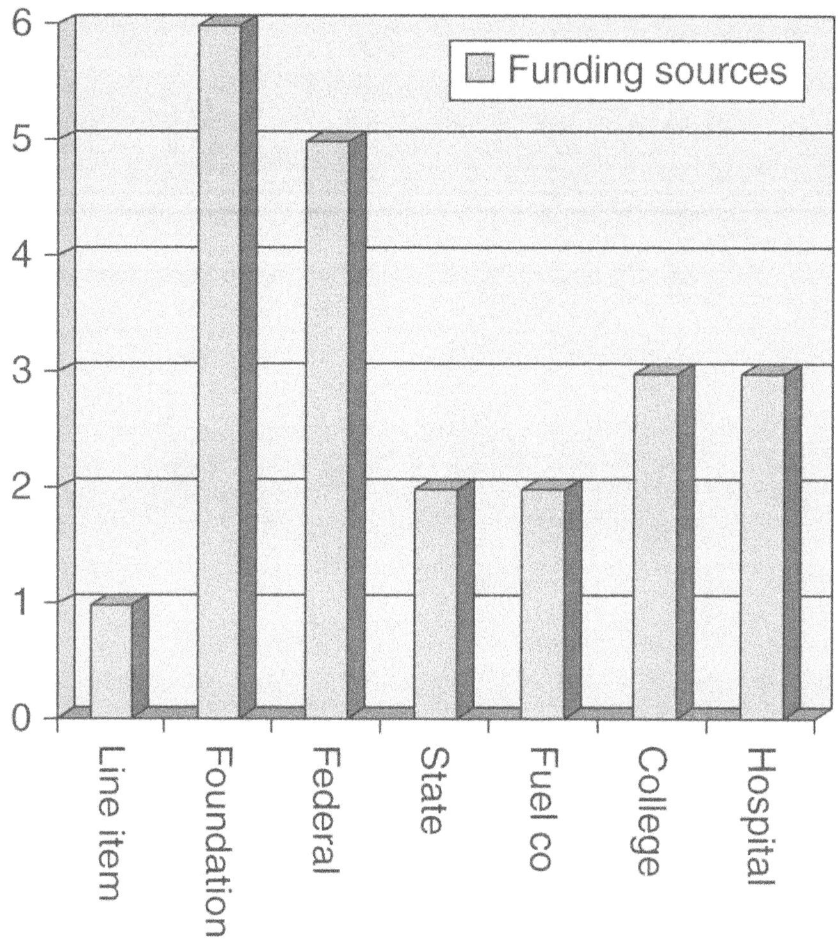

APPENDIX B

Populations Served

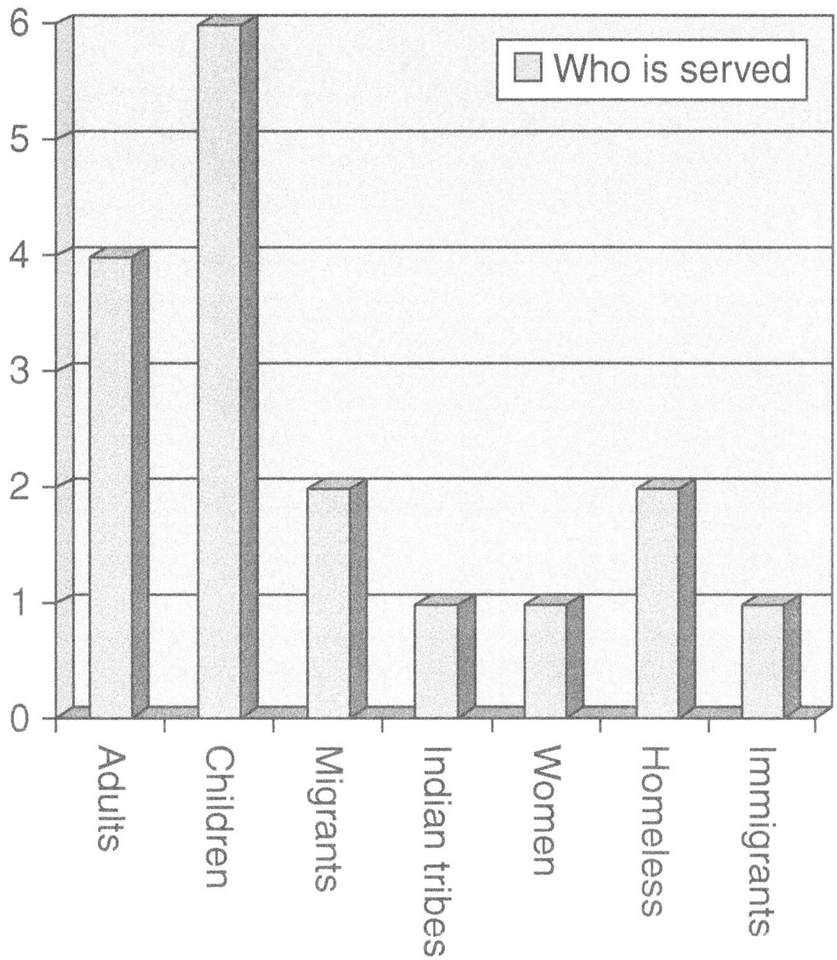

APPENDIX C

Services

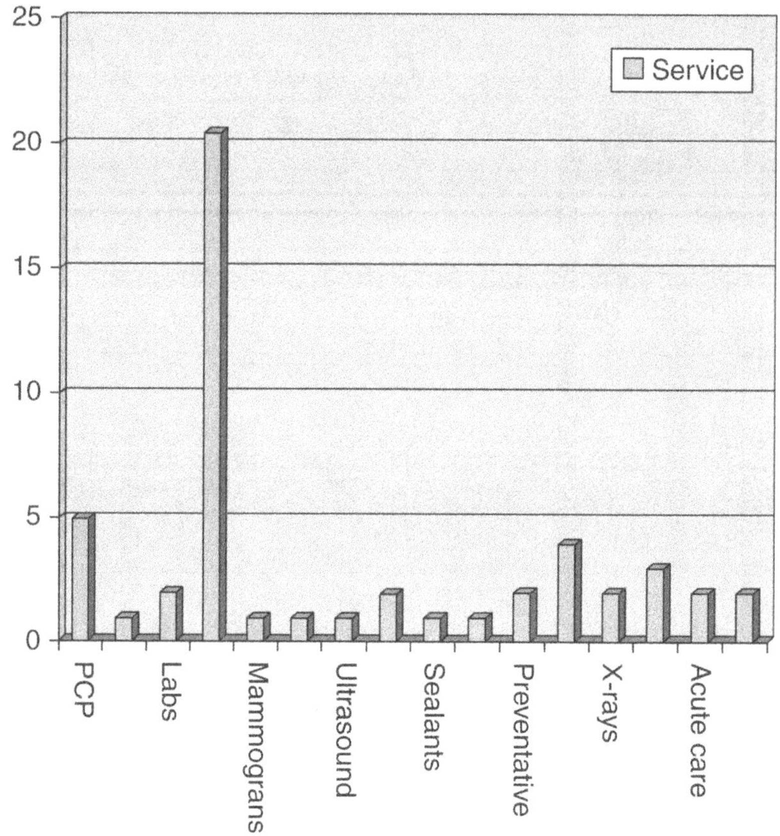

APPENDIX D

Staff

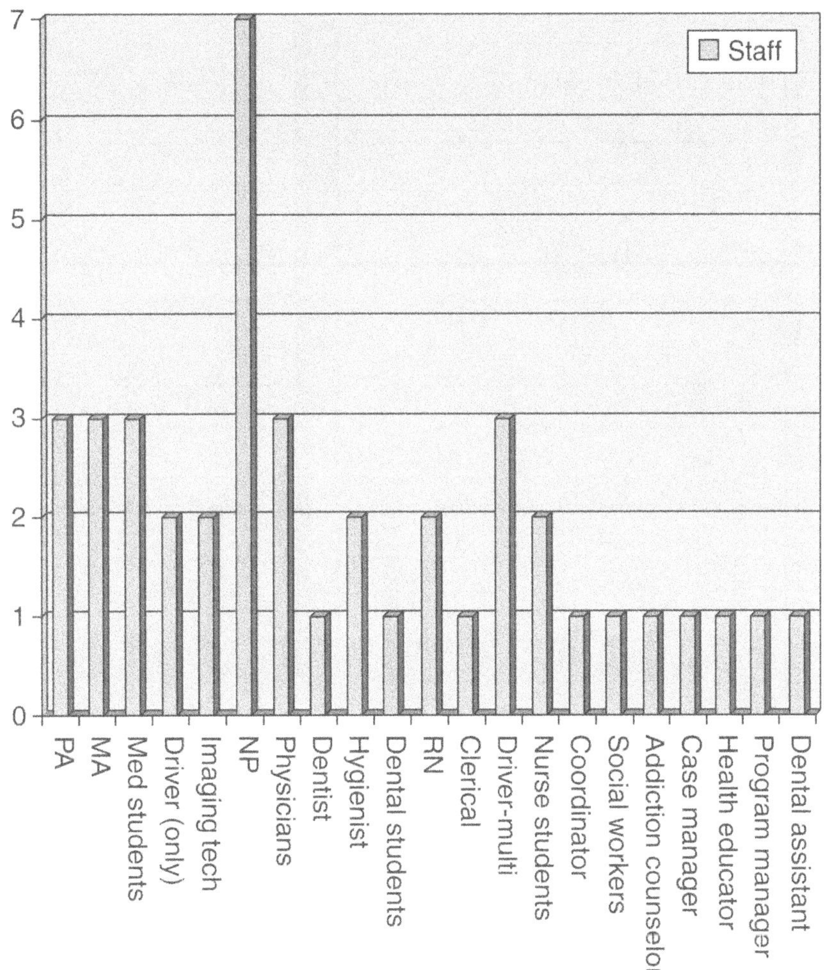

APPENDIX E

Challenges

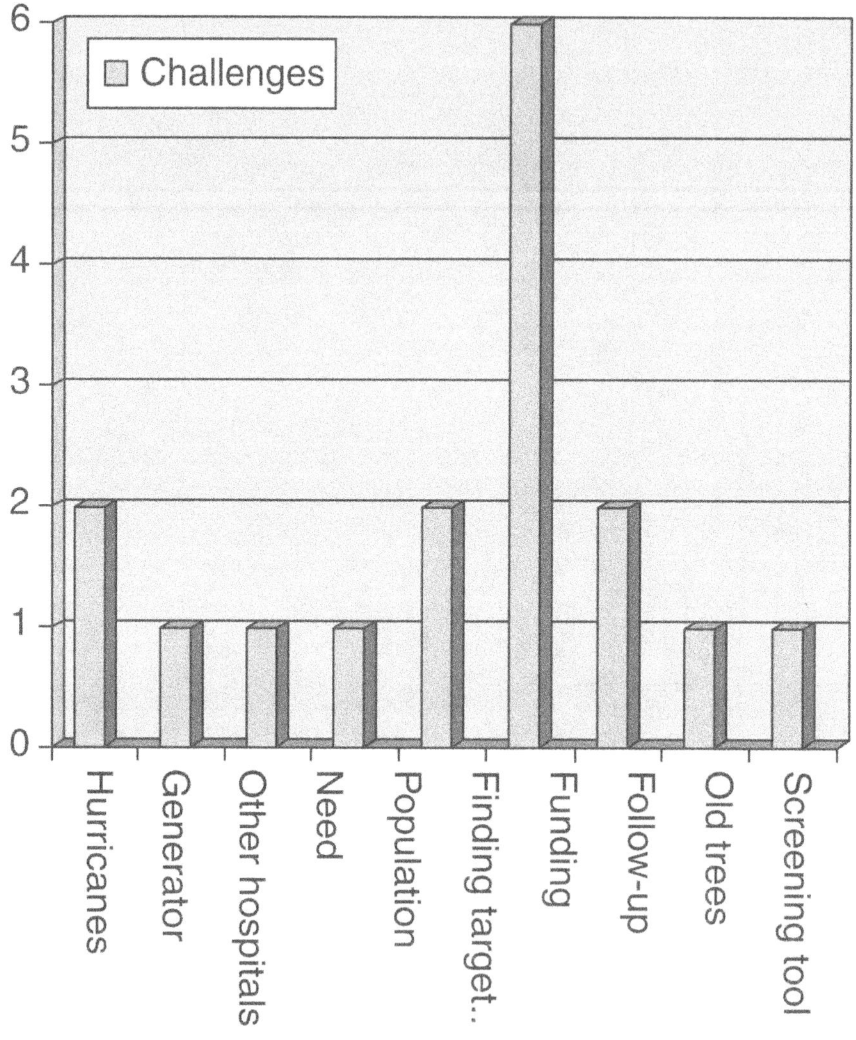

CHAPTER 18

Life Histories: Affluent Adolescents and Substance Abuse

Mary de Chesnay, Lisa Marie Walsh, Lacie Sezekes, Vicky Kronawitter, Kristin Cox, Suzanne S. Young, and Heather Payne

Objectives

At the end of this chapter, the reader will be able to

1. Describe the life history methodology as distinct from biography and autobiography.
2. Propose a methodology that can be used to collect life histories.
3. Compare and contrast the results of life histories with affluent adolescents and sexual abuse survivor.

INTRODUCTION

The first author's life history program of research on success in overcoming adversity began with a study of successful African American adults in the Southeast and was replicated in the Northeast and western United States. This study was reported in the first edition of this book (de Chesnay, 2005). During research courses with graduate students, she found that students became excited about the methodology and several completed graduate work using the life history methodology (de Chesnay, Rassilyer-Bomers, Webb, & Peil, 2008). Recently, an undergraduate course in vulnerable populations inspired a team of baccalaureate nursing students to collect life histories of young women who had successfully overcome addiction to drugs or alcohol. Another student in the class worked independently to collect the life history of a woman who had been sexually abused.

One of the most critical things nursing faculty can do is to inspire undergraduates by helping them realize that research can be fun, satisfying, and not as frightening as they usually perceive it to be, given the rigorous, yet dry way we tend to teach research in undergraduate programs. The life histories collected by these students were fun for them, cathartic for the key informants, and inspiring for the author to read.

Life histories are often collected during ethnographic research to tell the story of the culture through the eyes of those key informants most representative of the culture. There is a rich tradition of collecting life histories in anthropological research during long periods of fieldwork when the researcher lives within the community and develops relationships over time. Such long periods of fieldwork are not always possible in nursing research, however, so this chapter presents an abbreviated way to collect life histories from individuals who have much to teach nurses about living with their health conditions.

Life history differs from autobiography in that the agent of interpretation is the researcher, not the one whose life is being described. The informant tells his or her story to the researcher, who then interprets the story in light of the research questions and the cultural context in which the person lives (de Chesnay, 2005). Similarly, life histories differ from the life review techniques that are used therapeutically to help the elderly come to a sense of peace at the end of life and to leave a legacy of what they have learned for subsequent generations (Allen, 2009; Hrehocik, 2009; Thornton, 2008).

Many examples of detailed life histories can be found in the anthropological literature (Abrums, 2010; Davison, 1989; Early, 1993; Gmelch, 1986; James, 2000; Levy, 1988; Scheub et al., 1988; Sexton, 1981). These stories are usually drawn from the experiences of key informants during ethnography and comprise extensive histories of each cultural informant deemed to be a particularly interesting or expressive representative of that culture.

As nurses, social workers, and other health professionals developed research programs that focus on emic data, they adapted life history methods to better suit their own fields. However, because non-anthropologists bring diverse training and other traditions to their research, some confusion in the literature arises when authors equate life history with oral history. Life history is a story told by a researcher from data generated by a key informant and framing his or her life within the cultural context in which the person lived life. In contrast, oral history focuses on the historical context and is useful when the researcher wishes to document the historical evolution of a group, such as nurses who practiced in the military during the Vietnam War or survivors of the influenza epidemic of 1919.

At any rate, life history as a research design is gaining popularity internationally. Recent reports in the literature can be found in Brazil (Bellato et al., 2008; Bousso, Serafim, & Misko, 2010), Australia (Patching & Lawler, 2009; Wicks & Whiteford, 2006), the United Kingdom (Dyson, Goren, Hooper, & Cabral, 2008; Etherington, 2009; Hamilton & Atkinson, 2009; Monaghan & Cumella, 2009), Israel (Shrira & Shmoktin, 2008), the Netherlands (Yajima, van Huis, & Jiggins, 2010; and the United States (de Chesnay, 2005; de Chesnay et al., 2008; Moos, Schutte, Brennan, & Moos, 2010).

Life histories collected by nurses and social workers tend to be focused on specific topics, whereas those created by anthropologists as part of fieldwork tend to be full scale and tell the story of the whole life within that culture. For example, de Chesnay's (2005) research focuses on success at overcoming obstacles, whether these are trauma, racism, chronic diseases, or other specific stressors. Also targeting specific stressors are Yajima, van Huis, and Jiggins (2010), who studied members of farming communities in northern Malawi who have HIV/AIDS.

Nurses and social workers are practitioners, so they inevitably see their research as having the potential to inform their practices. In London, a team of social work researchers conducted life history interviews with 70 low-income families, including 9 Bangladesh immigrant families, to document the need for home-visiting services to the immigrants (Dyson et al., 2008). Similarly, Australian nurses who work with patients with eating disorders documented through life histories the critical need for appropriate training for healthcare professionals about this set of diseases (Patching & Lawler, 2009).

The flexibility of methods in life history is described nicely in a paper from Iceland. Life histories can be collected by individual researcher, teams, or even jointly with a key informant, as demonstrated by two people who met in an institution—one a patient, the other a staff member (Hreinsdottir & Stefansdottir, 2010).

THE METHODOLOGY

The methods for these studies were developed by de Chesnay in an attempt to refine the traditional anthropological techniques for nursing research. In traditional life history work framed within a year-long immersion in fieldwork, the stories can unfold over time as the ethnographer becomes part of the scene. For nursing research, the abbreviated version described here provides the nurse researcher with direction for active intervention that may not help the person but can be used to help people with the same condition. The original study was reported in the first edition of this book (de Chesnay, 2005). Subsequently, the students who coauthored the second-edition chapter were graduate students who completed life histories with individuals who had survived bereavement, colostomy, and multiple sclerosis (de Chesnay et al., 2008).

In the current edition, the three life histories of affluent adolescents with substance abuse problems were collected by a team of undergraduate students that was led by a student (Walsh) who is an experienced substance abuse counselor and who provided access to the key informants. Working with the same methodology, these students interviewed three young women who had conquered their demons and made new lives for themselves despite the overwhelming pull of substance abuse. The life history developed by Payne involved a woman who had been molested by a servant in her native country, India.

A method of focusing life history material for briefer reports was developed by Hagemaster (1992), who presented a clear outline for interviews conducted solely as life histories. The usefulness of such life narratives was described by Mattingly and Lawlor (2000). Beery, Sommers, and Hall (2002) used an adaptation of Hall's (1996) methodology of focused life stories to explore women's experience with pacemakers.

In the studies reported in this chapter, the life histories are abbreviated stories told by people who have something to teach others through the recounting of their path to success by overcoming the obstacles associated with their disease or condition. Success for each study was self-defined by the key informant, and refers to a sense of prosperity and general satisfaction with accomplishments and success at overcoming obstacles.

It is important to note that the data derived from this study are emic (from the person's viewpoint) rather than etic (from the researcher's viewpoint). Emic data are more powerful for the purpose of developing culturally appropriate interventions because of the increased likelihood of their relevance to the target audience.

Three methods of data collection may used in constructing life histories, in addition to participant observation: a series of semi-structured interviews, genograms, and time lines. The research question for the study on alcohol is this: How does a person achieve success in overcoming the obstacles associated with the condition of substance abuse and the particular challenges faced by affluent teenagers? Similarly, the research question for the study by Payne is this: How does a person successfully overcome the effects of the childhood trauma of molestation?

Key informants were recruited purposively. Genograms and specific demographic data for the sample are not presented here to protect participants' privacy. The genogram was originally developed as a clinical tool in family therapy, but is now widely used as an assessment tool in nursing and medicine. The genogram model developed for family therapy (McGoldrick & Gerson, 1986; McGoldrick, Gerson, & Shellenberger, 1999) was adapted by de Chesnay for use in her own clinical practice as a family therapist and as an instrument of research in an earlier study (de Chesnay, Marshall, & Clements, 1988). The purpose of the genogram was to streamline the analysis of family data.

Genogram questions involved gathering information about the family of origin and successful role models within the family. In the life history presented here, interviews included broad questions about the definition of success, facilitative factors and barriers, and stories from the informants' youth. Generally three or four interviews lasting approximately hours were necessary. Interviews were audio-taped to ensure accuracy.

The timeline data collection tool is simply a horizontal line on a blank page with "birth" at the left end and "present age" at the right end. Informants were asked to indicate on the line the critical events in their lives and the ages at which the events occurred. The timeline helped to clarify the sequence of events important to the person. Informants were given copies of the genograms and timelines, and were encouraged to change them as needed during the intervals between interview sessions.

After the institutional review board gave approval, the informants were recruited, the consent forms were explained and signed, and the interviews were scheduled, conducted, and analyzed. The first author (de Chesnay) served as a consultant and resource to the others, but the team worked with the data independently.

THE LIFE HISTORIES

Jennifer: "My Life Changed Completely"

Jennifer is a 23-year-old Caucasian female of Italian and German descent. She is approximately 5 feet 3 inches tall, weighs 125 pounds, and has shoulder-length blonde hair and brown eyes. She is very attractive, with light pale skin tone that is smooth and even and straight white teeth. She is also very well dressed and well spoken.

Jennifer was born to a 15-year-old mother from an affluent family in Los Angeles, California area. She was raised by her great-grandparents until she was 5 years old, then moved in with her mother and grandmother in Georgia. She was raised in an affluent area of metro Atlanta. Jennifer graduated from high school and has some college credits. Currently she is a manager of a retail cell phone store; she drives a very nice, new car on which she makes regular payments. Most importantly, she is able to live on her own and be independent for the first time in her life.

Genograms were collected to provide a picture of the family life of the key informant. The genogram data for Jennifer revealed that alcoholism ran in her family as far back as her grandfather. Her mother was an alcoholic schizophrenic with bipolar disorder who gave birth to her daughter at 15 years of age. Her father was an alleged meth (methamphetamine) addict who left her mother when she was pregnant. Her mother was also married three times. In one of the marriages, both her mother and her stepfather were physically and emotionally abusive to Jennifer. Jennifer herself is a recovering alcoholic and drug addict.

The purpose of the timeline is to identify critical events and the ages at which they occurred for each key informant. The critical events in Jennifer's life were being born to a 15-year-old mother with addictive and mental disorders. She began her life by residing with her great-grandmother until she was 6 years old. When she was 6, Jennifer moved in with her mother for the first time. From ages 6 to 11, she drifted in and out of her mother's household. At the age of 12, Jennifer had her first alcoholic drink and smoked marijuana for the first time. At 15, she realized that she had no self-respect after losing her virginity and felt "inhuman due to [my] lack of emotion." At 17, Jennifer used meth for the first time. She became engaged, but eventually her fiancé kicked her out due to her constant drug use. During this time, the realization of her inability to control her addiction occurred as well. At 18, Jennifer entered into recovery through Narcotics Anonymous. At 22, she began living independently while continuing the recovery process.

Stella: "I Finally Noticed the Clouds Again"

Stella is a 26-year-old Caucasian woman from an affluent community in Georgia. Her father, age 56, is a recovering alcoholic with an Italian–Lithuanian background; her mother, age 55, has a Welsh–Scottish background. Catholicism is the main belief system of the family, although Stella does not attend services. Stella is approximately 5 feet 4 inches tall, has short brown hair, and dresses very nicely. She has a great demeanor and is very well spoken. Stella has a high school diploma; she also graduated from a West Coast art school. She is currently working as a customer service representative for a supermarket chain.

The genogram data for Stella revealed that Stella's father was a recovering alcoholic. The critical events in Stella's life began at 6 years old, when Stella's father entered into recovery from alcoholism. When she was 7 years old, Stella's family moved from the West Coast to the Southeast, which really angered her. At age 14, she was sexually assaulted. At 17, Stella smoked pot and later in the year tried acid for the first time. When she was 18 years old, she started taking pain pills and tried Ecstasy for the first time. Also, she moved back to the West Coast. At 19, Stella tried cocaine, speed, and oxycontin for the first time. Stella, at age 20, attended a 12-step meeting on her own with no outside influence. At 21, she moved back to the Southeast and tried heroin for the first time. When Stella was 23, her older sister was raped. On May 11, 2007, at the age of 23, Stella entered into a recovery program to "get clean." At age 25, Stella had a child. Now 27 years old, Stella has been clean and sober for a little more than 3 years.

Emma "Just Happy to Be Alive"

Emma is a 21-year-old Caucasian female with long dark brown hair and brown eyes. She has an Italian heritage from her mother's side and is unsure of her father's heritage. She is 5 feet 6 inches tall and average weight. She is well dressed and well groomed, and spoke quietly during the interview. She has a high school education and is currently enrolled in college. The most significant genogram data for Emma revealed that all eight brothers of her father were alcoholics.

The critical events in Emma's life began when she was 1 year old, when her parents divorced due to her father's infidelity. At age 13, Emma found a bottle of oxycontin in her mother's closet and took the whole bottle over three days, For her, the event was the moment "it clicked": "I had found something that made me feel good." At 14, she started using heroin with her boyfriend, a habit that lasted for 6 years. At 15, Emma started dealing oxycontin in her affluent community. While she was between the ages of 18 and 20, six of her close friends died of overdoses. At this writing, she now has eight friends who have died of drug-related accidents.

At nineteen, she accelerated her deterioration by receiving an academic suspension from college, working at a strip club to pay for her drug habits, and passing out while smoking and setting the house on fire. At age 20, Emma hit rock bottom when she passed out at the wheel of her car and totaled it, became homeless as a result of burning the house down, and saw her weight drop to 90 pounds. Also, she overdosed on oxycontin, which prompted her mother to send her to a treatment program. Emma's successful resolution of her addiction began very recently—at age 20, when she entered treatment. At 21, she earned her 1-year sobriety chip, began college, and began living independently in an apartment.

Megna

Megna is a 34-year-old woman of "pure" East Indian descent. Megna is the survivor of multiple traumatic events: She was molested by a servant in her own home when she was of kindergarten age, she survived a violent car accident when she was 4 or 5 years old, and her father was an alcoholic throughout the entirety of her childhood. Today Megna lives in northwest Georgia and fulfills many of the criteria our society expects of "successful" people. She is willing to share her unique life experiences in the hopes of helping others.

Megna's genogram illustrates three generations of family, including both sets of Megna's grandparents, her parents, aunts, uncles, brothers, sister, and partner. In the genogram, Megna designated family members who lived together in India, all of whom were paternal kin. She noted that her maternal grandmother died when she was 4 years old, so she never got to know her; her mother was raised by her father as a "motherless child." Megna also discussed the disease history in her family, as well as the family's religious background.

Megna was molested each school day in kindergarten by the male servant who was tasked with preparing her for school. The servant who molested her did not remain in the house beyond her kindergarten year because he was caught stealing. Although Megna states that her family members were not as watchful as they should have been, her voice, words, and tone are not accusatory or bitter in making this admission. At the time of her molestation, Megna disliked what the servant was doing, and felt that it was wrong even at that young age. Megna points out that molestation is viewed in a very negative light in India, and notes that she felt shame over the events.

Megna's father was an alcoholic, which created a state of continual chaos for much of Megna's childhood. Megna's mother was always worried that the drinking would eventually kill her husband, but did not receive support from the other family members in the joint household, so this issue was a constant source of friction. The genogram identifies that only the paternal relatives were living in the household, so Megna's mother did not have her own set of family members there to support her on contentious issues. Megna remembers daily fighting, living in fear of fighting, "walking on eggshells," and coming to expect and even crave drama in a way. Her parents regularly split and got back together. Sometimes Megna would fall asleep in one town and wake up in another, because her mother had packed the children up in the night and taken them to a relative's house. Megna frequently had to stay with relatives when the upheaval was too great, and she was neglected at times. In addition, she had to act as a parent to her younger siblings. Megna's mother was a housewife, as was the tradition, and she did not have to work because the family was wealthy in India. Megna's mother was active in improving conditions for villagers when Megna was in her teenage years, which may have been a coping mechanism. Alcoholism is viewed negatively in much of India because it runs counter to the teachings of the ultra-religious factions there.

The entire family was involved in a major accident when Megna was 4 or 5 years old. Everyone was thrown from the car, and Megna's mother suffered an immediate miscarriage at the scene of the accident. Everyone survived with exception of the fetus, but Megna is still tense when she rides in cars to this day. She did learn to drive, but once she had her first accident driving, she "shut down."

CONCEPTS

Support from Loved Ones

If Megna could state in one word the pervasive theme in her interviews, that word would be "relationships." Megna's family and partner are the most important things in her life. Megna lived in a joint family until she moved to the United States at age 17, living under the same roof with all living grandparents, both of her parents, two uncles, four aunts, and all of her cousins. Everyone ate together and shared facilities. Megna stresses the closeness she feels and has always felt to her mother, sister, and youngest brother. She still speaks with her mother, sister, and youngest brother every day on the phone. She is deeply involved with her niece, and "base[s] her plans and the future kind of around her proximity . . . My goals do tend to be towards where I can make it to make sure that she's healthy, safe, and has everything, has all the resources she so she can do what she wants to do in her life." Megna lived with her sister at the University of Georgia, and has never lived alone. Cohabitation provides emotional resource continuity through changes.

Megna also has a very strong relationship with her monogamous partner, Salim, whom she has dated for 17 years and lived with for 15 years. Her daily life consists of spending the overwhelming majority of her time with Salim. "It's really more than words; it's been about the actions we have towards each other that have defined our relationship . . . we don't say what we are planning on doing with each other and things of that sort and promises and stuff—we just do what we feel and it works." Megna views this relationship as successful. She defines success in a relationship as consisting of mutual feelings, trust, having fun, and appreciation of small things such as "making the pot of coffee in the morning."

The three young women who used drugs and alcohol to cope did not have support systems in place that they could substitute for the drugs. They led lives of superficial relationships and social isolation despite their contacts with other drug users. Their support was limited to their drug use until they entered rehabilitation, where they could experience a supportive group and counseling staff.

Religion

Megna does not consider herself religious, but rather calls herself a "Muslim atheist," because she is an atheist but was raised as a Muslim and considers that her culture. While her father's side of the family were strictly observant, traditional Muslims of the small Indian Shia sect, her mother's side of the family were more permissive and diverse. The Shia sect was an "outcast" from the rest of the Muslim world because of its emphasis on education. Megna states that her family went to church every day when she was in India, and that it was like "Sunday school." Megna's maternal grandmother was of South African–Indian lineage, and her maternal grandfather was from the sizable city of Goa. Her maternal uncle converted to Hinduism. Her maternal aunt married a Catholic man and was not particularly religious. Megna attended Catholic school, because these schools were "the best" in the area for "correctly" raising young ladies. Salim's family are strict Baptists, but Salim is an atheist. Megna's family celebrates Christianity-based holidays with her young niece, such as the exchanging of presents on Christmas and egg hunts on Easter, but the focus is on family togetherness and lacks the religious component. Megna was caned at the convent school, which made her angry at the time, and she credits this caning with being the source of the anger response she sometimes has to people.

Coping

Megna copes by putting things out of her mind until she is prepared to deal with them. She repressed memories of her molestation until she was 13. During this time she was also attending Alateen, and had made a group of friends whom she felt accepted by and safe with; these factors may have contributed to the timing of her memories resurfacing. Today, Megna states that she puts worrisome issues out of her mind and distracts herself by watching television, getting on the computer, playing a game, or reading a "trashy" book. When she feels ready, she then discusses the anxiety-provoking issues with Salim or family members.

Initially, Megna told no one about having been molested. She told Salim before anyone else. Megna's sister and youngest brother were supportive when Megna informed them what had happened, as was Salim. Megna is only gently encouraged to talk about the things that have happened to her, but never pushed. Megna says that whatever Salim is doing, he stops, listens, and gives her unlimited time to talk. Salim "encourag[es] me to finish talking about it and actually dealing with it instead of pushing it to the back of my mind because that [is] going to hurt me so." Megna manages her negative feelings concerning being in a car by limiting who she rides with, making her fears known to persons driving her so they will be aware of her history, and avoiding riding on the interstate when possible. She says of her troubles: "It happened, so I'm going to deal with it, but I've definitely gotten support from every person I have told this to."

The adolescents who abused drugs and alcohol did so to cope, but their coping strategies were unsuccessful. It was only when they "hit bottom" and were forced to enter rehabilitation programs that they were able to look for different coping strategies.

Placing Value on Industry

When Megna's family moved to the United States in 1993, she was 17. The family experienced some culture shock at first, as they went from being wealthy in India to living in a one- to two-bedroom apartment. The deals they thought were in place vanished, and the already tight-knit family bonded even closer as they struggled to meet the common goal of survival. They no longer had servants to do things such as remove their shoes. Megna had not wanted to come to the United States because she did not want to leave her friends in India, but she found that she enjoyed cooking, doing her own dishes, and helping with homework. Her parents "leaned" on her, which gave her confidence and a new feeling of importance. Megna states, "The one thing I liked about coming to the United States [was that] it was the first time in my life I was going to be able to contribute financially to my family."

Megna's family and Salim supported her college education, which she says was "an extremely awesome time in my life, even as my parents were going through their separation and divorce." She has zest for her work, describing it as "very, very stimulating, constantly." She feels successful in her work. When she first arrived in the United States, her finances were so limited that she had to worry about buying a sandwich; now she buys whatever she wants: "I don't think about it twice."

Acceptance of Imperfection

Megna does not expect to erase the past or to pretend that it does not exist. She finished her interviews by saying, "I've moved on with my life, but in no way can I say that I'm completely healed. Really, there's no way for me to say that. There's no way I'm ever going to heal completely, [but] . . . your experiences become part of who you are and that's the way it is." She accepts that life and people are not perfect. She says, "I'm not going to sit here and put blame on whoever and what happened." Megna describes Salim as "just not motivated enough and . . . kind of lazy," yet is wholly accepting of him with his imperfections. Megna considers herself successful in key areas of her life such as relationships and career, despite her past.

One of the most important lessons that successful people learn is how to fail successfully. This step involves accepting themselves for who they are and not beating themselves up for who they are not. The affluent adolescents who fell into substance abuse grew up in environments in which no one was available to help them, perhaps due to their parents' own use of drugs as self-image boosters.

CONCLUSION

The data in this study were gathered by undergraduate students who had relatively little experience in both research and interviewing techniques. Even so, the students embraced the assignment with enthusiasm and dignity in the way they approached the participants. The young women interviewed for the affluent alcoholism life histories were not that different from some of the students in their cultural and ethnic backgrounds, yet vastly different in their purposefulness about life. The nursing students demonstrated great focus and determination to succeed and mastered their coursework as they progressed, without the need for the crutch that alcohol and drugs provide.

The common experience of conducting this research with respect—indeed, reverence—for the key informants perhaps will encourage these young women to continue their education beyond the baccalaureate degree they are earning now. As their teacher, I would like to think they will someday use what they learned in developing these life histories to earn their own doctorates and perhaps inspire their own students as they have inspired me.

WWW For a full suite of assignments and additional learning activities, use the access code located in the front of your book to visit this exclusive website: http://go.jblearning.com/dechesnay. If you do not have an access code, you can obtain one at the site.

REFERENCES

Abrums, M. (2010). *Moving the rock: Poverty and faith in a black storefront church.* Lanham, MD: AltaMira Press.

Allen, R. S. (2009). The Legacy Project intervention to enhance meaningful family interactions: Case examples. *Clinical Gerontologist, 32*, 164–176.

Beery, T., Sommers, M., & Hall, J. (2002). Focused life stories of women with cardiac pacemakers. *Western Journal of Nursing Research, 24*(1), 7–27.

Bellato, R., Santos de Araujo, L., Silva de Faria, A., Santos, E., Castro, P., Salome de Souza, S., & Maruyama, S. (2008). A historia de vida focal e suas potencialidades na pesquisa em saude e em enfermagem. Retrieved January 5, 2011, from www.fen.ufg.br/revista/v10n3a31.htm

Bousso, R., Serafim, T., & Misko, M. (2010). The relationship between religion, illness and death in life histories of family members of children with threatening diseases. *Revista Latino-Americana de Enfermagem, 18*(2), 156–162.

Davison, J. (1989). *Voices from Mutira: Change in the lives of rural Gikuyu women.* Boulder, CO: Lynne Reinner.

de Chesnay, M. (2005). "Can't keep me down": Life histories of successful African Americans. In M. de Chesnay (Ed.), *Caring for the vulnerable: Perspectives in nursing theory, practice and research* (pp. 221–231). Sudbury, MA: Jones and Bartlett.

de Chesnay, M., Marshall, E., & Clements, C. (1988). Family structure, marital power, maternal distance, and paternal alcohol consumption in father–daughter incest. *Family Systems Medicine, 6*(4), 453–462.

de Chesnay, M., Rassilyer-Bomers, R., Webb, J., & Peil, R. (2008). Life histories of successful survivors of colostomy surgery, multiple sclerosis and bereavement. In M. de Chesnay (Ed.), *Caring for the vulnerable: Perspectives in nursing theory, practice and research* (pp. 205–222). Sudbury, MA: Jones and Bartlett.

Dyson, C., Gorin, S., Hooper, C., & Cabral, C. (2008). Bangladeshi families living in hardship: Findings from research using a life-history approach. *Child and Family Social Work, 14*, 362–371.

Early, E. (1993). *Baladi women: Playing with an egg and a stone.* Boulder, CO: Lynne Reinner.

Etherington, K. (2009). Life story research: A relevant methodology for counselors and psychotherapists. *Counseling and Psychotherapy Research, 9*(4), 225–233.

Gmelch, S. (1986). *Nan: The life of an Irish traveling woman.* Prospect Heights, IL: Waveland.

Hagemaster, J. (1992). Life history: A qualitative method of research. *Journal of Advanced Nursing, 17*, 1122–1128.

Hall, J. (1996). Geography of childhood sexual abuse: Women's narratives of their childhood environment. *Advances in Nursing Science, 18*(4), 29–47.

Hamilton, C., & Atkinson, D. (2009). "A story to tell": Learning from the life stories of older people with intellectual disabilities in Ireland. *British Journal of Learning Disabilities, 37*, 316–322.

Hrehocik, M. (2009). Lives well-lived forever chronicled on video: The Legacies Project plans searchable archive to preserve life stories. *Long-Term Living for the Continuing Care Professional, 58*(7), 36–39.

Hreinsdottir, E., & Stefansdottir, G. (2010). Collaborative life history: Different experiences of spending time in an institution in Iceland. *British Journal of Learning Disabilities, 38*(2), 103–109.

James, D. (2000). *Doña María's story.* Durham, NC: Duke University.

Levy, M. (1988). *Each in her own way: Five women leaders of the developing world.* Boulder, CO: Lynne Reinner.

Mattingly, C., & Lawlor, M. (2000). Learning from stories: Narrative interviewing in cross- cultural research. *Scandinavian Journal of Occupational Therapy, 7*, 4–14.

McGoldrick, M., & Gerson, R. (1986). *Genograms in family assessment.* New York: W. W. Norton.

McGoldrick, M., Gerson, R., & Shellenberger, S. (1999). *Genograms: Assessment and intervention.* New York: W. W. Norton.

Monaghan, V., & Cumella, S. (2009). Support workers and people with learning disabilities: Participative and life history research. *Housing, Care and Support, 12*(3), 28–36.

Moos, R., Schutte, K., Brennan, P., & Moos, B. (2010). Late life and life history predictors of older adults' high-risk alcohol consumption and drinking problems. *Drug and Alcohol Dependence. 108*(1), 13–20.

Patching, J., & Lawler, J. (2009). Understanding women's experiences of developing an eating disorder and recovering: A life history approach. *Nursing Inquiry, 16*, 10–21.

Scheub, H., Mack, B., Schildkrout, E., Obbo, C., Wilks, I., & Romero, P. (1988). *Life histories of African women.* London: Ashfield.

Sexton, J. D. (1981). *Son of Tecún Umán: A Maya Indian tells his life story.* Prospect Heights, IL: Waveland.

Shrira, A., & Shmotkin, D. (2008). Can the past keep life pleasant even for old-old trauma survivors? *Aging and Mental Health, 12*(6), 807–819.

Thornton, J. E. (2008). The guided autobiographical methodology: A learning experience. *International Journal of Aging and Human Development, 66*(2), 155–173.

Wicks, A., & Whiteford, G. (2006). Conceptual and practical issues in qualitative research: Reflections on a life-history study. *Scandinavian Journal of Occupational Therapy, 13*, 94–100.

Yajima, M., van Huis, A., & Jiggins, J. (2010). Life history analysis of HIV/AIDS-affected households in rice and cassava-based farming communities in northern Malawi. *AIDS Care, 22*(10), 1195–1203.

CHAPTER 19

Staying with HIV/AIDS: A Compressed Ethnography of Zambian Women

Terra Grandmason

Objectives

At the end of this chapter, the reader will be able to

1. Review the literature on Zambian women with AIDS.
2. Evaluate the study on Zambian women with AIDS.
3. Evaluate the uses of ethnography with vulnerable populations in Africa and the United States.

OVERVIEW

As the leading cause of death in sub-Saharan Africa, HIV/AIDS results in severe physical, economic, and social disturbances. Women represent 57% of HIV infections in Africa, with Zambian women being 1.4 times more likely to be infected than men (United Nations General Assembly Special Session on HIV/AIDS [UNGASS], 2005). This study explores the experiences of women in Zambia, who face unique socioeconomic and sociocultural challenges while bearing the greatest disease burden.

This ethnography sought to increase understanding of how Zambian women living with HIV/AIDS survive in an environment where supports may be nonexistent or strained to the breaking point. The focal question asked was in which forms and to what extent support is present in the women's lives. The answer emerged as a detailed account of enduring and overcoming uncertainty and loss, drawing a picture of how nine impoverished Zambian women are "staying with HIV"—the local syntax used to describe their HIV-positive status, denoting a life permanently impacted by an incurable, impairing and fatal virus. The research question was this: In which forms and to what extent is support present in the lives of HIV-positive, low-income Zambian women?

REVIEW OF LITERATURE

In addition to social and emotional needs, support needs among women living with HIV in sub-Saharan Africa may include food, money, medicine, physical assistance, future orphan care, and health teaching (Harding, Stewart, Marconi, O'Neill, & Higginson, 2003; Plattner & Meiring, 2006). Meeting these needs is complicated amidst a deteriorating set of resources due to prolonged poverty, urbanization, and the impact of HIV/AIDS on local and national economies (Dyson, 2003; UNAIDS, 2004; World Bank, 2005). In South Africa and Zambia, monthly incomes typically fall 66% to 80% in households affected by AIDS (Barnett & Whiteside, 2002; Steinberg et al., 2002).

Because men were disproportionately affected early in the HIV/AIDS epidemic, single-parent households are now largely female headed (Moore & Vaughan, 1994; Niehaus, 1994; UNAIDS, UNFPA, & UNIFEM, 2004; World Bank, 2005). Marital rates in the region are decreasing, and widows may be unable to find new partners to help provide for them (Hunter, 2007; World Bank, 2005). Limited employment opportunities may be further hindered by HIV-related pain or fatigue, forcing women to rely on such uncertain work as selling produce or transactional sex (Hunter, 2007; Keogh, Allen, Almedal, & Temahagili, 1994).

The widespread stigma associated with HIV/AIDS is another obstacle to support for these women. The risk of eviction, rejection, or shame from social networks and the potential for discrimination in accessing financial, educational, and occupational resources often result in women hiding their HIV status (MANET, 2003; Plattner & Meiring, 2006). This factor increases their isolation and decreases the likelihood that women will access available supports (Ciambrone, 2002). Women often face blame, condemnation, and accusations of promiscuous sexual behavior if their HIV status is discovered (Panos Institute & UNICEF, 2001). Negative social consequences may also emerge from lifestyle alterations such as not breastfeeding or choosing not to have more children (Lawson, 1999).

Psychosocial support is important for dealing with the struggles of real and feared discrimination, unmet needs, and the difficult act of disclosing one's status (Chaava, 1990; Ciambrone, 2002; Kayawe, Kelly, & Baggaley, 1998; Uys, 2003). It also improves retention of HIV-related information, overall well-being, and performance of daily duties despite insomnia, pain or fatigue (Eisenberg, Kemeny, & Wyatt, 2003; Hughes, Jelsma, Maclean, Darder, & Tinise, 2004; Keogh et al., 1994; UNFPA, 2006). These considerations are important, as depression and suicidal ideation often occur following discovery of a positive HIV status (Keogh et al., 1994; Plattner & Meiring, 2006; Swindells et al., 1999). However, acceptance of one's own HIV-positive status and the establishment of a closer relationship with a higher power were found to contribute to well-being and a sense that there must be a purpose for one's HIV infection (Plattner & Meiring, 2006).

Although facing a unique set of obstacles due to their disadvantaged social and economic position, women share the wider African experience of lacking desperately needed resources and services. Women carry a greater burden of stigma surrounding HIV/AIDS, which limits their willingness to access supports. Despite general acknowledgment that support is beneficial, it is unclear to what extent different supports are present or affect the lives of these women.

In sub-Saharan Africa, where a variety of factors influence the existence of and access to support, few studies have explored the experience of support among HIV-positive women. For the purposes of this study, no published literature was found that focused on support among HIV-positive Zambian women.

METHODOLOGY

This research was conducted using a compressed ethnographic research design to accommodate a shortened research time frame (LeCompte & Schensul, 1999).

Sample

A purposive sample of 9 women was obtained. Women ranged in age from 38 to 48 years, with education levels ranging from grades 7 to 12. All participants were accessing outpatient services at the hospice. Further demographics are shown in **Table 19–1**. The women's experiences and perspectives of support were explored during their interviews, and their stories were analyzed for this study. Interviews with local nongovernmental organization (NGO) heads and HIV/AIDS services providers were also conducted to verify data interpretation and to provide a broader perspective of support available to the sample population.

Table 19-1 Study Participant Demographics

Marriage status	Widowed 78%	Married 11%	Unknown 11%
Work status	Unable 44%	Sporadic 33%	Stable Job 22%
Had children	Yes 100%	No 0%	Unknown 0%
Experienced the death of at least one child	Yes 56%	No 0%	Unknown 44%
Caring for orphans	Yes 33%	No 22%	Unknown 44%
Participated in community outreach	Yes 78%	No 11%	Unknown 11%
Taking antiretroviral medications	Yes 56%	No 22%	Unknown 11%
Disclosed status to more than one important friend or family member	Yes 78%	No 22%	Unknown 0%
Belonged to HIV/AIDS support group	Yes 78%	No 22%	Unknown 0%

Setting

One of the poorest nations in the world, Zambia has an AIDS rate of 16.5% among 15- to 49-year-olds (UNAIDS, 2004; UNDP, 2005). The median age of the general population is 16 years, and life expectancy is 37.5 years; over the past two decades, life expectancy has decreased by 14 years.

In 2003, Zambia instituted free HIV treatment. The semi-urban AIDS hospice in Lusaka Province, where this study was conducted, is one of many locations providing this free HIV treatment. Participants in this study resided in surrounding, densely populated compounds, which are illegally created shantytowns that are now largely considered legal residences and house the majority of Zambians (Kunda, 2004).

DATA COLLECTION AND ANALYSIS

Data were collected over 4.5 weeks through participant observation and open-ended interviews, allowing research to be guided by cultural concepts. Follow-up interviews were not conducted due to time constraints. Cultural informants and AIDS-based organizations and agencies provided feedback and assistance to ensure accurate data interpretation. Participant observations and informal discussions were recorded by note taking in a daily diary.

Interviews

A semi-structured questionnaire consisting of nine broad, open-ended questions guided interviews. Key cultural informants provided feedback on the interview approach, question design, and English syntax used in questions. Three pilot interviews were conducted in Nyanja with translation assistance, before the researcher decided to conduct interviews on a one-on-one basis in English to increase privacy, confidentiality, and control for how questions were asked and interpreted. It is critical to note that the interview guide in ethnographic research is almost never final; rather, each key informant is approached as an individual within her own immediate context. All interviews were conducted in a safe and private location and tape recorded as per consent.

Participants considering participation were provided the equivalent of $2 in the local currency, amounting to the cost of two local meals. This incentive was approved by cultural informants as an appropriate sum that was not so great that women would feel coerced to participate. It was clarified with women that compensation for considering the interview was theirs to keep, and they were not obliged to consent to or participate in the research.

Participant Observation

The researcher lived primarily with a local Zambian female-headed household, the residents of which were key cultural informants. She also resided part-time on hospice grounds, with patients and staff acting as key cultural informants. Participant observation occurred in both locations. At the hospice, observation took place during volunteer work, support group meetings, home care visits, and discussions and interactions with patients and staff. Away from the hospice, observation was conducted at social gatherings, meals, meetings with organizations, and walking or traveling daily on local buses.

Limitations

Given that the interviews were not conducted in the local languages, the depth and comprehensiveness of the data may be constrained. To maximize the ability of the researcher to conduct her own interviews, cultural informants and research participants with relatively high English proficiency were selected for the study, which resulted in a higher than average education level among participants. Also, the time allocated for data collection was sufficient to complete the research, but prevented follow-up interviews with the nine interviewees.

Data Analysis

Nine participant interviews were analyzed, at which point data saturation was reached. Using de Chesnay's (2005) qualitative data analysis format, transcripts and notes were confidentially coded for emerging categories, themes, and concepts. Coded and interpreted data were shared with cultural informants for further analysis and feedback. The data were not shared with the participants due to the short time frame and challenges in contacting and locating participants before the study ended. Triangulation through interviews, observations, and feedback from key informants helped ensure the accuracy of procedures and findings. Careful field notes were kept and reviewed regularly.

FINDINGS

Four major concepts emerged from interviews with the nine participants on the topic of support: uncertainty, encouragement, staying with HIV, and free mind.

Uncertainty

Uncertainty emerged as an ever-present threat and source of hope for women both before and after knowing their HIV status. Uncertainty is the constant awareness that one's situation can change rapidly and unexpectedly at any moment. In the case of the Zambian women, it complicated their struggle to secure food, housing, medical care, income, children's education, and children's futures. Women described uncertainty in their ability to control interactions with men, including husbands, and in predicting reactions to their HIV status. Institutional uncertainty was acknowledged in the form of corruption and unreliable service sectors. Although uncertainty appeared to afford hope that a situation could improve unexpectedly, it was most often described as contributing to loss, fear, and grief.

Loss was a significant component of uncertainty, including lost husbands, children, siblings, relationships, jobs, health and physical abilities, normalcy, and the will to live. The desire to prevent more loss was expressed by many participants, and past losses were described as painful reminders of needs no longer met. One woman described losing family members, and a critical support source, due to HIV:

> There are a number lost. All my elder brothers, they are all gone. Then my immediate brothers, they are all gone . . . I'm missing my sisters . . . The one who was so close to me, she was fond of me. When I saw her sick, I didn't want her to be sick. Even when she died, even now, because she used to go to South Africa, most of the time when I see these trucks I think, "Maybe she's coming." And I forget that she's dead, she's gone for good. So now I'm lonely. She used to encourage me. We used to play together most of the time. Whatever we used to do, she was there next to me.

Encouragement

Encouragement was described as an expression of concern, providing assurance that women's lives were valued and worth living. It was seen as an expression of faith that women could and should continue forward. Encouragement was derived from the physical presence of others, physical acts of support such as assistance during illness, supportive words, and material and financial gifts and loans. Self-encouragement was derived from personal resolve, prayer, faith, a connection with God, and a sense of purpose. Encouragement assisted women to seek information about their HIV status, and it reinforced their ability to stay with HIV.

Encouragement to Determine One's HIV Status

Encouragement to go for HIV testing was reported to be a factor influencing the decision to get tested. This type of support was provided through education about HIV symptoms and risk factors, and it included assurance that women would be supported or have a future if found to be HIV positive. Despite numerous factors influencing the decision to seek out HIV testing, the majority of women ultimately credited the encouragement of healthcare providers, who had informed them about symptoms and risks. Assurances were provided through free antiretroviral medications, an expanding service sector assisting those with HIV/AIDS, and a perceived decrease in stigma.

One woman shared her perception on the evolving social and medical context surrounding HIV/AIDS:

> That time when you used to hear about HIV/AIDS, [people] used to fear. We had that fear. You say, "Hah! I have to die" and you have to keep it to yourself. It's not like the way it is now . . . now it's open. A number of people, they want to help. . . Now I say, I do think if . . . free drugs were there that time when my brothers and sisters were sick, I think this time, they were going to be well . . . they were going to be there, they were going to be helped.

Encouragement to Stay with HIV

Encouragement was reported to contribute to self-acceptance of HIV-positive status, while assisting women to continue "staying with HIV" amid uncertainty, illness, pain, depression, and other daily struggles. Encouragement by family members was provided through physical, emotional, material, and financial support. Encouragement was also gained through faith, personal beliefs, supportive gestures, organizations, and supportive policies assisting women to seek testing, access treatment, learn about HIV, accept their status, implement self-care behaviors, and maintain hope and belief in their future. Support groups were highly valued sources of encouragement, as they focused on teaching women how to live with HIV, while providing a forum to share experiences and escape feelings of isolation or loneliness. One woman stated:

> When I joined the support group, life for me changed because I also receive encouragement from my fellow friends. When we meet together, you can see that we are not the only one going through it, this HIV virus—there are many. So, we encourage each other.

Women valued the encouragement during illness, particularly not being left alone with their thoughts, and being assisted to eat, walk, take medications, and maintain hygiene. Encouragement was also important to continue accessing health care and treatment despite ongoing challenges such as paying for transportation and enduring physical pain or side effects. One woman described the encouragement her father provided:

> My father encouraged me, in fact . . . when I started taking my drugs, I informed dad about it . . . Then he said, "Okay, it's okay. Look, continue. Maybe . . . your life will be prolonged. It's not you alone; there are a number of people . . . no, as long as you are well, it's okay. Because you'll continue doing things on your own . . . If you get better, it's better you do things—what you can manage, you'll be able to do . . . you'll be helping your children also. You'll raise up those children, you'll see that to the time when they grow up, and then when they will be married also."

Staying with HIV

"Staying with HIV" is the central concept emerging from this study. This term was used by participants to describe the process of living with HIV, with the understanding that the virus had moved permanently into their lives. This process began after women accepted their status, and involved piecing together support, normalizing life with HIV, and finding purpose.

Piecing Together Support

This process of seeking and accessing various resources promoted daily survival and helped women prevent or manage HIV-related complications. It occurred through the piecing together of financial, nutritional, shelter, physical, medical, educational, decisional, social, emotional, and spiritual/religious support. Women highlighted the necessity of being "open" to receiving support. They expressed gratitude for support received, yet felt frustration over their ongoing struggle and inability to provide for themselves. Many felt resented, and alluded to guilt or shame, for having to ask for help.

Although anyone could be a potential support, the sources identified by the interviewees are shown in **Table 19–2**. These resources were mentioned during the open interview process, rather than being derived from a comprehensive survey of support sources.

Short-term or temporary support came in the form of monetary or nutritional gifts and loans from family, friends, and churches; physical support during acute illness from family and healthcare providers; and "piece work" such as a one-day or week-long job. Long-term or ongoing support came from educational resources improving understanding of HIV, which consequently informed women's decisions and actions. Support groups, counselors, friends, and healthcare providers were identified as education sources:

> I get advice from the doctors; they teach us to look after ourselves carefully, to maintain a good diet. It's something that was difficult to know, to really know that a good diet would be helping someone [with HIV] be strong. We always said, "Since I get a low salary, I just buy whatever I buy, as long as the days are going."

Table 19–2 Identified Sources of Support

Support Sources ***(Number of Categories Identified as Support for)***	**Education/ Information**	**Emotional**	**Decisional**	**Social**	**Physical**	**Medical**	**Nutritional**	**Financial**	**Spiritual/ Religious**	**Shelter**
Family (9)	x	x	x	x	x	x	x	x		x
Church/congregation (7)		x		x	x		x	x	x	x
Friends (7)	x	x	x	x	x		x	x		
Spouse (7)	x		x	x		x	x	x		x
Support groups (6)	x	x	x	x			x		x	
Counselors (5)	x	x	x			x			x	
God/prayer (5)		x	x		x	x			x	
Income-generation (5)				x		x	x	x		x
Healing/recovery (4)	x	x	x						x	
Healthcare providers (4)	x		x		x	x				
Others with HIV (4)	x	x	x	x						
Children (3)		x		x	x					
Antiretroviral agents/ medicine (2)					x	x				
Media (1)	x									

> But this time I've learned that even some other foods do help . . . even keeping the home clean, even if that means [spending] money.

Family members were identified as sources of ongoing support, providing shared housing, transportation, money for medicines, food, and emotional comfort. Due to the financial struggle faced by families, their support was often described as erratic. As one woman shared, "I've got a sister who I stay with. When they told me to buy medicine, she buys medicine. Sometimes she can manage, sometimes she cannot . . . when she doesn't have money, I don't buy the medicine."

Dependence on others was reported to be necessary due to the difficulty in securing employment, attributed to HIV-related physical limitations, gender, or a lack of opportunity. All women pieced together informal work, although many were currently unable to work due to physical limitations. "Piece work" was heavily relied on, and described as often physically demanding activities such as cleaning; selling vegetables, fish, or beer; or transactional sex. One woman offered a reflection on trying to make ends meet:

> You wake up around 4 [A.M.] and you know that the following day you don't have anything [food] to give the children. You just start thinking, "What am I going to do?" Sometimes poverty, it can lead you into something bad. You plan of something which is not good, at the end of the day, you regret . . . for example, just a man. Yeah, a man asks you maybe to sleep with him, because here, women know that automatically if you sleep with a man, at the end of it, he will give you something . . . and that something is not that you are going to please yourself. Maybe you've got a family, you've got the children, you're a single parent. When you get that little money, you can buy something for the children at home.

There was consensus that the process of piecing together support was ongoing and always difficult. One woman stated, "It's a strange type of life. It's hard, but we have to continue in it; there's nothing else we can do." The mental and emotional strength to continue was attributed to prayer, social interactions, and support groups. All of the women identified God as a major source of support, providing them with hope and working through others to help them. Reflecting on it all, one woman stated, "Sometimes we're just surviving by God's grace."

Normalizing Life with HIV

Despite an ongoing struggle to survive and awareness that their life was now different than others' lives, the women in the study described a process of normalizing life with HIV. This process reportedly began after acceptance of their HIV status, and it evolved through connections with other HIV-positive persons.

Women described support groups as a setting where they shared the experiences and hardships of living with HIV, asked questions, and gained reassurance that they did not face HIV alone. While talking about her HIV support group, one woman stated, "It's a life that I've found [that is] something normal. Even though you are HIV positive, you are just like any other person; it's only that you are having the virus in your body."

Disclosure was also identified as an indirect component of normalizing life with HIV, as isolation and loneliness were reportedly exacerbated by hiding HIV status. Eight of the nine women interviewed eventually chose to disclose their status to important people in their lives. Some disclosed this information on the same day they received test results, whereas others waited two to three years to share their status. One woman was still unable to tell her family, despite the fact they were not identified as a source of support, for fear of being poisoned or otherwise harmed. Overall, disclosure was a positive experience resulting in increased support and understanding:

> I felt isolated by then. It was like I was living in another world. You know when you are keeping something from people, it's like you're in another world. . . . people don't really know who you are. But as for now, I don't really feel that way because I told them the secret that I have. You know when you are keeping something, it's like carrying a burden of which you don't even want anyone to know. But since now everyone knows, even when I get sick they know, "Oh, it's this [HIV]."

Finding Purpose

"Staying with HIV" was also described as a process of finding purpose and meaning in life despite having an HIV-positive status. Purpose was derived from the desire to stay alive to ensure the future of children. It was also obtained from contributing in some way to the well-being of others. The majority of women reported that HIV/AIDS outreach work provided purpose and gave their lives meaning. One woman stated:

> In my life I really wanted to help people who are sick . . . that's the kind of life I really like to lead. So for me to find myself here at the hospice, it's really a pleasure. I visit the people that are sick. I help them in any way they want me to help. So I think I'm trying to fulfill what I wanted.

Many of the women, whose physical deterioration had reversed following treatment, viewed themselves as proof to others that there is life after an HIV diagnosis. Community members reached out to them as HIV experts who could assist others potentially suffering from HIV. A number of the women also felt that HIV had taught them and their families a great deal. As one woman stated:

> I think it was for a purpose that I had to be HIV positive—so that I should know what other people are really going through. Ever since I knew that, I've come to learn a lot . . . it also helped my family to really know what's happening to some people, to really understand some diseases. That's a very good experience.

Finally, most women were assured through their belief in God that there was purpose in their disease status. One woman reflected, "I'm still around, maybe for a purpose. God preserved my life so that I can teach others also."

Free Mind

A free mind was desired by all women, and was broadly defined as freedom from worry and protection from uncertainty. Worry was attributed to lack of security and uncertainty over food and nutrition, finances, the future of their children, stable shelter, health, and life expectancy. A free mind was achieved in the short term through discovering their HIV status, understanding the ongoing illnesses suffered, having food for tomorrow, not being left alone during illness, getting treatment, or engaging in prayer. In the long term, a free mind was thought to be acquired through stability (stable finances, nutrition, shelter, and physical health), self-sufficiency (freedom from dependency through employment and physical health), and the knowledge that children's futures were secure (through a designated care provider to prevent orphanhood and ensure that children could complete their education).

Stability

Stability was described as the acquisition of financial security, food security, permanent housing, and the knowledge that a woman could manage her health so as to remain functional and productive. It was also identified as the ability to go to sleep at night without worrying about tomorrow—for example, whether the woman could pay school fees or feed her children.

Self-sufficiency

Although not seen as necessary to achieve stability (which could be provided by others), self-sufficiency was viewed as financial independence resulting in overall empowerment and freedom from dependency on others. Despite being in a stable relationship, one woman stated, "All I want is a job, so that I should take 100% responsibility for myself." Women largely envisioned opening their own business as the means to acquire and maintain their financial independence through income-generating activities, thereby allowing them to single-handedly maintain stability and secure the future of their children. One woman stated, "If I could create something, I can do business. Here if I can have a shop, I can do business." Each woman reported that getting a business started required up-front resources she could not secure.

Securing a Future for One's Children

The ability to secure their children's future was a long-term goal for the eight women who had living children. Although stability and self-sufficiency enabled women to create a stable future for children, if the women were to die before seeing children into adulthood, this responsibility was seen as falling to others.

All women felt that a permanent house to leave to children would protect them, particularly from a future on the street. Only one woman had a secure house, which she inherited from her deceased husband. All women felt that their children were too young to be on their own or caring for one another (children ranged in age from 2 to 19 years), but they agreed that if necessary, children could manage if they had secure housing. One woman stated:

> I must have a house. But whatever comes, if it's my death, those children must stay good, they should not suffer, they must be in one place . . . I'm staying with my mother, and that house of my mother is for my family. So, if I die, those children, they'll never keep them.

All women with living children also valued the education of their children, citing constant concerns over the struggle to pay school fees or assurances that future caregivers would continue to educate orphaned children. Education was described by many as a way to ensure their children had a successful future, especially female children.

DISCUSSION

Among the four emergent concepts (uncertainty, encouragement, staying with HIV, and free mind), the concept of staying with HIV was central to the findings, and imbued in each of the other concepts: It must proceed on a base of uncertainty, it is strengthened and fostered by encouragement, and it allows the pursuit of a free mind. The interrelationship of these concepts is illustrated in **Figure 19–1**.

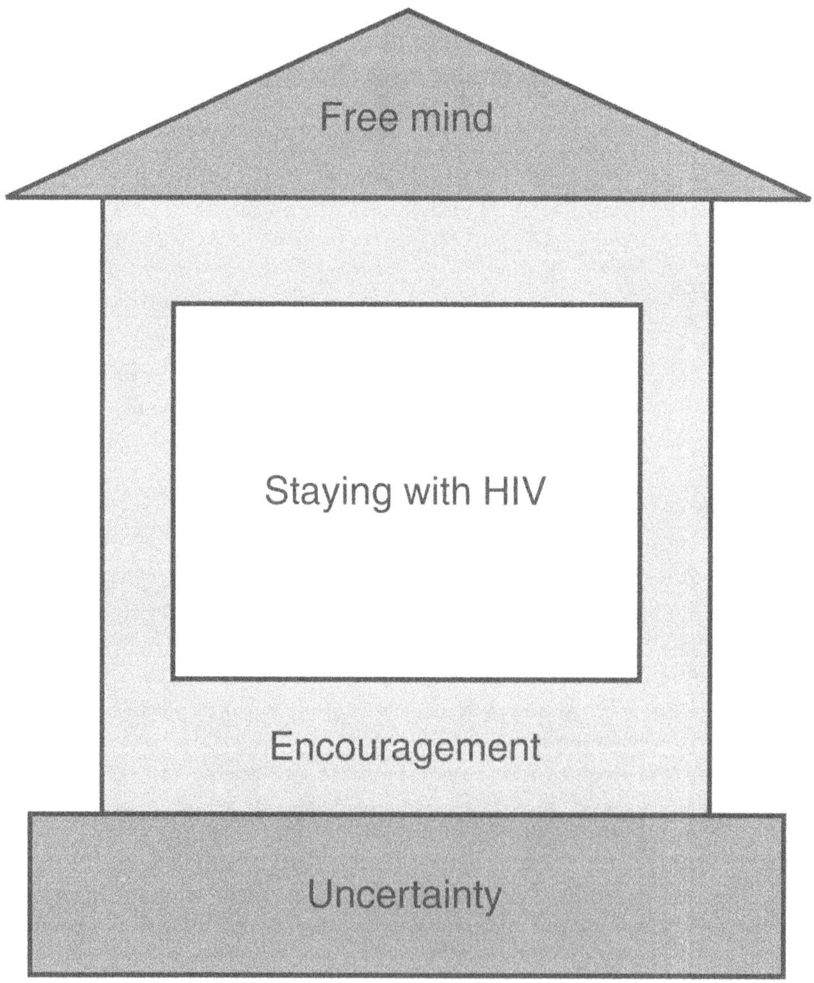

Figure 19–1 Structural components of staying with HIV.

Staying with HIV assumes the central position in the model. This concept represents the point at which women acknowledged and accepted that HIV had moved permanently into their lives (as represented in the model by a house or hut). For the women interviewed, it consisted of piecing together supports, normalizing life with HIV, and finding purpose in their illness. Consistent with the findings of Plattner and Meiring (2006), the Zambian study found acceptance of HIV status to be a factor contributing to overall well-being, as was the ability to find meaning in one's illness. It is important to note that the ability of women to stay with HIV was not realized in social isolation, but rather was greatly bolstered through internal as well as external encouragement.

"Encouragement" was an umbrella term used by women to describe the many internal and external supports that were both provided to and accessed by them. It contributed to the discovery and acceptance of their own HIV status, and it reinforced the process of staying with HIV and maintaining hope and a vision for the future. Whether attained actively or passively, encouragement appeared critical to fostering resiliency and resourcefulness, strengthening the willpower of women to continue staying with HIV despite the uncertainty that permeated their lives and their sometimes intense emotional and physical suffering.

Although a free mind is desirable to the majority of humanity, the free mind described and sought by participants in this study was not excessive in expectation, but was clearly challenging in the face of widespread poverty, gender inequality, and limited national or community infrastructure to aid in its realization. In a climate of uncertainty, there is wisdom in the desire to achieve self-sufficiency. Yet vehicles must be identified or expanded to boost women's ability to become self-sufficient.

CONCLUSION

This study looked at the role and experience of support among HIV-positive Zambian women. It discovered an array of support needs, and delineated a complicated interrelationship between support, culture, and poverty among women living with HIV. Among the women interviewed, "staying with HIV" emerged as a dynamic process that was key to survival, personal knowledge, gaining a sense of normalcy, and deriving meaning from life with HIV. To promote and strengthen the process of staying with HIV, the following conclusions are offered:

1. *The most acutely needed form of support is assistance to achieve self-sufficiency.* Women were hard-pressed to meet their daily needs and were unable to plan ahead for their future needs. They lacked control over the timing, type, quantity, and quality of support provided from any given source. Despite the high value placed on any existing support, they were limited in their reliability and capacity to assist themselves and others.

   Economic empowerment leading to self-sufficiency has been found to be a crucial component in enabling women to meet subsistence needs, provide for families, and acquire greater control over their lives and bodies (MANET, 2003; Pronyk et al., 2005; Sachs, 2005; SEF/RADAR, 2005).

2. *Encouragement can help promote earlier utilization of voluntary counseling and testing services (VCT) and ultimately decrease morbidity and mortality.* It is not news that barriers to testing still exist despite national policy supporting free testing and treatment. Women choosing to know their HIV status still reside in an environment that is perceived to be saturated with fear and stigma surrounding HIV (Guay et al., 1999; Maman, Mbwambo, Hogan, Kilonzo, & Sweat, 2001).

   In this study, the majority of women attributed their decision to be tested for HIV to encouragement and teachings received from healthcare providers. Most women did not discuss HIV or their plan to test with family or friends before their diagnosis, and most did not receive these parties' encouragement to seek testing. Due to the importance of emotional and decisional support from partners, family, and friends, their encouragement in directing women to seek testing is critical and must be promoted (Guay et al., 1999; Thabo, 2006).

   Most participants waited to undergo testing until they experienced the death of a husband or multiple acute or chronic illnesses. Encouragement to seek earlier testing can help decrease the suffering and financial toll inflicted by HIV-related illnesses, possibly prompting life-saving testing of partners or children, or preventing mother-to-child transmission.

3. *Fostering a sense of normalcy among HIV-positive women is necessary for well-being.* Most women interviewed highlighted stories about experiencing a sense of normalcy, times they did not feel alone in their struggle with HIV, or occasions when they did not feel "different" than others. This phenomenon was attributed to the creation and maintenance of relationships with other HIV-positive individuals, particularly within support groups providing ongoing support and counseling (Ciambrone, 2002; Krabbendam, Kuijper, Wolffers, & Drew, 1998).

4. *Finding purpose in life with HIV contributes significantly to meaning and self-worth.* Women appeared to derive significant purpose and meaning from their illness, which was attributed to a deepened understanding of suffering as well as the realization that they could help prevent HIV or minimize suffering in others. Women participated in community outreach and education on HIV prevention, education, and promotion of testing/VCT. Many women also volunteered to assist others during illnesses or death. The roles that most of the women played in their own communities as HIV outreach workers were crucial not only for their own sense of purpose and fulfillment, but had the added benefit of addressing stigma and increasing awareness within families and communities.

   This study supported the conclusions of Plattner and Meiring (2006), who found that belief in something greater than oneself contributes to of hope and meaning. Among these Zambian women living with HIV, this belief ultimately assisted them in going forward in life with both purpose and a vision of the future.

RECOMMENDATIONS FOR HEALTHCARE AND SERVICE PROVIDERS

Strengthen Support Groups

Support groups are a critical source of support that must be bolstered with greater informational, material, and financial resources to teach women about HIV and ways to live successfully with the virus, while providing a supportive setting that helps create a sense of normalcy. Support groups also have the potential to assist women in accessing other resources, finding purpose in their illness through organized outreach work, and potentially contributing to self-sufficiency by serving as a vehicle for microcredit, cooperative, or reimbursement ventures.

Increase Encouragement from Healthcare Providers

Encouragement from healthcare providers was effective when women were educated about HIV, symptoms, risks, treatment options, self-care, and medications. All women should be informed about the benefit of seeking early versus late testing, and those who are HIV positive should be continually educated about HIV and areas where they may be able to self-advocate (e.g., requesting pain medications, having company during illness, educating care providers or families, instituting behavior changes). Although women may not immediately seek VCT, encouragement empowers them with the knowledge necessary to recognize and act on symptoms and risks.

Promote and Provide Incentives for HIV-Positive Women to Engage in Community Outreach Work

Community outreach by these HIV-positive women provided a sense of purpose, and was often viewed as a personal or religious calling. By holding up their lives as examples for others, they increased community understanding of HIV, highlighted the needs of those infected, and demonstrated the prolonged and productive life possible when testing and treatment are sought in a timely manner. Incentives to engage in this work could foster the continuation of valuable outreach work, thereby increasing community awareness of HIV while simultaneously contributing to individual self-sufficiency. Such incentives might include financial, nutritional, or material reimbursement. Support groups offer a structure that can and is being utilized to provide such incentives.

CALL FOR FURTHER RESEARCH

This study serves as an initial investigation using a compressed ethnographic design. Further research is necessary to examine the role of support among women living with HIV/AIDS in Zambia from a variety of angles and at a deeper level. This study cannot be considered representative, as all participants were accessing medical services and 78% belonged to a support group. The median education level of study participants (10 years) was also higher than the national average for women in Zambia (6.6 years). These differences were likely the result of the decision to recruit women who were conversationally fluent in English and were accessing hospice services. Also, the participants' median age (41.3 years) was higher than that of most Zambian women affected by HIV/AIDS (30 to 34 years) (UNGASS, 2005). Future studies should be conducted with HIV-positive women from various educational levels and age ranges. Ideally, this study would be repeated in a rural location and an urban locale.

ACKNOWLEDGMENTS

Gratitude and deep appreciation are extended to the hospice counselor and the nine women who participated in this study. Special thanks must be given to Dr. Mary de Chesnay, an inspiring professor and exceptional research chair, and Dr. Barbara Anderson, the research committee member whose reviews and edits were invaluable in writing this study. A deeply personal "thank you" must also be expressed for the support and mentorship of Dr. Peter Kareiva, and the support and encouragement of Carol and Katy Mumba, Auntie Lillian, Michele Brommelsiek, Linda Lovick, Juan Sheenan, Leonard Haamunga, Sr. Stanislawa, Ida Mukuka, Malele Dodia, Thomas Kapakala, Beene, Karolina Sczpakowska, Mulenga Muleba, and Janelle Tuttle.

WWW

For a full suite of assignments and additional learning activities, use the access code located in the front of your book to visit this exclusive website: http://go.jblearning.com/dechesnay. If you do not have an access code, you can obtain one at the site.

REFERENCES

Barnett, T., & Whiteside, A. (2002). *AIDS in the twenty-first century: Disease and globalization.* New York: Palgrave Macmillan.

Chaava, T. (1990). Approaches to HIV counseling in a Zambian rural community. *AIDS Care, 2*(1), 81–87.

Ciambrone, D. (2002). Informal networks among women with HIV/AIDS: Present support and future prospects. *Qualitative Health Research, 12*(7), 876–896.

de Chesnay, M. (2005). "Can't keep me down": Life histories of successful African Americans. In M. de Chesnay (Ed.), *Caring for the vulnerable: Perspectives in nursing theory, practice and research* (pp. 221–231). Sudbury, MA: Jones and Bartlett.

Dyson, T. (2003). HIV/AIDS and urbanization. *Population & Development Review, 29*(3), 427–442.

Eisenberg, N. I., Kemeny, M. E., & Wyatt, G. E. (2003). Psychological inhibition and CD4 T-cell levels in HIV-seropositive women. *Journal of Psychosomatic Research, 54*(3), 213–224.

Guay, L., Musoke, P., Fleming, T., Bagenda, D., Allen, M., Nakabiito, C., . . . Jackson, J. B. (1999). Intrapartum and neonatal single dose nevirapine compared with zidouvodin for prevention of mother-to-child transmission of HIV-1 in Kampala, Uganda: HIVNET 012 randomized trial. *Lancet, 354*(9181), 795–802.

Harding, R., Stewart, K., Marconi, K., O'Neill, J. F., & Higginson, I. J. (2003). Current HIV/AIDS end-of-life care in sub-Saharan Africa: A survey of models, services, challenges, and priorities. *BMC Public Health, 3*(33), 1–6.

Hughes, J., Jelsma, J., Maclean, E., Darder, M., & Tinise, X. (2004). The health-related quality of life of people living with HIV/AIDS. *Disability and Rehabilitation, 26*(6), 371–376.

Hunter, M. (2007). The changing political economy of sex in South Africa: The significance of unemployment and inequalities to the scale of the AIDS pandemic. *Social Science & Medicine, 64*, 689–700.

Kayawe, I., Kelly, M., & Baggaley, R. (1998). HIV counseling and testing. *World Health, 51*(6), 12–13.

Keogh, P., Allen, S., Almedal, C., & Temahagili, B. (1994). The social impact of HIV infection on women in Kigali, Rwanda: A prospective study. *Social Science & Medicine 38*(8), 1047–1053.

Krabbendam, A., Kuijper, B., Wolffers, I., & Drew, R. (1998). The impact of counseling on HIV-positive women in Zimbabwe. *AIDS Care, 10*(suppl 1), S25–S37.

Kunda, M. (2004). Illegal compounds difficult to provide services-council. *LRF News, 48.* Retrieved January 9, 2007, from http://www.lrf.org.zm/Newsletter/january2004/features.html

Lawson, A. L. (1999). Women and AIDS in Africa: Sociocultural dimensions of the HIV/AIDS epidemic. *International Social Science Journal, 51*(3), 391–400.

LeCompte, M. D., & Schensul, J. J. (1999). *Designing and conducting ethnographic research: Ethnographer's toolkit, v.1.* Walnut Creek, CA: AltaMira Press.

Maman, S., Mbwambo, J., Hogan, N. M., Kilonzo, G. P., & Sweat, M. (2001). Women's barriers to HIV-1 testing and disclosure: Challenges for HIV-1 voluntary counseling and testing. *AIDS Care, 13*(5), 595–603.

MANET. (2003). *Voices for equality and dignity: Qualitative research on stigma and discrimination issues as they affect PLWHA in Malawi.* Lilongwe, Malawi: Author.

Moore, H., & Vaughan, M. (1994). *Cutting down trees: Gender, nutrition, and agricultural change in the northern province of Zambia, 1890–1990.* Portsmouth, NH/London: Heinemann/Currey.

Niehaus, I. (1994). Disharmonious spouses and harmonious siblings: Conceptualising household formation among urban residents in QwaQwa. *African Studies, 53*(1), 115–135.

Panos Institute & UNICEF. (2001). *Stigma, HIV/AIDS and prevention of mother-to-child transmission: A pilot study in Zambia, India, Ukraine and Burkina Faso.* London: Authors.

Plattner, I. E., & Meiring, N. (2006) Living with HIV: The psychological relevance of meaning making. *AIDS Care, 18*(3), 241–245.

Pronyk, P., Kim, J., Hargreaves, M., Makhubele, M., Morison, L., Watts, C., & Porter, J. (2005). Microfinance and HIV prevention: Emerging lessons from rural South Africa. *Small Enterprise Development, 16*(3), 26–38.

Sachs, J. (2005). *The end of poverty: How we can make it happen in our lifetime.* London: Penguin.

SEF/RADAR. (2005). The IMAGE Intervention. Retrieved February 15, 2007, from http://www.lshtm.ac.uk/genderviolence/reports/imagebrochforweb.pdf

Steinberg, M., Johnson, S., Schierhout, G., Ndegwa, D., Hall, K., & Russell, B. (2002). Hitting home: How households cope with the impact of the HIV/AIDS epidemic. A survey of households affected by HIV/AIDS in South Africa. Report compiled for the Henry J. Kaiser Family Foundation and the Health Systems Trust. Retrieved from www.hst.org.za/uploads/files/hittinghome.pdf

Swindells, S., Mohr, J., Justis, J. C., Berman, S., Squier, C., Wagener, M. M., & Singh, N. (1999). Quality of life in patients with human immunodeficiency virus infection: Impact of social support, coping style and hopelessness. *International Journal of STD and AIDS, 10*(6), 383–391.

Thabo, T. F. (2006) Social and psychological factors associated with willingness to test for HIV infection among young people in Botswana. *AIDS Care, 18*(3), 201–207.

UNAIDS. (2004). *2004 Report on the global AIDS epidemic.* Geneva, Switzerland: Author.

UNAIDS, UNFPA, & UNIFEM. (2004). *Women and HIV/AIDS: Confronting the crisis.* Geneva, Switzerland: UNAIDS.

UNDP. (2005). *Human development report 2005.* New York: Author.

UNFPA. (2006). *Sexual and reproductive health needs of women and adolescent girls living with HIV: Research report on qualitative findings from Brazil, Ethiopia, and the Ukraine.* New York: EngenderHealth/UNFPA.

United Nations General Assembly Special Session on HIV/AIDS (UNGASS). (2005). *Follow-up to the Declaration of Commitment on HIV/AIDS: 2005 Zambia Country Report.*

Uys, L. R. (2003). Aspects of the care of people with HIV/AIDS in South Africa. *Public Health Nursing, 20*(4), 271–280.

World Bank. (2005). *Zambia poverty and vulnerability assessment* (Report No. 32573). Human Development Division, Africa Region.

CHAPTER 20

Health Systems and Human Resources for Health: New Dimensions in Global Health Nursing

Capt. Patricia L. Riley

Objectives

At the end of this chapter, the reader will be able to

1. Discuss the need for a shift in thinking globally instead of nationally about health care.
2. Review issues related to changes in health systems in developing countries.
3. Identify key components of a plan for providing health services in low-income countries.

WWW

OVERVIEW

This chapter, which pertains to vulnerable populations in global settings, focuses on *health systems* and *human resources for health* (HRH)—topics that global research, policies, and programs are now embracing. Today's requirements for the global nurse practitioner necessitate that individuals have skills that go beyond competency in the provision of health services or sound management of healthcare programs and services. In addition to these abilities, relevant engagement in global health requires an understanding of the components making up a health system, as well as analytic capabilities for assessing, designing, and evaluating appropriate interventions. Because nearly every country—especially those designated as low-income countries—is experiencing a critical shortage of healthcare providers, competency in global nursing necessitates technical abilities that contribute to the HRH knowledge base, in addition to aptitude in interdisciplinary collaboration and communication, which are essential for working with a diverse range of national stakeholders in a variety of settings (Institute of Medicine [IOM], 2010b; Joint Learning Initiative, 2004; Reich, Takeni, Roberts, & Hsiao, 2008).

Over the past 30 years, there have been tremendous shifts and advancements in global health policies and initiatives. The past decade has introduced new paradigms that have revolutionized the way in which foreign assistance is provided. Governments are no longer the sole purveyors of health interventions. New players entering the arena include multilateral agencies (e.g., the World Bank), public–private partnerships (e.g., the Global Fund to Fight AIDS, Tuberculosis and Malaria), bilateral governmental initiatives (e.g., the U.S. President's Emergency Plan for AIDS Relief [PEPFAR]), the private sector (e.g., the Bill and Melinda Gates Foundation), and philanthropic trusts (e.g., the Wellcome Trust). Never before have there been so many global health initiatives supported with significant resources by such a wide array of donors. PEPFAR, which was reauthorized by the U.S. Congress in 2008, provides as much as $48 billion over a five-year period for addressing global HIV/AIDS, malaria and tuberculosis efforts (Henry J. Kaiser Family Foundation, 2008); the Obama administration's more recent Global Health Initiative (GHI) has increased this investment to $63 billion over the next six years. GHI's newer features include partnership frameworks between the U.S. government and national ministries of health that are focused on transitioning U.S. global assistance to local ownership and sustainable investment ("Implementation of the Global Health Initiative Consultation Document," 2010).

Another important factor influencing global health is the World Health Organization's (WHO) Millennium Declaration and its corresponding eight time-bound goals, known as the Millennium Development Goals (MDGs), which have brought increased attention to the health needs of the world's most vulnerable populations (WHO, 2005). The eight MDGs encompass overall themes for development such as poverty eradication, access to primary education, and promoting gender equality and the empowerment of women (**Table 20–1**). They also include specific health targets and related metrics regarding child and maternal mortality and reduction of HIV/AIDS, malaria, and tuberculosis. Benchmarks for environmental sustainability and global partnerships represent MDG 7 and MDG 8, respectively (WHO, 2005).

Each of these eight health targets is matched with corresponding health indicators, which serve as guideposts for global organizations, donors, and stakeholders alike, and provide an overarching framework for measuring progress with regard to commonly agreed-upon global priorities (WHO, 2005). Since the launch of this worldwide effort, the MDGs have garnered acceptance among rich and poor countries alike. Their ambitious timeline—targeted for attainment by the year 2015—has created momentum, if not a sense of urgency within the field of global health (Travis et al., 2004; WHO Maximizing Positive Synergies Collaborative Group, 2009). Increasingly, however, health systems constraints within low-income countries are seen as hindering attainment of the MDGs (Fryatt, Mills, & Nordstrom, 2010; Task Force on Health Systems Research, 2004; Travis et al., 2004). As noted in a WHO (2004b) report, "In countries with a high burden of HIV/AIDS, systems are often degraded and dysfunctional because of a combination of underfunding and weak governance. HIV/AIDS places additional burdens on these weakened health systems."

More specifically, inadequate infrastructure for providing service delivery, shortages of trained health workers, interruptions in the procurement and supply of health products, and poor governance—all elements of a dysfunctional health system—not only obstruct the global health assistance, but become a systematic problem unto itself (Hill, Mansoor, & Claudio, 2010; WHO Maximizing Positive Synergies Collaborative Group, 2009). Difficulty in producing reliable

Table 20–1 Health in the Millennium Development Goals

	Health Targets	Health Indicators
Goal 1: Eradicate extreme poverty and hunger		
Target 1	Halve, between 1990 and 2015, the proportion of people whose income is less than one dollar a day	
Target 2	Halve, between 1990 and 2015, the proportion of people who suffer from hunger	4. Prevalence of underweight children under five years of age 5. Proportion of population below minimum level of dietary energy consumption
Goal 2: Achieve universal primary education		
Target 3	Ensure that, by 2015, children everywhere, boys and girls alike, will be able to complete a full course of primary schooling	
Goal 3: Promote gender equality and empower women		
Target 4	Eliminate gender disparity in primary and secondary education, preferably by 2005, and at all levels of education no later than 2015	
Goal 4: Reduce child morality		
Target 5	Reduce by two-thirds, between 1990 and 2015, the under-five mortality rate	13. Under-five mortality rate 14. infant mortality rate 15. Proportion of one-year-old children immunized against measles
Goal 5: Improve maternal health		
Target 6	Reduce by three-quarters, between 1990 and 2015, the maternal mortality ratio	16. Material mortality ratio 17. Proportion of births attended by skilled health personnel
Goal 6: Combat HIV/AIDS, malaria and other diseases		
Target 7	Have halted by 2015 and begun to reverse the spread of HIV/AIDS	18. HIV prevalence among pregnant women and 15–24 years 19. Condom use rate of the contraceptive prevalence rate 20. Ratio of school attendance of orphans to school attendance of non-orphans and 10-14 years
Target 8	Have halted by 2015 and begun to reverse the incidence of malaria and other major diseases	21. Prevalence and death rates associated with malaria 22. Proportion of population is malaria-risk areas using effective malaria prevention and treatment measures

Continued

Table 20–1 Continued

		23. Prevalence and death rates associated with tuberculosis 24. Proportion of tuberculosis cases detected and cured under DOTS (Directly Observed Treatment Short-course)
Goal 7: Ensure environmental sustainability		
Target 9	Integrate the principles of sustainable development into country policies and programmes and reverse the loss of environmental resources	29. Proportion of population using solid fuels
Target 10	Halve by 2015 the proportion of people without sustainable access to safe drinking-water and sanitation	30. Proportion of population with sustainable access to an imported water source, urban and rural
Target 11	By 2020 to have achieved a significant improvement in the lives of a least 100 million slum dwellers	31. Proportion of population with access to improved sanitation, urban and rural
Goal 8: Develop a global partnership for development		
Target 12	Develop further an open, rule-based, predictable, non-discriminatory trading and financial system	
Target 13	Address the special needs of the least developed countries	
Target 14	Address the special needs of landlocked countries and small island developing states	
Target 15	Deal comprehensively with the debt problems of developing countries through national and international measures in order to make debt sustainable in the long term	
Target 16	In cooperation with developing countries, develop and implement strategies for decent and productive work for youth	
Target 17	In cooperation with pharmaceutical companies, provide access to affordable essential drugs in developing countries	46. Proportion of population with access to affordable essential drugs on a sustainable basis
Target 18	In cooperation with the private sector, make available the benefits of new technologies, especially information and communications	

Sources: "Implementation of the United Nations Millennium Declaration," Report of the Secretary-General, A/57/270 (31 July 2002), first annual report based on the "Road map towards the implementation of the United Nations Mellennium Declaration," Report of the Secretary-General, A/56/326 (6 September 2001); United Nations Statistics Division, Millennium Indicators Database, verified in July 2004; World Health Organization, Department of MDGs, Health and Development Policy (HDP).

morbidity and mortality data with which to benchmark progress on MDGs 4, 5, and 6 is also reflective of weakened health systems. Although select targeted initiatives have shown an overall trend of improved quality and equity with regard to access to health care (e.g., treatment for HIV/AIDS and tuberculosis), for low-income countries to ensure sustained steady progress in these areas, strengthened health systems are essential (WHO Maximizing Positive Synergies Collaborative Group, 2009). In its 2010 report titled *Preparing for the Future of HIV/AIDS in Africa: A Shared Responsibility*, the Institute of Medicine echoed similar themes regarding the importance of strengthening health systems by creating institutional and human resources capacity as an essential requirement for advancement in this area.

HEALTH SYSTEMS

Health Systems Overview

Due to weakened health infrastructure resulting from decades of neglect and insufficient investment, progress toward reaching the MDGs for health is compromised in most low-income countries (WHO Maximizing Positive Synergies Collaborative Group, 2009). Reasons for inadequate health infrastructure relate to the economic crises and political unrest that occurred in many developing countries during the 1980s, which were followed by restricted debt repayment and cuts in public health spending. These events, which negatively affected both health service delivery and health service providers, resulted in a dramatic rise in emigration of highly skilled, yet poorly paid healthcare providers. The exodus of the professional health workforce left the majority of developing countries unable to effectively respond to the HIV/AIDS epidemic by the time it was fully manifested in early 2000. As noted by the WHO Maximizing Positive Synergies Group (2009), the impact of HIV/AIDS resulted in further crippling of damaged health systems that were already overstretched. Put simply, the AIDS epidemic exacerbated the inability of low-income countries to effectively meet the health needs of their populations.

WHO (2007) defines health systems as the embodiment of "all organizations, people and actions whose primary intent is to promote, restore or maintain health." This definition encompasses both the determinants of health and the broader definition of health-improving activities, such as public health and contributions to health protection seen with legislation and government policy (WHO, 2007). The overall goals of health systems—to improve health and health equity for a national population—represent the best and most efficient use of available resources. Yet for many developing countries, this expectation exceeds their current reach (de Savigny & Adam, 2009). As noted in the 2000 World Health Report, *Health Systems: Improving Performance*, "every country has a health system however fragmented it may be among different organizations or however unsystematically it may seem to operate. Integration and oversight do not determine the system, but they may greatly influence how well it performs." (WHO, 2000). For these reasons, an understanding of this health systems approach is essential to effectively engage in global health.

WHO's Framework for Action characterizes the individual components of health systems into a set of discrete building blocks (**Figure 20-1**). Taken together, these building blocks make up a complete health system that—when functional—results in achievement of the overall goals

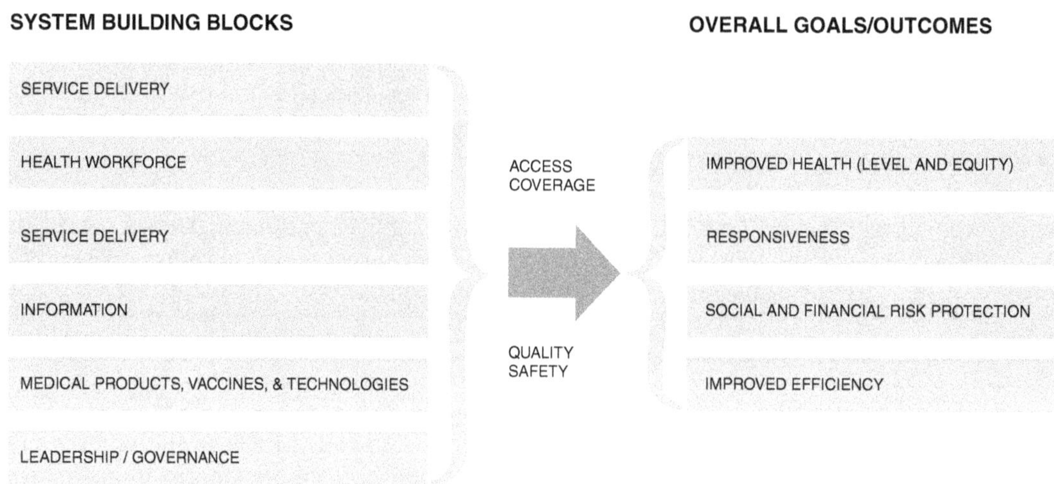

THE SIX BUILDING BLOCKS OF A HEALTH SYSTEM: AIMS AND DESIRABLE ATTRIBUTES

• Good health services are those which deliver effective, safe, quality personal and non-personal health interventions to those who need them, when and where needed, with minimum waste of resources.

• A well-performing health workforce is one which works in ways that are responsive, fair and efficient to achieve the best health outcomes possible, given available resources and circumstances. i.e. There are sufficient numbers and mix of staff, fairly distributed; they are competent, responsive and productive.

• A well-functioning health information system is one that ensures the production, analysis, dissemination and use of reliable and timely information on health determinants, health systems performance and health status.

• A well-functioning health system ensures equitable access to essential medical products, vaccines and technologies of assured quality, safety, efficacy and cost-effectiveness, and their scientifically sound and cost-effective use.

• A good health financing system raises adequate funds for health, in ways that ensure people can use needed services, and are protected from financial catastrophe or impoverishment associated with having to pay for them.

• Leadership and governance involves ensuring strategic policy frameworks exist and are combined with effective oversight, coalition building, the provision of appropriate regulations and incentives, attention to system-design, and accountability.

HEALTH SYSTEM BUILDING BLOCKS

To achieve their goals, all health systems have to carry out some basic functions, regardless of how they are organized: they have to provide services; develop health workers and other key resources; mobilize and allocate finances, and ensure health system leadership and governance (also known as stewardship, which is about oversight and guidance of the whole system). For the purpose of clearly articulating what WHO will do to help strengthen health systems, the functions identified in the World health report 2000 have been broken down into a set of six essential 'building blocks'. All are needed to improve outcomes. This is WHO's health system framework.

DESIRABLE ATTRIBUTES

Irrespective of how a health system is organized, there are some desired attributes for each building block that hold true across all systems.

Figure 20–1 The WHO Health System Framework.

Source: World Health Organization. (2007) *Everybody's Business: Strengthening Health Systems to Improve Health Outcomes-WHO's Framework for Action.* Geneva: WHO Press.

of improved health, responsiveness to the health needs of the community, social and financial equity, and improved efficiency (WHO, 2007).

Individual building blocks do not constitute a health system; rather, the health system comprises multiple relationships and interactions between the components. The ease with which each component interacts with the others determines the degree of functionality of the system. Most important, the interaction of the health system components can enable (or impede) health services to achieve the purpose for which they were created (de Savigny & Adam, 2009). Current approaches to furthering global healthcare development builds on systems concepts that include understanding the methods and processes of healthcare delivery, increasing the knowledge capacity of the health system, building and maintaining health information relationships, and encouraging a systems culture (de Savigny & Adam, 2009).

Health Systems Policy and Research

Over the past decade, global health policy has embraced two different strategies to advancing MDG attainment. One approach emphasizes disease-specific interventions, as illustrated by PEPFAR, the Global Fund to Fight AIDS, Tuberculosis and Malaria, and the Global Alliance for Vaccines and Immunizations; the other promotes a broad and integrated systematic approach to health improvement (de Savigny & Adam, 2009; WHO, 2000, 2007). **Table 20–2** contrasts a disease-specific intervention with the responses typically seen with health system interventions.

While disease-specific initiatives, such as PEPFAR and the Global Fund to Fight AIDS, Tuberculosis and Malaria (Global Fund), have been shown to improve health conditions in low- income countries, (Reich et al., 2008), some critics argue that targeted strategies have the potential to crowd out other health-promoting services within the health sector (Travis et al., 2004). For example, a WHO study of polio eradication reported that the majority of district-level staff noted a disruption of routine health service delivery during the period leading up to national immunization days (Møgedal & Stenson, 2002). Furthermore, a disease-specific lens can fragment an already weakened health system and prevent the development of other strategies that might enhance the sustainability of focused initiatives (Chan et al., 2010). As a result, the prevailing opinion in global health more recently has endorsed a balanced approach between disease-specific mandates and systems-based interventions and methodology (Reich et al., 2008). The Obama administration's GHI represents a good example of this new approach ("Implementation of the Global Health Initiative Consultation Document," 2010).

While WHO's health systems definition, framework, and essential building blocks are accepted tenets for global engagement, relatively little is known about the best approaches for systems improvement (Fryatt et al., 2010; Mgone, Volmink, Coles, Makanga, Jaffar, & Sewankambo, 2010; *Report from the Ministerial Summit on Health Research*, 2004; Sanders & Haines, 2006; Strengthening Health Systems: The Country Perspective, 2009; Task Force on Health Systems Research, 2004). This is partly due to the fact that until recently, support for health systems research was sparse—especially compared to the resources that have been made available for drug and vaccine discoveries (Mgone et al., 2010). Additionally, health systems research is a complex science, and the proven metrics for measuring impact are still

Table 20–2 Typical System Constraints and Possible Disease Specific and Health System Responses

Constraint	Disease-Specific Response	Health-System Response
Financial inaccessibility: inability to pay, informal fees	Exemptions/reduced prices for focal diseases	Development of risk-pooling strategies
Physical inaccessibility: distance to	Outreach for focal diseases	Reconsideration of long term plan facility for capital investment and siting of facilities
Inappropriately skilled staff	Continuous education and training workshops to develop skills in focal diseases	Review of basic medical and nursing training curricula to ensure that appropriate skills included in basic training
Poorly motivated staff	Financial incentives to delivery of particular priority services	Reward institution of proper performance review systems, creating greater clarity of roles and expectations regarding performance of roles, review of salary structures and promotion procedures
Weak planning and management	Continuous education and training workshops to develop skills in planning and management	Restructuring ministries of health, recruitment and development of cadre of dedicated managers
Lack of intersectoral action and partnership	Creation of special disease-focused cross-sectoral committees and tasks forces at national level	Building systems of local government that incorporate representatives from health, education, agriculture, and promote accountability of local governance structures to the people
Poor quality care amongst private sector providers	Training for private sector providers	Development of accreditation and regulation systems

Source: Travis, P., Bennett, S., Haines, A., et al. Overcoming health-systems constraints to achieve the Millennium Development Goals. *Lancet* 2004; 364, 900-906.

evolving. As a consequence, health systems and health system interventions are infrequently evaluated. In contrast to the vast amounts of resources that have been allocated to support disease-specific or targeted health interventions, to date there have been no robust prospective studies of the overall effects that targeted interventions have had upon local health systems. Thus there are insufficient data upon which conclusions can be drawn regarding the impact (either positive or negative) of disease-specific initiatives on health systems (Hill et al., 2010; WHO Maximizing Positive Synergies Collaborative Group, 2009).

A 2004 ministerial summit on health research, co-sponsored by WHO and the government of Mexico, identified the dearth of health system information as a major problem and cited the need for advancing a health systems research agenda (*Report from the Ministerial Summit on Health Research*, 2004). The information identified by these health ministers as critical to their decision making included integrated analyses that went beyond basic health statistics to capture key health system parameters, best practices, and other relevant information needed by policy makers, funders, managers, providers, and the general public (*Report from the Ministerial Summit on Health Research*, 2004). Equally important was the realization that few countries have information of sufficient quality to permit regular tracking of progress in health systems strengthening. The Task Force on Health Systems Research (2004) similarly noted this deficit and projected that that six out of eight MDGs would specifically benefit from increased investment in these areas.

Priority questions for low-income country researchers and decision makers include these:

- What are the best practices for integrating discrete health initiatives at the local level?
- What are optimal health management strategies, including the use of auxiliary (i.e., nonprofessionally educated) health workers?
- What are the costs and benefits analyses of different health care service models?

Investigating these questions requires improved data quality and availability, which in turn necessitate strengthened country capacity in collecting, processing, analyzing, and using health data (Mgone et al., 2010). It is in tackling the health information gap that answers to these and many other health systems questions can be answered—and answers to these questions will have a major bearing on the health and welfare of vulnerable populations, especially those at risk for morbidity, mortality, and the diseases of poverty.

HUMAN RESOURCES FOR HEALTH

HRH Overview

While global policies and resolutions in the early 2000s brought attention to the need for strengthened HRH capacity and HRH information systems in developing countries (Pan American Organization & WHO, 2001; WHO, 2004a), the first analysis of the impact of global workforce shortages on health services and health outcomes was reported by the Joint Learning Initiative—a consortium of more than 100 global health leaders launched by the Rockefeller Foundation with a supported secretariat at Harvard University's Global Equity Initiative (Chen et al., 2004; Joint Learning Initiative, 2004). As illustrated in **Figure 20-2** and **Figure 20-3**, their findings documented that workforce density can make a critical difference regarding mortality rates of vulnerable populations, such as mothers, infants and children younger than five years of age. A similar association was noted with regard to workforce density, health services, and the impact of MDG interventions, such as achieving 80% coverage of childhood

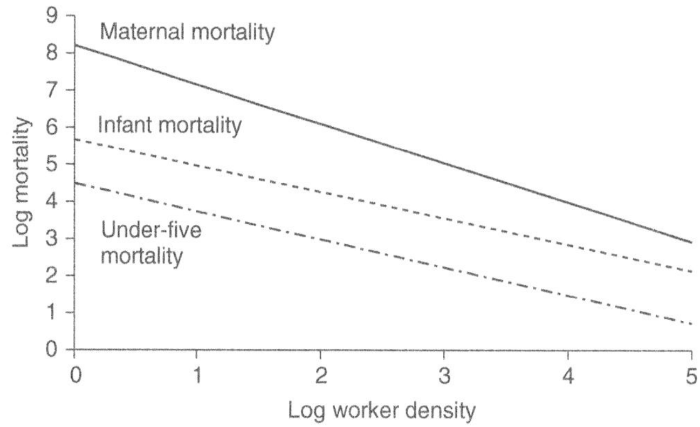

Figure 20–2 Association between workers density and mortality rates.
Source: Chen, L., Evans, T., Anand, S., et al. Human resources for health: Overcoming the crisis. *Lancet* 2004; 364; 1984-1990.

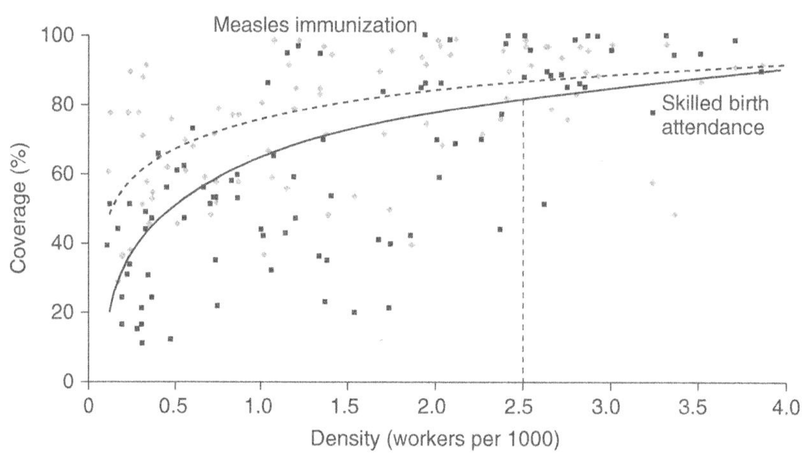

Figure 20–3 Association between health worker density and health service coverage.
Source: Chen, L., Evans, T., Anand, S., et al. Human resources for health: Overcoming the crisis. *Lancet* 2004; 364; 1984-1990.

measles immunization and ensuring the majority of births are attended by skilled providers (Chen et al., 2004).

Chen and his colleagues (2004) postulate that the critical minimum HRH coverage threshold is 2.5 workers per 1000 population. When the provider-to-population ratios fall below that level, health outcomes and preventive health services are significantly compromised. While some pregnancy-related services and life-saving child health services, such as immunizations or the provision of HIV/AIDS care, can be adequately provided by auxiliary staff, effective health workforce planning assumes a balance of professional, paraprofessional, and community health workers (WHO, n.d.). Based on these criteria, WHO has identified 57 HRH crisis countries (36 of which are in Africa) that have an estimated combined deficit of 2.4 million doctors, nurses, and midwives (WHO, 2006). HRH issues that challenge health service delivery to vulnerable populations include HRH out-migration, retention, and maldistribution. Each of these topics is briefly discussed here.

HRH Outmigration

While the majority of in-country health worker migration occurs when healthcare workers move from rural areas to urban centers, the most controversial migration stream entails the movement of highly skilled professionals from poorer countries to richer, more developed countries. The out-migration crisis largely pertains to physicians and nurse, who are able to achieve equivalency credentialing in destination countries (Joint Learning Initiative, 2004). Additionally, HRH studies suggest that professionals who out-migrate are among the countries' most qualified healthcare providers. For example, studies on Kenya's nursing workforce have documented that the majority of nurses who elect to out-migrate are typically RN or BScN prepared (Riley et al., 2007). Additionally, between the years 1999 and 2007, for every four nurses that Kenya added to its workforce through training, one existing nurse applied to out-migrate (Gross et al., 2010). Similar impacts to the healthcare system have been noted in the context of physician out-migration. While destination countries receiving physicians from low-income nations benefit from workforce additions, the United States', United Kingdom's, Canada's, and Australia's reliance on international medical graduates is reducing the supply of physicians in many developing nations (Mullan, 2005).

HRH Retention

In an attempt to offset the out-migration imbalance from HRH crisis countries, there is increased emphasis on identifying appropriate and effective workforce retention strategies. While current capacity-building approaches have focused on the production of health professionals as one way to address HRH shortages, some critics argue that this emphasis on producing new providers has the potential to overlook the solutions needed to retain those currently employed within the system (Haines & Sanders, 2005). PEPFAR's recently announced Medical Education Partnership Initiative (MEPI), a partnership with the National Institutes of Health (NIH) and the Health Resources and Services Administration (HRSA), is designed to provide a balance between transforming medical education within African medical schools and offering incentives for professional retention. Representing a five-year $130 million investment in pre-professional education, MEPI's goals include improving the quantity, quality, and retention of African medical graduates as well as improving Africa's medical research capabilities (Collins, Glass, Whitescarver, Wakefield, & Goosby, 2010). Of the current funding awards to African medical and nursing training institutions, 80% are directed toward incorporation of community-based education and/or rural training, in recognition of the fact that students who are recruited and training in rural settings are more likely to be willing to practice there. Seventy-three percent of MEPI awardees target nurses and nursing students for enhanced training (Collins et al., 2010).

Beyond this effort, however, there remains an unmet need to develop incentives that target HRH retention in rural and underserved areas. A recent literature review of motivational and retention issues affecting healthcare providers cited "limited career paths" and "promotion opportunities," in addition to the need for "improved working and living conditions," as being as significant in improving workforce retention as increasing employee wages alone (Willis-Shattuck, Bidwell, Thomas, Wyness, Blaauw, & Ditlopo, 2008). Similar themes are echoed in the Joint Learning Initiative's reports and the IOM report *Preparing for the Future of HIV/AIDS in Africa*. Both documents identify satisfactory remuneration, a positive work environment, and synchronization of support systems as core elements for sustaining an engaged and motivated workforce (IOM, 2010a; Joint Learning Initiative, 2004).

HRH Maldistribution

Within developing countries, structural imbalances often result in provider maldistribution. Examples include the placement of providers without regard to provider-to-population ratios, professional and specialty discrepancies (i.e., underinvestment in mid-level providers at the expense of physician specialty training), and geographic or "urban bias" whereby political or economic forces of a country reinforce provision of services and health investments in urban areas (Fritzen, 2007). Citing this issue as the most critical barrier for achieving universal healthcare coverage, Chen (2010) describes maldistribution of healthcare workers as "inextricably linked [to] workforce problems such as shortages and skill imbalances." According to this author, the shortages of healthcare coverage are exacerbated (if not caused) by the uneven supply of professional health providers in which excessive concentration of overly specialized professionals results in unnecessary tests and procedures, over-prescribing of drugs, and higher costs at the expense of the underserved.

In response to this problem, WHO convened an expert group that investigated issues pertaining to health provider access in remote and rural areas. After comprehensively reviewing evidence-based retention strategies specific to rural and remote areas, this expert group developed global policy recommendations tailored to ministries of health in which the maldistribution of providers impedes healthcare coverage. The intent is that these recommendations, which serve as an initial step for addressing HRH imbalances, will spearhead local implementation, monitoring, and evaluation of retention interventions (WHO, 2010a).

HRH Policy and Research

Global awareness of the indiscriminate recruitment of professional healthcare providers from low-income to high-income countries has resulted in the recent enactment of responsive global health policies. In a historic move in 2010, the 63rd World Health Assembly unanimously passed a resolution to adopt a voluntary global Code of Practice regarding the international recruitment of health personnel (WHO, 2010b). By committing to this Code, member states agreed to voluntarily adopt the principles and practices for the ethical international recruitment of health personnel, taking into account the responsibilities and rights of both the source (i.e., low-income countries) and the destination (i.e., high-income countries), other stakeholders, and those of the migrant health personnel themselves (WHO, 2008). In passing this resolution, the world's nations acknowledged the global dimension and complexities of the health workforce crisis and the interconnected nature of the problems and solutions.

Other recent policy developments affecting global HRH include the realignment of roles and responsibilities regarding healthcare delivery. Referred to as "task shifting," this process occurs when specific provider tasks are transferred (when appropriate) to mid-level health cadres or the auxiliary health workforces that generally have less professional training and fewer qualifications (WHO, 2008). The intent of this approach is to facilitate efficient use of existing human resources and ease bottlenecks common to service delivery in low-income countries. In situations where additional providers are needed, task shifting may also involve the delegation of some clearly delineated tasks to newly created cadres, such as advanced nurse practitioners. The 2010 IOM report *Preparing for the Future of HIV/AIDS in Africa* most recently elected to substitute "task sharing" for the "task shifting" terminology; the IOM contends that the former term more aptly describes the knowledge-based requirement in the provision of health care that must accompany any delegated performance skills. Used in this way, task sharing is neither "hierarchical [nor] territorial, and allows roles to expand or contract according to need" as befitting low-resource environments (IOM, 2010a).

In spite of the attention accorded to HRH, the field of global workforce research is still in its nascent stages, with more questions than available answers. The Mexico City Summit on Health Research identified HRH research as a priority, especially with regard to estimating workforce requirements for appropriate service delivery (*Report from the Ministerial Summit on Health Research*, 2004). Attendees' recommended global HRH research approaches include the following measures:

- Better balance between descriptive HRH studies, with those that are conceptual, policy driven, or designed to further the implementation science in this area. (To date there have been insufficient numbers of studies that develop theoretical models or metrics for measuring workforce activity.)
- More comparative HRH research that analyzes workforce dynamics within multiple contexts and countries, which is especially relevant for low-income settings.
- Integration of research findings with specific health workforce interventions so that documented country experiences can be assessed more systematically (WHO, 2006).

An example of this newer type of recommended research is a recent multicountry evaluation of policy interventions aimed at attracting nurses to rural areas, conducted by researchers from Kenya, South Africa, Thailand, and the United Kingdom (Blaauw et al., 2010). This study, which employed the discrete choice experiment (DCE) methodology—a quantitative technique for eliciting preferences in the absence of actual preference data—asked individuals to state their preference over hypothetical alternative scenarios (Mangham, Hanson, & McPake, 2009). The results revealed that for Kenyan and South African nurses, better educational opportunities or rural allowances would be most effective in increasing their retention within rural health posts; in Thailand, better health insurance coverage was shown to have the greatest impact in attracting nurses to rural installations. The introduction of DCE as a method for evaluating the effectiveness of workforce policies provides policy makers with an evidence base for selecting the most effective interventions to remediate personnel staff shortages. It also represents a promising methodological approach studying HRH issues (Blaauw et al., 2010).

Major challenges in undertaking studies on health workforce dynamics pertain to the absence of routine HRH data collection, data harmonization, and research (Joint Learning Initiative, 2004). More often than not, workforce data in developing countries are sparse; when data do exist, they are often fragmented. A recent systematic review of 63 national HRH information systems identified few instances in which HRH information was used for resource allocation and program planning. In particular, HRH-crisis countries—that is, those most in need of efficient utilization of scarce human and financial resources—were largely lacking accurate and timely data on workforce availability, qualification, deployment, and retention (Riley et al., 2010).

Current global health initiatives emphasize the need for human resources information systems (HRIS) that would facilitate the collection and dissemination of workforce information. When designed to operate within a health system, a national HRIS can provide information on health workforce size, composition, and deployment station. Such systems typically collect workforce "supply" data, such as professional registration, major qualifications, and continuing education, which are usually maintained by professional regulatory boards. Well-designed HRIS also have the capability to link supply data to workforce deployment data, which are typically maintained by an employer, such as the ministry of health. Functional HRIS provide current and accurate data that can be used for supporting HRH policy decisions. As an example, when Kenya's HRIS projected insufficient numbers of nurses available to replace those scheduled to retire within 5 to 10 years, the National Parliament voted to increase the mandatory retirement age of public health providers (all civil servants) from 55 years to 60 (Rakuom, Oywer, Arudo, Vidot, & Jones, 2010). Because many country HRIS remain in their infancy, the potential yield of information from HRIS has yet to be fully realized. Nevertheless, PEPFAR and other global initiatives identify the development HRIS and the strengthening of HRH data collection as a priority area of intervention (Dal Poz, Gupta, Quain, & Soucat, 2009; PEPFAR, 2009).

Increasingly, global HRH policy and research are being recognized as essential components of the global health agenda. While the importance of having adequate numbers of well-prepared providers has been well documented, there remain critical gaps within the scientific community regarding the best practices for addressing and responding to complex HRH issues. Given that nursing constitutes the largest health professional cadre worldwide, there is both the need and the opportunity for a new generation of global nurse investigators to uncover the solutions and strategies that can effectively address the workforce challenges largely experienced by the nursing profession. Expanding this knowledge base represents an important new direction for global nursing in the twenty-first century.

WWW

For a full suite of assignments and additional learning activities, use the access code located in the front of your book to visit this exclusive website: http://go.jblearning.com/dechesnay. If you do not have an access code, you can obtain one at the site.

REFERENCES

Blaauw, D., Erasmus, E., Pagaiya, N., Tangcharoensathein, V., Mullei, K., Mudhune, S., . . . Lagarde, M. (2010). Policy interventions that attract nurses to rural areas: A multicountry discrete choice experiment. *Bulletin of the World Health Organization. 88*, 350–357.

Chan, M., Kazatchkine, M., Lob-Levyt, J., Obaid, T., Schweizer, J., Sidibe, M.,. . . Yamada, T. (2010). Meeting the demand for results and accountability: A call for action on data from eight global health agencies. *PLoS Medicine, 7*, e1000223.

Chen, L. (2010). Striking the right balance: Health workforce retention in remote and rural areas. *Bulletin of the World Health Organization, 88*, 323. doi: 10.2471/BLT.10.078477

Chen, L., Evans, T., Anand, S., Boufford, J. L., Brown, H., Chowdhury, M., . . . Wibulpolprasert, S. (2004) Human resources for health: overcoming the crises. *Lancet, 364*, 1984–1990.

Collins, F., Glass, R., Whitescarver, J., Wakefield, M., & Goosby, E. P. (2010). Developing health workforce capacity in Africa. *Science, 330*, 1324–1325. Retrieved December 13, 2010, from http://www.fic.nih.gov/news/publications/Science-Article-Dec2010.pdf

Dal Poz, M. R., Gupta, N., Quain, E., & Soucat, A. (Eds.). (2009). *Handbook on monitoring and evaluation of human resources for health, with special applications for low and middle-income countries.* Geneva, Switzerland: WHO Press.

de Savigny, D., & Adam, T. (Eds.). (2009). *Systems thinking for health systems strengthening.* Geneva, Switzerland: Alliance for health policy and systems research. WHO Press.

Fritzen, S. (2007). Strategic management of the health workforce in developing countries: What have we learned? *Human Resources for Health, 5*, 4. doi: 10.1186/1478-4491-5-4. Retrieved December 13, 2010, from http://preview.human-resources-health.com/content/5/1/4

Fryatt, R., Mills, A., & Nordstrom, A. (2010). Financing of health systems to achieve the health Millennium Development Goals in low-income countries. *Lancet, 375*, 419–426.

Gross, J. M., Rogers, M. F., Teplinskiy, I., Oywer, E., Wambua, D., & Kamenju, A. (2010) *The impact of out-migration on the nursing workforce in Kenya*. Unpublished manuscript.

Haines, A., & Sanders, D. (2005). Building capacity to attain the millennium development goals. *Transactions of the Royal Society of Tropical Medicine and Hygiene, 99*, 721–726.

Henry J. Kaiser Family Foundation. (2008). Kaiser daily HIV/AIDS reports. http://globalhealth.kff.org/Daily-Reports/2008/July/31/dr00053609.aspx

Hill, P., Mansoor, G. F., & Claudio, F. (2010). Conflict in least-developed countries: Challenging the Millennium Development Goals. *Bulletin of the World Health Organization, 88*, 562–563.

Implementation of the Global Health Initiative Consultation Document. (2010). Retrieved from http://www.pepfar.gov/documents/organization/136504.pdf

Institute of Medicine (IOM). (2010a). *Preparing for the future of HIV/AIDS in Africa: A shared responsibility.* Washington, DC: National Academies Press.

Institute of Medicine (IOM). (2010b). *A summary of the February 2010 Forum on the Future of Nursing.* Washington, DC: National Academies Press.

Joint Learning Initiative. (2004). *Human Resources for health: Overcoming the crisis.* Cambridge, MA: Harvard University Press.

Mangham, L. J., Hanson, K., & McPake, B. (2009) How to do (or not to do): Designing a discrete choice experiment for application in a low-income country. *Health Policy and Planning, 24*, 151–158.

Mgone, C., Volmink, J., Coles, D., Makanga, M., Jaffar, S., & Sewankambo, N. (2010). Linking research and development to strengthen health systems in Africa. *Tropical Medicine and International Health, 15*, 1401–1406.

Møgedal, S., & Stenson, B. (2002). *Disease eradication: Friend or foe to the health system? Synthesis report from field studies on the Polio Eradication Initiative in Tanzania, Nepal and the Lao People's Democratic Republic.*

Geneva, Switzerland: WHO Press. Retrieved December 12, 2010, from http://www.who.int/vaccines-documents/DocsPDF00/www552.pdf

Mullan, F. (2005). The metrics of the physician brain drain. *New England Journal of Medicine, 353*, 1810–1818.

Pan American Organization & World Health Organization (WHO). (2001). *35th Session of the Subcommittee of the Executive Committee on Planning and Programming: Development and strengthening of human resources management in the health services.* Washington, DC. Retrieved December 13, 2010, from http://www.paho.org/english/gov/ce/ce128index-e.htm

President's Emergency Plan for AIDS Relief (PEPFAR). (2009). *Technical guidance for human resources for health: State of the program area.* Unpublished document.

Rakuom, C. P., Oywer, E. O., Arudo, J., Vidot, P., & Jones, T. (2010). *Health workforce information system: Kenya's nursing experience.* Report prepared for the Commonwealth Secretariat.

Reich, M., Takeni, K., Roberts, M., & Hsiao, W. (2008). Global action on health systems: A proposal for the Tokyo G8 summit. *Lancet, 371*, 865–869.

Report from the Ministerial Summit on Health Research, Mexico City, 15–20 November 2004. (2004). Geneva, Switzerland: WHO Press.

Riley, P. L., Vindigni, S. M., Arudo, J., Waudo, A. N., Kamenju, A., Ngoya, A., . . . Marum, L. H. (2007). Developing a nursing database system in Kenya. *Health Services Research, 42*, 1389–1405.

Riley, P. L., Zuber, A., Vindigni, S. M., Gupta, N., Verani, A., & Sunderland, N. (2010). *Information systems to monitor human resources for health (HRH): A systematic review.* Unpublished manuscript.

Sanders, D., & Haines, A. (2006). Implementation research is needed to achieve international health goals. *PloS Medicine, 3*, e186. doi: 10.1371/journal.pmed.0030186

Strengthening health systems: The country perspective. (2009). A global initiative to strengthen country health systems surveillance (CHeSS): Summary report of a technical meeting and action plan. Retrieved from http://www.who.int/healthsystems/healthsystems_thecountryperspective_1_09.pdf

Task Force on Health Systems Research. (2004). Informed choices for attaining the Millennium Development Goals: Towards an international cooperative agenda for health-systems research. *Lancet, 364*, 997–1003.

Travis, P., Bennett, S., Haines, A., Pang, T., Bhutta, Z., Hyder, A., . . . Evans, T. (2004). Overcoming health-systems constraints to achieve the Millennium Development Goals. *Lancet, 364*, 900–906.

Willis-Shattuck, M., Bidwell, P., Thomas, S., Wyness, L., Blaauw, D., & Ditlopo, P. (2008). Motivation and retention of health workers in developing countries: A systematic review. *BMC Health Services Research, 8*, 247, doi: 10.1186/1472-6963-8-247. Retrieved December 13, 2010, from http://www.biomedcentral.com/1472-6963/8/247

World Health Organization (WHO). (n.d.). Health workforce: Achieving the health-related MDGs. It takes a workforce! Retrieved December 13, 2010, from http://www.who.int/hrh/workforce_mdgs/en/index.html

World Health Organization (WHO). (2000). *The world health report 2000. Health systems: Improving performance.* Geneva, Switzerland: WHO Press.

World Health Organization (WHO). (2004a). World Health Assembly. International migration of health personnel: a challenge for health systems in developing countries. Retrieved December 13, 2010, from www.who.int/gb/ebwha/pdf_files/WHA57/A57_R19-en.pdf)

World Health Organization (WHO). (2004). *The world health report 2004: Changing history.* Geneva, Switzerland: WHO Press.

World Health Organization (WHO). (2005). Health and the Millennium Development Goals: World Health Organization. Retrieved August 18, 2010, from http://www.who.int/hdp/publications/mdg en.pdf

World Health Organization (WHO). (2006). *The world health report: Working together for health.* Geneva, Switzerland: WHO Press.

World Health Organization (WHO). (2007) *Everybody's business: Strengthening health systems to improve health outcomes: WHO's framework for action*. Geneva, Switzerland: WHO Press.

World Health Organization (WHO). (2008). *Task shifting: Rational redistribution of tasks among health workforce teams. Global recommendations and guidelines*. Geneva, Switzerland: WHO Press. Retrieved December 13, 2010, from http://www.who.int/healthsystems/TTR-TaskShifting.pdf

World Health Organization (WHO). (2010a). *Increasing access to health workers in remote and rural areas through improved retention*. Geneva, Switzerland: WHO Press.

World Health Organization (WHO). (2010b). *63rd World Health Assembly. International recruitment of health personnel: Global code of practice*. Geneva, Switzerland: WHO Press. Retrieved from http://www.who.int/workforcealliance/media/news/2010/codestatementwha/en/index.html

World Health Organization (WHO) Maximizing Positive Synergies Collaborative Group. (2009). An assessment of interactions between global health initiatives and country health systems. *Lancet*, *373*, 2137–2169.

CHAPTER 21

The Use of Community-Based Participatory Research to Understand and Work with Vulnerable Populations

Ellen Olshansky

Objectives

At the end of this chapter, the reader will be able to

1. Discuss community-based participatory action research as a methodology.
2. Describe how community action research meets the ethical standards for research with vulnerable populations.

INTRODUCTION

Health disparities and lack of access to health care among some disadvantaged populations have received increasing attention and concern among healthcare providers and health policy makers (Minkler, Blackwell, Thompson, & Tamier, 2003; U.S. Department of Health and Human Services, 2000). As healthcare providers and policy makers have become more concerned about the health of vulnerable populations, more research has been developed to better understand their plight. The goal of these research studies is to determine the most effective interventions. These studies, however, often fail to present the perspective of those who are vulnerable, resulting in less than optimal interventions. This chapter presents an overview of community-based participatory research (CBPR)—a more effective approach to learning about and working effectively with vulnerable populations.

Vulnerable populations encompass those groups with both decreased access to care and increased risk for illness and accidents. In trying to intervene with various vulnerable populations, it is imperative that healthcare providers understand their perspectives rather than imposing on them what we believe to be their experiences. Without such understanding, we may unwittingly exacerbate problems; moreover, community members who are vulnerable may feel that they are being given edicts, are disempowered, and lack a voice in deciding on the solution to their problems. An example is the exclusion of women from clinical trials, which has often had the disastrous results that findings related to men were simply applied to women without scientific evidence for the clinical significance of these findings. Women as a population became vulnerable by virtue of being excluded from research. Today, however, the National Institutes of Health mandates the inclusion of women in such investigations unless there is an obvious rationale for excluding them. Unfortunately, even the inclusion in clinical trials does not always guarantee that the perspectives and voices of women will be taken into account in the research. The issue of appropriate recognition of women's issues continues to be argued and debated (Parascandola, 2006).

Many researchers use open-ended approaches to understanding the experiences of others, including asking open-ended questions without imposing variables a priori. This approach yields important data that would not otherwise be generated. However, such research is done "on" the participants. CBPR takes a different approach, by actively involving the participants as co-researchers. This approach fills an unmet need; Clark and colleagues (2003), for example, have addressed the need for community members themselves to contribute to identifying the needs within their communities. This chapter presents an overview of the CBPR method and then describes why it is appropriate for working with vulnerable populations.

OVERVIEW OF COMMUNITY-BASED PARTICIPATORY RESEARCH

CBPR is an action-oriented research method that involves a team approach inclusive of all participants. "All participants" means that the researchers and the "researched" exist as equal members of the research team, all with an important voice in the research. Rather than referring to the process of doing research "on" people, this approach refers to doing research "with" people. The "people" are those members of a community of interest, those who are most directly affected by the phenomenon being studied. The members of a community also work in tandem with the researchers, leading to a collegial research effort within an environment of collaboration rather than the traditional hierarchical environment. One important goal of CBPR is to empower those who have not been empowered (e.g., those who are vulnerable) by helping them to eliminate oppressive situations or conditions that are contributing to their marginalization and vulnerability.

CBPR engages community members as active participants in the research. An important aim of this research is to generate an understanding of the community members' perspectives and needs so as to develop interventions that more effectively meet the needs of the community members. The concept of action is integral to CBPR (in fact, some refer to this kind of research as "participatory action research" or "action research") because the overt goal of this research is to take constructive action. CBPR is most appropriate for addressing the needs of vulnerable populations because it encourages the direct and active involvement of the members of those populations. Such an approach seeks to mitigate inequalities and oppression among vulnerable groups.

In recent years, CBPR has received increasing attention. Seymour-Rolls and Hughes (2000), Minkler et al. (2003), and Israel et al. (1998) have all addressed the importance of this approach to research in better understanding the nuances and complexities in communities of interest. Olshansky and colleagues (2005) described how CBPR can be used to understand and alleviate health disparities. At the Eastern Nursing Research Society (ENRS), a research interest group was recently formed with a specific focus on CBPR, reflecting the increasing interest in this approach to research.

Israel and colleagues (1998) have aptly described eight key principles of CBPR:

1. Recognizing that the community is the unit of study
2. Building on the strengths already present in the community
3. Continually facilitating collaboration and partnership in each phase of the research
4. Integrating knowledge and action (e.g., knowledge alone is not enough; it must be coupled with action for social change)
5. Promoting the alleviation of social inequality by co-learning
6. Using an iterative process
7. Focusing on wellness and an ecological perspective of health
8. Partnering in the dissemination of research findings

This chapter uses the framework presented by Israel and colleagues. The next section takes an in-depth look at each of these principles, followed by a focus on the applicability of each to working with vulnerable populations.

PRINCIPLES OF CBPR: APPLICABILITY TO VULNERABLE POPULATIONS

Recognizing That the Community Is the Unit of Study

This principle addresses the central focus of CBPR: the community and the factors that influence the community must be understood and addressed to understand the issues of the individual within the community. The concept is consistent with the ecological framework that addresses social, political, economic, environmental, and sociological factors as part of the community context and as contributors to the experience of individuals within the community. Although the experiences of each individual are important and each individual is unique, the focus is on the community in which the individual experiences situations and problems. Individual differences within communities are taken into account to develop a comprehensive understanding of the complexities within communities.

Building on the Strengths Already Present in the Community

This principle embraces the attitude that members of the community already have strengths despite the fact that they are vulnerable by virtue of unequal access to care and perhaps oppression by other dominant groups. In the spirit of empowerment, it is important to learn from these individuals how they view their strengths, how they would like to use their strengths to tackle the problems identified, and how they can improve on present strengths. It is imperative that the community members articulate these strengths and explain why they view them as strengths. Conversely, it is imperative that the members of the research team truly listen to and hear the community members' descriptions of how they cope with situations, how they have managed in the past, and what their views are in regard to how to continue to manage and move forward despite the vulnerabilities that they experience on a daily basis.

Focusing on strengths encourages empowerment among the members of the community. They feel that they have something to offer rather than being told what they should do by the researchers or health professionals. In addition, the researchers can learn from the community participants. Rather than imposing their views on the community participants (the traditional approach), the researchers can begin to understand what works best for the community participants.

Continually Facilitating Collaboration and Partnership in Each Phase of the Research

Collaboration and partnership are signature aspects of CBPR. To develop a collaborative partnership with the members of a vulnerable community requires much planning (Kelly, 2005). It takes time to develop a true partnership with members of the community, particularly when vulnerable community members have traditionally had a lack of trust of researchers from an academic or other institution. Taking the time initially to develop trust, thereby enabling the entrée of the traditional researcher into the community, is crucial to the success of the research. Strategies for achieving this trusting relationship include going into the community and conducting focus groups on site (as opposed to having the community members travel to the location of the researcher).

It is important that the researchers venture out of their "ivory tower." Community members, likewise, need to know that they have an open invitation to visit the researcher's location. Nevertheless, the point of overriding importance is for the researchers to enter the context of the community members. By doing so, they strive to understand the context, and to reverse the often stereotypical view of the ivory towers of academia. Gaining entrée into the community and developing trust among the community members are only the beginnings of this collaboration and partnership, however. Community members are considered equal partners in the research. They have an active voice in determining the research question, in designing the research method, in contributing to the data collection and analysis, and in disseminating the research results. They work in partnership as equal members of the research team.

It is important to recognize the unique skills and contributions made by each member of the research team. The community members are the experts in the actual phenomenon under study. The traditional researchers are the experts in research methodology, including collection and analysis of data, and writing up or presenting research results. Therefore, each member of the research team contributes to the overall effort based on his or her area of expertise, but all members of the research team are involved in all the steps of the research process to greater or lesser degrees.

Focus groups are commonly used in CBPR as a way to involve all members of the research team and to elicit perspectives from the various members of the research team. Focus groups are a way of facilitating discussion within an atmosphere of openness, where the goal is to hear the various perspectives and views of community members and the traditional research members. The focus group serves several purposes. First, it helps members of the team get to know one another and allows them to hear each person's perspectives and description of his or her own experiences. Second, it helps the members come together in a collaborative manner as they begin to understand each person's experiences, focusing on the differences among them while also looking for and eventually being able to define commonalities. Third, the focus group allows the members to more clearly define the research problem, establish the focus of the research, and identify the goals and outcomes of the research.

Integrating Knowledge and Action

A crucial component of CBPR is action, in the form of developing and implementing interventions within the community that will help to alleviate the problems identified by the research group. CBPR is a form of research with the overt purpose of making social change to alleviate disparities, oppression, and other factors that lead to vulnerability. CBPR is true "translation research," in that the translation into practice occurs in an immediate and ongoing fashion from the moment the research commences and throughout the entire process. By working closely and collaboratively with community members who desire constructive social change, the emphasis on action to achieve this constructive change is paramount in CBPR. This approach is especially germane to nursing education, as nursing students are a strong voice for social change necessary to improve health disparities among vulnerable populations (Reimer-Kirkham, Van Hofwegen, & Hoe-Harwood, 2005).

Promoting the Alleviation of Social Inequality by Co-learning

The principles discussed in the previous subsections contribute to alleviating social inequality. The principle of promoting the alleviation of social inequality by co-learning is directly related to the principle of integrating knowledge and action. To alleviate social inequality, it is imperative that constructive social change leads to social emancipation and alleviation of oppression. Such social change will truly be useful only if those less fortunate (those who are vulnerable) are empowered. Integrating this principle into CBPR reflects the complexity of this research approach. This research process encompasses developing collaborative partnerships, involving all members of the community actively in the research project, overtly seeking to make social change in a constructive manner, and doing all of this while empowering those less fortunate. In fact, without such empowerment, the other aspects of the research will not be achieved. Lofman, Pelkonen, and Pietila (2004) have aptly described the importance of the involvement of the community members as a means to address unequal power relationships.

Using an Iterative Process

An iterative process is one in which each of the phases of a study is conducted in a circular, as opposed to a linear, fashion. A phase is not a discrete part of the process; rather, each phase informs the next phase, and subsequent phases may lead to returning to previous phases to make changes based upon continuous learning throughout the CBPR process. This iterative process is central to all qualitative research. CBPR employs qualitative research methods through focus groups, eliciting perspectives of informants in their own words, and approaching data in an interpretive manner.

The research begins in an inductive manner, as the research question is open-ended and the goal is to learn the perspectives of the members of the community without imposing preconceived variables on the investigation. As the research continues, certain variables that are generated through the research process receive greater focus based on the presence of continuing data to support these variables. In qualitative terms, this practice is referred to as saturation of data (Strauss & Corbin, 1998). At this point, data collection becomes more deductive—that is, focused on looking for further evidence of both predetermined and emerging variables. Previously collected data are reanalyzed with the explicit purpose of looking for data or evidence to support the existence of these variables. This iterative process involves going back and forth with data collection that influences data analysis, which then furthers data collection.

Focusing on Wellness and an Ecological Perspective of Health

CBPR proposes that multiple and interacting factors within the social context influence and are influenced by health. This ecological perspective embraces the notion that context is a key factor in understanding how to promote wellness. The context includes biological, psychological, environmental, social, and interpersonal factors. Health and wellness occur within this context. Using CBPR, the research team seeks to understand the factors in this ecological perspective. These factors are uncovered by open-ended questions and participant observation.

Partnering in the Dissemination of Research Findings

As noted earlier, in CBPR all members of the research team are involved in all aspects of the research process, including the dissemination of research findings. Traditionally, the dissemination of research has consisted of researchers writing for publication or presenting their findings at conferences. These publications and conferences are typically refereed—that is, reviewed by a panel of experts who are also researchers and scholarly peers. In CBPR, those peer reviews continue, but research findings are also disseminated in magazines and meetings of the lay public. Those publications that are sent to peer-reviewed journals will, ideally, include the lay community members are co-authors. The research data and findings are “owned,” in a sense, by all members of the research team—a key aspect of CBPR.

CBPR AND VULNERABLE POPULATIONS

Vulnerable populations often lack a voice in regard to what they need and how these needs could best be met. Traditionally, presumed “experts” from health care and other arenas have dictated solutions to vulnerable populations—a one-way flow of information. This dominant attitude, while perhaps well meaning, is usually counterproductive, because it keeps vulnerable populations in vulnerable positions, and they continue to lack a voice. A CBPR approach seeks to address these limitations of the traditional approach to assisting vulnerable populations. It aims to assist the vulnerable in attaining and maintaining a voice, to recognize those who are vulnerable as the true "experts" about the issues they are experiencing, and to ultimately enable them to forge a partnership in social change.

Implementing a CBPR Approach with Vulnerable Populations

Even after establishing the critical need for CBPR in alleviating inequalities and oppressions suffered by vulnerable groups, it remains difficult to implement such an approach. Although many barriers exist, one goal of nurses and other healthcare providers and researchers is to work actively to overcome those barriers. This section presents strategies for implementing CBPR in research and healthcare settings.

In academic research settings, support for such an approach is sorely needed. The National Institutes of Health clearly recognizes of the need for CBPR, reflected in its recent call for research proposals that incorporating CBPR. In educational settings, this approach should be included in research courses in undergraduate and graduate programs.

Academic researchers and healthcare clinicians should partner with one another to develop research programs that include community members. An ideal CBPR project would include academic researchers, clinicians, and community members. In addition, health policy experts and members of health insurance companies could be included in such research. All of these participants in the research process will contribute important perspectives. When the research team is expanded to include the voices of the community members, those individuals will then have the opportunity to voice their concerns to the various members of the healthcare team.

For a full suite of assignments and additional learning activities, use the access code located in the front of your book to visit this exclusive website: http://go.jblearning.com/dechesnay. If you do not have an access code, you can obtain one at the site.

REFERENCES

Clark, M. J., Cary, S., Diemert, G., Ceballos, R., Sifuentes, M., Atteberry, I., . . . Trieu, S. (2003). Involving communities in community assessment. *Public Health Nursing Journal, 20*, 456–463.

Israel, B. A., Schulz, A. J., Parker, E. A., & Becker, A. B. (1998). Review of community-based research: Assessing partnership approaches to improve public health. *Annual Review of Public Health, 19*, 173–202.

Kelly, P. J. (2005). Practical suggestions for community interventions using participatory action research. *Public Health Nursing, 22*(1), 65–73.

Lofman, P., Pelkonen, M., & Pietila, A. M. (2004). Ethical issues in participatory action research. *Scandinavian Journal of Caring Science, 18*, 333–340.

Minkler, M., Blackwell, A. G., Thompson, M., & Tamier, H. (2003). Community-based participatory research: Implications for public health funding. *American Journal of Public Health, 93*, 1210–1213.

Olshansky, E., Sacco, D., Braxter, B., Dodge, P., Hughes, E., Ondeck, M., . . . Upvall, M. J. (2005). Participatory action research to understand and reduce health disparities. *Nursing Outlook, 53*, 121–126.

Parascandola, M. (2006). From exclusion to inclusion: Women and minorities in clinical trials. *Research Practitioner, 7*(2), 52–64.

Reimer-Kirkham, S., Van Hofwegen, L., & Hoe-Harwood, C. (2005). Narratives of social justice: Learning in innovative clinical settings. *International Journal of Nursing Education Scholarship, 2*(1).

Seymour-Rolls, K., Hughes, I. (2004). Participatory action research: Getting the job done. *Action Research E-Reports, 4*. Retrieved from http://www.fhs.usyd.edu.au/arow/arer/004.htm

Strauss, A., & Corbin, J. (1998). *Basics of qualitative research: Techniques and procedures for developing grounded theory* (2nd ed.). Thousand Oaks, CA: Sage.

United States Department of Health and Human Services. (2000). *Healthy people 2010: Understanding and improving health*. Washington, DC: Office of Disease Prevention and Health Promotion.

CHAPTER 22

Immigrant Vulnerability: Does Capitalism in the United States Matter?

Jenny Hsin-Chun Tsai

Objectives

At the end of this chapter, the reader will be able to

1. Identify key factors that contribute to vulnerability in immigrants.
2. Describe a plan for a qualitative study on Chinese immigrants.
3. Describe how United States society can shape the lives of Chinese immigrants.

WWW

International migration (or immigration) is an ancient phenomenon. With globalization, this old phenomenon is happening faster and becoming more diversified than ever before. In 1997 in the United States alone, 25.8 million persons—9.7% of the total U.S. population—were immigrants (Schmidley & Gibson, 1999). In 2000, the number of immigrants increased to 28.4 million, representing 10.4% of the nation's total population (Lollock, 2001). The most recent American Community Survey estimates (U.S. Census Bureau American FactFinder, 2008) suggest that there are 37.9 million immigrants, accounting for 12.5% of the total U.S. population, and showing a steady increase in all areas of in the United States. Schmidley and Gibson's (1999) projection indicates that from 1995 to 2050, 40% of the total immigrant population will be Hispanic, 30% will be from Asia and the Pacific Islands, 20% will be non-Hispanic whites, and 10% will be African American. As a result, demand for culturally competent care is knocking on the doors of clinicians, educators, researchers, and healthcare administrators harder than ever before.

Scientists believe that as a result of the extensive upheavals involved in immigration, the health of immigrants is threatened and their risk for poor health is increased after resettlement. In other words, changes experienced during transition add to the vulnerability of immigrants

(Meleis, 1996). With regard to mental health, Ödegaard's (1932) investigation in the United States regarding mental illness in adult immigrants; Rutter et al.'s (1974) survey of children in the United Kingdom; Munroe-Blum, Boyle, Offord, and Kates' (1989) study of children in Canada; Baider and colleagues' (1996) work with Russian immigrants in Israel; Barnes' (2001) screening of recent refugees in the United States; Griffin and Soskolne's (2003) cross-sectional study of Thai migrant agricultural workers' psychosocial distress in Israel; Sundaram, Oin, and Zøllner's (2006) investigation of suicide risks among foreign-born individuals in Denmark; Anbesse and colleagues' (2009) qualitative study of mental health issues of Ethiopian female domestic migrants to Middle Eastern countries; and many other works show various kinds and degrees of adverse mental health consequences for immigrants and refugees.

Studies from other scholars further show factors that are associated with the health status and vulnerability of immigrants. For example, Anderson's study (1985) with Indo-Canadian and Greek women in Canada found that the women's help-seeking experiences were affected by their own perceptions of health, inability on the part of health professionals to grasp the circumstances of their lives, and their experiences of discrimination. Studies with Polish immigrants (Aroian, 1990), Iranian immigrants (Lipson, 1992), and Korean immigrants (Nah, 1993) in the United States showed that language and occupational accommodation were two key factors for successful resettlement. The existence of ethnocultural communities in the area where immigrants move was also found to be important for immigrants' psychosocial adaptation and health (Baker, Arseneault, & Gallant, 1994; Tsai, 2006). Weitzman and Berry's work with poor immigrant women in New York (1992) indicated that being poor and being an immigrant contributed to these women's limited use of U.S. medical care and poor health status. Notably, these women faced even greater barriers to health care than poor and uninsured Americans did.

The transition during immigration and resettlement adds to the vulnerability of immigrants. Nevertheless, this vulnerability is not a static, self-contained entity. Immigrant vulnerability is produced through ongoing interactions with social, economic, political, and cultural structures of the receiving country. Chopoorian (1986) reminded members of the nursing profession that a lack of consciousness about social, political, economic, and cultural factors prevents nurses from arriving at a comprehensive view of human health. Such a lack of consciousness about these issues keeps the profession in a peripheral role in the larger arena of social, economic, and political affairs of the United States. To promote the health of immigrants, health professionals need to "acquire, through their education, a theoretical base that allows them to analyze the socioeconomic and political factors that influence health care delivery" (Anderson, 1991, p. 716) and other aspects of everyday life.

Partial findings of a critical ethnographic study (Tsai, 2001) are presented in this chapter to highlight the effects that the receiving country's economic structure has on the vulnerability of immigrants. These effects are illustrated through events of these individuals' daily lives, their psychosocial reactions, and the adaptive strategies they used during resettlement in the receiving country. The implications of these findings for U.S. health professionals are then discussed.

DESCRIPTION OF THE STUDY

This critical ethnographic study took place in a metropolitan area in the northwest region of the United States between 1998 and 2000. It was designed to explore how immigrant families' lives are shaped by the larger societal context of the receiving country. Data were collected from nine Taiwanese immigrant families recruited through community snowball referrals. Participants were protected through compliance with the university-approved procedures for human subjects.

Sample

A total of 29 participants, representing these 9 families, contributed to the overall data. Of the 29 participants, 16 were parents with a mean age of 45.3 years (standard deviation [SD] = 2.4). Nine had completed college (16 years) in Taiwan, and four had advanced education (3 master's degrees and 1 doctorate) in North America. As for the 13 children, they were between 8 and 21 years of age, with a mean of 16.1 years (SD = 3.7). Their education ranged from second grade to first year of college.

These families arrived in the United States as immigrants between January 1989 and August 1998 through three mechanisms: own employment ($n = 3$), sponsored by siblings who were naturalized U.S. citizens ($n = 4$), and returning to the United States ($n = 2$) (in which case, one of the key family members already had permanent resident status or citizenship in the United States). Most families ($n = 8$) lived in middle-class areas.

Data Generation

Participants were interviewed one to three times, alone or with other family members. All interviews were semistructured and were conducted primarily in Chinese. English was occasionally used with children who were limited in Chinese proficiency or to convey certain ideas. All of the interviews were conducted at home, with the exception of one participant who chose to meet at a restaurant because his parents and sibling did not participate. The length of visit for each interview ranged from 1.5 to 10 hours. Interviews were recorded on audiotape with the consent of the participants. During the interview visits, observations were undertaken to learn about family dynamics, family structure, family affect, daily family activities, the physical home environment, network contacts, and opinions about extrafamilial environments.

In addition to interviews and observations, each participant completed a demographic and immigration questionnaire at the end of the first interview. The children's version had 21 items and collected each child's demographic information. The adult version had 41 items that gathered each adult participant's individual information and his or her family information. Both Chinese and English versions were available. Assistance was available at the scene to help participants complete the questionnaires.

Data Analysis and Scientific Rigor

Descriptive statistics (frequency, mean, and SD) were used to analyze the questionnaire data.

Narrative analytical technique (Riessman, 1993) guided the analysis of the interview data. In the first step, interviews were transcribed from audiotapes to paper (in Chinese).

Both verbal and nonverbal communications were preserved in the Chinese transcripts. After close examination of the Chinese transcripts, portions of the Chinese language transcripts (i.e., narrative segments) were selected, translated, and preserved in the English-language transcripts for in-depth analysis.

Substantive and methodological codes were written next to the highlighted narrative segments. Other analytical notes were also written next to the related narrative segments. Ongoing comparisons of stories across different family members in the same family and across families were made during the analysis process. Ongoing consultation with senior researchers and colleagues with diverse backgrounds, as well as confirmation with participants, refined the analysis. Fewer and fewer new codes were generated with each newly analyzed interview after half of the interviews were analyzed. Codes gradually merged and became more abstract and analytical. HyperRESEARCH (Version 2.03), a computer-assisted qualitative software, was used to manage the data and emerging codes.

FINDINGS

The in-depth analysis revealed that four aspects of U.S. societal context shaped the everyday lives of immigrants. One of these was economic—that is, the norms, values, and practices defined by U.S. capitalism; the other aspects were immigration policy, Western imperialism, and social class. Marketing culture, insurance, and credit were the three themes of the economic context identified in the data related to U.S. capitalism.

Marketing Culture

Marketing culture refers to "the degree [to] which the norms and practices of business for selling products and making profits for business owners influence immigrants" (Tsai, 2001, p. 168). Similar to what occurs in the rest of the U.S. population, families in this study received multiple phone calls, mailings, or in-person visits for various product sales and donations. Taiwan is a capitalist country, yet its economic structure and culture differ from those found in the United States. In particular, the United States emphasizes individualism and the free market, whereas Taiwan emphasizes collectivism and tighter government control.

Participant families had different cultural knowledge about and conceptions of telecommunications and product sales. Many of them complained about their contacts with sales representatives in the United States. "Ordering magazines is the same [problem]. They knock on your door all the time. Ask you to order, ask you for donation. Many of this type of problem," said one family (Tsai, 2001, pp. 168–169). They were distressed, bothered, and frustrated by these practices and the hassles derived from these practices. As one participant said, "We only called Taiwan for a few minutes. Why it cost so much?! We later knew the reason [because we did not sign up for any long-distance promotion plan]. There is only one phone company in Taiwan. You just need a phone and then you have everything" (mother of two, living in the United States for 18 months at the time of the interview) (Tsai, 2001, p. 168).

Some families were concerned and worried about being cheated or having financial or even legal complications because "there are charges against some wrongdoing all the time in

America. Lawsuits are everywhere" (Tsai, 2001, p. 169). The levels of frustration and worry were found to be higher within the participant families who were less proficient in English or who did not have friends or relatives in the area to which they moved.

Families usually thought of strategic solutions to decrease their stress level and protect themselves after a few bad experiences with sales people. For instance, some families chose to say no to everything and stick with whatever (telephone company, magazine subscription) they had at the time. After learning from friends or relatives with knowledge about the U.S. marketing culture, another strategy was sometimes adopted by the immigrants: speaking with a strange foreign accent or improper grammar in hopes that this behavior would stop salespersons from further explaining their products. Some families adapted to the U.S. marketing culture by adjusting their personal perceptions. They treated the money lost to purchasing products they regretted as the "tuition" they had to spend as part of their immigration journey. "Be careful" was the phrase used by some participants throughout the interviews.

Insurance

Insurance is "the types and amounts of insurance necessary to adequately protect the families" (Tsai, 2001, p. 171). Health and life insurance were exported from the United States to Taiwan decades ago. Thus Taiwanese are familiar with the concepts of health and life insurance. Because of the increasing use of cars in Taiwan, car insurance was adopted in Taiwan in the mid-1990s. After participant families immigrated, they began to realize that many more types of insurance existed in the United States. As one participant said, "Everything needs to be insured." The expense of insurance was much higher than they had expected.

The participant families' greatest concern was the cost of health insurance. Taiwan has a universal healthcare system. Having to purchase one's own health insurance when not employed was an unfamiliar concept to families who were new to the United States. In one family who immigrated as an investment, members did not realize that they needed to purchase individual health insurance until they became involved in the local Taiwanese community. Families felt helpless in the face of the high cost of health insurance; at the same time, they could not go without insurance. Unfortunately, the road to finding a health insurance plan was not straightforward. There are many insurance plans offered by different companies. Before participant families could even make a decision, they had to learn about copayments, deductibles, preferred doctors, prevention, and so forth. For participant families who spoke limited English, choosing an insurance plan was challenging. They had to rely on relatives or friends in the area (more so than did those families who were comfortable with English) to resolve the insurance issues.

To overcome the problems with insurance, the first step was staying as healthy as possible to avoid healthcare expenses while the family was looking for jobs that offered benefits. One family said, "When we just got here, we had no insurance. Could not get sick! We bore with it for half a year. Took some over-the-counter drugs [when we're sick]" (Tsai, 2001, p. 173). Some families flew back to Taiwan for their healthcare needs, usually the nonemergency kind, because as one participant said, "Add a round trip ticket on top of [the treatment cost], I still have plenty left. It's still cost-effective" (Tsai, 2001, p. 172). A few families would just pay for the insurance regardless of the cost because they knew the importance of having insurance in the United States.

Credit

Credit refers to "the degree of which the value of credit affects immigrant families in the [United States]" (Tsai, 2001, p. 174). In capitalism, credit means money and profits (Weber, 1992). Credit history—a widely used concept in the United States—is employed to assess a prospective customer's potential for profit making for the business owner. A good credit history means a potential for making profits from this prospective customer. However, credit history is not a concept that exists in Taiwan. Thus families living in the United States for the first time were surprised and confused when apartment managers asked about credit history and requested investigation fees. Although families in the study were lucky enough to have the investigation waived, some had friends who could not even rent an apartment because they had no credit history at the time. One family said that a friend had to pay six months' rent in advance in cash to secure a place to live.

The lack of credit history not only presented problems for immigrants' access to housing, but also hampered their ability to get loans and credit cards and, ironically, chances to build up their credit history. In the area of loan and credit card applications, no family was lucky with these services. As one unhappy family described their experience: "American banks were not willing to loan to us because he wants you to use credit as deposit, right? Chinese use properties as deposit for loans. That's the difference" (Tsai, 2001, p. 128). Families eventually turned to Chinese-owned banks for help. Regardless of the fact that the process with Chinese-owned banks was not completely smooth, families at least got the loan or credit card from the bank as a start.

DISCUSSION

Decades of studies of immigrant experiences have informed us of the resettlement experience and its accompanying threats to immigrant health in countries such as Canada, the United Kingdom, and the United States. Analysis of the stories of nine Taiwanese immigrant families reveals that immigrants' everyday life is inseparable from the economic structure of the receiving country. Three capitalist practices—the marketing culture, insurance, and credit—create a living context that increases immigrants' vulnerability in the United States.

The financial burden, potential legal ramifications, and limited access to housing, loans, and health care are not the kinds of experiences that immigrants to the United States anticipate before their immigration. Literature has shown that when people move into a new country they have to adapt, to varying extents, to the language used by the receiving country, the physical environment, the culture, the systems, the loss of social support, and economic survival (Aroian, 1990; Baker et al., 1994; Lipson, 1992; Sam & Berry, 1995; Tsai, 2001). These adaptive processes can last from years to a lifetime. Such unexpected experiences represent additional stressors that place individuals in the United States at risk while they are attempting to manage the other demands they must face as immigrants. Moreover, as part of the capitalist environment or economic structure, people in the United States are always bombarded with sales promotions for new products, business changes, new insurance coverage, and increases in healthcare costs. Even Americans who were born and raised in the United States struggle to understand the changes and choices available to them and to deal with these economic practices.

Immigrants—and particularly new immigrants—can easily get lost in the massive amount of information thrown at them. Making an informed decision is a much more challenging and stressful process for new immigrants than for native-born Americans and established early-wave immigrants. In other words, immigrants' vulnerability exists along a continuum. The degree of the vulnerability increases when the receiving country's economic structure intersects with immigrants' language challenges, unfamiliarity with the systems, or limited access to local social networks for support. In this study, the participant families (who had been in the United States no more than 10 years) discussed their self-doubt about the decisions they made; they revealed their worries and frustration about the financial and legal consequences of their decisions. Unlike those citizens born in the United States, immigrants can face deportation for numerous legal issues (e.g., not reporting an address change to the immigration authority, speeding tickets, credit problems, or crime). Thus, not only are immigrants concerned about the same financial and legal consequences as the people of the receiving country, but they also need to worry about the legal consequences specifically tied to their immigration status.

Navarro (1993, 2003) argues that the problems of the U.S. healthcare system cannot be understood without including capitalism—the moving force behind the financing and delivery of health services in the United States—in the discussion. Health insurance companies are controlled by corporate owners and have a tremendous power over how services are provided by health care providers. Profit and efficiency are the bases for their decision. Insurance premiums are raised to cover growing medical costs and ensure profits. In response, employers shift the cost of insurance premiums to their employees or provide limited choices of insurance plans or no insurance at all. More people become uninsured and face greater barriers to access health care for treatment and illness prevention (Asplin et al., 2005; Himmelstein, Woolhandler, & Hellander, 2001; Kleinke, 2001; McCollister, Arheart, Lee, Fleming, Davila, & LeBlanc, 2010; Taylor, Larson, & Correa-de-Araujo, 2006). Capitalism in the United States has an intimate relationship with immigrants' everyday experience: This economic framework not only shapes the nation's healthcare system, but also drives the production of goods and marketing, the creation of insurance policies, and access to those things which fill basic needs. To decrease immigrants' vulnerability and promote their health, it is absolutely essential to include capitalism in the discussion.

IMPLICATIONS FOR HEALTH PROFESSIONALS

Health professionals have ample opportunities to work with immigrants: in acute care settings, primary care settings, long-term care facilities, community clinics, workplaces, home settings, and schools. In fact, health professionals are in a valuable position to ensure health equity for immigrants.

This section offers some ways for health professionals to be true health advocates for this often vulnerable population.

As a micro-level approach, during visits health professionals should include questions that can help them better understand the effects of the U.S. capitalist economic structure and practices on the stress levels and well-being of immigrant clients. Because immigrant clients are already using their individual resources (e.g., personal intelligence and knowledge, social networks) to develop sufficient strategies to overcome those stressors, health professionals can (and should) serve as another resource for these clients. If immigrant clients do not have adequate individual resources to develop effective adaptive strategies, health professionals should then initiate the discussion and collaborate with the clients to formulate some potentially practical and successful strategies.

In addition to changing their own practices, health professionals should share their knowledge with their colleagues and policy makers to heighten their awareness of the effects of the receiving country's economic structure on immigrants' vulnerability and health status. With such greater awareness, fewer health professionals and policy makers will use culture or language barrier as a catch-all category to explain all immigrant experiences (McGrath, 1998; Tsai, 2003). Instead, more will have a more comprehensive understanding of immigrants' experiences and healthcare needs. As a result, more health professionals and policy makers will provide relevant interventions for the immigrant population and engage in the reconstruction of social and health policies that are driven by U.S. capitalism—a system that is beyond immigrants' control, yet has tremendous effects on their everyday lives.

CLOSING THOUGHTS

Immigrants are at a higher risk for poor health. Nevertheless, their risk is not solely a result of their language skills, education, levels of assimilation to the receiving country, or knowledge about the systems of the receiving country. The country's own historical, sociocultural, economic, and political structures play significant roles in shaping immigrants' everyday experiences and health status. This chapter has provided some preliminary insights into the effects of the U.S. economic structure on immigrant vulnerability. To provide culturally competent care to the immigrant population, further investigation into each of these structural effects and their interactions with immigrants' vulnerability is crucial. Cross-national comparison is needed as well. Of course, it is also necessary for more health professionals and policy makers to recognize that the health experiences and stresses that immigrants identify are, indeed, products of complex social processes. Immigrants then will not be blamed for their problems while the "causes" of the problems lie in the larger societal context.

ACKNOWLEDGMENTS

This chapter is based on the author's dissertation study. The study was supported in part by the American Nurses Foundation, the Psi-Chapter-at-Large of the Sigma Theta Tau International, the Robert Gilbert Foundation of the Association of Child and Adolescent Psychiatric Nurses, and the Hester McLaws Nursing Scholarship Fund of the University of Washington School of Nursing. An earlier version of this chapter was presented at the 2nd State of Science Congress in Washington, D.C., in September 2002.

For a full suite of assignments and additional learning activities, use the access code located in the front of your book to visit this exclusive website: http://go.jblearning.com/dechesnay. If you do not have an access code, you can obtain one at the site.

REFERENCES

Anbesse, B., Hanlon, C., Alem, A., Packer, S., & Whitley, R. (2009). Migration and mental health: A study of low-income Ethiopian women working in Middle Eastern countries. *International Journal of Social Psychiatry, 55*, 557–568. doi: 10.1177/0020764008096704

Anderson, J. M. (1985). Perspectives on the health of immigrant women: A feminist analysis. *Advances in Nursing Science, 8*(1), 61–76.

Anderson, J. M. (1991). Immigrant women speak of chronic illness: The social construction of the devalued self. *Journal of Advanced Nursing, 16*, 710–717. doi: 10.1111/j.1365-2648.1991.tb01729.x

Aroian, K. J. (1990). A model of psychological adaptation to migration and resettlement. *Nursing Research, 39*, 5–10.

Asplin, B. R., Rhodes, K. V., Levy, H., Lurie, N., Crain, A. L., Carlin, B. P., & Kellermann, A. L. (2005). Insurance status and access to urgent ambulatory care follow-up appointments. *Journal of the American Medical Association, 294*, 1248–1254.

Baider, L., Ever-Hadani, P., & DeNour A. K. (1996). Crossing new bridges: The process of adaptation and psychosocial distress of Russian immigrants in Israel. *Psychiatry, 59*, 175–183.

Baker, C., Arseneault, A. M., & Gallant, G. (1994). Resettlement without the support of an ethnocultural community. *Journal of Advanced Nursing, 20*, 1064–1072. doi: 10.1046/j.1365-2648.1994.20061064.x

Barnes, D. M. (2001). Mental health screening in a refugee population: A program report. *Journal of Immigrant Health, 3*, 141–149.

Chopoorian, T. J. (1986). Reconceptualization the environment. In P. Moccia (Ed.). *New approaches to theory development* (pp. 39–54). New York: National League for Nursing.

Griffin, J., & Soskolne, V. (2003). Psychosocial distress among Thai migrant workers in Israel. *Social Science and Medicine, 57*, 769–774.

Himmelstein, D., Woolhandler, S., & Hellander, I. (2001). *Bleeding the patient: The consequences of corporate health care.* Monroe, ME: Common Courage.

HyperRESEARCH (Version 2.03) [Computer software]. Thousand Oaks, CA: ResearchWare.

Kleinke, J. D. (2001). *Oxymorons: The myth of a US health care system.* San Francisco, CA: Jossey-Bass.

Lipson, J. G. (1992). The health and adjustment of Iranian immigrants. *Western Journal of Nursing Research, 14*, 10–29. doi:10.1177/019394599201400102

Lollock, L. (2001). *The foreign-born population in the United States: March 2000, current population reports* (U.S. Census Bureau, Current Population Reports P20–534). Washington, DC: U.S. Census Bureau.

McCollister, K. E., Arheart, K. L., Lee, D. J., Fleming, L. E., Davila, E. P. LeBlanc, W. G., . . . Erard, M. J. (2010). Declining health insurance access among Hispanic workers: Not all jobs are created equal. *American Journal of Industrial Medicine, 53*, 163–170. doi: 10.1002/ajim.20720

McGrath, B. B. (1998). Illness as a problem of meaning: Moving culture from the classroom to the clinic. *Advances in Nursing Science, 21*(2), 17–29.

Meleis, A. I. (1996). Culturally competent scholarship: Substance and rigor. *Advances in Nursing Science, 19*(2), 1–16.

Munroe-Blum, H., Boyle, M. H., Offord, D. R., & Kates, N. (1989). Immigrant children: Psychiatric disorder, school performance, and service utilization. *American Journal of Orthopsychiatry, 59*, 510–519. doi: 10.1111/j.1939-0025.1989.tb02740.x

Nah, K. (1993). Perceived problems and service delivery for Korean immigrants. *Social Work, 38*(3), 289–296.

Navarro, V. (1993). *Dangerous to your health: Capitalism in health care.* New York: Monthly Review Press.

Navarro, V. (2003). Policy without politics: The limits of social engineering. *American Journal of Public Health, 93*, 64–67.

Ödegaard, O. (1932). Emigration and insanity. *Acta Psychiatrica et Neurologia*, Suppl 4, Copenhagen, 11–206.

Riessman, C. K. (1993). In P. Manning, J. Van Maanen, & M. Miller (Eds.), *Narrative analysis.* Newbury Park, CA: Sage.

Rutter, M., Yule, W., Berger, M., Yule, B., Morton, J., & Bagley, C. (1974). Children of West Indian immigrants—I: Rates of behavioral deviance and of psychiatric disorder. *Journal of Child Psychology and Psychiatry, 15*, 241–262.

Sam, D. L., & Berry, J. W. (1995). Acculturative stress among young immigrants in Norway. *Scandinavian Journal of Psychology, 36*, 10–24. doi: 10.1111/j.1467-9450.1995.tb00964.x

Schmidley, A. D., & Gibson, C. (1999). *Profile of the foreign–born population in the United States: 1997* (U.S. Census Bureau, Current Population Reports P23–195). Washington, DC: U.S. Government Printing Office.

Sundaram, V., Oin, P., & Zøllner, L. (2006). Suicide risk among persons with foreign background in Denmark. *Suicide & Life-Threatening Behavior, 36*(4), 481–489.

Taylor, A. K., Larson, S, & Correa-de-Araujo, R. (2006). Women's health care utilization and expenditures. *Women's Health Issues, 16*, 66–79.

Tsai, J. H. C. (2001). *One story, two interpretations: The lived experiences of Taiwanese immigrant families in the United States.* Unpublished doctoral dissertation, University of Washington, Seattle.

Tsai, J. H. C. (2003). Contextualizing immigrants' lived experience: Story of Taiwanese immigrants in the United States. *Journal of Cultural Diversity, 10*, 76–83.

Tsai, J. H. C. (2006). Xenophobia, ethnic community, and immigrant youths' friendship network formation. *Adolescence, 41*(162), 285–298.

U.S. Census Bureau American FactFinder. (2008). *2008 American Community Survey 1-year estimates.* Retrieved from http://factfinder.census.gov/home/saff/main.html?_lang=en

Weber, M. (1930/1992). *The protestant ethic and the spirit of capitalism* (A. Giddens, Trans.). London: Routledge.

Weitzman, B. C., & Berry, C. A. (1992). Health status and health care utilization among New York City home attendants: An illustration of the needs of working poor, immigrant women. *Women and Health, 19*(2/3), 87–105. doi: 10.1300/J013v19n02_05

UNIT IV

Practice

The ones who are crazy enough to think they can change the world are the ones who do.

—Steve Jobs
www.quotationspage.com

Predisposition to Non-insulin-dependent Diabetes Mellitus Among Former–Soviet Union Immigrants

Nataly Pasumansky

Objectives

At the end of this chapter, the reader will be able to

1. Explain why immigrants from the former Soviet Union might be at risk for diabetes.
2. Describe a cultural approach to intervention with diabetic immigrants from the former Soviet Union.
3. Compare and contrast the uses of natural remedies with diabetic immigrants from the former Soviet Union.

Scientific articles and media reports have documented the existence of a worldwide epidemic of diabetes. Likewise, surveys about prevalence of diabetes in the United States have reported that diabetes increased 33% between 1990 and 1998, with rates continuing to increase steadily (Levetan, 2001). According to a report published by the Centers for Disease Control and Prevention (CDC), diabetes is currently the sixth leading cause of death in the United States.

Prevention and treatment of diabetes are difficult tasks that require both a cultural and an individual approach. The National Diabetes Information Clearinghouse (NDIC, 2003) emphasizes that certain ethnic groups have an increased incidence of diabetes among adults 20 years old and older. Many cultural groups, new immigrants among them, are also known to have an increased incidence of diabetes. Given the stress of immigration and the associated changes of lifestyle and diet, new immigrants are more prone to diabetes. One such group, former–Soviet Union immigrants, needs special attention because it includes many elderly and chronically ill persons.

Former–Soviet Union immigrants often have poor dietary habits and sedentary lifestyles that put them at risk of developing obesity—a major risk factor for diabetes. With the collapse of the former Soviet Union, many people there became poor and resorted to the only diet that they can afford, usually high in calories and carbohydrates with few fresh fruits and vegetables. In addition, with little emphasis on prevention, former–Soviet Union immigrants have little awareness of healthy diet and lifestyle options; therefore, diabetes is often diagnosed late, when the disease is already in progress. After immigration, persons with diabetes and prediabetes have a difficult time learning a new language and finding a job, causing them to pay less attention to their health. In addition, these immigrants often are poor and have no access to basic health care.

Healthcare access for former–Soviet Union immigrants is also complicated because of their diversity. Those who immigrate to the United States often come from different republics of the former Soviet Union, though the majority come from Russia and the Ukraine. Most know the Russian language; however, some immigrants who came from other places, such as Latvia or Uzbekistan, may not know or be not fluent in Russian. In addition, immigrants from these areas have different customs and religions. Even though interpreter services may be helpful, it is still not easy to accommodate the diverse cultural groups in this vulnerable population.

Nurse practitioners (NPs) who manage former–Soviet Union immigrants require understanding of specific cultural behaviors and dietary habits. Advanced practice nurses may be particularly appropriate to care for Russian-speaking immigrants because they usually spend more time with patients than physicians. In addition, advanced practice nurses focus on developing individualized, cost-effective treatment plans. NPs may have more expertise at gaining patients' trust because of the additional time spent with patients and their traditional education to treat the whole patient, including lifestyle modifications. With an increased knowledge of health practices and the historical background of immigrants, NPs may have higher adherence rates among their patients.

A culturally sensitive approach to diabetes education and treatment has been suggested in many publications (London, 2002; Public Health Seattle and King County, 2001). Diabetes treatment depends on many factors, including as stress, diet, and healthy lifestyle; therefore, cultural aspects and trends are building blocks for understanding how to treat diabetes in Russian-speaking immigrants. Unfortunately, little is known about Russian-speaking immigrants and diabetes. Thus NPs will need to assess risk factors and develop customized plans for prevention of diabetes and diabetic complications in the immigrant population from the former Soviet Union.

LITERATURE REVIEW

A cultural approach in diabetes treatment and prevention is important for NPs and other healthcare providers. The existing body of literature addresses diabetes in different ethnic groups such as Chinese, Vietnamese, Cambodians, and Latinos (Adams, 2003; Mull, Nguyen, & Dennis, 2001; Rankin, Galbraith, & Huang, 1997). The increased mortality rate among Russian immigrants from chronic diseases including diabetes was a major concern for Israel and has been studied from a variety of perspectives (Ben-Noun, 1994, 1995; Rennert, Luz, Tamir, & Peterburg, 2002). The incidence of chronic diseases has been reported to be significantly higher in Russian Jewish immigrants than in Israeli veterans (Brodov, Mandelzweig, Boyko, & Behar, 2002; Rennert et al., 2002). This problem of chronic diseases among Russian immigrants significantly influenced Israeli mortality statistics and required changes in the Israeli medical system. However, little is known about diabetes among the community of former–Soviet Union immigrants in the United States.

Preventive Care Practices Among Former–Soviet Union Immigrants

The literature indicates that in Russia, health promotion is poor, with people usually going to their provider only if they have health problems, especially in the middle-age group (Aroian, Khatusky, Tran, & Balsam, 2001; Mehler, Scott, & Pines, 2001). Female Russian immigrants tend not to use health screening resources such as blood pressure checks, cholesterol screening, Pap smear, mammography, and breast self-examination. According to Ivanov and Buck (2002), former–Soviet Union immigrants do not believe in health prevention and usually do not visit a clinic for screening exams. In addition, women do not receive information about the need for such screening measurements (Ivanov & Buck, 2002).

Heavy cigarette smoking, high alcohol consumption, poor dietary intake, and little attention to physical fitness have contributed to chronic health problems in the Russian population (Duncan & Simmons, 1996; Mehler et al., 2001). A major problem identified in the former Soviet Union was the absence of basic health screening measurements such as cholesterol testing, high blood pressure screening, Pap smear, and mammogram (Duncan & Simmoms, 1996). Authors did not mention the importance of glucose screening for this population with multiple risk factors, however.

Russian articles about diabetes say that people are aware of healthy lifestyle, healthy diet, and health promotion, but they pay more attention to those aspects of health when they already have a health problem. According to the Russian Federation Ministry of Health, there is no appropriate preventive care for diabetes. When the Ministry of Health did an investigation in Tumen (a medium-size city in Russia) in 2000, however, millions of patients were diagnosed with diabetes. Those patients already had serious cardiac problems as a result of hidden diabetes (Ministry of Health, Russian Federation, n.d.). Manvelov (1999), a Russian physician, noted in his article that 50% of patients who suffered a cerebral vascular accident (CVA) in Russia may have had diabetes as a risk factor before the CVA occurred. He also stated that the diabetes rate in Russia is in the range of 4% to 5%, but in some populations may be as high as 20%. This high prevalence of diabetes among Russians suggests that the genetic component of diabetes plays a role in this population, making it a unique problem for Russian immigrants in the United States or elsewhere in the world.

The adverse effects of diabetes, similar to the situation with some other chronic conditions (e.g., cardiovascular diseases), may be minimized with appropriate nonmedication care. "Medical nutritional therapy, exercises and diabetes education" can treat diabetes and prevent complications (Levetan, 2001). In addition, Colagiuri et al. (2010) note that social support is a most important factor for prevention of diabetes complications. Russian families can be very supportive, but they may not understand the importance of prevention or early treatment of diabetes. Even though former–Soviet Union immigrants are usually highly educated, they have little disease prevention knowledge. A CDC task force recommended diabetes education information be made widely available in communities (CDC, 2003). Unfortunately, because of language and cultural barriers, Russian-speaking immigrants often do not attend community education meetings. Thus education on a one-on-one basis by NPs may be more beneficial for them.

Diet and Obesity Among Russian-Speaking Immigrants

Dietary habits vary within different cultural groups. Russian-speaking immigrants are a diverse group, and they have different eating patterns. Nevertheless, knowing the most common Russian diet patterns is important for NPs so that they can discuss dietary changes with these clients if needed. Brown (2003) emphasized that more studies are needed to examine nutritional habits among ethnic groups and highlighted how important it is for healthcare providers to understand their patients' specific cultural diet and help people adjust for a healthier lifestyle.

Diet habits depend on cultural differences and vary from country to country within the former Soviet Union. Diets in Russia are typically high in carbohydrates and fat and low in vegetables. Oystragh (1980), a Russian-speaking physician practicing in Australia, conducted a study on Russian Jewish immigrants in Australia. In his practice, he performed routine urine and serum glucose tests on new patients; he found that in his case load, there were 15 diabetic patients among the total 158 patients—9.49%, a much higher rate than the average Australian incidence of 3.0%. He attributed the increased diabetes rate to two main factors: the high-stress period of immigration and a diet "extremely high in starches, where potatoes, bread, cakes, biscuits are eaten in almost every meal" (Oystragh, 1980, p. 270). The author observed only a small group of immigrants but he believed that this small group provided an accurate picture of the dietary habits of many Russian immigrants.

Obesity as a result of poor dietary habits is a major risk factor for developing non-insulin-dependent diabetes mellitus (NIDDM). Nikitin (1989) found that people who migrated to the eastern region of the Soviet Union, Siberia, increased their risk of developing diabetes, with obesity being an important risk factor in this trend. More than half of woman who migrated to Siberia experienced a rapid weight gain during the first years of migration (Nikitin, 1989). A more recent study of 644 Russian immigrants in New York found that they were also at increased risk of development of diabetes. Thus former–Soviet Union immigrants are "invisible minorities" with high diabetes risk, and the main predisposition factor among them is obesity (Hosler, 2003).

In Popkin's study (1998), data were collected from a Russian longitudinal monitoring survey. Analysis of these data revealed a consistent increase in adult and particularly elderly obesity. Popkin (1998) found that the overall increase in the total obesity rate was more than 5 percentage points per 10-year period in Russia. The same author also emphasized that prevalence of NIDDM and many cardiovascular conditions related to NIDDM, such as hypertension, dyslipidemia, and atherosclerosis, is increasing rapidly in poor countries.

Another study conducted in Russia by Zabina et al. (2001) observed that in Russia, as in the United States, the cause of chronic deseases is typically related to lifestyle risk factors such as poor diet and inadequate physical activity. According to these researchers' survey of 542 men and 1,151 women living in Moscow, more than half of men were currently smoking at the time of the study, and more than half of men and women had a body mass index (BMI) greater than 25, signifying that they were overweight (Zabina et al., 2001). These results are consistent with the findings of Duncan and Simmons (1996), who used physical assessment data of 30 Russian immigrants to show that 65% of participants were overweight, yet only 14% were advised to lose weight. Duncan and Simmons (1996) questioned whether former–Soviet Union immigrants are aware of obesity as a health problem. In contrast, studies carried out by Ministry of Health of Russian Federation showed that Russian immigrants who have been diagnosed with diabetes are aware of the importance of diet in the treatment of diabetes, because many studies published in Russian focus on the need for a healthy diet in diabetes (Sharafertdinov, Mesheryakoba, & Plotnikova, 1997). Nevertheless, a review of the Russian-language literature did not show any encouraging information about diabetes prevention and suggestions for diet change prior to disease onset.

Medication Versus Natural Remedies

In the former Soviet Union, as in other countries, including the United States, a variety of medications are available for treatment of diabetes. However, the use of natural remedies in Russian cultures remains open to discussion. In an older article by Wheat et al. (1983), former-Soviet Jewish patients were found to consider all drugs to be poison and to believe more in natural remedies. Today the extent to which natural remedies are used for diabetes treatment in the Russian community is unknown. As in many other countries, urban and highly educated people may not even be aware of natural remedies; in contrast, the rural population may believe natural remedies to be best choice of treatment. NPs, as primary care providers, need to know the risks and benefits associated with these natural remedies.

Multiple studies in Russia focusing on the use of natural remedies have shown an increased interest in natural remedies. One of those studies about green coffee was done in Moscow Center for Modern Medicine, Russian Ministry of National Defense. Green coffee contains 55% chlorogenic acid, which is an antioxidant. Green coffee volunteers received 90 mg/day of either chlorogenic acid or placebo. Results showed that blood glucose levels dropped 15% to 20% in participants who received chlorogenic acid compared to those who did not. The researchers concluded that chlorogenic acid has a potential role in management of diabetes (Fields, 2003).

Another study used blueberry leaves tea (known as "chai cherniki" in Russian) for gastric colic and diabetes. Blueberry leaves extract contains caffeoylquinic acid and hydroxicinnamic acids (Jimenez del Rio, 2003). The study, which was conducted in the Moscow Center for Modern Medicine (the same center that performed the research about green coffee), showed that blueberry leaves extract "possesses physiologically significant glucose-reducing potencies" (Jimenez del Rio, 2003).

It is not known from the literature review whether those remedies are used often by Russian-speaking patients in the former Soviet Union or by immigrants. More studies are needed in the United States for detecting risks and benefits of these natural remedies, as they are not currently in wide used in this country.

Stress and NIDDM

Former–Soviet Union immigrants, like other immigrants, experience high levels of psychological stress. Smith (1996) noted that Russian immigrants leave to escape very poor living conditions and joblessness, but often face the same problems after entering the United States. They tend to end up in inner-city apartments in areas characterized by crime problems, have low status, and obtain low-paying jobs. With the stress of adapting to these multiple factors, Russian immigrants pay little attention to their health. Brodov et al. (2002), in studying 13,742 patients of two cohorts (Soviet Union and Israeli born), found a statistically significant difference in mortality rates after a 7-year follow-up to the heart disease screenings in the 1990's between the two groups (14.7% and 18.5%, respectively; $p < 0.001$). The main cause of mortality rates in this study were chronic diseases, especially coronary artery disease (CAD). However, the authors suggested that the reason for those chronic diseases was psychological stress: Stress has an adverse effect on many chronic diseases, including NIDDM.

Many Russian-speaking immigrants may consider stress to be a major risk factor for NIDDM onset (Meyerovich, 2003; Resick, 2008; Sidorov, Novikova, & Solov'ev, 2001). Multiple studies have demonstrated that stress affects glycemic control negatively in clients who already have type 1 or type 2 diabetes. Little research evaluating the relationship between stress and diabetes onset exists, however. Peyrot et al. (1999) found that stress affected glycemic control mostly because it leads to poor compliance with the treatment regimen; these authors suggested that there may also be a connection between stress and diabetes onset.

A study carried out by Fukunishi et al. (1998) with a sample of 600 persons indicated that poor utilization of social support is associated with the onset of glucose tolerance abnormality. These authors suggested that lack of social support from family, relatives, and friends as well as other stress-related factors are negatively correlated with glucose tolerance tests in persons not known to have diabetes.

Despite these findings, stress is rarely discussed as a risk factor for diabetes onset during healthcare visits. With Russian-speaking immigrants, who might believe in the relationship between diabetes and stress, this issue should be discussed by NPs during office visits.

CASE STUDIES

The case studies presented in this section illustrate the problems in caring for former–Soviet Union immigrants with diabetes. These case studies were recorded following the telephone interviews with the chosen participants. The names and some identifying details were altered to protect the privacy of the participants.

WWW Case Study 1: Boris

Boris S., a 75-year-old male refugee, emigrated with his family from Sverdlovsk, a large city in Russia, to the United States 8 years ago. Before emigrating, Boris worked as an engineer in a factory, where he sat most of the day. He had almost no physical activity after work. He was overweight, liked to eat foods rich in simple sugars, and had no family history of diabetes.

Boris was diagnosed with diabetes in Russia 10 years ago. Initially, he noticed that he was thirsty all the time. Boris asked people around him what the problem could be, and they recommended that he be checked by an endocrinologist. Boris went to a local endocrinologist, who did a blood sugar exam and sent Boris home, stating that Boris had no problem with his sugar. He continued to suffer from excessive thirst, however, and people around him started to notice that he was drinking water all the time. Boris went to endocrinologist once more, at which point the endocrinologist sent him to another place for glucose tolerance test. "They let me drink sugar and then tested my blood every hour," stated Boris. After this test, the physician diagnosed him with type 2 diabetes. The endocrinologist told Boris that the first time he visited he had pre-diabetes, but now his diagnosis was diabetes. According to the endocrinologist, his diabetes was caused by working in the stressful environment at the factory; the physician did not mention that Boris was overweight.

The endocrinologist gave Boris some diabetic Polish medication, enough to last for one month. Boris did not receive any specific education regarding his diabetes and was sent home without a glucometer. Every month he came to endocrinologist to check his blood sugar and to receive his diabetic medications. He knew that he should avoid simple carbohydrates in his diet, however, although that challenge remains very difficult for him. Every once in a while Boris eats food not recommended in his diabetic diet.

After Boris came to the United States, he was diagnosed with hypertension and CAD, which required open heart bypass surgery. In addition, he has spinal stenosis, making it difficult for him to do any exercises because of the back pain. "Physicians here recommend physical activity such as walking and bicycling, but I can't do anything because shooting pain in my spine and legs and in addition I walk like on pillows and cannot feel my legs well because of my diabetes neuropathy, so I continue to be overweight. When my son came to visit me, I noticed that he is getting big, and I suggested him immediately start to lose weight," said Boris.

Now Boris is visiting his primary care provider every three months. He checks his blood glucose at home. Boris does not believe in natural remedies. His diet now consists of mostly vegetables, some fruits, oatmeal, buckwheat, and all kind of meats. His primary care provider gives him instruction regarding a diabetic lifestyle, and he tries very hard to follow those instructions.

WWW Case Study 2: Marina

Marina P., 67 years old, emigrated to the United States as a refugee from Kiev, Ukraine. She was diagnosed with diabetes 14 years ago in Ukraine. Before emigrating, she worked as an accountant in a sewing factory. At work, she sat most of the time and did not have time for physical activity. As a result, she became overweight, although she did not perceive that it was a health problem.

For two years before she was diagnosed with diabetes mellitus, Marina felt thirsty all the time and had urinary urgency. Despite her symptoms, she did not seek medical help and continued to live with this "discomfort." Marina's friend, who was a physician, noticed that Marina frequently went to the restroom and suggested that she have her blood sugar checked.

When Marina went to the clinic and healthcare providers checked her blood and urine, it was determined that she already had diabetes. The physician suggested that there was something wrong with Marina's pancreas, but failed to mention her weight and her lifestyle as factors. Initially, her physician suggested consuming a low-carbohydrate diet and taking prescribed medications. When this regimen did not make Marina feel better, she started to take a Hungarian medication for diabetes. She did not have a glucometer at home; instead, she checked her blood sugar once in a month in a local clinic.

At the time of her immigration to the United States 9 years ago, Marina had very high blood glucose, kidney problems, arthritis, neuropathy, and poor vision. It was suggested that she take insulin, but she insisted on oral medications. As a first step, Marina was referred to a dietitian, with her daughter helping her with translation. She received prescriptions for three different types of diabetic medications, and now her blood sugars are stable and within normal limits.

Marina received education from her primary care provider and dietitian and decided not to go to diabetes support groups. For now, her diet consists mostly of a lot of vegetables, buckwheat, and meat. She likes potatoes and used to eat them in every dish before, but the dietitian asked her to reduce amount of potatoes to preserve a healthy diet. She still needs to reduce her weight but finds it difficult because of severe arthritis and diabetic neuropathy. "Diabetes is distorting everything," said Marina.

WWW Case Study 3: Tatiana

Tatiana, a 52-year-old female, emigrated from Yarkutsk, a city in northern Russia. She was diagnosed with diabetes in Russia about 15 years ago, shortly after she moved to Novosibirsk, in the southern part of Russia. While she had resided in the north, Tatiana had stopped eating fresh fruits and vegetables because no fresh products were available at the market; only during summertime could she eat fresh products that grew in her backyard. She also gained weight at that time. After her diagnosis, Tatiana did not take any some medications for diabetes and checked her blood sugar every month in a local clinic. At that time Tatiana had not received any education or information about diabetes, but she did read literature on her own to find out more about the disease.

In the 5 years after her initial diagnosis, Tatiana moved to the United States. At the time of her emigration, her diabetes was not under control. Tatiana also discovered that she had hyperlipidemia and hypertension, and that the multiple aches in her legs and arms actually were signs of diabetic neuropathy. Tatiana also was getting many ear and other bacterial infections, which she learned may be because of her diabetes, rather than a weak immune system as she was told in Russia.

In the United States, Tatiana started to take new medications for diabetes, hypertension, and hyperlipidemia and was referred to diabetic education. She refused to go to a diabetic education program, but did read a lot of books and articles about diabetes. Tatiana believes in natural remedies and uses them for her condition.

Recently Tatiana was informed that her diabetes is not under control and she needs to start insulin injections. She has refused to begin the recommended treatment. She has been under a lot of stress and believes that why her diabetes is not under control. In fact, she is sure that stress is a major factor in ensuring diabetes control.

Tatiana read about a new injectable medication and asked to start to use Byeta injections, but not insulin. Her blood sugars are now under better control, and she feels better and fewer body aches. Nevertheless, she refused to accept the fact that she may need to have insulin injections in the future.

Case Study 4: Svetlana

Svetlana, 70 years old, emigrated from Novosibirsk in Russia. She was diagnosed with diabetes 15 years ago in Russia. Her mother was also a diabetic; she died from diabetes complications. Svetlana was very anxious to discover that she has diabetes. In Russia, she was told to change her diet by not eating any sweets but did not receive any specific treatment for diabetes. Once a month, she went to a local clinic to check her blood sugar.

When Svetlana moved to the United States, she already had hypertension, coronary artery disease, and hyperlipidemia. She started a complex medication treatment and went with an interpreter to a diabetes education program. Svetlana learned a lot about lifestyle modifications and healthy diet and tried to lose weight. She started to eat a lot of vegetables, healthy grains that she used to eat in Russia, and limited amounts of potatoes, white bread, and sweets.

Despite all attempts to keep Svetlana's blood sugars within the recommended range, her diabetes was still not controlled and she started to develop neuropathic pain in her legs. Svetlana was told that she needed to initiate insulin treatment. She was very reluctant to do, because she did not want to use insulin like her mother for the rest of her life. With proper explanation that included cultural awareness of Svetlana's concerns, she finally agreed to start insulin treatment and went to diabetic education center to learn how to start insulin initiation.

Case Study 5: Oleg

Oleg, a 44-year-old male, immigrated to the United States from a small city at Ukraine 10 years ago. Oleg is a truck driver. On his annual physical exam, measurement of his HgbA1c led to the discovery that he has diabetes already in progress. A blood test also showed that he has hyperlipidemia. Oleg was invited for a follow-up and diabetes treatment initiation. He was overweight, but had no symptoms of polyuria, polyuria, polydipsia, or polyphagia. Oleg's diet consisted of a lot of white bread, potatoes, and other starches that he was taking from home to eat on his journeys. He did not visit fast-food restaurants while on the road, because he did not like the food there. As a truck driver, Oleg spent a lot of time sitting; he did not have time for physical activity after work.

Oleg was shocked when he was told that he has diabetes. He said that he had been under a lot of stress at his work, which he believed was the reason for his diabetes diagnosis. He agreed to start medication treatment for his diabetes. However, he also asked for natural remedies that were readily available and indicated that possibly he would be able not to take "all those chemicals that are harmful for my body." He also was sure that he will be cured with medications, lifestyle, and diet; with reduced stress, he suggested, he will not need any treatment in the future. Oleg refused to go to diabetes education program and asked a Russian-speaking provider to educate him on a one-on-one basis.

Case Study 6: Anna

Anna, a 56-year-old female, immigrated to the United States from Kharkov, a large town in Ukraine. She was diagnosed with NIDDM soon after immigration. Anna does not believe in any medications; therefore, she started to increase her physical activity and follow a strict diet after her diagnosis. Her diet consisted mostly of vegetables and some meat. Anna stated that she ate a lot of cabbage. In addition, she started to take natural remedies that were sent to her from Ukraine; later she found some natural remedies, similar to the Ukrainian versions, in the United States. Her blood sugars were still not under control, however, and she was also diagnosed with hyperlipidemia. Anna tried medication for her cholesterol, but the medication "destroyed her liver" and she stopped taking it.

Now Anna is not overweight but her blood sugars are not under control. Despite all attempts from several physicians, she refused to take any prescription medications for diabetes and hyperlipidemia, instead taking only natural remedies. Anna also refused to go to a diabetes education center, claiming that she knows everything about diabetes. Recently her ECG showed some changes and she was referred to a cardiologist.

The preceding case studies described urban, educated immigrants who were diagnosed with diabetes before or after immigration to the United States, with the exception of the fifth and sixth case studies. In the latter instances, the patients were diagnosed with diabetes after they had been living in the United States for some time; they were included here because after immigration, the individuals continued to maintain a similar diet and lifestyle than to their diet and lifestyle before immigration. Because of their diabetes, the individuals profiled here have multiple complications. In the United States, they are receiving complex treatment, including blood glucose control and prevention efforts directed at avoiding further complications of diabetes. Despite the fact that these people are from different cities and countries of the former Soviet Union, Russia and Ukraine, their stories share certain commonalities.

The case studies presented here demonstrate the patients' generally poor awareness of diabetes, and highlight the lack of preventive measurements that followed their diagnosis with diabetes in their home countries. Although most of the case study participants believed that natural remedies are the appropriate first line of treatment for diabetes and that all "chemicals" are harmful for them, some of them had no any awareness of natural remedies. All case study participants believed that they had developed diabetes because of their stressful situations or that a stress has significant impact on developing diabetes. Most participants were reluctant to attend group education at diabetic education centers and preferred education to be conducted on a one-on-one basis with the healthcare provider. Before diabetes education by healthcare providers, they had paid little attention to diabetes risk factors such as poor diet and sedentary lifestyle. With proper education after diagnosis, however, all case study participants changed their lifestyle, but continued to include in their diet healthy products that they were familiar with before immigration. In the United States, they became more aware of their condition and achieved better glycemic control, but sometimes it was too late to prevent many of their diabetic complications.

Consistent with the reports in the case studies, a Russian article by Sharafertdinov et al. (1997) described the typical diet for many former–Soviet Union diabetic patients as consisting of cereals such as buckwheat and grains (e.g., rye wheat) or whole-wheat bread as a main dish. Nurse practitioners need to be aware that Russian-speaking immigrants may prefer their specific type of diet and be prepared to help them find healthy alternatives that will meet their ethnic preference—for example, encouraging them, in addition to eating healthy grains, to consume more vegetables and other healthy products that are available at the market. In addition, NPs may inform their former–Soviet Union clients that although U.S. restaurants, including fast-food restaurants, may have healthy meals, those places often offer large portions—too large for people who are trying to reduce their weight. Referral to a dietitian who is knowledgeable about this ethnic group may be very helpful for Russian immigrants in trying to manage the lifestyle changes necessary as part of diabetes treatment.

These case studies paint a general picture of former–Soviet Union immigrants with diabetes, but the description is limited to these several cases only. The diversity of Russian-speaking immigrants is an important aspect that needs to be taken into consideration in any study addressing this cultural group.

IMPLICATIONS FOR PRACTICE

As the worldwide incidence of diabetes increases, multiple studies are needed to examine the various facets of this disease. In particular, researchers should pay attention to cultural factors. Prevention and treatment of diabetes require a culturally sensitive approach because diet and lifestyle—the major risk factors in diabetes—have strong cultural components. Studies conducted in the United States and other countries receiving Russian-speaking immigrants have confirmed an increased risk of type 2 diabetes in this population. However, with proper diabetic education, diabetic complications may be prevented. Prevention of diabetes and diabetic complications is essential for new immigrants, who are often poor and have limited access to health care. Nurses need to emphasize the importance of diabetes prevention and educate patients about issues such as stress, diet, lifestyle, pre-diabetes, metabolic syndrome, and other risk factors for diabetes and about the complications related to late diagnosis of existing problem.

From this literature review of Russian clients and diabetes, two specifics related to this culture were identified: use of natural remedies as a treatment and stress as a perceived etiology. The NP might be surprised that a Russian patient would refuse to accept the standard treatment for diabetes and instead prefer to take natural remedies. However, with appropriate cultural understandings and knowledge about those natural remedies, the NP will be better able to explain how natural remedies may be more helpful when combined with other treatment plans.

In Russian culture, stress is considered to be a main risk factor for diabetes onset. NPs may forget to discuss stress as a risk factor because they are more concerned about obesity and sedentary lifestyle factors that seem more important in preventing or treating diabetes. Most Russian-speaking patients, however, would appreciate the NP's exploration of stress-related risk factors with them. It is reasonable to discuss stress in this context because these immigrants have moved to another country to begin a new life and usually have to learn a new language and way of life, which leads them to experience tremendous stress.

Smith (1996) makes another important point for nurses who are providing care for this population. She explains that Russian immigrants often ask to see only physicians, rather than nurses or nurse practitioners. They may even become angry if they are assigned to spend time with a nurse, instead of a physician. This reaction is understandable: In the former Soviet Union, the role of the nurse is mainly to obey the commands of physicians; the nurses in those countries are usually not allowed to make decisions regarding patient care. In addition, immigrants may not understand the role of nurse practitioners, because this specialty does not exist in their former countries. Thus NPs may need to discuss with patients the role of nurses and nurse practitioners first, before they delve into the patients' health issues.

The literature review and case studies presented in this chapter aim to help NPs understand why Russian-speaking patients need unique approaches in terms of health care. It may be very useful for the prevention of diabetes or diabetic complications if Russian-speaking immigrants, when visiting the clinic for any health problems, also receive education or screening for diabetes. In addition, when NPs are educating their patients about healthy lifestyle habits, including a healthy diet, a key element is for client to be seen as part of the care management team in selecting health promotion and maintenance strategies.

The literature about Russian-speaking immigrants and diabetes reveals that little is known about diabetes prevention among the Russian-speaking ethnic groups, even those who clearly have a predisposition toward diabetes. More studies are needed about diabetes rates among Russian immigrants, their diet patterns, and the effect of specific diets on the development of diabetes.

WWW

For a full suite of assignments and additional learning activities, use the access code located in the front of your book to visit this exclusive website: http://go.jblearning.com/dechesnay. If you do not have an access code, you can obtain one at the site.

REFERENCES

Adams, C. R. (2003) Lessons learned from urban Latinas with type II diabetes mellitus. *Journal of Transcultural Nursing*, *14*, 255–265.

Aroian, K., Khatusky, G., Tran, T., & Balsam, T. (2001). Health and social service utilization among elderly immigrants from the former Soviet Union. *Journal of Nursing Scholarship*, *33*(3), 265–271.

Ben-Noun, L. (1994) Shchihutmahalot chroniot vemaafyanim sociodemografiim ecel olim hadashim mihever haamim beshana harishona. [Chronic diseases in immigrants from Russia (CIS) at a primary care clinic and their socio-demographic characteristics]. *Harefuah, 127,* 441–445.

Ben-Noun, L. (1995). Hergeley natilat trufot neged yeter-lahaz-dam vemahalot lev klilit ezel' olim mihever-haamim. [Use of medication for hypertension and coronary heat disease by Russian immigrants]. *Harefuah, 129,* 392–394.

Brodov, Y., Mandelzweig, L., Boyko, V., & Behar, S. (2002). Is immigration associated with an increase in risk factors and mortality among coronary artery disease pat? A cohort study of 13,742 patients. *Israel Medical Association Journal, 4,* 326–329.

Brown, D. (2003) More studies need to examine habits within ethic groups. *Journal of the American Dietetic Association, 103,* 706.

Centers for Disease Control and Prevention (CDC). (2003, January 17). Diabetes public health resource. Retrieved November 6, 2003, from http://www.cdc.gov/diabetes/projects/community.htm

Colagiuri, S., Vita, P., Cardona-Morrell, M., Singh, M., Farrell, L., Milat, A., . . . Bauman, A. (2010). The Sydney Diabetes Prevention Program: A community-based, translational study. *Biomed Central Puyblich Health, 10*(328), 1–7. Retrieved September 16, 2010, from www.biomedcentral.com/1471-2458/10/328

Duncan, L., & Simmons, M. (1996). Health practices among Russian and Ukrainian immigrants. *Journal of Community Health Nursing, 13,* 129–137.

Fields, C. (2003). Applied food sciences announces weight loss benefits to its green coffee antioxidant extract. Natural Product Industry Center. Retrieved July 8, 2003, from www.npicenter.com/index.asp?action=NBViewDoc&DocumentID=4388

Fukunishi, I., Akimoto, M., Horikawa, N., Shirasaka, K., & Yamazaki, T. (1998). Stress coping and social support in glucose tolerance abnormality. *Journal of Psychosomatic Research, 45,* 361–369.

Hosler, A. (2003). Diabetes among immigrants from former Soviet Union: International diets. Retrieved June 5, 2003, from www.dietconsuitants.com/russian-diet.html

Ivanov, L. L., & Buck, K. (2002). Health care utilization patterns of Russian-speaking immigrant women across age groups. *Journal of Immigrant Health, 4,* 17–27.

Jimenez del Rio, M. (2003). Blueberry leaves extract: Diabetes and more. Retrieved July 8, 2003, from www.annieappleseedproject.org/blubleavexm.html

Levetan, C. (2001). Diabetes prevention. How about now? *Clinical Diabetes, 19,* 34–38.

London, F. (2002). Improving compliance. What we can do. In *2002 PDR diabetes disease management guide* (2nd ed., pp. 501–505). Montvale, NJ: Thomson PDR. Manvelov, L. C. (1999). Saharnyi diabet kak factor riska celebrovaskulyarnyh zabolevanii. [Diabetes as a risk actor for cerebro-vascular accidents]. *Lechashii vrach, 9,* 1–9. Retrieved July 8, 2003, from http://www.osp.ru/doctore/1999/09/09.htm

Mehler, P., Scott, J., & Pines, I. (2001). Russian immigrant cardiovascular risk. *Journal of the Poor and Underserved, 12*(2), 224–235.

Meyerovich, M. (2003). Somatic symptoms among recent Russian immigrants. American Medical Association. Retrieved July, 7, 2003, from www.ama-assn.org/ama/pub/article/8401-1959.html

Ministry of Health, Russian Federation. (n.d.). Phederal'naya celevaya programa: Saharnyi diabet. Retrieved July 17, 2003, from http://www.minzdrav-rf.ru/in.htm?rubr=130

Mull, D. S., Nguyen, N., & Dennis, J. M. (2001). Vietnamese diabetic patients and their physicians: What ethnography can teach us? *Western Journal of Medicine, 175,* 307–311.

National Diabetes Information Clearinghouse (2003, May 3). National diabetes statistics. Retrieved November 4, 2003, from http://diabetes.niddk.nih.gov/dm/pubs/statistics/index.htm

Nikitin, Y. P. (1989). Problemasaharnogo diabeta v regionah Sibiri. [The problem of diabetes mellitus in the Siberian regions]. *Vestnik Akademii Meditsinskikh Nauk, 5,* 35–39.

Oystragh, P. (1980). Diabetes mellitus in Russian Jewish immigrants. *Australian Family Physician, 9*, 269–270.

Public Health Seattle and King County. (2001, October 19). Public health news release: New community-based diabetes activities will help bridge the health gap for minority communities. Retrieved November 17, 2003, from http://www.metrokc.gov/health/news/01101801.htm

Peyrot, M., McMurry, J. F. Jr., & Kruger, D. F. (1999). A biopsychosocial model of glycemic control in diabetes: Stress, coping and regimen adherence. *Journal of Health and Social Behavior, 40*, 141–158.

Popkin, B. M. (1998). The nutrition transition and its health implications in lower-income countries. *Public Health Nutrition, 11*, 5–21.

Rankin, S. H., Galbraith, M. E., & Huang, P. (1997). Quality of life and social environment as reported by Chinese immigrants with non-insulin–dependent diabetes mellitus. *Diabetes Educator, 23*, 171–176.

Rennert, G., Luz, N., Tamir, A., & Peterburg, Y. (2002). Chronic disease prevalence in immigrants to Israel from the former USSR. *Journal of Immigrant Health, 10*(4), 29–33.

Resick, L. (2008). The meaning of health among midlife Russian-speaking immigrant women. *Journal of Nursing Scholarship, 40*(3), 248–253.

Sharafertdinov, K. K. Mesheryakoba, V. A., & Plotnikova, O. A. (1997). Izmenenie poslepishevoi glikemii pod vliyaniem nekotoryh uglevodosoderzhashih produktov u bol'nyh saharnym diabetom. [Change of postprandial glycemia under effect of some carbohydrate containing food in patients with type 2 diabetes]. *Lechebnoe pitanie, 1*, 27–30.

Sidorov, P. I., Novikova, I. A., & Solov'ev, A. G. (2001). Rol' negativnyh social'nyh i psichologicheskih factorov na poyavlenie i kurs lechenia saharnogo diabeta. [The role of unfavorable social and psychological factors in the onset and course of diabetes mellitus]. *Terapevticheskii Archiv, 73*, 68–70.

Smith, L. (1996). New Russian immigrants: Health problem, practices, and values. *Journal of Cultural Diversity, 3*, 68–73.

Wheat, M. E., Brownstein, H., & Kvitash, V. (1983) Aspects of medical care of Soviet Jewish émigrés. *Western Journal of Medicine, 139*, 900–904.

Zabina, H., Schmid, T. L., Glasunov, I., Potemkina, R., Kamardina, T., Deev, A., . . . Popovich, M. (2001). Monitoring behavioral risk factors for cardiovascular disease in Russia. *American Journal of Public Health, 91*, 1613–1614.

CHAPTER 24

Barriers to Healthcare Access for Latino Service Workers in a Resort Community

Caroline Cogan

Objectives

At the end of this chapter, the reader will be able to

1. Describe some of the key factors in providing health care for Latino workers in a resort community.
2. Compare and contrast the issues in health care for Latinos who work in resprt areas versus in other types of regions.
3. Provide examples of how health care might be provided to Latinos in resort communities.

INTRODUCTION

Many traditionally underserved populations in rural communities have difficulty accessing health care due to the lack of medical facilities. Access is especially problematic in affluent resort communities in which there is great disparity between the "haves" and "have-nots." The purpose of this chapter is to identify the barriers and proposed strategies to improve access to health care by Latino service workers in an affluent resort community in the western United States. During the winter, the area is a major ski resort. In summer, hikers and others interested in the great outdoors enjoy the peace and splendor of the mountains.

The study described here examined the healthcare resources in the community for the Latinos who provide a major role in the service industry. These people work in low-paying jobs that are critical to the smooth operation of a resort area. Despite the importance of their functions, the people who function as housecleaners, maids in hotels, restaurant workers, and so on are often "invisible" in the sense that, if they do their jobs well, they are not really noticed by the wealthy individuals they serve. The project was inspired by the author's commitment to the community as a part-time resident and as an advanced practice nurse with a strong sense of social justice regarding the poor and underserved.

Little research has been conducted in resort communities. Barriers to health care exist in these locations that are sometimes politically determined. For example, one cannot open a healthcare clinic in this resort area and receive federal funding based on the physician-to-population ratio because the ratios do not accurately reflect the number of physicians available to provide health care for this population. Based on the U.S. Census Report (USCR, 1990–2004) report, there are 71 physicians employed in this area. However, these numbers do not actually depict the number of physicians actually providing care in the community. For example, the only local community hospital has just 31 physicians on its medical staff. According to the Wood River Medical Society, approximately half of the physicians work on a part-time basis and, therefore, are not available to assume a full patient load (Smith, personal communication).

Most of the resort's 21,000 residents live there on a part-time basis. According to local officials, there are 2,400 housing units in the primary resort area, of which 1,600 are second homes, reflecting the affluence of the community (Foley, 2004). An overwhelming financial disparity exists between the permanent residents, who range from minimum-wage workers to the wealthy elite. Like many famous tourist destinations, the resort in question is known for its lush golf courses and snow-covered mountains. Because of the remote geographic area, however, the businesses rely on local residents to work in the service industry. The harsh winters and treacherous mountain terrain make long-distance commuting from outlying towns difficult. Most of those who work in the service sector earn minimum wage or less and commute from outlying cities 40 miles away.

THE LITERATURE

The first section of the chapter consists of a literature review on access issues in the United States. The second part is a description of a ski resort in the western United States that struggles to serve the healthcare needs of the underserved residents of the community.

Barriers to Health Care

Barriers to healthcare access were a major theme in many articles reviewed for this chapter (Anderson, 1995; *Healthy People 2010*, 2006; Probst, Moore, Glover, & Samuels, 2004; Solis, Marks, Garcia, & Shelton, 1990). Individual barriers particularly relevant to Latino service workers include economic issues, immigration status, transportation, and language. Individual barriers are distinct from cultural barriers, which include beliefs, norms, customs, and rituals that prevent particular groups from seeking health care (Hunter, Gaylord, Britnell, & Ashford-Works, 1998).

Economic Issues

The cost of healthcare services is a major barrier. Latinos often forego treatment because they do not have the money to pay for services and are unable to obtain health insurance. This issue is especially problematic for immigrants who do not have legal status (Anderson, 1995) or who do not speak English (Lee & Choi, 2009). For example, in a study of Hispanic women immigrants to the United States, the findings revealed that these women do not seek prenatal health care due primarily to language barriers and the issues of cultural competence that arise when healthcare providers simply use interpreters (Shaffer, 2002).

As Johnson (2001) notes, vulnerable people often cannot afford the cost of health care. The lack of financial resources was cited throughout the research literature as the number one reason for not accessing health care. Even those individuals who have insurance may not have enough money for the copayments or deductibles, even with the reduced rates offered by some clinics. A related barrier is the lack of medical clinics and providers who accept Medicaid or who offer sliding-scale fees to care for the large number of uninsured and indigent people (Kaiser, 2003). Failure to be flexible on payments leads to longer appointment times, waiting room delays, and excess usage of emergency departments by individuals who do not want to wait for appointments.

The median income for the vulnerable group examined in this chapter is less than $44,000 annually (Kaiser, 2003). This rural town's service-worker population does not have the disposable income to pay for insurance premiums or healthcare cost. Low-income wage earners do not earn enough money to purchase health insurance and cover the cost of basic needs. Although these workers recognize the importance of health insurance, they choose to pay bills, obtain food, and cover rent rather than purchase insurance. They have little, if any, discretionary income. Some fear that if they already owe previous bills, they may not be able to receive additional medical assistance. If the medical bills remain unpaid, many fear retribution by authorities, particularly immigration officials.

Immigration Status

Although the issue of undocumented Mexican Americans is particularly timely given the attention currently being paid to the U.S. border problems, it is unclear how many of these people have found their way to the community of interest. It is likely that the workers who are employed by the major facilities have legal immigration status; in contrast, the many landscapers and construction workers who come and go might not be legal immigrants. One model program in Chicago was created to help newly legalized immigrants learn the intricacies of the healthcare system, as this issue often flummoxes émigrés to the United States (McElmurry, Park, & Busch, 2003).

Transportation

Barriers such as transportation and language also were a common theme in reports of obstacles to obtaining health care (Casey, Blewette, & Call,2004). Transportation was an issue because many immigrants do not have driver's licenses or even know how to drive. Rural areas do not have public transportation. The service workers rely on friends who have cars, but the friends who have cars are more likely to work during clinic times and are not available to drive them to appointments. Additionally, because of the enormous costs of housing, local service workers are forced to live 25 to 40 miles outside of town and carpool or shuttle into work each day. Scheduling a medical appointment requires them to take a day off from work to see a primary care provider in another town.

Language

Because Spanish is the primary language among Latino service workers and most Anglos do not speak Spanish, communication is often difficult. In the resort area, 90% of the population is Caucasian and English-speaking, with 10% being Spanish-speaking or speaking another language as their first language (USCR, 1990–2004). The Latinos in the resort area find it difficult just trying to make a doctor's appointment, let alone understand all that was said to them during their appointments. The language barrier for Latinos who are not fluent in English if the providers do not speak Spanish is enormous (Johnson, 2001).

Cultural Values

For some of the Latino service workers, who are mainly from Mexico, a strong cultural value is to be tough and not need health care. Illness in the Latino population is perceived as a weakness (Anderson, 1995). The practice of waiting until the health problem has reached a crisis point appears to contribute to the difficulty Latinos face when accessing health care. Although Latino adults may wait and postpone their own health care, however, they do not have the same expectation of toughness for their children. Parents put the needs of their children before themselves at any financial cost.

Another cultural barrier is that some Latinos rely on *curanderos* (traditional healers) or friends for advice. *Curanderos* treat their clients with home remedies, herbs, and over-the-counter medications (Doty & Ives, 2002; Najm, Reinsch, Hoehler, & Tobis, 2003). Sometimes the advice of *curanderos* and friends or family members may conflict with that given by the healthcare establishment.

Denial also plays a role in access, in that young people might see themselves as invincible and believe that nothing bad can happen to them. Like youth in many cultures, young Latinos might minimize their injuries or symptoms. Denial might happen on two levels: they might not attend to dangerous or unhealthy practices or they might "tough it out" when they become ill. This reaction is consistent with Anderson's (1995) work on the cultural value of being tough and traditional notions about machismo (Galanti, 2003).

Healthcare Literacy

Additional healthcare barriers found in the literature (Vezeau, 2005) include the complexity of the healthcare forms, which leads to two major problems. The first problem is inability to complete medical forms, leading to frustration and avoidance of medical services (Anderson, 1995). The second problem is that individuals with little or no recorded health history are the ones least able to provide accurate medical information in times of crisis (Mercer, 2001).

Another problem identified in the literature is the lack of clinics with a Spanish translator. In a study conducted by the Association of Community Organization for Reform (2004), hospitals were contacted to determine whether a Spanish-speaking interpreter was available. The law requires that all hospitals provide an interpreter upon request, yet more than 50% of these facilities did not offer this assistance (Association of Community Organization for Reform, 2004). The problems associated with incomplete or inaccurate communication about health history and status are obvious and critical.

Demographic Trends

The United States is experiencing a shift in its demographic trends, including an increase in cultural diversity. Demographers predict that the next two decades will bring racial and ethnic minority populations to a numerical majority in the United States (Sue & Sue, 1999). The reality is that African Americans, American Indians, Alaska Natives, Asian Americans, Pacific Islanders, and Latinos accounted for 30% of the total U.S. population in 2000 (U.S. Department of Health and Human Services [HHS], 2001). The shares of these population groups are projected to increase to 40% of the total population by 2025 (HHS, 2001). Social workers and medical professionals have attempted to prepare for the coming population shifts by creating initiatives and standards related to cultural diversity and practice. These professional responses have yielded mixed results, however.

The Latino population in the United States is characterized by its rapid growth, with this group projected to increase to 97 million by 2050, representing one-fourth of the total U.S. population. Mexican Americans account for almost two-thirds of Latino Americans, with the remainder being of Puerto Rican, Cuban, South American, Central American, Dominican, and Spanish origin. Latinos are highly concentrated in the southwest United States; 60% of all members of this group live in California, Arizona, New Mexico, Colorado, and Texas. However, other states have also seen increases in their Latino populations. From 1990 to 2000, the number of Latinos more than doubled in Arkansas (170%), North Carolina (129%), Georgia (120%), Nebraska (108%), and Tennessee (105%), for example (USCR, 1990–2004).

Many of North Carolina's county departments of health, social services, and other community service agencies are experiencing a steady rise in the number of Latino families they serve, and with good reason. North Carolina has the fastest-growing Latino population in the United States.

It is a mistake to assume that Latinos are a homogeneous culture, however. In fact, Latinos are an extremely diverse group. They include individuals with a wide range of characteristics from many different countries, regions, socioeconomic backgrounds, cultures, and races. For example, Spanish-language nuances can dramatically affect interpretation from country to country.

Cultural Competence

Nurse practitioners continue to strive to achieve cultural competence. McPhatter (1997) viewed cultural competence in terms of transforming knowledge and awareness of culture into interventions that support and sustain healthy functioning within the appropriate cultural contest. More recently, de Chesnay, Wharton, and Pamp (2005) have described cultural competence in terms of acting in a way that is respectful of the values and traditions of the patient while performing nursing actions.

The Sociopolitical Environment and Unresponsive Professions

The broader sociopolitical environment affects the practitioner's work with culturally diverse groups. As Sue and Sue (1999) pointed out, traditional medicine may sometimes serve to oppress multiethnic groups. The ethnocentric bias of the medical establishment values compliance or adherence with its own regimens and protocols. If patients do not comply or adhere with these rules, they risk receiving punitive messages from their healthcare providers.

Sue and Sue (1999) speculated that the underutilization of health and mental health services is related to the cultural insensitivity and inappropriateness of formalized services for culturally diverse groups. Findings from the Commonwealth Fund Minority Health Survey (LaVeist, Diala, & Jerrett, 2000) support this contention. Data from this survey revealed that of 43% of African Americans and 28% of Latinos, in comparison with 5% of white people, believed that because of their cultural background, a healthcare provider treated them poorly. The lack of professionals' ability to practice in a culturally competent way further oppresses their patients who face biased behavior within the larger society.

High-Need Populations

Latinos are relatively under-represented among people who are homeless or have children in foster care. However, they are present in high numbers in several other vulnerable populations who experience health disparities. For example, Latino Americans are 9% more likely to be incarcerated, compared to 3% of non-Latino Americans. Latino men are nearly four times as likely as white men to be imprisoned at some point during their lifetime (Weich & Angulo, 2000).

Latinos who served in the U.S. military services during the Vietnam War were at higher risk for war-related post-traumatic stress disorder than were black and non-Latino white veterans. Many suggest refugees from Central America experienced considerable civil war–related trauma in their homelands. Studies have found rates of post-traumatic stress disorder among Central American refugee patients ranging from 33% to 60% (Weich et al., 2000).

In general, Latino Americans have rates of alcohol use similar to non-Latinos. However, female Latinas usually have lower rates of alcohol and drug use than their male counterparts. Rates of substance abuse are higher among U.S.-born Mexican Americans compared to Mexican-born immigrants. Specifically, substance abuse rates are twice as high for U.S.-born Mexican American men than for Mexican-born men, but—somewhat surprisingly—are seven times higher for U.S.-born Mexican American women than for Mexican-born women (Weich et al., 2000).

Latinos with diabetes are at higher risk of heart disease, but they can reduce that risk, according to a new national health awareness campaign unveiled recently by the National Diabetes Education Program (NDEP) during the National Council of La Raza's annual conference. By controlling blood sugar, blood pressure, and cholesterol, people with diabetes can live longer, healthier lives (*Healthy People 2010*, 2006). In 2004, Health and Human Services Secretary Thompson announced a campaign, titled *Si Tiene Diabetes, Cuide Su Corazon*, which is aimed at helping Latino Americans better understand the need to control all aspects of their diabetes.

AVAILABILITY OF MENTAL HEALTH SERVICES

In 1990, approximately 40% of Latinos either did not speak English at all or did not speak it well. While the percentage of Spanish-speaking mental health professionals is not known, only 1% of licensed psychologists who are also members of the American Psychological Association identify themselves as Latino. Moreover, there are only 29 Latino providers compared to 173 non-Latino white providers per 100,000 population (LaVeist et al., 2000). If these proportions of Spanish-speaking to non-Spanish-speaking providers hold true for other healthcare professionals, then the problems of communication are clearly enormous for Latino clients.

Access to Mental Health Services

Nationally, 37% of Latinos are uninsured, compared to 16% of all Americans. This high proportion is driven mostly by Latinos' lack of employer-based coverage—only 43% compared to 73% for non-Latino whites (LaVeist et al., 2000). Although Latino service workers in the community of interest might value insurance, they view it as discretionary and have no room in their meager budgets for spending on luxuries such as health insurance.

Appropriateness and Outcomes of Mental Health Services

Few studies on the mental health resources of Latinos are available. One randomized study found that members of low-income, Spanish-speaking families were more likely to suffer a significant exacerbation of symptoms of schizophrenia in highly structured family therapy than in less structured case management. Several studies have found that bilingual patients are evaluated differently when interviewed in English as opposed to Spanish, thereby influencing outcomes (Johnson, 2001).

One national study found that only 24% of Latinos with depression and anxiety receive appropriate care, compared to 34% of whites. Another study found that Latinos who visited a general medical doctor were less than half as likely as whites to receive either a diagnosis of depression or antidepressant medicine (LaVeist et al., 2000). The extent to which Latinos attempt to access mental health services is unclear, but these services might be considered a luxury for people who are not well educated.

Need for Mental Health Care

There was no difference in the frequency of mental disorders among Latino Americans living in the resort community compared to non-Latino white Americans (Kaiser, 2003). Adult Mexican immigrants typically have lower rates of mental disorders than Mexican Americans born in the United States, and adult Puerto Ricans tend to have lower rates of depression when they are living on the mainland (HHS, 2001). It is not clear that the methods of measurement used to compile these statistics are standardized, however, so the existing studies have limited applicability.

Some researchers have found that Latino youth experience proportionally more anxiety and delinquency behaviors, depression, and drug use than do non-Latino white youth. Among older Latinos, one study found that more than 26% of the sample were depressed. When depression was related to physical health, only 5.5% of those without physical health problems were depressed (HHS, 2001).

Culture-bound syndromes seen in Latino Americans include *susto* (fright), *nervios* (nerves), *mal de ojo* (evil eye), and *ataque*, which may include screaming uncontrollable, crying, trembling, verbal or physical aggression, dissociate experiences, seizure-like or fainting episodes, and suicidal gestures (HHS, 2001).

In 1997, Latinos had a suicide rate of approximately 6%, compared to 13% for non-Latino whites. However, in a national survey of high school students, Latino adolescents reported more suicidal ideation and attempts proportionally than non-whites and blacks (HHS, 2001).

STATE OF THE ART OF THE LITERATURE REGARDING HEALTHCARE ACCESS

Areas of Agreement

The major area of agreement in the research literature is that the Latino population is in crisis when trying to access health care. Latinos often encounter language difficulties when trying to make appointments because the clinic personnel do not speak Spanish (Mercer, 2001). If they are able to explain that they need an appointment, they still have difficulty expressing their symptoms and the nature of the medical problem. Latinos state that sometimes when they are trying to access healthcare clinics, they are confronted with humiliation and embarrassment at not being able to speak English and are treated disrespectfully. This makes it difficult and anxiety producing to try to access health care.

The literature documents that there is a critical need for federal and state policy makers to acknowledge Latino health disparities and lead the way to better health and quality of life for this population. For example, research with significant funding conducted under the auspices of federal agencies is lacking for this population. Although there are strong disparities among income levels, differing rates of uninsured individuals, and a generally low education level for this population, only recently have federal agencies begun to take notice. For example the resort community of interest described in this chapter recently received a large amount of funding from the Department of Health and Welfare to help meet the community's needs (Mason, 2005).

The sources reviewed seem to reach consensus in stating that Latino individuals face many unique challenges when trying to access health care—namely, cost of services, inability to access services, and cultural and language barriers. Johnson (2001) also pointed out other issues repeatedly mentioned in the literature, including long waits, inconvenient clinic hours, and disrespectful treatment from healthcare providers. Hunter et al. (1998) urged providers to remember not to generalize rural communities, but rather to embrace the differences of the communities and ethnic populations. This idea is particularly relevant to policy makers.

Areas of Disagreement

There is disagreement as to whether individual resort communities or large suburban areas should be studied in future research when addressing the healthcare needs of Latinos and the underinsured. One study by Mercer (2001) points out that this population is highly diverse and varies greatly from county to county across the United States. Thus studying the needs of larger populations would not address the needs of Latinos from specific rural resort areas. Other studies do not mention this issue, implying that individual communities are not different enough to warrant studying each for to determine culturally based solutions to problems of healthcare access. Both arguments have some value. If the statement by Mercer were true—that is, the diversity between counties is great—then it would be prudent to do further research within subgroups to develop health guidelines for populations from each country of origin.

Another area of disagreement in the literature is concerned with the relative importance of different types of barriers to health care. Johnson (2001) found that the number of clinics was a larger barrier to accessing health care than language differences between providers and patients (Carson, Jenssen, & Synder, 2004). However, most of the studies report language to be the number one barrier.

A final area of inconsistency relates to the effect of long wait times in the clinic. According to Johnson (2001), while it is necessary to do further research, development of a standardized method for retrieving data is necessary before additional studies should be conducted. The lack of standardized methods for collecting data is a source of confusion in the literature and makes interpretation of results difficult and generalizability limited.

Gaps

A major gap in the literature is the lack of information on barriers to health care for Latinos in affluent communities. This chapter attempts to address this problem by focusing on a specific rural community and the needs of that population. However, the nature of resort communities might indicate that the problems faced by Latinos in the ski resort described here might be similar to those issues in other types of resorts with affluent and disadvantaged groups.

Overall, the published research on the healthcare barriers facing Latino populations in the United States, particularly in rural areas, is lacking or suspect. Some workers do not have immigration papers and so avoid contact with government agencies; thus they remain unaccounted for in any research (Carson et al., 2004).

The Latino population continues to grow. It is already the largest minority group in the United States, and it is becoming more difficult for the healthcare system to ignore the needs of this population. There is an abundance of reports and articles based on observation and trends relating to the healthcare needs of Latinos, but only a limited amount of actual research has been conducted in this area. Most publications seem anecdotal or theoretical. On the positive side, the amount of research in this field is likely to increase because of the rapid growth and critical needs of this population. The sheer numbers of people who are uninsured will create the demand for more research and new models to address their unmet needs for health care.

COMMUNITY DESCRIPTION: THE RESORT COMMUNITY

An attempt to create a new model was inspired by the author's involvement in the community of a ski resort in a western state. This rural area has many Latino service workers who hold menial jobs, yet are critical to the local economy. The community of interest is a summer and winter resort area located in the western United States. This resort, which is considered by many to be one of the most desirable and exclusive vacation destinations in the United States, attracts people of means and influence. The mountain community has a beautiful setting located at 6,000 feet elevation in the Pioneer Range of the Rocky Mountains and is home to many famous people. It is not uncommon to shop at local supermarkets and stand beside celebrities who are also shopping for groceries.

The area was first developed as a mining town in the 1800s, and its successes and failures were dependent on the productivity of the mines—a statement also true for many similar towns of this region. In 1936, Averill Harriman chose this specific resort area as the location of the first ski resort in the United States. The Union Pacific Train line was extended to the region and the main lodge was built in 1936. Since that time the area has flourished with the rapid expansion of the ski industry and other sports activities. Summer recreation, such as golfing, tennis, hiking, and bicycling, have become extremely popular and attract even more tourists than the traditional winter sports.

A stable, but small population of people live year-round in the vicinity and support the local economy. Full-time residents include wealthy retirees, professionals such as attorneys and real estate developers, small business owners, and low-wage service workers. The average income for this county is $44,000, exceeding the average per capita income for the United States as a whole, which was $14,000 in 2001 (Rogers, 2006). The resort community itself has a per capita income of $31,000, with 8% of the population in the county living below the poverty level (USCR, 1990–2004). The county also has the highest cost of living compared with the surrounding communities. The high cost of living makes it difficult for service workers to afford housing in the town itself, so they live outside and commute to work.

The service workers in particular are extremely important to the economy of the resort area. They serve as the principal labor force for the businesses that flourish here. However, there is great disparity between the income of the tourists and part-time residents in comparison with the income of the full-time workers, even professionals. For example, registered nurses have a starting wage of $19 per hour in this area, compared to the starting wage of $24 per hour found in the state of Washington (USCR, 1990–2004). The salaries of nannies, restaurant workers, construction workers, and other service workers vary depending on their employers. Although the salaries or hourly wages might be slightly better than their counterparts in a middle-class urban neighborhood, the cost of living is so much higher that proportionately, they do not keep as much of their wages.

Since 2000, this resort community had one of the largest population increases in the region, with the robust growth expected to continue (USCR, 1990–2004). Ownership of a vacation home is a growing trend in ski resorts, although it remains controversial. The second-home debate centers on whether the part-time residents contribute to the community's wealth or burden it. In this community, 36% of the residents are part-time residents. Amazingly, approximately 70% of the jobs in this resort community are in the heart of the local ski resort, although half of the service workers live elsewhere (USCR, 1990–2004).

The argument that vacation home owners in resort communities have detrimental effects on the local economy is based on the rationale that these part-time residents displace full-time residents on fixed incomes, consume unnecessarily large quantities of resources, drive up real estate prices, and do not contribute to local businesses (Foley, 2004). Herein lies one of the complex issues when trying to create free clinics to support the total community.

The affluence of the residents skews the basis upon which federal funds are allocated. The mean income appears much higher than usual due to the extreme wealth of the few versus the low income of the many permanent residents. This resort community ranks 44 on the list of the 50 counties in the state of study in terms of receiving federal monies; it currently receives $205 in tax dollars for every man, woman, and child residing in this community compared to the statewide average of $839 per capita (Mason, 2005). These statistics are staggering and explain the vast disparity in income and resources in this area.

As a long-term visitor to the region, the author has become concerned about the healthcare options available to the large segment of the population who are either uninsured or underinsured. Although there are many physicians and other healthcare professionals and a new, modern hospital in this area, they appear to primarily serve the more affluent members of the community. In discussions with community members, it was mentioned that, while access to health care is available through the local emergency department, the fee schedule is not adjusted for the poorer patients. Thus an unplanned trip to the emergency department for something as minor as a sinus infection can become a financial burden, which serves as a deterrent to most of the Latino service workers who might otherwise seek out health care.

This area is not unlike many successful resorts in that the popularity and success of the resort area cannot continue to grow unless the needs of the large working population are met. The local political leaders in of the area are cognizant of this looming problem, but have thus far not been successful in developing affordable and easily attainable health care for all.

It is quite apparent that there are gaps about what is known concerning access to health care for Latino service workers in resort communities. There is great diversity among the resort communities as well as among the Latinos who work in them. Therefore, it is imperative to examine a specific community in depth, because the research indicates that each community is so diverse that generalizing an implementation plan is impossible (Association of Community Organization for Reform, 2004). Each community needs to develop its own plan for providing access to service workers, but monies are rarely allocated to turn this goal into reality.

The Ski Resort

Community leaders in this area recognize that there is a problem with access to care for the Latino service workers. For example, a prominent figure within the local hospital stated that he recognized the extent of the problem but offered no solutions. In fact, he mentioned that the hospital is not interested in developing a free or low-cost clinic for this segment of the population. Although the emergency room and clinics are available to all members of the community, the substantial costs involved in accessing them limit their use by low-income individuals.

Members of the major medical group in the community were contacted, but also had no interest in developing more facilities for this population of patients. The hospital has recently closed its medical staffing, which means that a new physician moving into the area cannot obtain hospital privileges until a current member of the medical staff retires, dies, or moves. This decision was made to protect the income of the current physicians practicing in the area and to prevent physician turnover. While this policy makes for a successful medical practice, it deters new physicians from moving to the area—physicians who may be willing to see more low-income and underinsured patients.

The ski resort community likewise does not meet the requirements of a medically underserved area (MUA). The resort had 74 physicians in 2002, compared to 54 in 1996. This figure represents 3.6 physicians per 1,000 patients for this community (American Medical Association, 1996–2002). Based on these data, one might think that there is no need for more physicians to support the population. However, the report does not detail which of the 74 physicians work part-time, which work seasonally, which accept charity cases, or which use a sliding scale for payments. Although these data make the physician coverage seem adequate, in reality there are large gaps in the medical care delivered to this community. For example, the new local hospital and various clinics do not offer sliding-scale fees for underinsured patients.

Random phone calls were made to the hospital emergency department and several independent clinics to inquire about the availability of services for individuals without insurance. The clinics contacted stated that, if patients are willing to accept a lengthy wait and make regular monthly payments at the standard fee, they would be able to see the patient.

The demographic data are alarming for this resort community. While there appears to be an adequate number of physicians to serve the population, this is an illusion: The majority of physicians will not see uninsured or underinsured patients, and an adequate medical center is not available to serve this portion of the population. Thus these people are forced to leave the community to obtain basic health care. However, because they live far away from the community, they would not be able to work on the days they need to see a provider.

This community is not designated as a medically underserved area because of the physician-to-population ratio, so the area would not qualify for federal funds to support a new clinic. As stated previously, the number of physicians available is quite misleading because many physicians work part-time and are completely unavailable to the service workers and indigents. Although it may be still possible to qualify for some federal funding, the process could be quite lengthy with no guarantees for success. This situation is a "Catch-22" for the service workers, who must choose between accessing care in their home towns or working.

Other Resorts

Like the ski resort just described, other recreation resort areas experience similar situations when trying to deliver health care to underserved or underinsured members of their community. Although not rural in the same sense as the ski resort, the resort community of Hilton Head Island, South Carolina, experienced the same healthcare disparities as the ski resort, but one local physician found an answer. Dr. Jack McConnell, a retired physician on Hilton Head Island, observed the disparity of health care for the service workers of the island. Committed to making a change, he met with a group of local retired physicians to share his vision of opening a free clinic; 13 of the 29 physicians agreed to join forces and help. At the time, although all of the physicians agreed with the concept, many were very skeptical that such a clinic could open (Graves, 1996).

McConnell convinced the state that the clinic would be supported entirely by donated funds. High malpractice insurance and medical license renewal fees were a deterrent for many retired physicians, who declined to participate on that basis. After convincing the state legislators to pass a special exception from state requirements for the new clinic, McConnell purchased malpractice insurance at a reduced fee. Likewise, South Carolina allowed an exemption of medical license fees, which allowed the retired physicians to practice medicine at this free clinic. In July 1994, the doors opened to this healthcare clinic for the needy. The Hilton Head clinic is a model of how a community that does not meet the state and federal requirements for a MUA can nevertheless support the underserved population with volunteers who offer a wealth of experience in health care.

Aspen, Colorado, is another wealthy ski resort, claimed by many to be the fourth richest town in the United States. With demographics similar to the community of interest in this paper, Aspen has a population of 14,000 people. Of those, 90.5% are considered white and 6.5% are Latino. Service workers maintain the viability of this ski resort; indeed, without these people, the economy of Aspen would be severely compromised.

In recent years, Aspen and other Colorado ski resorts such as Vail and Breckenridge have faced a decline in revenues related to less retail consumerism, according to the Aspen Retail Study (BBC Research & Consulting, 2003). The population of Aspen has decreased by 1.2% since 2004 (USCR, 1990–2004). With one local hospital willing to see the indigent population and additional hospitals located 30 miles away, healthcare access has become a factor in providing health care for the entire community.

Aspen has reported a loss in revenue for three consecutive years. Owing to the lack of support systems to provide for the working population, people are choosing to move to areas where housing and services are affordable. An extensive report by the city's planning committee does not mention other possibilities for this loss, such as lack of service workers to provide for the seasonal influx of tourists.

DISCUSSION

Two issues stand out as particularly significant in the literature on vulnerable populations and health care: access to healthcare facilities and inadequate numbers of healthcare facilities available to the most vulnerable members of the population. These shortfalls must be addressed if the needs of the working poor are to be served. In the resort described in this chapter, the community residents were not aware that the hospital functions as a closed medical unit. This concept of staffing is of particular interest when discussing issues of healthcare access. Although a closed medical unit does not discourage physicians to practice independently in the community, only a designated number of physicians are given privileges to the hospital. Therefore, highly qualified physicians are not able to open practices in this town because of their inability to gain admitting privileges.

The vulnerable population of interest in this chapter is Latino service workers: residents who commute from outlying towns to work in service-oriented jobs in the ski resort. In this resort community, 10.7 % of the population is Latino. The average household income for a Latino family in the community is $44,000 (HHS, 2004). The community is 90% white and 10.7% Latino, with an average age between 25 and 44 years of age. Its unemployment rate is 4%, though it fluctuates during seasonal activities (HHS, 2004). The community relies on this particular population to maintain its businesses' operating status. Without this population, many of the businesses would not be able to function, particularly during the high season.

The services offered to the community focus on the elite tourist population, with few services being devoted to the Latino population. For example, a single local hospital serves the resort community, theoretically providing access to health care for all individuals, even as it warns some away because the fee for service does not vary depending on income. There are no discount stores to purchase low-cost basic needs such as undergarments. To purchase these items, one would have to travel 25 to 40 miles outside the resort community. This need for long-distance travel is a huge burden in the winter season, when it is not uncommon to have 2 to 3 feet of snow fall in one night and 12-foot drifts, making the roads impassible even if one had a car.

The term "rural" has no single accepted definition. For the purpose of this chapter, the following are commonly viewed as rural indicators: low population size and density, distance from urban areas, low degree of urbanization, and few types of economic activity (HHS, 2004). One of the difficulties in receiving federal monies is the inability to designate this community as medically underserved (MUA). Due to the number of wealthy residents who live there on a full- and part-time basis, the statistics do not show a need for designation as underserved. The economic separation of this town is significant, with an enormous gap separating the wealthy elite from the working poor, with a relatively small middle class in between the two extremes. The working poor are defined here as individuals who spend at least 27 weeks in the labor force, but whose income falls below the official poverty line, which for this community is $31,000 annual income or less (HHS, 2004).

The economic disparity in this population leads to one of the major problems for the Latino residents—namely, lack of accessible health care. In this community with a population of 21,000, 8% earn less than the federal poverty level, meaning less than $31,000 per year (USCR, 1990–2004). This is an important problem on many levels, not only from an economic standpoint, but also in terms of the resources related to the ability to purchase health insurance. Addressing the problem of health care for the vulnerable population of Latino service workers in this rural town is critical for the growth of the community. The number of residents earning less than the federal poverty level may not be significant in itself, but when one considers that this community has a higher cost of living than any other local region, the number of poor people becomes highly relevant.

Owing to the lack of healthcare facilities or existing resources in the community, many of the underserved workers eventually relocate, leaving the resort community without support workers. Each year there are more unopened businesses and longer wait times at the local restaurants and lodging cafeteria due to a lack of workers. In December 2006, the local ski mountain did not open at the desired time due to a shortage of employees.

Ideally, studies will be undertaken to help determine the reasons for the current decline in the number of available workers. If specific causes were isolated to explain the loss of low-income support workers, the community could then focus on solutions to ensure that all groups within this community receive adequate care from local resources. In addition, and more importantly, restructuring the community services would help the entire community by reducing the crime rate and providing a better society in which to live and significantly improve the economy.

CONCLUSION

Preliminary results of this community examination indicated that there is a need for affordable and convenient healthcare services for Latino service workers. Potential solutions addressing the lack of facilities include reallocating existing services, adding needed services, analyzing the success of similar resorts, and developing a new model for this community. The disparity between the income and financial status of the two major groups is profound and will not change. Ultimately, the success of the community will depend on the availability of low-income workers, so a solution must be found to accommodate their needs. Expecting them to travel back to the outlying towns in which they live for needed health care is neither fair nor economically practical.

A more reasonable approach to this problem is to develop a private clinic staffed by a physician and two or three nurse practitioners. Much of the clinic's funding could be obtained from fees generated from patients on a sliding scale. When public awareness of this effort increased, contributions could be obtained. The local hospital raises approximately $1 million per year in donated funds from this small but affluent community. Public funding from the City Council and county health department may also be available. For as little as $250,000 for the first year, a model program could be opened and expanded with donated services, a sliding-scale fee-for-service structure, and grant funding.

SUMMARY

This chapter has raised questions about how a resort community can support Latino service workers' needs for affordable health care. The literature review revealed that specific types of barriers exist for this population in accessing health care. Once the relevant healthcare barriers are understood, appropriate solutions may be considered. These solutions might include the creation of a free clinic with both public and private funding and volunteer services from retired physicians and nurse practitioners. In lieu of this model, expanding the attractiveness of the existing facilities to the lower-income population through improvements in transportation, communication, and access may be possible. Either alternative will provide much-improved health care for this underserved community.

As the diversity of these small rural resort towns increases, so too will the need for highly specialized physicians and nurse practitioners. Communities such as this resort will need to restructure services or risk losing workers due to decreased productivity related to illness. A plan to eliminate health disparities among Latinos and underserved populations will require a comprehensive and coordinated approach by health and human service organizations, commitment from different levels of government, and full participation of the private sector.

For a full suite of assignments and additional learning activities, use the access code located in the front of your book to visit this exclusive website: http://go.jblearning.com/dechesnay. If you do not have an access code, you can obtain one at the site.

REFERENCES

American Medical Association. (1996–2002). Physician distribution in the U.S. Retrieved February 3, 2006, from www.AMA.org

Anderson, R. M. (1995). Revising behavior model of access to medical care. *Journal of Health and Social Behavior, 36*, 1–10.

Association of Community Organization for Reform. (2004). Speaking the language of care: Language barriers to hospital access in American cities. Retrieved November 27, 2004, from http;//www.acorn.org

BBC Research & Consulting. (2003). The Aspen retail study. Retrieved May 12, 2006, from www.aspenpitkin.com

Carson, K. L., Jenssen, L., & Synder, A. (2004). The health and nutrition of Latino migrant and seasonal farm workers. Center for Rural Pennsylvania, pp. 1–20.

Casey, M. M., Blewett, L. A., & Call, K. T. (2004). Providing health care to Latino immigrants: Community-based efforts in the rural Midwest. *American Journal of Public Health, 94*(10), 1709–1711.

De Chesnay, M., Wharton, R., & Pamp, C. (2005). Cultural competence, resilience and advocacy. In M. de Chesnay (Ed.), *Caring for the vulnerable: Perspectives in nursing theory, practice and research* (pp. 31–42). Sudbury, MA: Jones and Bartlett.

Doty, M. M., & Ives, B. L. (2002). Quality of health care for Latino population: Finding from the Commonwealth Fund 2001 health care quality survey. Commonwealth Fund, pp. 1–12.

Foley, G. (2004, September 1). Can our valley find a balance? Retrieved May 11, 2006, from www.mountainexpress.com

Galanti, G. (2003). The Hispanic family and male–female relationships: An overview. *Journal of Transcultural Nursing, 14*(3), 180–185.

Healthy people 2010. (2006). Retrieved January 26, 2006, from www.HealthyPeople2010.org

Hunter, R., Gaylord, S., Britnell, M., & Ashford-Works, C. (1998). *Making a difference in rural communities: A guide for trainees in the health professions.* Chapel Hill, NC: University of North Carolina at Chapel Hill, Department of Medicine, Program on Aging.

Johnson, M. D. (2001). Meeting the health care needs of a vulnerable population: Perceived barriers. *Journal of Community Health Nursing, 18*, 24–28.

Kaiser, H. J. (2003). State the facts on-line: Idaho minority heath median family income by race/ethnicity. Retrieved April 18, 2005, from http://www.statehealthfacts.kkf.org

LaVeist, T. A., Diala, C., & Jerrett, N. C. (2000). *Minority health in America.* Baltimore, MD: Johns Hopkins University Press.

Lee, S., & Choi, S. (2009). Disparities in access to health care among non-citizens in the United States. *Health Sociology Review, 18*(3), 307–320.

Mason, R. (2005, July 15, 2005). Blaine County benefits from $4.3 million dollar investment from the Department of Health and Welfare. Retrieved May 12, 2006, from www.healthandwelfaredept.org

McElmurry, B. J., Park, C. G., & Busch, A. G. (2003, March 6). The nurse–community health advocate team for urban immigrant primary health care. *Journal of Nursing Scholarship, 35*(3), 275–281.

McPhatter, A. R. (1997). Cultural competence in child welfare: What is it? How do we achieve it? What happens without it? *Child Welfare, 76*, 225–278.

Mercer, M. M. (2001). Initiatives to improve access to rural health care services: A briefing paper. Arizona Health Care Cost Containment System, pp. 1–55.

Najm, W., Reinsch, S., Hoehler, F., & Tobis, J. (2003). Use of complementary and alternative medicine among the ethnic elderly. *Alternative Therapies, 9*(3), 50–57.

Probst, J. C., Moore, C. G., Glover, S., & Samuels, M. E. (2004). Person and place: The compounding effects of race/ethnicity and rurality on health. *American Journal of Public Health, 94*(10), 1695–1703.

Rogers, G. (2006, January 2006). Blaine County profile. Retrieved May 11, 2006, from www.cl.idaho.gov

Shaffer, C. (2002). Factors influencing the access to prenatal care by Hispanic women. *Journal of the American Academy of Nurse Practitioners, 14*(2), 93–96.

Solis, J. M., Marks, G., Garcia, M., & Shelton, D. (1990). Acculturation, access to care, and use of preventive services by Hispanics: Findings from HHANES 1982–1984. *American Journal of Public Health.* (Dec; 80 Suppl), 11–19.

Sue, D., & Sue, D. (1999). *Counseling the culturally different.* New York, NY: John Wiley & Sons.

U.S. Census Report (USCR). (1990–2004). Blaine County, Idaho. Retrieved January 26, 2006, from www.quickfacts.census.gov

U.S. Department of Health and Human Services (HHS). (2001, February). *Mental health: Culture, race, and ethnicity: A supplement to Mental health: A report of the U.S. Surgeon General.* Rockville, MD: Author, pp. 20–27.

U.S. Department of Health and Human Services (HHS). (2004). The 2004 HHS poverty guidelines. Retrieved April 16, 2006, from Http://aspe.hhs.gov/poveryt/04.shtml

Vezeau, T. (2005). Literacy and vulnerability. In M. de Chesnay (Ed.), *Caring for the vulnerable: Perspectives in nursing theory, practice, and research* (pp. 407–418). Sudbury, MA: Jones and Bartlett.

Weich, R., & Angulo, C. (2000). Justice on trial: Racial disparities in American criminal justice system. Retrieved April 16, 2006, from www.HRW.org/backgrounder/usa/race

CHAPTER 25

Navy Nurses: Vulnerable People Caring for Vulnerable Populations

Capt. Mary Ann White

Objectives

At the end of this chapter, the reader will be able to

1. Describe the work of Navy nurses and how they are vulnerable.
2. Compare and contrast the issues related to Navy nurses working in high-risk areas versus nurses in other types of disaster conditions.
3. Identify a researchable problem based on the chapter that involves military nurses.

INTRODUCTION

Imagine the vulnerability of a wife and mother of two keeping her ready bag packed in the corner and waiting for the phone to ring, bringing news as to where she will be sent in support of the war that just began in Kuwait. This takes little imagination for the writer, as it was her experience as a Navy Reserve nurse during Desert Storm. Nurse Corps officers in the Navy Reserves face unique challenges as they balance their military obligations with the many competing priorities imposed by their civilian careers. They could be considered vulnerable due to their multifaceted circumstances. Their stories of providing care whenever and wherever called upon illustrate beautifully several of key concepts proposed by de Chesnay and Anderson (2008) to be particularly useful in caring for people who are vulnerable: cultural competence, resilience, and advocacy.

To appreciate these accounts, it is critical to understand more fully Navy nursing and how it differs from its civilian counterparts. Therefore, these stories will be preceded with an

The views expressed in this chapter are those of the author and do not necessarily reflect the official policy or position of the Department of the Navy, Department of Defense, nor the U.S. government.

overview of nursing in the Navy to enhance the reader's understanding. Vignettes will then be provided as vivid examples of how these nurses have applied their skills in caring for vulnerable people in an array of global environments: deployed to war in Afghanistan, aboard the U.S. hospital ship *USNS Comfort* (T-AH 20) during humanitarian relief in Haiti, and in medical centers state-side and in Europe. All of the vignettes are slices from the life of these Reserve officers.

NAVY NURSING

Mission

Each Navy Nurse Corps officer begins a career in the Navy by taking a statutory oath of office. This promise and covenant is made to the nation: "to support and defend the Constitution of the United States, against all enemies foreign and domestic." The oath implies an affirmation of the officer to be ready to deploy anytime, anywhere to meet the mission. The Navy medicine mission is constantly changing in response to evolving world events and politics. Humanitarian missions to Haiti following a devastating earthquake, wartime deployments to Iraq, nation building in Afghanistan, or counterterrorism in the horn of Africa are to name but a few of these operations. To meet these missions, Navy nurses provide nursing care beyond the scope of traditional care, treating vulnerable individuals and populations worldwide. Their career journey includes many experiences beyond the confines of a bricks-and-mortar hospital or clinic.

Clinical Competence

The Navy nurse must be clinically competent to serve in hospitals, the operational theater, on humanitarian missions, and in joint environments. The global geographic environment in which these nurses serve creates the need for them to be multitalented, with cross-training for skills in disaster nursing. Disparate circumstances necessitate a certain amount of expertise in pediatrics, obstetrics, and nonbattle disease processes. Both clinical and cultural competence are essential for them to meet the healthcare needs they will encounter on their diverse assignments.

Reserve Nurses

Nurses in the Reserves have a parallel mission: They must be clinically competent in all these arenas, yet they may not necessarily perform these skills in their civilian role. They must also be ready to perform these clinical duties immediately upon recall for a mission, often with short notice. Moreover, these nurses must accomplish their clinical and operational training on a part-time basis—that is, one weekend per month and two weeks per year. Additionally, as mentioned earlier, they face multiple challenges as they balance their military obligations with the many competing priorities imposed by their home life and civilian career. These struggles are encapsulated in one Reserve nurse officer's conclusion that being mobilized for an active-duty assignment would actually simplify her life:

> I believe that the most difficult challenges for a reservist is that full-time active personnel fail to recognize that we do not work just one weekend a month and two weeks a year. For the most part we all have full-time jobs plus our military

> commitment, plus family obligations and general-life errands and tasks. Time is of the essence and requires much organization to make all this work. This allows for just six days off a month to manage family plus [run] errands plus [take] personal time—not to mention the time spent preparing for a drill weekend (paperwork, courses, and presentations that are a part of our weekend). I, for one, would like to have this remembered, recognized, and appreciated. Being mobilized greatly simplified time management.

VIGNETTES

Deployed to War

Currently, Navy nurses are serving in the Iraqi and Afghanistan war zones. Such a wartime mission requires evacuating the injured from the battlefield, sending the severely injured back for higher levels of definitive care, and returning the less injured to duty as soon as possible. These nurses are providing care for their own forces as well as for forces of other coalition countries, local civilians caught in the crossfire of war, and insurgents brought for care (Wynd, 2006.

This Reserve nurse's story is about caring for children caught in the chaos of war in Afghanistan:

> One day in early October, a group of children including two little Afghan girls went out to play in their village, as I'm sure they had done many times before. One child stepped the wrong way, and in a split second her life was changed forever. An improvised explosive device (IED) planted by their countrymen to kill and maim the enemy had blown up two of their own innocent girls. The girls were related to each other. One was approximately eight years old and the other four years old (they don't celebrate birthdays in Afghanistan). I can't use their real names, so I will call the older girl Grace and the younger one Hope.

The nurse then recounted caring for Grace and explained how hope was instilled in the midst of pain:

> Grace had abdominal surgery to remove shrapnel that was blown into her little belly. She survived her surgery and did quite well. Once she could breathe on her own and was stable, she was moved to the acute care ward, where she recovered for several weeks. She was incredibly stoic and never smiled at first. Our staff of nurses and corpsmen worked tirelessly to break through that wall of fear, confusion, and mistrust. She had to endure some painful dressing changes and the usual post-op pain associated with the type of surgery she had undergone.
>
> One day, one young female corpsman broke down the wall, and it was the beginning of a joy-filled relationship with the ward staff. Each day she became stronger and bolder in her interactions with us. Initially, she would reluctantly hold hands. Eventually her interactions expanded to the point of hugs for everyone. She enjoyed being carried around by the female staff and sitting on our laps

> as we did our work. Her smile lit up the ward and she became quite the popular young lady. She remained with us long after her recovery time because she had to wait for her cousin to work through her ongoing problems.

Her saga continued, as Grace's advocate worked closely with the father who would soon provide the child's care:

> Hope is younger and smaller than Grace, and so the explosion caused her to suffer a severe head injury. The trauma team was not sure that she would survive at all, and if she did, what her quality of life would be. It is a harsh world in the villages here if you have any sort of physical disability, and chances for survival are slim.
>
> Hope survived her initial brain surgery and went to the ICU. She was in critical condition for a long time. After several days, the decision was made to remove her breathing tube. She was able to breathe on her on own. She clearly had significant brain damage and the outlook was grim. She came to the ward for ongoing therapy and care. Her father was at her bedside throughout her hospitalization. We worked hard to get Hope to overcome her brain injury. It still didn't look good. There are no rehab centers in Afghanistan . . . no brain injury units . . . no Bryn Mawr Rehabs! This little girl had a significant brain injury and had the front part of her skull removed and sewn into her abdomen for replacement later. We finally had to face the reality that this child could not survive outside of our hospital.
>
> We had a tearful conference with the doctors and nurses and the father. It was decided that we would pull her feeding tube and see if we could get Grace to swallow any liquids or foods. Slowly, she began to swallow her own secretions, and then we were able to give her some liquids through a syringe. We taught her father how to feed her and he did a great job. Thanks to some timely donations of Jell-o and applesauce and Pediacare formula, we advanced her diet ever so slowly and things were looking up. Hope was beginning to move her left side and already had full use of her right side. She was whispering words but nothing that made any sense. She cried every time we looked at her, let alone changed her bandages, but we could get the occasional smile.

The officer concludes with an acknowledgment of respect for all of her patients, regardless of their differences:

> I was not prepared to care for the children who are victims of this war. It is not an easy balance to deliver First World care in a Third World nation. We treat all lives here as sacred and provide the finest care to all who land on our doorstep.

During wartime, nurses work in hostile environments, often in harm's way.

Humanitarian Mission

Peacekeeping, nation building, and humanitarian missions throughout the world are often additional Navy assignments. These missions may take the form of a planned medical readiness and training exercise (MEDRETE) or they may occur in response to a natural disaster, as in the deployment of the *Comfort*. Navy Reserve nurses involved in these humanitarian activities provide medical assistance to host nations ranging from "sick call" services to assisting in advanced surgical procedures. In these missions, it is necessary to have an understanding of the country and area-specific endemic diseases. Language barriers are also a concern, so all missions require medically trained translators.

A Reserve Nurse Corps officer who volunteered to go on the *Comfort* to Haiti recalled:

> I am extremely proud of my career as an officer in the Navy Nurse Corps. Part of the joy of being a Navy nurse has been the opportunity to serve on many different platforms, more so than my civilian counterparts. As an adult critical care nurse, I have taken care of a variety of patients, including burn, trauma, and open heart surgery patients as well as many others. When the earthquake hit Haiti on 12 January 2010, I felt that I had to be there and had to use my experience to help take care of my people. (Etienne, 2010)

She continued:

> As I reported to the very busy intensive care unit (ICU) for further instructions, I quickly realized that my close to 30 years' nursing experience was not enough to prepare me for what I would face. Wake-up call #1: There were many injured children fighting for their life in the ICU. My relationship with children is usually all about hugs and kisses, food and fun activities. Reality #2: I was the only health professional in the ICU who understood and spoke Creole.
>
> As I walked in the ICU that day, I was taken back by the cry of an eight-year-old boy. "I want my father! I cannot live without my father! I don't want anything except for my father!" The depth of sorrow expressed and the choice of words by this young boy would give you the impression that he was certain that he would not see his father again. Realizing that I was the only one who understood what he was saying, I was drawn to him to try to provide comfort. My offers for any comfort measures, like pain medicine, food, and liquid, were rejected by this child, who continued to repeat, "I don't want anything but my father!' I translated what was going on to the nurse who was taking care of him. (Etienne, 2010)

She recalls her role as advocate for her patients:

> I was glad that I was useful the minute that I stepped foot onto the *Comfort*. I had many collateral duties during my month on the *Comfort*, and although many were unofficial, they were very necessary. I was a patient advocate for many, with limited understanding of their medical condition. As a member of the ethics committee, we discussed best approaches to challenging cases. As a Haitian American and a senior officer, I was sought after for guidance in special circumstances. I responded to codes when possible. I worked as a liaison promoting dialogue between the translators, the ICU, and medical staff. I made rounds

> on the wars to visit patients who were in the ICU. I guess that you can say I was a nurse by day and ethical/social support by night. (Etienne, 2010)

Hospital Mission

Much of military nursing in these settings is characterized by the independent and autonomous nature of the work. Military nurses are often the leaders of patient care teams and, therefore, must have management and organization skills.

This Reserve nurse worked in the operating room (OR) of a major military hospital in the United States during her weekend duty. She recalls:

> One morning I was assessing a soldier who was having his tenth surgical procedure. He explained that no one was with him because his father had to go back to work in Pennsylvania. I immediately went into parent mode. What a difficult decision. Even though this young man, in his early twenties, was an adult, he was very vulnerable. He leg was still stabilized by an external fixation device. He was still unsure of his future due to the injury from the IED explosion to his leg. He shared that he hoped this would be his last surgery prior to being sent to a medical facility closer to home. We started talking about his hometown, and about the time that the orthopedic resident walked up. The fact that our soldier and the resident had grown up in the same hometown felt serendipitous. Although they hadn't attended the same high school, they were able to establish a bond that added to the caring environment.
>
> I did get to speak with his father prior to the surgery. I know that it made me feel better that I was able to communicate our plan, answer his questions, and assure him that we would call him after the surgery to update him on his son's condition.

She continued with another encounter:

> Despite my extensive experience in the OR, the greatest challenge was caring for a soldier from Texas who had over a period of three months lost all of his extremities. This patient was in the ICU on contact precautions due to the complexity of his injuries. We were going to be doing washouts and wound evacuation changes on three extremities.
>
> We got our handoff from the ICU nurse and then went to meet the patient. He was awake. Introducing oneself and looking directly into the eyes of what had once been a strapping Marine was surreal in some ways. His eyes probed mine, and I felt an overwhelming need to say something profound that would somehow make things better. What I did was introduce myself, perform my safety check and assessment, and help transport him to the OR, thankful that the Versed had been given. The pictures on his bedside table showed him and his wife prior to his deployment. They were both smiling, as were the children in the pictures.

She concluded:

> I remember what a Navy Nurse friend of mine returning from Landstuhl shared. She had a patient with a similar injury while serving in Germany. She put her heart and soul into a soldier who lost all of his extremities. She met the family and was able to share a love of horses with the patient over time. A few months after his transport stateside, she received a picture in the mail of this soldier riding a horse, held in place by a device made by his father. Life is amazing.

Another Reserve Nurse Corps officer mobilized to a hospital in Germany reported:

> This has been my first deployment, as I am a "late-comer" to the Navy Nurse Corps. The team I work on is equally divided between Army, Navy, Air Force, and civilian nurses.
>
> I would like to share one story with you that touched me during my stay here. A young officer was injured in an IED blast. His body was fine, but his head and face were badly injured, swollen, and disfigured, and he lost one eye. Through his time here (which was longer than usual, as he was Canadian), we became accustomed to his appearance so that he became normal to us. When it was time for him to leave us, we were rolling him out on the stretcher to return home. He stopped me and signed that he needed a blanket, so I ran back to the room. (He was unable to speak but could use sign language.) I wondered why he wanted the blanket and discovered that he was not asking for it for himself, but instead because he realized that he might be difficult to look at and wanted to prevent others from being upset by his appearance—so he had me cover his face. I was amazed. In his time of great pain, sacrifice, and illness, he took the time to think of others and their feelings.
>
> I will tell you this is not an isolated incident but rather happens many, many times. Having the opportunity to provide care in Europe—I could never have imagined how wonderful it would be to serve our nation in Europe.

CONCLUSION

These personal accounts from nurses working as Reserve nurses on the battlefield, on the hospital ship, and in a hospital setting allow us to look into the reactions and concerns of nurses as they experience vulnerable individuals and populations. Their stories provide examples of cultural competence in nursing—that is, care that embraces the cultural differences that exist between the nurse and the patient while meeting the healthcare needs of culturally diverse patients. These nurses demonstrate the ability to be open to different cultures and show the utmost respect for their patients, who were different than themselves. Inherent in their care was the need to infuse hope into their patients' despairing situations and to act as an advocate by simply informing the patient and then supporting whatever decision he or she makes.

For a full suite of assignments and additional learning activities, use the access code located in the front of your book to visit this exclusive website: http://go.jblearning.com/dechesnay. If you do not have an access code, you can obtain one at the site.

REFERENCES

De Chesnay, M., & Anderson, B. A. (2008). *Caring for the vulnerable: Perspectives in nursing theory, practice, and research*. Sudbury, MA: Jones and Bartlett.

Etienne, F. (2010). Twice the service. *The Lantern: The Journal of Nursing Stories*, *2*, 2.

Wynd, C. (September 30, 2006). A proposed model for military disaster nursing. *OJIN: The Online Journal of Issues in Nursing*, *11*(3), Manuscript 4. doi: 10.3912/OJIN.Vol11No03Man04

CHAPTER 26

Ethics of End-of-Life Care

Lois R. Robley

Objectives

At the end of this chapter, the reader will be able to

1. Compare and contrast issues related to dying in the industrialized world versus the developing world.
2. Describe palliative care in terms of key concepts and techniques.
3. Provide examples from research that illustrate best practices in palliative care.

VULNERABILITY OF THE DYING

Schroeder and Gefenas (2009) offer the following definition of vulnerability: "To be vulnerable means to face a significant probability of incurring an identifiable harm while substantially lacking ability and/or means to protect oneself" (p. 117). While it is important to be cautious when using the label of vulnerability because "labeling individuals as 'vulnerable' risks viewing vulnerable individuals as 'others' worthy of pity" (Ruof, 2004, p. 412), vulnerability remains an important concept that calls our attention to those in most need and for whom we have a unique moral responsibility.

In keeping with this carefully crafted definition, those persons who are living with chronic, debilitating, and life-threatening illness are considered vulnerable, as are their families. Persons face harm to the self (from the ravages of disease, disability, and existential threat) while often requiring special protection because of frailness; weakness; pain; symptoms such as nausea, immobility, and dependence; being unable to speak; lack of dignity; and distress. Families often encounter unresolved grief, feelings of guilt, and the burdens of caring. The moral obligations of healthcare professionals are heightened for those who are dying expressly because they often lack the ability or means to protect themselves and one another.

DYING AROUND THE WORLD

Dying is a common experience for all humans, but when and how we die vary widely among people across the world and within populations. Worldwide, more than 57 million people die each year (Central Intelligence Agency [CIA], 2010). The leading causes of death depend on income level within societies. Coronary heart disease is consistently listed as a leading cause of death for all societies. Within lower-income countries, however, infectious diseases such as lower respiratory infections, diarrheal diseases, and human immunodeficiency virus (HIV)/acquired immune deficiency syndrome (AIDS) are the most frequent causes of death. Among middle-income countries, other leading causes of death are stroke and chronic obstructive pulmonary disease (COPD). Among high-income countries, stroke and upper and lower respiratory cancers abound as causes of death (World Health Organization [WHO], 2008).

In countries with low income, 80% of deaths occur in the age span of 0 to 69 years, whereas in counties with high income 70% of deaths occur among people age 70 or older. Children and adults who live on the continent of Africa fare far worse than those who live in other regions of the world. For example, African children ages 0 to 4 years have double the rate of death (37 deaths per 1,000 live births) when compared to the region with the next highest number of deaths in this age group, the eastern Mediterranean (WHO, 2008). As many as 1.5 million children in predominantly developing countries die of diarrhea, which accounts for more deaths worldwide than AIDS, malaria, and measles combined (Wardlaw, Salama, Brocklehurst, Chopra, & Mason, 2010). Correspondingly, average life expectancy ranges across the world from 83 years in Japan and San Marino to 42 years in Zimbabwe and Afghanistan (WHO, 2010).

These disparities regarding cause of death are cause for global concern. In addition, disparities also arise based on the varying degrees within a population of attentiveness to the needs of the dying. The elements of concern in this setting include the lack of availability of standard medication used to provide comfort for the dying; inadequate or absent public policy about end-of-life care; varying cultural, sociological, and ethical issues surrounding death and dying; geographical dispersion of populations; and lack of adherence to internationally proclaimed quality standards of palliative care. For example, despite the WHO (1986) call for healthcare professionals around the world to provide analgesia for their patients in pain, it is known that the "vast majority of cancer and AIDS patients in the developing world . . . still lack access" to opioids for pain relief (Joranson, Ryan, & Maurer, 2009, p. 194). Morphine, an inexpensive and effective treatment for pain and breathlessness, is disproportionately used. When the International Narcotics Control Board published data on the per capita use of morphine around the world, its report revealed that six nations accounted for 79% of all morphine use. In contrast, countries whose residents made up 80% of the world's population consumed only 6% of morphine for patient pain relief (Gwyther, Brennan, & Harding, 2009).

The solutions to many of these thorny problems related to end-of-life care lie in the development of targeted palliative care and hospice programs in all countries.

PALLIATIVE AND HOSPICE CARE

The word "palliative" arises from the Latin *palliare*, meaning "to cloak" or to make "symptoms of a disease less severe without removing the cause" (*Oxford English Dictionary*, 2006). As Meier, Isaacs, and Hughes (2010) state, "Palliative care focuses on the relief of suffering for patients with serious and complex illness and tries to ensure the best possible quality of life for them and their family members" (p. 4). This kind of care is delivered wherever the patient may be (e.g., hospital, home, nursing home, assisted living facility) and is delivered simultaneously with curative treatments. It involves management of the person's symptoms holistically, addressing physiologic, psychologic, social, and spiritual needs. The National Consensus Project on Palliative Care (2009), states that the goals of palliative care are as follows:

> [To] prevent and relieve suffering and to support the best possible quality of life for patients and their families, regardless of the stage of the disease or the need for other therapies. Palliative care is both a philosophy of care and an organized, highly structured system for delivering care. Palliative care expands traditional disease-model medical treatments in the hospital and home to include the goals of enhancing quality of life for patient and family, optimizing function, assisting with decision making and providing opportunities for personal growth. As such, palliative care can be delivered concurrently with life-prolonging care or as the main focus of care. (p. 4)

Early palliative care (provided at the time of diagnosis of a life-threatening or serious illness) has been shown to improve longevity, quality of life, and mood (Temel et al., 2010). In a randomized controlled study of patients diagnosed with metastatic non-small-cell lung cancer (Temel et al., 2010), those patients who received early palliative care, as compared to those who received standard oncology care, had statistically better quality of life, received less aggressive treatment, and lived longer.

Hospice is a type of palliative care that is targeted to those individuals who are near death (Jennings, Ryndes, D'Onofrio, & Baily, 2003). Typically persons are referred to hospice when curative therapy no longer provides benefit or when the harms or drawbacks to treatment outweigh the benefits. The Medicare hospice benefit in the United States (and often private insurance) covers the predicted last six months of life, although many persons can and do receive extensions of the hospice benefit.

In recent years, nurses and physicians have connected with colleagues across the globe to foster palliative care and hospice development. Countries such as the United Kingdom, under the direction of the passionate leadership of the late Dame Cicely Saunders, have been willing ambassadors for palliative care and hospice around the world, disseminating information, fostering standards of care, and encouraging new development of palliative care and hospice (Praill & Pahl, 2007). Yet much work needs to be done, particularly in sub-Saharan Africa, where cancer and HIV/AIDS mortality is increasing (Harding & Higginson, 2005). Hospice and palliative care services policies differ widely across the globe, ranging from those countries with no known hospice/palliative care activity to those countries where hospice and palliative care activities are approaching integration with the wider health system. According to latest figures, approximately half of the countries around the world (117) have at least some palliative care/hospice services. Only 35 countries (15%), however, fall into the category labeled as "approach integration of palliative care services with their mainstream health care systems" (International Observatory on End-of-Life Care, 2006, p. 7).

The "Quality of Death Index" is a recent report that ranks nations on the quality of care and infrastructure support for palliative and end-of-life care (The Economist Intelligence Unit, 2010). This study, which was conducted by the Economist Intelligence Unit and funded by the Lien Foundation (a Singaporean philanthropic organization), measured the basic end-of-life healthcare environment, availability of end-of-life care, cost of end-of-life care, and quality of end-of-life care. In its development of the rankings, it used such measures as life expectancy, healthcare expenditures per gross domestic product (GDP), availability of hospice and palliative care programs, public awareness of palliative care, training availability for palliation, access to pain medications, doctor–patient transparency about end of life, and status indicators (e.g., existence of national strategies for quality palliative care). In the report, the authors state that "while more than 100 million people would benefit from hospice and palliative care annually (including family and carers [sic] who need help and assistance in caring), less than 8% of those in need access it" (p. 5). Out of 40 countries analyzed, the United Kingdom ranked number 1 and India ranked 40 in overall quality of death.

DYING IN THE UNITED STATES

Despite its status as having one of the world's best healthcare systems and the visible emergence of palliative care and hospice in recent years, the United States ranks ninth among the 40 nations analyzed in the Quality of Death Index (The Economist Intelligence Unit, 2010). In 2007, 2,423,712 persons died in the United States (Centers for Disease Control and Prevention [CDC], 2010). What was death like for those individuals? Has the experience of dying and death improved since the landmark studies on death and dying were reported?

WWW A Case in Point

A recently documented case in the United States illustrates the fact that this country has a long way to go before it provides optimal end-of-life care for all of its residents. Mr. Tomas Nagunu (a pseudonym), a 69-year-old husband and father of five adult children, was diagnosed with stage IV metastatic non-small-cell lung cancer after surgery for repair of an avulsion (metastatic) fracture of the right hip. Tomas elected to pursue radiation therapy, which was the only treatment choice predicted to help reduce the size of the tumor in his lung and "give" him six months to one year of life. He was counting on his family—particularly his daughter Janice, who was a seasoned registered nurse—to care for him at home. The entire family, including grandchildren, agreed to assist in his care. At the time of her father's discharge from the hospital, Janice asked the physician and social worker about hospice care and was told, "We can handle this. We don't need hospice yet." Fentanyl patches were prescribed for the often, spasmodic and severe metastatic bone pain. The family went through 11 weeks of turmoil trying to lovingly care for

Tomas. They were repeatedly forced to deal with anxiety, agitation, hallucinations, increasing breathlessness, decubiti, and increasing pain, calling the physician again and again for advice and prescriptions. Not until two days before his death did the family receive the support of hospice. When Tomas died, the family wondered aloud if his death could be attributed to the transfer to hospice.

MAJOR STUDIES

Three major scientific studies illustrated the plight of the dying in the United States: the Study to Understand Prognosis and Preferences for Outcomes and Risks of Treatment (SUPPORT, 1995), an Institute of Medicine (IOM) study published in 1997 (Field & Cassel, 1997), and the 2002 study from Last Acts known as "Means to a Better End."

The SUPPORT study was conducted in five medical centers and involved more than 9,000 patients across the United States. Shortcomings documented in this research included poor communication between doctor and patient/family despite targeted interventions intended to improve such communication. Forty-six percent of do not resuscitate (DNR) orders were written within two days of death. For 50% of conscious patients who died in the hospital, family members reported that they experienced moderate to severe pain at least half the time.

The IOM study (Field & Cassel, 1997) demonstrated that in the United States, death is fought with steel-like determination. Also, while people generally desire to die at home, the overwhelming majority die in institutions. The IOM study also revealed that there is frequent use of aggressive curative treatments in advanced disease. The average length of stay in hospice reported in this study was less than one week, denying the patient and family the opportunity to reap the benefits of more appropriate holistic care.

In 2002, Last Acts' "Means to a Better End" study was published under the auspices of the Robert Wood Johnson Foundation. It rated states on the basis of eight elements of good end-of-life care: the strength of advance care planning legislation, the proportion of deaths that occurred at home, how well hospice was recommended and used, how often hospitals included pain and palliative care services, how often elderly received ICU care in the last six months of life, how well nursing homes managed their residents' pain, the adequacy of state policies regarding good pain management, and the number of nurses and physicians trained in palliative care. This study revealed serious deficits in most states and the urgent need to improve end-of-life care in all eight quality criteria.

In addition to these three studies, other analyses of the state of palliative care have been done. In 2008, report cards were published by the Center to Advance Palliative Care (CAPC) that rated states on the quality of their palliative care. The 50 states were given an overall grade of "C" with regard to the prevalence and access to palliative care programs and professionals within hospitals. The study authors state:

> Approximately ninety million Americans are living with serious and life-threatening illness, and this number is expected to more than double over the next twenty–five years with aging of the population. Yet, studies show that most people living with a

> serious illness experience inadequately treated symptoms; fragmented care; poor communication with their doctors; and enormous strains on their family caregivers. [See also Radwany, Albanese, Clough, Sims, Mason, & Jahangiri, 2009.]

Research has also been conducted to determine the factors considered important at the end of life by chronically ill patients, family, physicians and other care providers. Steinhauser et al. (2000) found that certain commonalities are identified as essentials for good end-of-life care. The most important of these considerations were being kept clean, naming a decision maker, having a nurse with whom one feels comfortable, knowing what to expect about one's physical condition, having someone who will listen, maintaining one's dignity, trusting one's physician, being free of pain, and saying good bye to important people. This study, and others completed since its publication (e.g., Bonin-Scaon, Sastre, Chasseigne, Sorum, & Mullet, 2009) illustrate that while the physical needs must be met, psychosocial and spiritual considerations need attention as well.

ETHICS OF CARE FOR THE DYING

Claims are made that excellent care for the dying is a moral act. Justification is based upon a triptych of ethical approaches that can be applied to this issue: the principle of justice (including social justice), appeals to human rights, and ethics of care.

The Principal of Justice

Using biomedical ethical principles—particularly justice—as a guide to treatment of the vulnerable such as the dying, both similarities and differences become apparent around the globe. In American bioethics, four principles (Beauchamp & Childress, 2001) have assumed preeminence within biomedical ethics: autonomy (self-rule), beneficence (doing good), nonmaleficence (avoiding and preventing harm), and justice (fair, equitable, and appropriate treatment in light of what is due or owed to persons). Autonomy calls for improved education about and the writing of advance directives. Distributive justice drives the need for guidelines and standards for treatment of all who are dying.

In European bioethics and biolaw, the principles of vulnerability, autonomy, dignity, and integrity have risen to the status of collective importance (Rendtorff, 2002). Of these four principles, vulnerability is said to be "ontologically prior to the other principles; it expresses better than all other ethical principles in the discussion the finitude of the human condition, and therefore it might be the real bridging idea between moral strangers"—that is, between the patient and the healthcare professional (Rendtorff, Kemp, & Commission of the European Communities, 2000, p. 46). Responsibility to care for the vulnerable is the philosophy behind universalizing hospice and end-of-life care within European communities.

In ancient Chinese medical ethics, concepts similar to the Western principles of beneficence and nonmaleficence—that is, doing good and avoiding harm—take precedence over autonomy. The good of the whole society is preeminent. Yet, guided by the Confucian philosophy humaneness (*jen*), Chinese medical ethics calls for equal treatment and justice, particularly for the worst-off individuals (Tsai, 1999).

On the African continent, the traditional concept of personhood has an ecological, biological, and communitarian orientation (Tangwa, 2000). People in Africa traditionally believe that humans are interdependent throughout the life span with plants, other animals, inanimate objects, forces, and spirits. "Within this world view, transmigration, reincarnation, transformation and transmutation, within and across species, are believed to be possible" (Tangwa, 2000, p. 42). Consequently, there is "a deep-seated attitude of live and let live, be and let be," which calls for collective decision making about anything in life. Community consensus rules (Tangwa, 2000, p. 42). The emergent development of an African nursing ethics (Arries, 2009) has its roots in an ethics of justice and care, but also incorporates this sense of community. The concept of individual is an individual in and through others, is called variously "ubuntu" (South Africa) or "maat" (Egypt). As Desmond Tutu (2000) explains, "Ubuntu is the essence of being a person. It means that we are people through other people. We cannot be fully human alone. We are made for interdependence, we are made for family. When you have ubuntu, you embrace others. You are generous, compassionate" (p. 12). Metz (2009) expresses this concept in normative ethics terms by saying that "an action is wrong insofar as it fails to honour relationships in which people share a way of life and care for one another's quality of life" (p. 183).

Human Rights

In addition to the principle of justice, human rights are invoked as justification for palliation and excellent end-of-life care. A human right is founded on duty: that which is owed to another in all circumstances and under all conditions solely on the basis of the other being human. Appeal to human rights can also be justified using utilitarian theory, which states that a society is better off if palliation and pain management are seen as rights because relief of suffering and providing benefit meet the health goals of society. Palliation is also cost-effective in developed nations, primarily through its ability to produce shorter lengths of stay in hospital and lower costs per day per patient. Thus this approach to end-of-life care protects scarce resources (CAPC, 2010). Recently published evidence points to the fact that use of palliative care early after diagnosis of serious illness significantly increases longevity and improves quality of life (Temel et al., 2010). Social justice is pivotal to the public health arena (of which palliative and end-of-life care are a part) because the distribution of goods and the bearing of burdens ought to be evenly distributed (Gostin & Powers, 2006).

Palliative care and pain management are pivotal to the health of a society. According to the National Consensus Project for Quality Palliative Care (2009) in the United States, "Palliative care teams should work toward equitable access to palliative care across all ages and patient populations, all diagnostic categories, all healthcare settings including rural communities, and regardless of race, ethnicity, sexual preference, or ability to pay" (p. 10). Lohman, Schleifer, and Amon (2010) decry the fact that "tens of millions of people around the world suffer moderate to severe pain each year without treatment" (p. 1741); they challenge states and nations to abide by WHO's "analgesic ladder" (found at http://www.who.int/cancer/palliative/painladder/en/) and, through legislation and in practical ways, to make opioids available for severe pain management. As these authors note, "the right to be free from torture, cruel, inhuman and degrading treatment or punishment is also a fundamental human right that is recognized in numerous international human rights instruments" (p. 6).

Claiming that palliative care and human rights are based on principles of universality and nondiscrimination, Gwyther, Berman, and Harding (2009) cite the International Bill of Rights and the International Covenant on Economic, Social and Cultural Rights, General Comment 14, as laying out those rights for all people. Within the United States, the National Consensus Project for Quality Palliative Care (2009) has as its mission the provision of consistent, high-quality care to all who are in need of palliative care. Its Clinical Practice Guidelines address the multidimensional aspects of palliation, including the domains of structures and processes of care; the physical aspects of care; the psychological and psychiatric aspects of care; the social aspects of care; the spiritual, religious, and existential aspects of care; the cultural aspects of care; care of the imminently dying patient; and the ethical and legal aspects of care. Efforts are also under way to develop an international minimum data set for assessing the quality of end-of-life care provided by nations (Casarett, Teno, & Higginson, 2006).

Ethics of Care

An ethics of care, as articulated by a number of authors well cited in the nursing literature, often is portrayed as standing in juxtaposition to an ethics of justice (Gilligan, 1982, 1987; Noddings, 1986, 2002). Nevertheless, there are many ways in which justice is enveloped in an ethics of care. The pivotal focus of an ethics of care is the "attending to and meeting the needs of the particular others for whom we take responsibility" (Held, 2006, p. 10). Emotions are valued and relations to others are practical and become the focus of critical attention. The person who cares as well as the recipient of care is affected and influenced by the relation with others, colleagues, friends, family, and patients. This mutual interdependence is understood by nurses around the world when they say they gain personally and professionally from giving care to others. Ethics of care involves action—that is, paying close attention to the feelings, needs, desires, and thoughts of the one cared for. It involves understanding the other's point of view (Noddings, 1986).

An ethics of care addresses and challenges unequal relationships and dependency—those related to socioeconomic, aging, life circumstances and power differences, for example. It does not compel us to view individuals as autonomous beings (with individual rights), but rather as complex, situated humans in relations with one another.

Demonstrating an ethics of care includes being just. Treating others fairly and with equality is caring ethics in practice. For example, a nurse who provides excellent end-of-life care to a 43-year-old mother dying of ovarian cancer would also provide excellent end-of-life care to an 83-year-old unmarried woman dying of end-stage stroke (although the actual action may be different). Held (2006) maintains, however, that an ethics of care and an ethics of justice ought to be kept conceptually distinct from each other, and applied as the event or situation warrants. An ethics of care is seen as applicable globally when, for example, rulers and legislators are persuaded to identify with and attend to their connections with the public they serve. There is acknowledged a place for human rights and justice, but an ethics of care may be more effective in dealing with society's problems (Tronto, 1993, 1996) and could be conceptualized as the underpinnings of conflict management where difficulties over opioid policies, for example, arise.

EFFORTS TO ADDRESS IMPROVED CARE AT THE END OF LIFE

In 2008, only 1.4 million deaths in the United States, representing 38% of all patient deaths in this country, occurred while patients were receiving hospice services; the median length of stay in hospice was 20.3 days (National Hospice and Palliative Care Organization [NHPCO], 2009). There are only 394 certified palliative care nurse practitioners in the United States—that is, 220 dying persons per nurse, a number that does not include other patients who required palliative care. Thus there is a wide gap between the services actually needed and the number and preparation of nurses to provide leadership in the competent care of seriously ill and dying patients. One of the obstacles to excellent and timely end-of-life and palliative care at all levels, however, continues to be the lack of palliative and hospice care education for all nurses and those in undergraduate and graduate nursing programs (Paice, Ferrell, Virani, Grant, Malloy, & Rhome, 2006a, 2006b).

A national nursing education program to correct this problem among nurses has been under way since February 2000, spearheaded by the American Association of Colleges of Nursing (AACN) and the City of Hope (AACN, 2010a). The End-of-Life Nursing Education Consortium (ELNEC), as it is named, provides education in palliative care for undergraduate and graduate nursing faculty; continuing education providers; staff development educators; specialty nurses in pediatrics, oncology, critical care, and geriatrics; and other nurses with training. The recipients of ELNEC education teach this essential information to both nursing students and practicing nurses (ELNEC, 2010). More than 11,375 nurses and other healthcare professionals, representing all 50 U.S. states plus 65 international countries, have received ELNEC training to date (ELNEC, 2010). The program involves nine modules: nursing care at the end of life; pain management; symptom management; ethical/legal issues; cultural considerations; communication; grief, loss, and bereavement; achieving quality care; and preparation and care at the time of death (AACN, 2010b). A corresponding educational program for physicians was launched called Education in Palliative and End of Life Care (EPEC, 2010). Hospice and palliative medicine was recognized as a subspecialty within the American Board of Medical Specialties (ABMS, 2010) and board certification became available in 2008.

Those who have been educated in such programs have taken their knowledge and skills to others. It is likely that millions of students, nurses, and patients have been affected by these educational efforts.

Until recently, there was a serious lack of palliative and end-of-life care information in nursing textbooks (Ferrell, Grant, & Virani, 2001; Ferrell, Virani, Grant, & Borneman, 1999; Kirchhoff, Beckstrand, & Anumandla, 2003). Today, however, there are two leading U.S. textbooks in palliative care for nursing: *Palliative Care Nursing: Quality Care to the End of Life* by Matzo and Sherman (2009), now in its third edition, and the *Oxford Textbook of Palliative Nursing* by Ferrell and Coyle (2010), also in its third edition. These are superior resources for nurse education and reference. Other classic nursing texts in all specialties are including more content on palliative and end-of-life care. The book (available free of charge) entitled *Children's Palliative Care in Africa* addresses many aspects of childhood palliative care in the African continent (Avery, 2009). Comprehensive palliative nursing texts have been written in by United Kingdom authors as well (e.g., Payne, Seymour, & Ingleton, 2008).

Teaching Nurses and Nursing Students

Most nurses have had little education in palliative and end-of-life care. In fact, a recent study found that senior nursing students near the completion of their program claimed only "little" or "some" knowledge of palliative care (Demitropoulos, 2007). Advanced practice nursing students who were not yet introduced to ELNEC equated palliative care solely with end-of-life care and perceived the role as prolonging life rather than maintaining quality of life (Shea, Grossman, Wallace, & Lange, 2010).

Through the efforts of ELNEC education for nurse faculty, and under the leadership of the AACN (2008) through its accreditation criteria ("The Essentials of Baccalaureate Education for Professional Nursing Practice"), that situation is now changing. For example, Virani, Malloy, Ferrell, and Kelly (2008) report that nurses in California who participated in ELNEC education, when surveyed before the ELNEC program and again 12 months after the program, showed highly significant improvement in their perceived effectiveness while caring for dying patients. Model examples of excellence in end-of-life care emerged from this education and the work of individual educators. Oncology-ELNEC, partnering with the Oncology Nursing Society, has been effective in disseminating knowledge, improving the care delivered in clinical practice, and enhancing the knowledge and effectiveness of oncology nurses (Coyne, Paice, Ferrell, Malloy, Virani, & Fennimore, 2007). ELNEC has also partnered with the Association of Pediatric Oncology/Hematology Nurses (APOHN) to spread the education of palliative care to pediatric nurses. Success in these arenas has also led to the development of a funded program in partnership with the Department of Veteran Affairs to educate its workforce (AACN, 2010c).

Mallory (2002) found that even one-time education can have a positive effect on nursing students' attitudes toward care of the dying. Additional studies are currently being conducted to examine the effect of ELNEC education on student knowledge, attitudes, and skills in providing palliative care, both in the United States and elsewhere.

Driven by the clear need for quality palliative and end-of-life care around the globe, the ELNEC leaders have adapted their program for nurses in countries other than the United States. The need for such care is overwhelming among vulnerable suffering and dying populations. The first five-day ELNEC Consortium International training conference provided education and support materials for nurses in leadership positions from countries in Eastern and Central Europe and the former Soviet and Central Asian countries (Paice, Ferrell, Coyle, Coyne & Callaway, 2007). A program evaluation indicated the feasibility of working with a sample of nurses from diverse countries and revealed excellent reception and knowledge building among the participants. Palliative care for children was identified as a special need in countries where the death rate among those 0 to 2 years of age is high. To date, ELNEC trainers have provided education for nurses in 65 countries (ELNEC, 2010).

Public Policy Initiatives

Despite evidence that palliative care enhances quality of life and reduces hospital costs (Morrison et al., 2008) and that access to both palliative care and hospice is beneficial to patients and their families, it is not yet a given that patients and their families are routinely provided these services (Campbell, 2010). Access, delivery, and financing of palliative care are the foci of public policy initiatives (including national cancer control policies) often spearheaded by international organizations such as the World Health Organization, the American Society of Clinical Oncology, the Institute of Medicine (Stjernsward, Foley, & Ferris, 2007), and the International Council of Nurses (2006). The Hospice and Palliative Nurses Association in the United States, through its membership in a consortium made up of national professional organizations, has helped develop the National Consensus Project (Ferrell et al., 2007), which sets the standards for quality palliative care—an important first step in policy development. In addition, national dialogue is currently under way to address the following issues:

- Increasing per diem rates for Medicare hospice reimbursement
- Improving national communication about death and dying
- Demonstrating measurable quality in end-of-life care
- Creating incentives for dialogue about palliative care between patients and healthcare providers
- Changing support for caregivers in the home
- Increasing funding for nursing and medical research in palliative care
- Creating demonstration projects that improve access for patients with serious and chronic disease
- Improving the impetus and funding for nurse and physician education and certification programs (Field & Cassel, 1997; Last Acts, 2002b; Reb, 2003)

THE ALLEVIATION OF SUFFERING

In a recent article, Ferrell and Coyle (2008) carefully examined suffering and nursing's role in witnessing the multiple ways in which people, particularly those with cancer, suffer. These authors maintain that the actions of nurses ease the suffering of patients and their families as they live through the often devastating effects of diagnosis, treatment, and its aftermath. Such ethical actions include providing timely pain and symptom relief, being fully present, modeling gentle care giving that is often emulated by family members, and acknowledging and discussing losses and suffering. The nurse treats each person as a unique individual, understanding that suffering is very personal. The nurse focuses on the whole person—the physical, psychological, social, and spiritual. This whole-person approach is the foundation of care provided by palliative and hospice programs.

Ethics of Care in Practice

While paying attention to these facets of suffering among all of their patients, nurses practice what is necessary care for the dying. In the case of Tomas Nagunu (the example given earlier in this chapter), the suffering of the patient and family could have been alleviated if the ethics of care were applied. An ethics of care involves work and energy on the part of the ones caring—in this case, the nurse in the primary care office or the advanced practice nurse within the oncology service. It must be recognized that a daughter who is a nurse is a daughter first: She reacts and cares as a daughter first, and as a nurse second. Nurses who are caring family members without specialist education in palliative/hospice care will use their knowledge and skills in familiar ways, but these approaches may not be the most advantageous in a given situation of serious illness and dying.

To apply the ethics of care to the case of Tomas, it would be imperative to recognize the meaning of each nursing encounter with the patient and to establish significant connections with him and his family, despite the complex and fast moving pace of today's nursing world. Citing the work of Gilligan (1987), Fairchild (2010) states: "caring in nursing has been viewed as a moral way of being, focused upon concern for self and others, goodness, responsibility and connectedness, and, ultimately, an intentional unity and being with self and others" (p. 354). If the first and subsequent encounters with Tomas and his family were seen in this light, the nurse would quickly attempt to understand the situated "big picture" of the family, their desires for Tomas, and their goals for his care. An ethics of care would employ the skills of dialogue and exchange. Establishing meaningful connections in this case would lead the nurse to consider the family's expectations in light of the available resources among its members in the home.

It would be important to understand the challenges for Janice of caring for her own father while bearing this responsibility for the family. Nurses caring for their own family members have dual responsibilities and specific needs (Aubeeluck, 2006) that may best be understood by other nurses. A nurse knows about the burdens and benefits of caregiving in the family. He or she knows that this experience will have lasting effects on the quality of life of the caregivers and often will cause "anxiety, depression, physical symptoms, restrictions of roles and activities, strain in marital relationships and diminished physical health" (McMillan, 2005, p. S133). It will leave a permanent impression of end-of-life care upon all who witness it.

The nurse also recognizes that patient suffering has a profound effect on the family and its cohesion (Hebert & Schulz, 2006; Roscoe, Osman, & Haley, 2006). Anticipating all of the various factors involved in this family's unique situation, the office nurse knows there will be need for support and information particularly about symptom management.

The caring nurse has knowledge of the multifaceted nature of palliative and hospice care and the assistance it can provide to Tomas, Janice, and the entire family. The nurse would explore those benefits with them in light of the family's goals and the family's need to care for their husband and father. In a caring ethic, interventions are tailored to the individual needs of the family (Hebert & Schulz, 2006). Working to sustain healthy connections between the family members and between nurses and their patients may be a challenge, but it is nonetheless a caring act worth the effort (Roscoe et al., 2006). Nurses who subscribe to an ethics of care would initiate conversations about evidence-based practice and empower women in this family to access the assistance needed to properly care for Tomas (MacKinnon, 2009). Because referral to palliative or hospice care requires a physician order, convincing the physician of the benefits of either approach in this situation would be the advocate's responsibility. The nurse would wish to use language that demonstrates concern for the physician, who may have a difficult time addressing the transition from curative therapy to comfort and end-of-life care.

Once a referral is made, or if the family seeks out hospice independently, communication between the hospital/office nurse and the hospice/palliative care nurse would be enormously beneficial to ensure the needed continuity of care (Cohen, 2009) and to facilitate the transition. It would also provide a sense of unity for nurses. Over time and after establishing a caring relationship, the nurse in palliative care/hospice who is skillful at communication will gently address with the patient and family the transition toward acceptance of their impending loss (Lowey, 2008).

CLINICAL ETHICS IN END-OF-LIFE CARE

The ethical issues arising in end-of-life care are not limited to the troubling lack of access to hospice, care of those suffering, and caregiver burden. They also include dilemmas over pain management, decision making about withdrawal of life support, requests for nondisclosure of diagnosis, and artificial nutrition and hydration.

As palliative care consultation increases in hospitals, more aggressive pain and symptom management ensues. Nurses and family members may question whether administering opioids will hasten death. First, as medication for the alleviation of pain is begun, the lowest possible dose is prescribed to alleviate pain, dyspnea, and attendant suffering. Then, as needed and as the patient develops tolerance to the medication, the dose is often titrated upward. Mental confusion and somnolence may occur before respiratory depression and death, triggering staff to taper or discontinue the opioid.

Veatch, Haddad, and English (2010), discuss the ethical issue of direct versus indirect killing. Using the concept of death as "evil," they cite the widely accepted moral principle of "indirect or double effect":

> To be acceptable, the evil must not be intended. Also, the good that is done, such as the relieving of pain, must be at least as great as the evil. Finally the evil cannot be the means to the good end. (p. 185)

Thus, when the nurse intends to comfort the dying patient, and pain and symptom relief are imperative, even if respiratory depression may occur, the nurse is doing good. He or she is not using the morphine drip, for example, as a means to killing. Although one person will administer the last dose of an opioid, the seeming causal effect between that last dose and the death, while emotionally laden, is likely to be spurious.

Much has been written about futility (Sibbald, Downar, & Hawryluck, 2007) and decision making at the end of life, particularly in light of the use and application of technology (e.g., Amella, Lawrence, & Gresle, 2005; Meeker & Jezewski, 2008). To what extent does aggressive curative treatment improve outcomes? How might these same treatments add to symptom burden and prolong the dying process? Early palliative care, counseling, and ethics committee consultation can anticipate and negotiate these issues, teaching and guiding families through the decision-making process.

In Eastern cultures (e.g., Schwartz, 2010) and among well-intentioned individuals, a request for nondisclosure of diagnosis or prognosis may be asked of the healthcare team. The moral question is whether anyone has the authority to override the patient's claim to such information. In a society that values autonomy, authority resides solely with the patient: He or she is generally asked, "To what extent do you want to know?" The patient may defer to a family member, who is considered a morally ascribed surrogate. Evidence exists, however, that patients often know more than the family or healthcare provider assumes (Kendall, 2006) and wish to know information about their illness, treatment, and prognosis (Coyle & Sculo, 2003). Collective silence generally results in heightened anxiety for patient, family, and nurse. A request for nondisclosure may not necessarily bring up an ethical dilemma if the nurse and physician would attempt to understand the point of view of the family, invoke flexibility, respond with care to the family's distress, and employ negotiation skills (see Hallenbeck & Arnold, 2007).

The Terri Schiavo case, which became a prominent fixture in the news and was discussed at length in the professional literature, focused national attention on the burdens and benefits of artificial nutrition and hydration (ANH) as well as decision making for patients in persistent vegetative states. The question remains: Is providing artificially delivered nutrition prolonging life or prolonging death—that is, providing comfort or causing discomfort—at the end of life? There are specific situations when ANH will be clinically beneficial: delirium, opioid toxicity and severe dehydration.

Fast Facts information about tube feedings (Hallenbeck, 2005), a summary statement of the extant evidence related to the artificial administration of food and fluid near the end of life, summarizes the situation in this way: "Although commonly used, current data does not provide much support for the use of artificial enteral nutrition in advanced dementia, or in patients on a dying trajectory from a chronic illness" (p. 1). It has been shown that there is no advantage to ANH in preventing aspiration or improving survival (Hospice and Palliative Care Nursing Association [HPNA], 2003). Actively dying persons do not experience hunger or thirst, and tube feedings cause considerable discomfort. Being sensitive to the values and cultural/religious perspectives of the decision makers is equally important. Nurses can focus on relaying factual information to the patient's surrogate(s) and providing support and counseling as they suffer through making decisions about what is considered a nurturing and caring act (Eggenberger & Nelms, 2004).

CONCLUSION

This chapter has discussed the vulnerability of the dying person and his or her family. A global and national picture of end of life leads to acknowledgment of the considerable disparities in care and need for improvement in this area of practice, particularly in pain management. Ethical principles and theoretical approaches—particularly social justice, human rights, and ethics of care—may be used to analyze and incite action toward improved care for the dying. The ongoing efforts to improve professional education are one way that hospice/palliative care can be expanded and ethical issues prominent in nursing care at the end of life can be addressed.

For a full suite of assignments and additional learning activities, use the access code located in the front of your book to visit this exclusive website: http://go.jblearning.com/dechesnay. If you do not have an access code, you can obtain one at the site.

REFERENCES

Amella, E. J., Lawrence, J. F., & Gresle, S. O. (2005). Tube feeding: Prolonging life or death in vulnerable populations? *Mortality, 10*(1), 69–81.

American Association of Colleges of Nursing (AACN). (2008). Essentials of baccalaureate nursing education for professional nursing practice. Retrieved from http://www.aacn.nche.edu/education/pdf/BaccEssentials08.pdf

American Association of Colleges of Nursing (AACN). (2010a). End of life care. Retrieved from http://www.aacn.nche.edu/elnec

American Association of Colleges of Nursing (AACN). (2010b). ELNEC core curriculum. Retrieved from http://www.aacn.nche.edu/elnec/curriculum.htm

American Association of Colleges of Nursing (AACN). (2010c). Veterans Administration awards contract to the City of Hope to expand the End-of-Life Nursing Education Consortium (ELNEC) program to improve palliative care at U.S. Veterans Hospitals. Retrieved from http://www.aacn.nche.edu/Media/NewsReleases/2010/elnecveterans.html

American Board of Medical Specialties (ABMS). (2010). Subspecialties. Retrieved from http://www.abms.org/who_we_help/physicians/specialties.aspx

Arries, E. J. (2009). Is an African nursing ethics possible? *Nursing Ethics, 16*(6), 681–682.

Aubeeluck, M. J. (2006). Nurses' experiences of caring for their own family members. *British Journal of Nursing, 15*(3), 160–165.

Avery, J. (2009). *Children's palliative care in Africa*. New York: Oxford University Press.

Beauchamp, T. L., & Childress, J. F. (2001). *Principles of biomedical ethics* (5th ed.). New York: Oxford University Press.

Bonin-Scaon, S., Sastre, M. T. M., Chasseigne, G., Sorum, P. C., & Mullet, E. (2009). End-of-life preferences: A theory-driven inventory. *International Journal of Human Development, 68*(1), 1–26.

Campbell, M. L. (2010). When will "usual care" in advanced illness be "palliative care"? *Journal of Palliative Medicine, 13*(8), 934–935.

Casarett, D. J., Teno, J., & Higginson, I. (2006). How should nations measure the quality of end-of-life care for older adults? Recommendations for an international minimum data set. *Journal of the American Geriatrics Society, 54*, 1765–1771.

Center to Advance Palliative Care (CAPC). (2008). *America's care of serious illness: A state-by-state report card on access to palliative care in our nation's hospitals*. New York: Author. Retrieved from http://www.capc.org/reportcard/state-by-state-report-card.pdf

Center to Advance Palliative Care (CAPC). (2010). Hospital quality assurance: Estimated cost savings. Retrieved from http://www.capc.org/building-a-hospital-based-palliative-care-program/financing/cost-savings

Centers for Disease Control and Prevention (CDC). (2010). Deaths and mortality. Retrieved from www.cdc.gov/nchs/fastats/deaths.htm

Central Intelligence Agency (CIA). (2010). The world fact book. Retrieved from https://www.cia.gov/library/publications/the-world-factbook

Cohen, M. Z. (2009). Loss of continuity and lack of closure in therapeutic relationships were associated with feelings of abandonment at the transition to end of life care. *Evidence-Based Nursing, 12*(4), 128.

Coyle, N., & Sculco, L. (2003). Communication and patient/physician relationship: Phenomenological inquiry. *Journal of Supportive Oncology, 1*, 206–215.

Coyne, P., Paice, J. A., Ferrell, B. R., Malloy, P., Virani, R., & Fennimore, L. A. (2007). Oncology End-of-Life Nursing Education Consortium training program: Improving palliative care in cancer. *Oncology Nursing Forum, 34*(4), 801–807.

Demitropoulos, S. M. (2007). *The extent of knowledge on the death and dying process as perceived by senior nursing students.* Unpublished master's thesis, University of Nevada. ProQuest Information and Learning, UMI #1451073.

The Economist Intelligence Unit. (2010). The quality of death: Ranking end-of-life care across the world. Retrieved from http://www.lifebeforedeath.com/pdf/Quality_of_Death_Index_Report.pdf

Education in Palliative and End of Life Care (EPEC). (2010). The EPEC project. Retrieved from http://www.epec.net/EPEC/Webpages/index.cfm

Eggenberger, S. K., & Nelms, T. P. (2004). Artificial hydration and nutrition in advanced Alzheimer's disease: Facilitating family decision-making. *Journal of Clinical Nursing, 13*, 661–667.

End-of-Life Nursing Education Consortium (ELNEC). (2010). Fact sheet. Retrieved from http://www.aacn.nche.edu/elnec/factsheet.htm

Fairchild, R. M. (2010). Practical ethical theory for nurses responding to complexity in care. *Nursing Ethics, 17*(3), 353–362.

Ferrell, B., Connor, S. R., Cordes, A., Dahlin, C. M., Fine, P. G., Hutton, N., . . . Zuroski, K. (2007). The national agenda for quality palliative care: The National Consensus Project and the National Quality Forum. *Journal of Pain and Symptom Management, 33*, 737–744.

Ferrell, B. R., & Coyle, N. (2008). The nature of suffering and the goals of nursing. *Oncology Nursing Forum, 35*(2), 241–247.

Ferrell, B. R., & Coyle, N. (Eds.). (2010). *Oxford textbook of palliative nursing* (3rd ed.). New York, NY: Oxford University Press.

Ferrell, B. R., Grant, M., & Virani, R. (2001). Nurses urged to address improved end-of-life care in textbooks. *Oncology Nursing Forum, 28*(9), 1349.

Ferrell, B., Virani, R., Grant, M., & Borneman, T. (1999). Analysis of content regarding death and bereavement in nursing texts. *Psycho-Oncology, 8*, 500–510.

Field, M. J., & Cassel, C. K. (Eds.). (1997). *Approaching death: Improving care at the end of life.* Washington, DC: Institute of Medicine, National Academy Press.

Gilligan, C. (1982). *In a different voice: Psychological theory and women's development.* Cambridge, MA: Harvard University Press.

Gilligan, C. (1987). Moral orientation and moral development. In E. F. Kittay & D. T. Meyers, (Eds.), *Women and moral theory* (pp. 19–33). Lanham, MD: Rowman and Littlefield.

Gostin, L. O., & Powers, M. (2006). What does social justice require for the public health? *Health Affairs, 25*(4), 1053–1060.

Gwyther, L., Brennan, F., & Harding, R. (2009). Advancing palliative care as a right. *Journal of Pain and Symptom Management, 38*(5), 767–774.

Hallenbeck, J. (2005). Tube feed or not tube feed? *Fast Facts and Concepts, 2*, 10. Retrieved from http://www.eperc.mcw.edu/fastfact/ff_010.htm

Hallenbeck, J., & Arnold, R. (2007). A request for nondisclosure: Don't tell mother. *Journal of Clinical Oncology, 31*(25), 5030–5034.

Harding, R., & Higginson, I. J. (2005). Palliative care in sub-Saharan Africa. *Lancet, 365*, 1971–1977.

Hebert, R. S., & Schulz, R. (2006). Caregiving at the end of life. *Journal of Palliative Medicine, 9*(5), 1174–1187.

Held, V. (2006). *The ethics of care: Personal, political, and global.* New York: Oxford University Press.

Hospice and Palliative Care Nursing Association (HPNA). (2003). HPNA position paper: Artificial nutrition and hydration in end-of-life care. *Journal of Hospice and Palliative Nursing, 5*(4), 231–234.

International Council of Nurses (ICN). (2006). Position statement: Nurses' role in providing care to dying patients and their families. Retrieved from http://www1.icn.ch/PS_A12_NursesroleDyingPatients.pdf

International Observatory on End-of-Life Care. (2006). *Mapping levels of palliative care development: A global view.* Lancaster, UK. Retrieved from http://www.eolc-observatory.net/global/pdf/world_map.pdf

Jennings, B., Ryndes, T., D'Onofrio, C., & Baily, M. A. (2003). Access to hospice care: Expanding boundaries, overcoming barriers. *Hastings Center Report, Special Supplement,* S3–S7, S9–S13, S15–S21.

Joranson, D. E., Ryan, K. M., & Maurer, M. A. (2009). Opioid policy, availability, and access in developing and nonindustrialized countries. In J. Ballantyne, S. Fishman, & J. P. Rathmell (Eds.), *Bonica's management of pain* (4th ed., pp. 194–208). Philadelphia: Lippincott, Williams & Wilkins.

Kendall, S. (2006). Being asked not to tell: Nurses' experiences caring for cancer patients not told their diagnosis. *Journal of Clinical Nursing, 15*(9), 1149–1157.

Kirchhoff, K. T., Beckstrand, R. L., & Anumandla, P. R. (2003). Analysis of end-of-life content in critical care nursing textbooks. *Journal of Professional Nursing, 19*(6), 372–381.

Last Acts. (2002a). *Means to a better end.* New York: Author. Retrieved from http://www.rwjf.org/files/publications/other/meansbetterend.pdf

Last Acts. (2002b). Proposed policy changes to improve access and financial viability. *State Initiatives in End-of-Life Care, 17,* 6.

Lohman, D., Schleifer, R., & Amon, J. J. (2010). Access to pain treatment as a human right. *BioMed Central, 8*(8). Retrieved through Open Access at http://www.biomedcentral.com/1741-7015/8/8

Lowey, S. E. (2008). Letting go before a death: A concept analysis. *Journal of Advanced Nursing, 63*(2), 208–215.

MacKinnon, C. J. (2009). Applying feminist, multicultural and social justice theory to diverse women who function as caregivers in end-of-life and palliative home care. *Palliative & Supportive Care, 7*(4), 501–513.

Mallory, J. L. (2002). The impact of a palliative care educational component on attitudes toward care of the dying in undergraduate nursing students. Doctoral dissertation, North Carolina State University. *Dissertation Abstracts International, 63*(12A), 4188 (UMI No. ATT3076731).

Matzo, M. L., & Sherman, D. W. (2009). *Palliative care nursing: Quality care to the end of life* (3rd ed.). New York: Springer.

McMillan, S. C. (2005). Interventions to facilitate family caregiving at the end of life. *Journal of Palliative Medicine, 8*(suppl 1), S132–S139.

Meeker, M. A., & Jezewski, M. A. (2008). Metasynthesis: Withdrawal of life-sustaining treatments: The experience of family decision-makers. *Journal of Clinical Nursing, 18,* 163–173.

Meier, D. E., Isaacs, S. L., & Hughes, R. G. (Eds.). (2010). *Palliative care: Transforming the care of serious illness.* San Francisco: Jossey-Bass.

Metz, T. (2009). The final ends of higher education in light of an African moral theory. *Journal of Philosophy of Education, 43*(2), 179–201.

Morrison, R. S., Penrod, J. D., Cassel, J. B., Caust-Ellenbogen, M., Litke, A., Spragrens, L., & Meier, D. E. (2008). Cost savings associated with United States hospital palliative care consultation programs. *Archives of Internal Medicine, 168*(16), 1783–1790.

National Consensus Project for Quality Palliative Care. (2009). *Clinical practice guidelines for quality palliative care.* Pittsburgh, PA: Author.

National Hospice and Palliative Care Organization (NHPCO). (2009). *NHPCO facts and figures: Hospice care in America.* Alexandria, VA: Author.

Noddings, N. (1986). *Caring: A feminine approach to ethics and moral education.* Berkeley, CA: University of California Press.

Noddings, N. (2002). *Starting at home: Caring and social policy.* Berkeley, CA: University of California Press.

Oxford English Dictionary. (2006). Palliate. New York: Oxford University Press.

Paice, J. A., Ferrell, B. R., Coyle, N., Coyne, P., & Callaway, M. (2007). Global efforts to improve palliative care: The International End-of-Life Nursing Education Consortium Training Programme. *Journal of Advanced Nursing, 61*(2), 173–180.

Paice, J. A., Ferrell, B. R., Virani, R., Grant, M., Malloy, P., & Rhome, A. (2006a). Appraisal of the graduate end-of-life nursing education consortium training program. *Journal of Palliative Medicine, 9,* 353–360.

Paice, J. A., Ferrell, B. R., Virani, R., Grant, M., Malloy, P., & Rhome, A. (2006b). Graduate nursing education regarding end-of-life care: Solutions to an urgent need. *Nursing Outlook, 54,* 46–52.

Payne, S., Seymour, J., & Ingleton, C. (2008). *Palliative care nursing: Principles and evidence for practice.* New York, NY: Oxford University Press.

Prail, D., & Pahl, N. (2007). The worldwide palliative care alliance: Networking national associations. *Journal of Pain and Symptom Management, 37*(5), 506–508.

Radwany, S., Albanese, T., Clough, L., Sims, L., Mason, H., & Jahangiri, S. (2009). End-of-life decision making and emotional burden: Placing family meetings in context. *American Journal of Hospice & Palliative Medicine, 26*(5), 376–383.

Reb, A. M. (2003). Palliative and end-of-life care: Policy analysis. *Oncology Nursing Forum, 30*(1), 35–50.

Rendtorff, J. D. (2002). Basic ethical principles in European bioethics and biolaw: Autonomy, dignity, integrity and vulnerability: Towards a foundation of bioethics and biolaw. *Medicine, Health Care and Philosophy, 5*(3), 235–244.

Rendtorff, J. D., Kemp, P., & Commission of the European Communities, Biomedical and Health Research Programme (Eds.). (2000). *Basic ethical principles in bioethics and biolaw, Vol 1.* Copenhagen: Centre for Ethics and Law.

Roscoe, L. A., Osman, H., & Haley, W. E. (2006). Implications of the Schiavo case for understanding family caregiving issues at the end of life. *Death Studies, 30,* 149–161.

Ruof, M. C. (2004). Vulnerability, vulnerable populations, and policy. *Kennedy Institute of Ethics Journal, 14*(4), 411–425.

Schroeder, D., & Gefenas, E. (2009). Vulnerability: Too vague and too broad? *Cambridge Quarterly of Healthcare Ethics, 18,* 113–121.

Schwartz, P. Y. (2010). Good death in the Chinese culture: A relational perspective. *Death Studies, 34*(3), 278–284.

Shea, J., Grossman, S., Wallace, M., & Lange, J. (2010). Assessment of advanced practice palliative care nursing competencies in nurse practitioner students: Implications for integration of ELNEC curricular modules. *Journal of Nursing Education, 49*(4), 183–189.

Sibbald, R., Downar, J., & Hawryluck, L. (2007). Perceptions of "futile care" among caregivers in intensive care units. *Canadian Medical Association Journal, 177*(10), 1201–1208.

Steinhauser, K. E., Christakis, N. A., Clipp, E. C., McNeilly, M., McIntyre, L., & Tulsky, J. A. (2000). Factors considered important at the end of life by patients, family, physicians, and other care providers. *Journal of the American Medical Association, 284*(19), 2476–2482.

Stjernsward, J., Foley, K. M., & Ferris, F. D. (2007). Integrating palliative care into national policies. *Journal of Pain and Symptom Management, 33*(5), 514–520.

SUPPORT Investigators. (1995). A controlled trial to improve care for seriously ill hospitalized patients: The study to understand prognoses and preferences for outcomes and risks of treatments (SUPPORT). *Journal of the American Medical Association, 274,* 1591–1598.

Tangwa, G. B. (2000). The traditional African perception of a person. *Hastings Center Report, 30*(5), 39–43.

Temel, J. S., Greer, J. A., Muzikansky, A., Gallagher, E. R., Admane, S., Jackson, V. A., . . . Lynch, T. J. (2010). Early palliative care for patients with metastatic non-small-cell lung cancer. *New England Journal of Medicine, 363*, 733–742.

Tronto, J. C. (1993). *Moral boundaries: A political argument for an ethic of care.* New York, NY: Routledge.

Tronto, J. C. (1996). Care as a political concept. In N. J. Hirschmann & C. Di Stefano (Eds.), *Revisioning the political: Feminist reconstructions of traditional concepts in Western political theory* (pp. 139–156). Boulder, CO: Westview Press.

Tsai, D. F. (1999). Ancient Chinese medical ethics and the four principles of biomedical ethics. *Journal of Medical Ethics, 25*(4), 315–321.

Tutu, D. (2000). *No future without forgiveness.* New York, NY: Doubleday.

Veatch, R. M., Haddad, A. M., & English, D. C. (2010). *Case studies in biomedical ethics.* New York, NY: Oxford University Press.

Virani, R., Malloy, P., Ferrell, B. R., & Kelly, K. (2008). Statewide efforts in promoting palliative care. *Journal of Palliative Medicine, 11*(7), 991–996.

Wardlaw, T., Salama, P., Brockelhurst, C., Chopra, M., & Mason, E. (2010). Diarrhoea: Why children are still dying and what can be done. *Lancet, 375*, 870–871.

World Health Organization (WHO). (1986). *Cancer pain relief.* Geneva, Switzerland: Author.

World Health Organization (WHO). (2008). Fact sheet: The top ten causes of death. Retrieved from http://www.who.int/mediacentre/factsheets/fs310/en/index.html

World Health Organization (WHO). (2010). Global health observatory: Life expectancy. Retrieved from http://apps.who.int/ghodata

CHAPTER 27

The Samfie Man Revisited: Sex Tourism and Trafficking

Mary de Chesnay

Objectives

At the end of this chapter, the reader will be able to

1. Differentiate between sex tourism and sex trafficking.
2. Discuss the health implications of the sex tourism and trafficking industries.
3. Describe the roles of specialty nurses (psychiatric-mental health, community health, and nurse practitioners) in helping people who have been trafficked.

www

INTRODUCTION

This chapter calls attention to some key issues related to the growing problem of modern-day slavery—in particular, sex slavery. Sex tourism and sex trafficking are described and clinical reports presented that illustrate some of the health issues encountered by the vulnerable women and children who are the major victims of the traffickers and tourists.

It is important to distinguish between prostitution and the subset of prostitutes who are slaves (Butcher, 2003). Some confusion persists in the literature and media about the two, and Cusick et al. (2009) warn that prostitution is not always a result of trafficking. Some would argue that there is a population of prostitutes who are consenting adults and that they should not be viewed as criminals, but this is a discussion for another place.

This chapter focuses on those sex workers who are the victims of traffickers and those who are in the business of providing sex to tourists. The term "samfie man" is used to capture the essence of those who prey on people around the issues of sex. "Samfie man" is a Jamaican word meaning "con man," often one who pretends to use witchcraft to trick people. This chapter was inspired by meeting one of these individuals who happened to come from Jamaica, but the term can easily be used to describe any scam artist. In this chapter, it may be difficult to tell the difference between the samfie man and his prey, as some of the victims eventually become the exploiters.

Sex tourism refers to travel for the express purpose of engaging in sexual encounters with people of different races, with individuals of different ethnicities, or, frequently, with underage partners. Sex trafficking is modern slavery functioning as a global business that promotes exploitation of men, women, and children primarily for sex but also as a source of cheap labor. For the purposes of this chapter, the samfie man is the villain in each of the case studies—the man or woman who introduced the person to a life of exploitation and abuse.

SEX OFFENDERS

There would be no market for sex tourism and trafficking if there were not a huge number of sex offenders worldwide. Whether they are pedophiles, rapists, wife beaters, or just sociopaths who indulge their own needs at the expense of others, consumers of sex trafficking and sex tourism create both victims and opportunities for the criminal organizations that make money by selling sex. In a bizarre twist of logic, however, victims of child sex trafficking are often treated as criminals because they are trained to be seducers and the "johns" are seen as customers instead of child sex predators (Jayasree, 2004; Raymond, 2004: Williamson & Prior, 2009). Thus child prostitutes are placed in juvenile detention facilities, while their customers go free.

One argument made in the literature is that legalizing prostitution might be one answer to decriminalizing the victims. Similar to those who advocate legalizing certain drugs (marijuana, for instance), proponents of this view suggest that legalization of prostitution would not only decriminalize "consensual" prostitution but also remove the need for involvement of criminal organizations in the sex industry and decrease the level of violence associated with prostitution. This argument seems to assume that prostitutes engage in selling sex for money because they prefer to earn a living this way. While sex between consenting adults is one thing, it is difficult to view women engaged in prostitution as choosing prostitution as a career, when the stories they tell about how they entered the life so obviously focus on coercion—that is, coercion by family or friends who destroy their sexual innocence, cons by people they meet who take advantage of their gullibility to pretend to help them meet their dreams of modeling or acting, and kidnapping by organized rings of traffickers.

SEX TOURISM

Sex tourism refers to vacations to destinations where the primary purpose of the trip is to have sex with people far away from home—that is, away from the home-based rules of conduct and social controls. In some cases, the prostitutes are "consenting adults"; often, however, they are current or former victims of predators who have coerced or finessed them into a life of selling sex for the profit of their handlers.

The Caribbean has experienced shifts in mobility of locals from agricultural jobs in isolated rural areas to cities and resort areas that support a growing tourism industry. The shift has accounted for some residents' increased vulnerability to foreigners looking for sex. These rural people come to the city looking for work, which is often unavailable, so they sell their bodies to survive. They are transformed from what they grew up believing they were (traditionally heterosexual) to what the market demands (homosexual or bisexual.) In one study in the Dominican Republic, interviews with 72 Dominican male sex workers with male clients revealed how they maintain their own sense of masculinity in what the researchers called "staged authenticity" to counteract the negative stereotypes of homosexuals and increased risk of HIV/AIDS (Padilla, 2008).

In Peru, tourists come not just to look at Machu Pichu (Bauer, 2008), but also to engage in sex with locals who are different from themselves. The phenomenon of "bricherismo," which is practiced in Cuzco, exploits the Incan culture for the purpose of sex with foreigners who favor men with long hair who speak Quechua and claim to be descended from the Inca. This practice creates new disease trends in isolated areas and a need for public health education for hospitality employees.

The people whom the tourists seek for sex are often minors. This demand for minors, in turn, creates a market for trafficking in children both in the United States and abroad (Kotrla, 2010; Williamson & Prior, 2009). The preference of customers for young victims feeds the virginal fantasies of the johns (Dickson, 2004).

SEX TRAFFICKING

A conservative estimate is that approximately 50,000 women and children are trafficked into the United States each year for the purposes of sex slavery (Miller, Decker, Silverman, & Raj, 2007). Others are trafficked for labor but will not be discussed here, as this chapter focuses on the sex trade. The estimated number of people who are trafficked throughout the world exceeds 2.5 million. Although trafficking is increasingly recognized by governments as a serious problem, few have found ways to help the victims (Svrivankova, 2006).

ORIGINAL FIELDWORK

The clinical cases presented in this chapter resulted from fieldwork in Jamaica to examine family structure (de Chesnay, 1986a, 1986b). At that time, the author was conducting doctoral research on family variables as part of a cognate in anthropology. In the course of field trips and subsequent visits to Jamaica and later Central America, she came across individuals who were involved in sex work. As a nurse, she found that people felt comfortable talking to her about the most intimate details of their lives. They often shared problems and issues spontaneously, similar to what nurses and physicians experience at social gatherings when people tell them about their ailments.

THE CLINICAL REPORTS

The cases reported here were inspired by real people but have been disguised quite a bit to protect their privacy, to the extent that the clinical reports are essentially fictional and represent the stories of hundreds of people who have been victimized by the traffickers and tourists. It is important to stress that these people were telling their stories openly but not within the context of research. The institutional review board (IRB) permission covered the family structure study; the clinical cases were outside that context. However, over the years, the author has had interactions in other parts of the world that have focused her attention on the extent of the problems of sex workers and victims of the traffickers. As a nurse, the author wants to call attention to the health issues of people, but the wider social context is social justice health policy.

Ideally, presenting these stories will call attention to the necessity for governments to do more to protect their citizens. The implications for nurses include the critical need to take thorough histories for people who present with any indications they might have been sex workers at some point.

The dangers of the sex trade inhibit people from calling the authorities. People who are sold are commonly told that they or their families will be killed if they tell, resist, or try to escape. Therefore, it is imperative that nurses and other health professionals who treat these patients do so within a climate of safety and security , protecting not only their confidentiality under privacy laws, but also shielding them from further abuse at the hands of the predators.

WWW Magda

Magda is a 25-year-old woman from Russia who entered a contest at the age of 13 in Moscow to fulfill her dream of becoming a high-paying fashion model. From a poor family, she had three younger siblings and yearned to help her parents provide a better life for them. Her family was happy and hard-working but poor, and she wanted to ease the financial burden on her parents. Magda was told that she had made the contest finals and would be flown to Paris, where she would be photographed by a famous fashion photographer whose name she recognized from the magazines she and her friends read at the library. She was escorted on an airplane by a "husband and wife," who told her that they had her parents' permission for the trip, but that she could not see them to say goodbye because they had to make the next flight in order to meet with the busy photographer. The couple also said that she must pretend to be their daughter because she did not have her own passport. If she refused to play along, they said, her own parents "would get in a lot of trouble with the police." Magda was told how pretty she was and how much money she would make as a model, and the couple promised to help her set up a bank account to send the money back to her parents.

Once she arrived in Paris, Magda was placed in a warehouse with a dozen other women of many nationalities. The woman who escorted her learned she was a virgin and let slip that she would earn much money but she had to be "prettied up." She had her hair styled and cosmetics applied, and she was given beautiful clothes to wear for the photo shoot by a man who said he was an assistant to the famous photographer. Then she was placed in a locked room separate from the other women. By the time she realized she had been sold to traffickers, she had no way to communicate and no one to ask for help.

Magda was sold to a wealthy man who treated her well at first but tired of her when she reached her fifteenth birthday. At that point, he gave her to his friend, who preferred teenagers. She was passed around until she became so sick from sexually transmitted diseases (STDs) and malnutrition that she was sold to a pimp who turned her out on the street. Repeated beatings and threats to kill her if she tried to escape or return home were successful at intimidating her, to the point that Magda lost the will to resist. She was told that her parents and younger siblings would be killed if she did not cooperate. Eventually rescued by an aid organization, Magda was malnourished, diseased, and broken in spirit. Her prognosis for recovery is minimal without help beyond what the organization can provide.

Rita

Rita and David prey on affluent men and women from the United States and Europe who go to the Caribbean as sex tourists looking for partners of a different race. They specialize in heterosexual activities but are not averse to homosexual encounters if the price is right. As attractive people, they command a high price. They save their money with the idea of retiring early and leaving the business. They dream of a life in Europe, living among the jet set.

Rita is David's partner both in life and in crime. She is a beautiful, light-skinned black woman who keeps fit and wears expensive clothes and jewelry that she can well afford or that are given to her as gifts by her regular clients. Her story begins at the age of 20, when her parents disowned her after they discovered she was servicing the wealthy American and European men who came to the Caribbean. Rita was making enough money to support herself and then became involved with David, who rescued her from a pimp. The two became business partners and backed each other up as well as designing their cons for the tourists.

Rita is not retired. She states that she is young and beautiful enough to attract the wealthiest clients and that she can afford the luxury of accepting only men (or women) she can tolerate in bed. Her body is fit, and she maintains her sexual health. She becomes angry at any thought that she is vulnerable, preferring to view herself as completely in control of her life.

David

David is a handsome man in his mid-thirties with dark hair, soft brown eyes, and extremely polite manners that mask his contempt for most people. He describes himself as a sex worker who specializes in affluent white American women who come to the Caribbean as sex tourists to have sex with black men. He is independent but works with a partner (Rita). David emphatically refuses to work with pimps—individuals whom he sees as the lowest form of humanity. He is very protective of Rita and backs her up when she is with a client. At the same time, he reports that he has no difficulty taking advantage of the wealthy women he services since "they get what they deserve and I give them their money's worth."

David takes good care of himself and sees a doctor regularly for STD check-ups. His presenting problem to the nurse is gastrointestinal pain and frequent diarrhea for which he takes Imodium and ibuprofen, but he is beginning to think there is something more seriously wrong than indigestion. When he learns that his diagnosis of Crohn's disease could seriously affect his business, he begins a series of doctors' visits in an attempt to find someone who can "make this go away" without surgery. During the period of doctor shopping, he becomes severely depressed and considers suicide. David's income and lifestyle depend on his clients seeing him as desirable sexually, and he is terrified of living with Crohn's disease with its unpredictable and embarrassing flare-ups.

WWW Luisa

Luisa is a young woman in her late teens from Guatemala who was sold to sex traffickers at the age of five by her parents, who were desperate for money to feed their 10 other children. The contrast between the poverty of her family's life and her own lifestyle as a sex worker often makes her wonder whether she would have been better off at home with her parents, yet she does not blame them for selling her. She views the sale of their oldest daughter as her parents' desperate attempt to save the family, and she has convinced herself that she is tough enough to handle the 20 to 25 men she is expected to service daily. If she falls short, she is beaten and deprived of what little food the handler gives her.

Luisa was five years old when she was first sent to a brothel, where she was brutally raped by a man whose job was to prepare her for her new life. She was hurt, confused, and terrified not only at the brutality but at the whole of her world crumbling. She had been starved for lack of food at home, but her family treated her with kindness to the extent that they were able. She held onto the idea that she is saving her family, which allowed her to tolerate her unbearable life.

At the age of 12, Luisa was swept up in an undercover sting operation. A police officer posing as a "john" was able to arrest her current handler, but he was part of a ring with major financial backing and the ringleaders went free. Luisa was placed in a juvenile detention facility because her family could not be found. Even if they could be found, authorities would not have released her back to the people who sold her to the traffickers. In a misguided attempt to convince her that her lifestyle was her parents' fault for selling her, the "therapist" assigned to her by the aid organization paradoxically took away the only comforting thought that had maintained Luisa during her years of abuse—that she was helping her deserving family. Immediately after this session with her therapist, Luisa succeeded in killing herself with an overdose of aspirin.

HEALTH ISSUES

HIV/AIDS and STDs

Perhaps not surprisingly, trafficking is largely responsible for the AIDS pandemic at least in China. In China, for example, commercial sex workers and injection drug users have introduced HIV into the population of Yunnan province, which has a higher rate of HIV than other provinces (Xiao, Kristensen, Sun, Lu, & Vermund, 2007).

Mental Health Issues

Post-traumatic stress disorder (PTSD) is an obvious effect of sexual exploitation, but perhaps even more insidious is the destruction of self-esteem. Women and children who have been trafficked view themselves as worthless and experience a kind of numbing of the soul. Some might call this clinical depression, and some of these women do try to kill themselves. Others find the strength to live on in the hope that their lives will change.

INTERVENTION

In January 2006, President George W. Bush signed the Trafficking Victims Protection Reauthorization Act (H.R. 972), after receiving unanimous congressional approval for the legislation. This law reauthorizes and expands the original 2000 law focused on international human trafficking by targeting the purchasers of illegal sex acts—that is, the customers and traffickers who exploit domestic victims. That provision, known as the End Demand for Sex Trafficking Act, focuses on halting the trafficking of people, primarily women and children, in the United States for purposes of sexual slavery. The End Demand measure is designed to help police investigate and prosecute sex trafficking cases. It also will provide funds to assist trafficking victims, including the establishment of residential care centers for underage children. Under the legislation, studies and conferences to ascertain progress in this area will be conducted regularly (Strode, 2006).

While the United States' legislation centers around helping the victims, it is first necessary to identify and define them as victims. Similar to the treatment of rape and child molestation, it is useful to define them as "survivors" during treatment and when interacting with them, but make no mistake-these people are victims and if defining them as victims helps to obtain scarce resources for them, it is not only acceptable, but preferable to do so.

Child victims of traffickers are clandestine and may be hard to reach. Identifying victims becomes easier when one realizes that the behaviors of victims are similar to the behaviors linked with substance abusers (since they are sometimes drugged by their handlers in order to control them.) Other indicators are missing school (if they are even allowed to attend school) and worldly knowledge, gained by being shipped around or having contact with "johns" who move around and talk about their work.

The United States focuses on providing a safety net for victims through shelters, PTSD treatment, medical intervention for trauma and disease, psychological help, and medications. These interventions are obviously needed, but we need to go further in decriminalizing the victims of trafficking. What is wrong with the picture when a child like Luisa is locked in a juvenile detention center and the traffickers to whom she was sold go free?

ACKNOWLEDGMENTS

This chapter was derived from a paper presented to the Society for Applied Anthropology in Santa Fe, New Mexico, during the conference held April 5–10, 2005.

For a full suite of assignments and additional learning activities, use the access code located in the front of your book to visit this exclusive website: http://go.jblearning.com/dechesnay. If you do not have an access code, you can obtain one at the site.

REFERENCES

Bauer, I. (2008). "They don't just come for Machu Pichu": Locals' views of tourist–local sexual relationships in Cuzco, Peru. *Culture, Health and Sexuality, 10*(6), 611–624.

Butcher, K. (2003). Confusion between prostitution and sex trafficking. *Lancet, 361*, 1983.

Cusick, L., Kinnell, H., Brooks-Gorden, B., & Campbell, R. (2009). Wild guesses and conflated meanings: Estimating the size of the sex worker population in Britain. *Critical Social Policy, 29*(4), 703–719.

De Chesnay, M. (1986a). Jamaican family structure and sex roles. *Journal of the Alabama Academy of Sciences, 57*(3), 153.

De Chesnay, M. (1986b). Jamaican family structure: The paradox of normalcy. *Family Process, 25*, 293–300. doi: 10.111/j.1545-5300.1986.00293.x

Dickson, S. (2004). *Sex in the city: Mapping commercial sex across London.* London: The Poppy Project, Eaves Housing for Women. Retrieved from www.womeninlondon.org.uk

Jayasree, A. (2004). Searching for justice for body and self in a coercive environment: Sex work in Kerala, India. *Reproductive Health Matters, 12*(23), 58–67.

Kotrla, K. (2010). Domestic minor sex trafficking in the United States. *Social Work, 55*(2), 181–187.

Miller, E., Decker, M., Silverman, J., & Raj, A. (2007). Migration, exploitation and women's health: A case report from a community health center. *Violence Against Women, 13*(5), 486–497.

Padilla, M. (2008). The embodiment of tourism among bisexually-behaving Dominican male sex workers. *Archives of Sexual Behavior, 37*, 783–793.

Raymond, J. (2004). Prostitution on demand: Legalizing the buyers as sexual consumers. *Violence Against Women, 10*(10), 1156–1186.

Strode, T. (2006). President Bush signs bill targeting sex trafficking, says U.S. has duty in fight. Retrieved from http://erlc.com/article/president-bush-signs-bill-targeting-sex-trafficking-says -us-has-duty-in-fig

Svrivankova, K. (2006). Combatting trafficking in human beings. *International Review of Law, Computers and Technology, 20*(1–2), 229–232.

Williamson, C., & Prior, M. (2009). Domestic minor sex trafficking: A network of underground players in the Midwest. *Journal of Child and Adolescent Trauma, 2*, 46–61.

Xiao, Y., Kristensen, S., Sun, J., Lu, L., & Vermund, S. (2007). Expansion of HIV/AIDS in China: Lessons from Yunnan province. *Social Science and Medicine, 64*(3), 665–675.

UNIT V

Programs

There can be no vulnerability without risk; there can be no community without vulnerability; there can be no peace, and ultimately no life, without community.

—M. Scott Peck
www.thinkexist.com

CHAPTER 28

Developing Population-Based Programs for the Vulnerable

Anne Watson Bongiorno and Mary de Chesnay

Objectives

At the end of this chapter, the reader will be able to

1. Describe the importance of creating a business plan when designing new programs to serve the vulnerable.
2. Discuss the importance of stakeholders when proposing new programs.
3. Develop an idea for a new program that serves a vulnerable population.

WWW

Population-based programs can strengthen communities by increasing the amount of resources available to promote social justice. This unit focuses on how nurses can structure programs to serve large numbers of vulnerable people. To maximize effectiveness, community health programs should serve populations by implementing the best practices related to the health issue that is the focus of the program and doing so in a cost-efficient way. Here we discuss the importance of a common vision, using a business plan and creating partnerships with major stakeholders. We also share ideas to consider when designing programs so as to maximize their impact with scarce resources. This unit covers the multiple components to successful program planning.

FOCUS OF THE PROGRAM

Problem Statement

The problem statement captures the significance of the health issue in relationship to the focus of the program, clearly defines the purpose of the program, and identifies the population served by the program. When beginning a program, start with the problem and be sure that major stakeholders agree on the problem statement and measures of success (Lewis, 2008).

Stakeholders

Programs targeting vulnerable populations implicitly seek to reduce health disparities. As part of program development, the program planner needs to learn how who the stakeholders are and how to identify them. Stakeholders are representative of community engagement in the project. They are those members of the community who function as the power brokers of the program. Stakeholders often include nonprofit organizations or political entities that can help establish and sustain the program; they also encompass individuals who will be affected by the program or are the target of the program (Issel, 2004).

Stakeholders traditionally are quite invested in the program and should demonstrate diversity in their perspectives. For example, when one of the authors of this chapter (Bongiorno) was involved in organizing a statewide coalition for lung health, she looked for a wide variety of representation that would create a powerful basis for action. Stakeholders in this situation included representatives of service organizations, widely respected research scientists in the state, government officials such as the Attorney General, elected local- and state-level officials, and people with diagnoses of lung illness. She sought to develop a board that was representative of the ethnicity, gender, and geographic location of those with lung disease and those interested in its prevention. The goal with this stakeholder representation was to create a broad base of scientific expertise and basis for action. Bongiorno considered human service potential, political will, economic acumen, and media attention to the issue of lung health to be key factors in selecting coalition members.

Programs built with a broad stakeholder base clarify the values being espoused, the sociopolitical and economic factors at play, and the scientific merit of interventions that can make or break a program. A cohesive stakeholder group develops synergy through the influence of its members.

Gatekeepers

Closely related to stakeholders are gatekeepers—those people who have power and authority, usually by way of their positions within the setting. They can use this authority in one of two ways: to facilitate a project they support or to create barriers to those programs they do not support. It does not matter whether the program is a service program or a study; gatekeepers need to be identified early in the process and persuaded to support the plan of action.

A positive example of gatekeepers was described in the first edition of this book, when the second author and colleagues (Colvin, de Chesnay, Mercado, & Benavides, 2005) designed a research project in a barrio of Managua, Nicaragua. Early in the process of beginning the study on mothers' access of health care in the barrio, the research team met with a key community leader. The woman who was the lead *brigadista* (community health worker) welcomed the team into her home, where we described the study and planned how to approach the community. She gave the researchers many helpful tips on the interview instrument, women to invite first, timing, and culturally appropriate incentives to participate in the study.

In contrast, a negative gatekeeper can effectively halt a program. Consider the doctoral student who planned a study in which she would access a rural African American sample through a local church. She obtained the permission of the pastor, who was enthusiastic in supporting her. When she arrived for data collection, however, the student was told by the deacon that he had not given his permission to collect data through the church and he would not allow her to enter. Inability to resolve the power struggle between the pastor and the deacon cost the student months of work, in that she needed to revise her entire methodology.

Values

The values section is a list of the core values held by the designers of the program. For example, for those who work with vulnerable populations, a key value is social justice. The values section might include statements like the following examples:

> For a program to reduce violence against children: *Every child has the right to live free of abuse.*
> For a public education campaign to prevent HIV/AIDS: *The public has a right to know the risks of sharing needles.*

Mission

The mission statement is an opportunity for the program designers to clearly say what they plan to do and why they believe it is important. The following example is a mission statement for a mobile free clinic designed to provide primary care:

> The North Country Mobile Health clinic provides access to affordable primary care for indigent, rural residents of the tri-county area.

DESIGN PROCESS

Recruiting the Team

A useful place to start designing a program is to obtain help from like-minded people who share a concern about the issue and the population. It is very important to partner with members of the community who will be affected by the program.

For example, in upstate New York, a tri-county coalition was formed to assess chronic disease prevention after a community assessment showed significantly high rates of diabetes, cancers, and heart disease in the region. The faculty of the community health program joined with other key health members, industry, legislators, and those affected by the problem to develop a strategic plan. Nursing faculty and students assessed levels of obesity, tobacco use, and lack of physical activity, and they consulted on multiple projects as an ongoing resource to the coalition. Key leaders and community members formed the Action for Health Committee. In just three years, the committee garnered significant grant funding for projects to improve the built environment. A greenway project was begun and clean outdoor air policies were passed in multiple municipalities. Other projects have been initiated to promote increased physical activity and healthy nutrition as the new norm. A free Disk Golf course was constructed as one of the first projects, as it was a popular request among community residents. Representation from the group who are the recipients of the program has been vital to the ongoing success of this project.

Feasibility Study

The proposed program must be realistic, be cost-effective, and have the potential to achieve its goals. The feasibility study defines the skills and resources needed to implement the program and offers alternative solutions. It asks the question, how viable is this program? The existing need and the proposed service are examined for practicality and usefulness. The feasibility study highlights strengths and weaknesses of the proposal, and its capacity to deliver the program (Stanhope & Lancaster, 2010).

In one rural elementary school, the nurse determined that few of the students who were identified as having poor vision via annual vision screenings subsequently saw an optometrist for follow-up and correction. A student public health nursing project was developed in collaboration with the university, local health department, and area optometrists to examine potential solutions to this problem. Although theory and evidence supported the need for a program to provide access to optometry services, the initial solution of providing free transportation, free vision screening at the optometrist, and free glasses was impractical in relation to the capacity of the community to deliver the program. An alternative solution agreed upon by five area optometrists was for each to provide four free eye exams and glasses to children each month—an affordable solution.

This example highlights the importance of considering how to prioritize scarce resources so that programs will be sustainable over time. It brought the problem to individuals who had the ability to offer a solution and gave them the opportunity to act.

Capturing Data

Informal talks and formal interviews may yield important data about a particular need in a community and often serve as the catalyst for action. For example, a tobacco prevention coalition had a goal to decrease tobacco use in upstate New York. Part of its strategic work plan was to encourage women of low socioeconomic status to access the statewide Quit Line. In an informal discussion, the director mentioned that that few women in this target group from one particular county accessed the Quit Line. A quick interview with the director resulted in a more systematic approach to health communication in the organization. The director acknowledged that although the use of the materials fit the organizational goal, the current materials had not been formatively tested and media outlets were not well researched. Because the key to effective health communication is to understand the audience, the coalition developed a plan to test the usefulness of current products and develop ideas for greater appeal and better placement of materials.

Surveys and focus groups provide rich data about a population problem from the emic point of view. In the New York example, the coalition determined that with the new tobacco prevention communication program, it needed to know how to strategically place messages that would attract attention of women of low socioeconomic status. Specifically, the coalition needed to know what was and was not appealing in print media to this group. Nursing students used this opportunity to develop a qualitative service learning project. They recruited community members to participate in focus group discussions. Students developed a written survey and conducted anonymous curbside surveys in places where the women congregated. Data showed that print information was at a reading level beyond the capabilities of the target group and did not resonate with the audience. New, simplified outreach materials were then developed, tested, and placed in areas where the women congregated—thereby bridging a gap in previous outreach efforts.

Participant observation is an important data-gathering technique to use with vulnerable populations because the data collected in this manner are nonlinear, are contextual, and provide salient information about a problem whose dimensions cannot be gleaned from quantitative methods. For example, in a student project about accessibility in the built environment, street crossings were observed by nursing students. They counted how many people in a given period of time crossed the street and observed driver behavior, difficulties encountered by pedestrians, and conditions of the built environment. Throughout the semester, students also gained information about perceptions of accessibility by conducting community discussions. The results of the project were used to improve walkability of area townships.

Good programs directed toward vulnerable populations are built upon a foundation of evidence that creates a compelling story of need, a gap in service, and the ability to develop an effective strategy to improve the health of the population. Hence, program planners must also elucidate the scientific underpinnings for their proposal. The epidemiology of the health issue should be clearly and succinctly communicated. The cultural congruence of the program intervention needs to be addressed when gathering data, as well as the bicultural diversity of the program recipients.

A BUSINESS PLAN

Definition and Role in Seeking Funding

Experienced grant writers know all too well that funding will be awarded only for ideas that are feasible and sustainable. Funding agencies want to be assured that the grantee is functioning within the limits of his or her ability and experience. The business plan is the document that provides funding agencies with this kind of valuable information. A business plan is a vital tool in a grant proposal to identify and prioritize the resources needed to implement the program (Longest, 2004). It highlights both the strengths and the weaknesses of the proposal. In addition, it explains how the grantee will allocate resources to meet the current and future needs of the program.

At a minimum, the business plan should define the mission and goals of the program and outline how the grantee plans to conduct business to match the purpose of the program. Traditionally, the business plan describes the program, product, and purpose, and discusses the market for the program now and in the future. The plan provides a detailed financial analysis, management plan, and a personnel plan with dates and budget.

Business plans may range from simple to complex, depending on the scope of the program and request for funding. For example, one school of nursing wanted students to learn first-hand the role of advocacy for vulnerable populations. Nursing leaders developed a simple business plan for the proposed program. The mission of the program was to increase nursing students' awareness of advocacy as a nursing mandate for vulnerable populations. Two objectives of the program were to increase knowledge of lobbying practices and to apply knowledge of the legislative process to a vulnerable population. The market analysis indicated an extreme knowledge deficit regarding the role of population-based advocacy among current students. Grant writers then outlined a specific strategy and implementation plan to meet the mission of the program.

In the program, students spent a semester investigating a vulnerable population, learning the legislative process, and preparing for a visit to the state capital and their legislator to share their concerns. The management team included faculty and administrators. The financial plan included a detailed budget of costs to the university and students, and a projected cash flow from grants and other sources of funds.

Costs and Budget

Anticipating costs is an important part of any business plan. Project financing should be identified, including accountability and communication regarding costs, and current and projected revenues, surplus, and deficits. It is critical to the success of any program in staying within its budget to project the cash flow and create a balance sheet. Expenses, personnel costs, indirect costs, and issues such as inflation or market adjustments need to be factored into more complex program plans. The proposed budget must realistically match the amount of funds a grant agency is willing to award. The program developer's vision of the program and budget must be realistically aligned for a funding agency to consider the proposal. Matching ideas to funding is a vital element in grantsmanship.

Sources of Funding

People who believe strongly in the programs they develop can be quite creative at seeking funding. *Grants and contracts* serve as an excellent way to seek funding, although writing and submitting the grant can sometimes take several months. Grants directories are valuable resources in this quest, as they detail the focus of the grant-sponsoring organization, contact information, guidelines for grant writing, and much other useful information.

Public campaigns can generate large amounts of money targeted to the program of interest. Sometimes it is possible to designate a program as a new United Way agency. If not, creating a similar public campaign is not difficult if the team recruits the support of the local media. For example, the KSU Community Clinic Program is a nurse-managed clinic at Kennesaw State University under the WellStar College of Health and Human Services and staffed by the WellStar School of Nursing. After the clinic received favorable publicity in the local media during its new building dedication, KSU faculty and staff responded to requests for funding by asking that their Capital Campaign donations be designated for the clinic. Walk-a-thons are another popular way of raising funds. Student nurses' groups in many universities employ this method to raise money for their organizations or for health promotion awareness.

Grass roots fundraising should not be overlooked if relatively small amounts of funds are needed. Students often use bake sales and car washes to raise funds for airplane tickets to developing countries where they combine learning community health nursing with service. *Formal dinners* with highly visible speakers combined with *raffles* can earn thousands of dollars if the right community leaders are invited. For example, John Walsh (host of the *America's Most Wanted* television program) agreed to be the featured guest at a fundraiser for Prescott House, the Children's Advocacy Center of Jefferson County, Alabama.

EVALUATION

Evaluation of programs can be accomplished through traditional research methods. Quantitative measures include tools designed to collect stakeholder demographic data and identify the satisfaction of participants, such as surveys and questionnaires. Qualitative measures for this purpose might include interviews and focus groups.

EXAMPLES

Swarovski Worksite Wellness Program

Swarovski Worldwide Lighting in Plattsburgh, New York, partnered with State University of New York (SUNY) nursing faculty and the Clinton County Health Department to launch the first worksite wellness program in the county. All collaborators are partners with the local Action for Health Committee.

The Swarovski facility lacked wellness resources for its employees, yet had a workforce who expressed interest in prevention services. To address this need, a multiyear project was planned that would be implemented by sequential cohorts of preselected senior-level nursing students. Stakeholders were identified, including workers from all shifts, senior management, and the local healthcare providers and the health department. Nursing students worked with Swarovski to recruit a wide variety of staff to form a worksite wellness committee. The wellness committee met multiple times to establish a common purpose. Initial goals were to develop a common set of short- and long-term objectives and establish mission and vision statements. Students conducted a needs assessment and laid the groundwork for policy development and sustainable change.

A survey and worksite index assessment were completed. Seventy percent of the workforce completed the instruments ($n = 239$). Results of the needs assessment indicated that employees had poor access to healthy lifestyle choices in the workplace, which in turn led to increased health disparity and decreased quality of life. Nursing students are currently helping to achieve Swarovski's goals of implementing a walking program, revising existing tobacco policies, and implementing a healthy-food vending machine policy. Long-term goals will be to establish a weekly farmer's market and to establish screening and intervention programs to reduce risks of chronic disease.

Prescott House

In the mid-1980s, the second author of this chapter (de Chesnay) was involved in working with the district attorney to set up a children's advocacy center in Jefferson County, Alabama (de Chesnay

& Petro, 1989). The intention of this program was to reduce further victimization of child sex abuse survivors through the criminal justice system and to improve prosecution rates of offenders. The team had been concerned about the extreme emotional distress experienced by children and their non-offending family members as prosecution of the offenders proceeded through the slow-moving justice system. Grant funds became available for a project to model a center after one that had been started by the district attorney in Huntsville, Alabama.

To assess the need for such a program in Jefferson County, the team conducted interviews with a variety of stakeholders. The most powerful finding from this research was that children were required to tell their stories over and over to many professionals in intimidating circumstances, such as in police stations and courthouses with big, adult furniture. The short-term goal was to require all individuals who needed to interview children to find a quiet, private place; the long-term goal was to create a new space with age-appropriate furniture and anatomically correct dolls.

On a short-term basis, the team designated a quiet space in the police station that was equipped with smaller furniture for children. Dolls and coloring materials were brought to the room to enhance the interviews. All interviewers came to the child. The effectiveness of this plan was limited, however, in that the child still needed to tell the story many times. With each subsequent telling of the story, many children become confused or numb and the story sounded false.

The long-term solution was to acquire a building that would be dedicated to interviewing the children. Funds were raised through private donations, and the house was named Prescott House in honor of the local citizen who donated the building. Prescott House is located away from the courthouse, in a residential neighborhood. The former residential space was renovated to accommodate a large conference room upstairs with age-appropriate interview rooms for young children and adolescents. The arrangement of rooms with closed-circuit television enables the child to be in the interview room with one interviewer who wears an earpiece. All other professionals are required to watch from the conference room and feed their questions to the interviewer.

SUMMARY

This chapter has offered some basic ideas about program development. Nurses are in a unique position to provide such programs for vulnerable populations, and the following chapters offer examples of the fine work they do. With appropriate planning and involvement by stakeholders, programs at the local level can make great contributions to their communities.

For a full suite of assignments and additional learning activities, use the access code located in the front of your book to visit this exclusive website: http://go.jblearning.com/dechesnay. If you do not have an access code, you can obtain one at the site.

REFERENCES

Colvin, S., de Chesnay, M., Mercado, T., & Benavides, C. (2005). Child health in a barrio of Managua. In M. de Chesnay (Ed.), *Caring for the vulnerable: Perspectives in nursing theory, practice, and research* (pp. 161–70). Sudbury, MA: Jones and Bartlett.

De Chesnay, M., & Petro, L. (1989). The accountability of incest offenders. *Medicine and Law*, *8*, 281–286.

Issel, L. M. (2004). *Health program planning and evaluation: A practical, systematic approach for community health*. Sudbury, MA: Jones and Bartlett.

Lewis, J. (2008). *Mastering project management* (2nd ed.). New York, NY: McGraw-Hill, pp. 108–109.

Longest, B. (2004). *Managing health programs and projects*. San Francisco, CA: Jossey-Bass, pp. 64–73.

Stanhope, M., & Lancaster, J. (2008). *Public health nursing: Population-centered health care in the community* (7th ed.). St. Louis, MO: Mosby/Elsevier.

CHAPTER 29

Childhood Autism in a Rural Environment: Reaching Vulnerable Children and Their Families

Ellyn Cavanagh

Objectives

At the end of this chapter, the reader will be able to

1. Define autism spectrum disorder (ASD) in terms of key identifiers.
2. List the symptoms of ASD.
3. Describe the cultural components of ASD.

WWW

INTRODUCTION

Autism spectrum disorder (ASD) is a neurodevelopmental medical condition associated with unique abnormalities in brain development. Autism exposes children to many risk factors, such as loss of important relationships. Affected children do not experience typical human interaction with the outside world in a natural manner. Internal protective factors such as temperament, coping skills, good parenting, and supportive environment may all increase the child's ability to interpret and adapt to the stimuli from the external environment, however.

This chapter covers inherent vulnerabilities of autism, resilience, and implications for professional nursing practice. The term "resiliency" is most often used to describe the protective process that results in a more positive outcome for individuals who are at risk for either social or psychological factors (**Figure 29–1**). It is often thought of as the opposite of risk or vulnerability. The social confines of autism make affected individuals dependent upon family support as they go from social isolation to social perplexity. Resilience as an outcome in autism is a measure of the individual child's strengths, which depend on the physical and social capital of the family and the larger community. Therefore, the focus of this chapter is on nursing

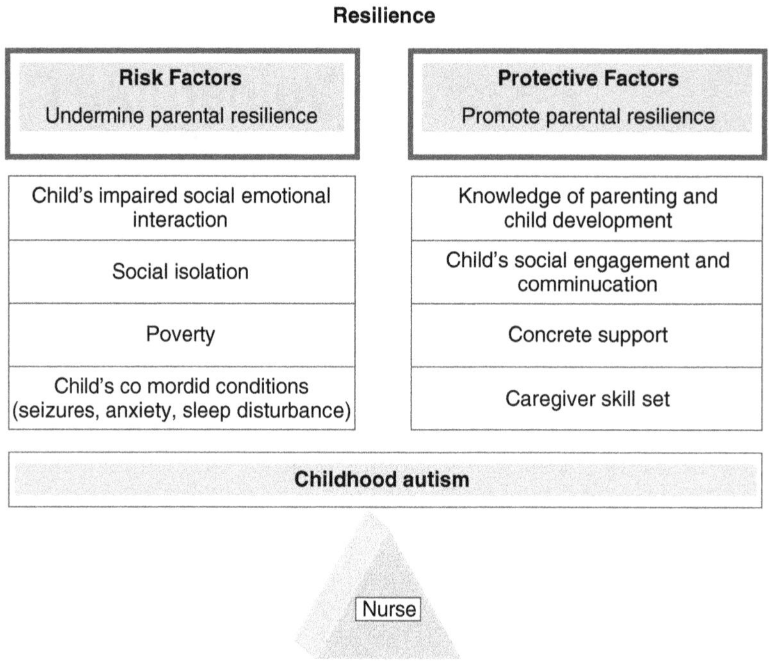

Figure 29–1 Resilience.

interventions to support the family network through an understanding of the full range of potential resources that might protect the child from risk.

Individuals who have autism seem to manage well if they are identified early in childhood, if their families are taught to differentiate normal from abnormal behaviors and are given specific strategies to enrich the child's early experiences and cognitive development, and if the child is enrolled into an intensive educational program. The needs of children with ASD straddle the education and healthcare systems. Nursing priorities include recognition of autism as disordered development, an understanding of the autistic nervous system, and family-focused care. The interplay between vulnerability and resilience will be illustrated through case examples of children living in rural New England communities.

THE AUTISM NERVOUS SYSTEM

The autistic nervous system is best understood according to symptoms. Common symptoms of ASD include delayed language, social unrelatedness, and unusual sensitivity to the environment. Unusual and restricted behaviors may also be observed such as a need for rigidity and highly structured routines, preoccupation with sameness, repetitive body movements, insensitivity to pain or temperature, and apparent deafness. Although commonly associated with mental retardation, autism differs from other developmental disorders in that the behavioral features are distinctive and do not simply reflect developmental delay but rather a disordered development. Social and adaptive abilities, language level, and nonverbal intelligence are important predictors of independence and long-term prognosis. Most typically developing children will exhibit nonverbal communication and joint attention skills before the age of one year. Children with autism fail to develop social engagement and suffer impairments in social interaction and communication (Myers, Johnson, & American Academy of Pediatrics Council on Children with Disabilities, 2007).

Theoretically a congenital disorder, autism is often characterized by symptoms that appear during early infancy. Four basic trajectories represent the potential outcomes for children who are diagnosed in early childhood:

- Recovery of language and development of compensatory social skills
- Failure to develop proficient language and persistent poor social interaction
- Progressive developmental gains and acquisition of maladaptive behaviors with variability in communicative skills
- Developmental regression and nonfunctional behaviors

These developmental pathways are established during childhood and operate across the life span. The goal is to establish the diagnosis within the first two years of life and begin treatment immediately. The American Academy of Pediatrics' Council on Children with disabilities states that the primary goals of treatment are (1) to maximize the child's ultimate functional independence and quality of life by minimizing the core features; (2) to facilitate development and learning; (3) to promote socialization; (4) to reduce maladaptive behaviors; and (5) to educate and support families (Myers et al., 2007).

Children with autism also face much higher comorbidity. Cognitive impairment or an intelligence quotient (IQ) equal to or less than 70 has been reported for 40% to 62% of children whose conditions were consistent with the case definition for ASD. Seizure disorders occur in 25%, central nervous system malformations occur in 20%, significant dysmorphology in 25%, microcephaly in 5% to 15% and macrocephaly in 30%. In addition, sleep problems are common in children and adolescents with ASDs at all levels of cognitive functioning (Myers et al., 2007).

VULNERABILITY AND RESILIENCE

The level of vulnerability is defined by the constellation of symptoms in the autism spectrum. Resilience, in the setting of ASD, comprises the capacity of family to navigate its way to the necessary resources and to sustain well-being in the face of this diagnosis. Parents are typically ill prepared for the challenges of having a child with autism, so they need resilience to deal with the unexpected diagnosis.

For example, one of the precursors of positive childhood development is attachment. Parents' first clue to their child's condition is often the social disconnect experienced by the child and their difficulty in establishing a reciprocal relationship with the child. Social impairment is the central vulnerability, the defining feature of the disorder, and not explicable in terms of cognitive delay alone. The social dysfunction in autism is distinctive and disabling. Autism interferes with the ability of the child to recognize faces, use language, possess emotions, or develop self-awareness (Martinez-Pederast & Carter, 2009). In addition, children, adolescents, and adults with ASD often have comorbid psychiatric difficulties, with the most common being anxiety and depression (Howlin, 2005).

Resilience is the family's response to the need to create and protect the child's core social skills. The child with social deficits relies on his or her primary social group—the family—to cope with the uncertainty of the outside world. The child may have difficulties with social reciprocity, appropriate conversational skills, and other higher-order language ability, such that his or her behaviors are perceived as bizarre or strange.

Each family arrives at the starting line of parenting through the autism diagnosis with different equipment, and each child with autism presents with a variation in strengths and weaknesses. Families are required to recognize and exploit the child's strengths and create a relationship of mutual stimulation and elevation. The goal is to for the family to eventually tap into those higher-order needs for affiliation, belonging, esteem, and efficacy, rather than mere survival or comfort. Families build daily interactions around their child and rely on professionals for expert opinion, anticipatory guidance, measurement, troubleshooting, and simple support. ASD has no cure, and there has been little examination of which factors might decrease parental perceptions of vulnerability after the diagnosis. The earlier the diagnosis is made in the child's life, the more likely it is to affect the parents' developing view of their child; thus it is most important that practitioners recognize the disorder early and develop a long-term management plan.

Seltzer and colleagues (Seltzer, Kraus, Osmond, & Vestal, 2000; Seltzer, Shattuck, Abbeduto, & Greenberg, 2004) describe three ways in which families are affected by having a child with autism. First, compared to parents of children with other developmental disabilities, these families face greater stress, depression, anxiety, and other negative mental health outcomes. Second, the consequences of ASD are pervasive and lasting, changing from childhood through adolescence. In earlier childhood years, families welcome intervention programs and extensive treatment regimens. As the child reaches adolescence, however, families recognize that the child's level of functioning or capacity for transition to independent living may not change dramatically. Third, social support and the use of specific coping strategies can ameliorate or buffer the magnitude and impact of stress among family members. The social ecology must provide the necessary resources, and resilience is measured by the ability of individuals, their families, and communities to negotiate culturally meaningful ways for resources to be shared. Resilience is best understood as a process of adaptation to adversity that is scaffolded by environmental, cultural, social, psychologic, and physiologic processes (Cameron, Ungar, & Liebenberg, 2007).

ELEMENTS OF RESILIENCE

Environmental Components

One of the most insidious and insurmountable environmental vulnerabilities is resource insufficiency. The treatment plan for ASD involves intensive educational support and behavior therapy in all settings. Unfortunately, educational services are underfunded, sometimes grossly so. Without funds, it is difficult to build any kind of service system for autism treatment. Resource insufficiency inevitably leads to shortages in skilled staff and difficulties in training and recruiting appropriate personnel. Such shortages energize the search for treatment modalities that might be more cost-effective but are not as effective as more costly options and, in some cases, are actually harmful.

The availability of educational services depends on local tax revenue—a key problem in rural communities, which often have a high poverty rate. The environmental vulnerability is that services for children with ASD need to be delivered in the immediate present, not years down the line. The problem with rural poverty in this sense is not only the dependence on limited tax-based revenue, but also the further limitation of philanthropic or community resources. Environmental resources for local, early intervention, which are generally paid for through the educational system, affect timely identification of and intervention with children with autism; inevitably, different jurisdictions make critical choices on the utilization of these education resources.

WWW *Case: The Preschool Environment—Thomas and Educational Support*

Thomas was diagnosed with autism at age 30 months, at which point early intervention services were started on a schedule one hour per week. Thomas was eligible for preschool at 36 months and enrolled at the local elementary school. He was nonverbal, so he was assigned a one-on-one paraeducator who was well meaning but not skilled with autistic children. The role of the paraeducator is to support the child in a classroom, as a human attachment, but this role is typically a low-paying position with a minimal skill set expected.

Thomas's mother stepped in and asked the educational team and school board for financial support to receive training in applied behavioral analysis (ABA). ABA methods are used to teach social skills, enhance communication, and reduce interfering maladaptive behaviors. They agreed, and his mother became Thomas's paraeducator. The role evolved and today she is a leader within the small rural elementary school. For a year her son was the only child in the school system with autism. When a second child was diagnosed a year later, the school was ready for immediate intervention. Through her training, Thomas's mother enlisted a certified ABA therapist to travel from the southern part of the state once a month to consult on both children. The cost is shared between the school and two families. This intervention resulted in less disruption in the children's education and brought a collective gain in therapies for both children. In this way, the rural district provided ABA at the preschool level and effectively started a program for managing ASD.

Schools have the potential to support children with ASD at both policy and practice levels. The National Research Council, in its report titled *Educating Children with Autism* (Lord,

McGee, & Commission on Educational Interventions for Children with Autism, 2001), recommends at least 25 hours per week of intensive early intervention be provided as soon as a child is diagnosed. If diagnosis occurs prior to age three years, the Family, Infant and Toddler Program (FITP) is responsible for coordinating services for the child and his or her family. However, 25 hours per week of active engagement in intensive instructional programming is considerably more service than children in FITP generally receive in rural communities. Essential Early Education programs typically provide three to five half-days per week of a preschool program and some additional home visiting for parent education or support. A preschool program may or may not be an intensive program and is frequently less than the recommended minimum of 25 hours per week (Lord et al., 2001).

In Thomas's case, he was an autistic child living in a rural community school with 87 students in kindergarten through fifth grade, and there was no therapist available to provide the recommended educational support. Such rural environments tend to have more single-parent families and young workers lacking a higher education and, therefore, are more vulnerable to income inequality. However, Thomas's mother—a single mother on a limited income—developed a cooperative agreement with the school board, negotiated a role for herself, and created an environment for justice and reduction of vulnerability.

Cultural Components

In New Hampshire, home to the famous "Live free or die" motto, the culture is inherently anti-tax. Local governments are lean and, as a result, more efficient. However, rural healthcare settings are challenged by the limitations placed on providers. Vulnerability occurs when professionals are stretched beyond their comfort levels in caring for individuals with developmental disabilities. In an urban setting, a wider choice of healthcare providers exists because more providers are available in a concentrated area. In contrast, for rural families, there is often no choice in selecting a provider, and if the provider has a limited skill set, the family has no recourse. Further, it is a cultural expectation among these rural populations not to question the expertise or skill sets of their healthcare providers.

Case: Cultural Factors in the Early School Age Period—The Reynolds Family and Delayed Diagnoses

The Reynolds family has three children younger than the age of seven years and a limited income. Two of the children have developmental delays. The family receives its primary care through a rural-based family practice group. When the children presented for well-child care, they were fearful and uncooperative, and saw a different provider each time. The providers within the group had limited experience with children who fall along the autism spectrum and did not refer the children to early intervention.

When the children entered kindergarten and first grade, the educators identified their developmental problems. Both children had challenging behaviors and were not able to be taught in a group setting. The educational team requested a development evaluation, and the healthcare provider referred the children to a tertiary center. The parents had no money to travel to a tertiary center, the small health practice had no coordinator to help them fund the referral, and the family was left to negotiate with a tertiary health system on their own. After a conversation with the children's mother, an administrative assistant at the tertiary referral center recognized the dilemma and arranged a relatively simple intervention: a gas card and a two-day stay at the tertiary center housing alternative. This action preserved the family's independence and did not require clinical expertise, just an empathetic approach using para-clinical skills. In this case, the cornerstone for stability was laid by the para-clinical person who understood the challenge and made a decision to strengthen the system of care delivery.

The cultural milieu can present challenges for families with ASD-affected members. Not only are special educators, therapists, and psychologists less available in small, rural communities, but teachers' expectations for education of the child can be lower. The follow-up on the Reynolds children illustrates a cultural synergy of both risk and protective factors. One of the Reynolds children received the diagnosis of ASD with the recommendation for an individualized educational program. The parents were not willing to have the child labeled with this diagnosis because teachers in the community had expressed the opinion that autistic behavior occurred secondary to poor parenting. Further, in this rural community, the parents were well known, and in the past each had experienced a rebellious relationship with the local teachers. The parents were defensive, neither having completed high school, and they were not comfortable entering into a meeting with the teachers. The school district did not have a special education advocate available.

The nurse practitioner at the tertiary referral center offered to be present at the meeting by teleconference. During the meeting, they used critical thinking as well as professional decision making to support the child's educational program. This intervention helped clarify expectations. The educational team was resourceful and made offers for accommodations. The parents expressed feelings of empowerment, and the child gained an individualized educational plan. The cost of this intervention was billed as a follow-up appointment and covered by the state health program.

A cultural risk in a small rural community is that the family is rarely anonymous when it seeks care. In this environment, individuals often arrive in the professional offices with a past that is well known. This prior knowledge can present barriers at multiple levels. It is important for practitioners to understand the subtle nuances that may derail a treatment plan. In the preceding case, the mother articulated the humiliation she felt about living on public assistance with an unemployed partner. She felt judged by the community at large and as a result approached any gesture of help with suspicion. As a consequence, she was not able to take advantage of the local community resources.

The nurse practitioner recognized that resilience in not an individualized cultural phenomenon. Children do not rise up phoenix-like above adversity; rather, the community must share resources to provide the opportunity for the child to flourish first within the family circle. In this case, the gas card, housing, and a teleconference call buffered the risk in this child's life and built capacity for his parents. Later, a second nudge came from the nurse practitioner, who alerted the community mental health team about needed respite services. The system rallied around the family as community members offered services to repair the car and improve the living situation. This nurse created change and addressed vulnerability by working across disciplines and embedding culturally appropriate family-centered care into work settings, the home, and the classroom. Ultimately, the cultural strengths of the community contributed toward making necessary changes to foster attachment with this autistic child.

Social Components

Dealing with a child with ASD at any age can be extremely time-consuming for families. Thus a key vulnerability associated with this diagnosis is parenting role stress. The types of parental stress experienced generally change over the child's life span, and families may have complications that challenge their ability to handle the additional stress load. Initially, parents must deal with the emotional aspects of discovering that their child has a significant developmental disability (Beatson, 2008). As the child grows older, areas of weaknesses are likely to persist, even as areas of strength emerge that, when nurtured, buffer the vulnerabilities. Nevertheless, because of the high level of daily stress, crises can overwhelm the family and create dangerous situations. The child with autism has a very narrow range of attachment behaviors and when threatened often regresses developmentally, manifesting anxious behaviors.

Crisis situations develop when behavioral challenges become too great for the family to manage. In addition, if the family is facing disruption owing to changing roles, housing, or finances, the child's stability is threatened and crises can develop rapidly. In a rural community, the availability of services outside of the educational system is often limited; thus, when a family's social situation changes, it may not be easy to obtain backup care.

Case: Social Factors and the School Age Child—Phillip and Sleep Disorder

Phillip is a nine-year--old nonverbal youth with ASD and a chronic sleep disturbance. He has difficulty getting to sleep at night and often wakes after two to three hours. When awake, he screams and requires constant supervision. His parents have been taking turns responding to this dilemma. They stay awake in four-hour shifts at night, and they sleep during the day when Phillip is at school.

Recently, Phillip has been getting physically aggressive during the wakeful periods and his behavior at school is worsening. He has bitten his mother and she has difficulty controlling him while she is alone, so the father is frequently called upon to intervene. There is no quality sleep for anyone. The insular nature of the problem is causing a decline in the well-being of the entire family owing to their lack of sleeplessness and irritability. Phillip has gotten into a pattern of falling asleep in the early morning; if awakened for school, he becomes combative. The parents often decide to let him sleep and keep him home from school—a pattern that is repeated day after day. Because the child is not being taught, the problem has evolved from a sleep disturbance into an education failure.

The solution to this social dilemma involves an ecological approach. Foremost, the physical aggression is socially unacceptable. Parents who encounter this problem are usually not forthcoming in describing the situation until the risk of injury or actual harm occurs. In this case, the questions asked to parents were pivotal: "What is your threshold of calling for help?"

and "Who would you call?" The threshold for alerting others was if Phillip bit his mother hard enough to draw blood, and the agency or person they would call was the police. When queried about why they did not consider the primary care provider, mother said that her past experience was that healthcare providers were uncomfortable with the behavior and unable to come up with a solution, even on a short-term basis. When queried about using any health facility, such as an emergency room, the response was even more negative: The parents stated that this practice would create a larger problem. In small communities, public servants such as the police and fire personnel play a vital role in managing crises, because they make house calls and have a level of understanding about how to assess risk and de-escalate a situation.

The solution in this case involved the regional child development team. The child needed an assessment and a two-tiered approach to the problem.

Having a child with autism imposes a higher level of social isolation on the family. The risk is that the social isolation and the behaviors may reach a critical level rapidly because parents are working at maximum capacity, and that they then become helpless. In a rural setting, informal networks of support may not be in close proximity, or may be unavailable, overburdened, or unsuitable; thus the only option for parents becomes the ultimate call for help in a crisis. It is important for practitioners to have a clear understanding of the social connectedness of the family. It is also imperative that professionals who have philosophic differences acknowledge the problems and either resolve them or not get involved with the case. The addition of a complicated professional relationship is counterproductive.

The informal network of caregivers is the first line of defense, followed by alliances built through community involvement, such as clergy or sheltered programs, and finally more skilled caregiving and respite care. The formal network, defined as community health professionals, regional programs, and at the extreme residential care, is another alternative. If a child's primary social network is failing, as in this case, it is imperative to reduce the parenting stress and work toward stability.

Phillip responded to sleep medication, but the treatment required almost two weeks to achieve a complete six-hour sleep cycle. In the interim, the mother was hospitalized with chest pain and the father was left as sole provider for a week.

Psychological Components

Psychosocial quality of life is predicted by autism severity. As a student with autism works to change behaviors or learn difficult skills, it is essential that the reward for this effort be substantial enough for him or her to extend this effort. Individuals with autism need a consistent approach in education and teaching/learning strategies. Some families do not show an interest in being interventionists on behalf of the child, some are already extended close to their psychological limits, and some have other family responsibilities. Some parents expect the school to do total care. Thus some families do not accept a family-centered philosophy as an option. These cases are challenging for providers, and the practitioners need to accept the situation, using a positive tone laced with compassion. Such families may be in an evolutionary process, and they may become more supportive on a psychological level with time and patience.

Case: The Adolescent Period—Sara, an Adolescent with Attention and Aggression Issues

Sara is an adolescent with autism. When educators noted a decrease in Sara's attention span and an increase in problem behaviors in school, the practitioner assessed the situation and prescribed central nervous system stimulants. Over the next few weeks, Sara had severe anxiety and became increasingly resistant to school. The medication to increase her attention span was not effective and Sara's behavior deteriorated. Her mother had no recourse except to agree to let Sara stay home because she believed the school was not providing her daughter with an appropriate education.

Treating a target symptom alone—rather than a target symptom within a disorder, such as autism—often creates secondary problems. As demonstrated by this case, providers in rural areas have less training in handling mental health issues and the chronic needs of individuals with autism. The result for Sara was an exacerbation of her core symptoms of obsessive anxiety. Sara regressed and developed secondary problems related to her ASD. In general, individuals with autism have a higher degree of internal distractibility that can manifest as inattention. Although the medication prescribed for Sara was intended to make her more internally driven (i.e., hyper-focused), it actually caused her to develop heightened anxiety. This anxiety was manifested as refusal to participate in school. She was no longer willing to put forth the effort because the rewards were not great enough, and she reverted to self-stimulatory behavior. Once such behaviors overwhelm a rural educational system, few alternatives are typically available because there are few trained behavior specialists who can break down the problem in a systematic manner.

Sara was evaluated at the regional center, and started on medication to help reduce her aggression and school avoidance. The central nervous stimulants were discontinued and a low-dose selective serotonin reuptake inhibitor was started. While stimulant medications are prescribed to treat inattention and hyperactivity symptoms, they may exacerbate stereotypic behaviors, such as hand flapping, tic-like behaviors, and a paradoxical response, resulting in increased hyperactivity, obsessive behaviors, and mood liability (Di Martino, Melisa, Cianchetti, & Zuddas, 2004; King & Bostic, 2006).

Autism is three to five times more common in boys than in girls, but girls with autism are more likely to be severely intellectually impaired (Fombonne, 2005). When children with ASD move beyond the elementary school programs, it is necessary to focus on behavioral regulation. In adolescence, the term *transition* is used to describe movement from child-centered activities to adult-oriented activities. For some youth, the hormonal contribution of puberty makes this period even more challenging. Problematic emotional reactions and behaviors such as aggression and self-injury are common in older individuals with ASD. Recent surveys indicate approximately 45% of adolescents and as many as 75% of adults with ASD are treated with psychotropic medications. Increasing age, lower adaptive skills and social competence, and higher levels of maladaptive behaviors are associated with greater likelihood of medication use (Tsakanikos, Costello, & Holt, 2006).

The most common use of medications is for managing disruptive behaviors, such as self-injury, aggression, compulsions (repetitive behaviors), hyperactivity, mood lability, anxiety, and sleep disturbances (Kanne, Christ, & Reisersen, 2009). Such medications do not cure autism, however. Rather, the goal of treatment is to alleviate the most troublesome behavioral symptoms that impair or distress the child and/or interfere with therapeutic efforts, such as intensive education and socialization (Witwer & Lecavalier, 2005).

Nurses need to recognize the social challenges that occur as a result of adolescence. The youth with autism is much more vulnerable, and at higher risk for regressive behaviors as a result of the physiology involved. Such behaviors may, in turn, overwhelm the family system. Teens with autism need individually focused care to minimize the anxiety and social disorganization that threaten their ability to achieve inclusion. At this point in development, the adolescent with autism needs to have a certain level of independence; any regression is problematic. A team approach during this critical period is absolutely necessary.

Physiological Components

The communication impairments characteristic of ASD may lead to an unusual presentation of atypical signs of common disorders; most prevalent are gastrointestinal and sleep disturbances. In a nationally representative sample, researchers found that children with ASD spent twice as much time with the physician per outpatient visit compared with children in control groups. A wide variety of physical illnesses and aberrant physiologic states in ASD can produce pain and discomfort that, in turn, generate high rates of problem behavior and impede psychosocial and educational development (Carr & Owen-DeSchryver, 2007).

Case: Physiological Comorbidities—Camus, a Preschooler with a High Lead Level and Seizure Disorder

Camus is a three-year-old child diagnosed with autism. Prior to his third birthday, he was mouthing objects as one of his self-stimulatory behaviors. His blood level of lead, as measured at the child development center shortly after diagnosis, was 40 µg/dL. Camus lived in a 200-year-old farmhouse, and the source of lead poisoning was lead paint in the window frames. The home was owned by the family, who had lived there for many generations. However, the family was delinquent in its property taxes, so was not eligible for state funding for lead abatement until the balance was paid. The child remained in the house and received oral iron treatment, but his lead level remained toxic and his behavior worsened. This financial dilemma affected both the quality of his education and his ability to learn because of the lead toxicity. Nurses were involved at the state and regional levels, but the interventions were ultimately determined by the ability of parents to complete their financial obligation. In consultation with the nurse practitioner at the tertiary level, the family was able to assess their situation and make the decision to tear down the house and live in a temporary house on the property. The cost of property taxes far exceeded the cost of a new modular home. This solution left them in the same situation of owing taxes, but the child was in a safer environment.

Camus continued to demonstrate behavioral regression as the lead was slowly absorbed into his system. He was diagnosed with a seizure disorder when his pica progressed to the self-injurious behavior of biting. He was excluded from his preschool program because his unpredictable biting injured the paraeducator. The nurses involved in his care collaborated across several agencies and coordinated efforts with parents as case managers. The family lived in rural isolation but had daily contact with a web of providers to improve their child's behavior to the point where he could safely be reintroduced to his school environment.

CONCLUSION

Development in children with ASD is not merely delayed, but also different and disordered. Autism affects development by interfering with socialization, communication, and learning. The goal of intervention is to potentiate human development through collaborative and responsive family partnerships with the educational and healthcare teams. Interventions should focus primarily on improving good parenting practices, as they represent the most important factor in the adjustment of children. A focus on resilience calls for attention to be paid to building capacities in children through family-centered care by developing a flexible and responsive system in health care and education. At the level of clinical work, the focus is on well-child care and early identification of social impairment. Deficits in social interaction in autism change over the course of development but remain an area of great disability even for the highest-functioning adult with autism.

To manage patients with ASD, the nurse must be knowledgeable about normal and abnormal development, recognize developmental milestones, and be able to use a validated screening tool. General developmental screening at 9, 18, and 24 months of age will identify most children with autism. The early signs for an ASD diagnosis include concerns regarding a child's social skills, communication, and restricted or repetitive patterns of behavior, interests, and activities (American Psychiatric Association, 2000). A child should respond to his or her name by one year of age, and the lack of this pivotal social skill is concerning for ASD. An infant who presents with a relative lack of social interest and an over-concern with environmental (nonsocial) change is considered to be at high risk for such disorders. Various rating scales and checklists may aid in diagnosis but do not replace the need for thoughtful and careful assessment (Greenspan & Brazelton, 2008). **Table 29–1** highlights some key points about ASD for healthcare providers.

Developmental or behavioral regression describes a significant loss of previously acquired milestones or skills. It is generally assumed that regression occurs in a minority of children with autism. The mean age at which parents report regression is 20 months. The most frequently reported aspect of regression is loss of language, followed by loss of social–emotional connectedness. Some groups of children are at risk for later diagnosis, especially those who have many primary care providers, those who live in a rural area, and those who live in poverty (Mandell, Maytali, & Zubritsky, 2005).

Resilience in ASD is a dynamic social process that is supported by the family. To promote resilience, it is necessary to have resources available that provide a structure through which individual capacity may flourish.

Practitioners working in rural areas should have additional training to understand how to implement and manage a family-centered plan of care. All families should have explicit support

Table 29–1 Five Points Every Provider Should Know About Autism Spectrum Disorder

1. The medical home model is the ideal model for ASD service delivery; however, the care of an individual with autism is highly dependent upon the professional profile of the provider.
2. Sometimes not all of the diagnostic features of ASD are present by age three years. Many children do not show clear repetitive behaviors at two years of age. Between three and four years of age, preschool children with autism exhibit the more classical picture.
3. Early and continuous intervention in ASD is highly desirable and has measurable effects on later intellectual and communicative abilities.
4. Parental stress is significantly greater for mothers of children with autism than for mothers of children with mental retardation or physical disabilities. Family life can end up revolving around the needs of the child with autism. Concerns may arise about taking the child into the community due to behavior challenges. ASD can be particularly challenging because the child appears "normal" physically, but may exhibit extreme behavior problems that are not understood by community members.
5. There is the need for constant vigilance for children who have no understanding of danger. As the child grows bigger and stronger, some families struggle with addressing behavior challenges such as aggression.

plans in place to address problem behaviors exhibited by their ASD-affected members. In addition, practitioners should partner with emergency responders, educators, and community activists to create a safety net for families (Carbine, Behl, Azor, & Murphy, 2010). Nurses will find themselves faced with issues beyond their expected roles when dealing with the complex problems of these families. It is critical to remain authentically connected with families and willing to respond to their most pressing needs. A continuum of services from birth to death is needed for individuals on the autism spectrum (Carbine et al., 2010; Elder & D'Alessandro, 2009). **Table 29–2** lists resources available to nurses regarding ASD.

Finally, nurses working with the families must have a flexible repertoire and willingness to connect with the parents. Parenting an autistic child is an isolating experience, simply because of the nature of the disorder, (Elder & D'Alessandro, 2009). A skilled and resourceful nurse can regulate the level of stress so that it becomes motivating rather than overwhelming. Home visits, teleconferences, and regularly scheduled clinic appointments create space and time to discuss hopes and aspirations as well as the reality of daily challenges. In addition, the nurse must establish partnerships with the educational team for interdisciplinary care. Reliable partnerships help prevent distortion of information. Moreover, the nurse should create communities that can function as sustaining circles of mutual support.

Be realistic with parents about the long journey that lies ahead. Explain that families need a supportive, collaborative team to help their child reach his or her fullest potential. By putting these approaches into action, the nurse frees the family from the illusion that they could or should accomplish these goals alone or that they have to carry the load alone. Emphasize that the family can share the care of their child with others and focus on what they do well.

Table 29–2 Autism Spectrum Disorder Resources for Nurses

Autism: Caring for Children with Autism Spectrum Disorders: A Resource Toolkit for Clinicians—American Academy of Pediatrics: http://www.aap.org/healthtopics/autism.cfm
Center for Social Emotional Foundations for Early Learning: http://www.vanderbilt.edu/csefel
Developmental Screening Policy Statement: http://www.medicalhomeinfo.org/screening/indexx.html
Enhancing Developmentally Oriented Primary Care (EDOPC): http://www.illinoisaap.org/medicalhome.htm, http://www.illinoisaap.org/DevelopmentalScreening.htm
National Center of Medical Home Initiative for Children with Special Needs: http://www.medicalhomeinfo
Pathways to Independence Natural Supports Project: http://www.waisman.wisc.edu/naturalsupports
Public Awareness Program on Early Childhood Development: http://www.cdc.gov/ncbddd/autism/actearly
Understanding Autism Spectrum Disorders—American Academy of Pediatrics: http://www.aap.org/hea;thtopics/autism.cfm
Zero to Three: http://www.zerotothree.org

By adopting an empathetic perspective with working with families with an ASD-affected member, the nurse can gain an understanding of vulnerability and the resilience of the human spirit. There is hope in this situation, as reflected in the following passage from an autistic adult who was diagnosed with autism in infancy and experienced comorbid seizure disorder:

> I'm amazed to think how much my parents did for me even as they must have gotten so little back at the time. Hearing my parents' recollections of my earliest years has been a magical experience for me: to see for myself in hindsight the extent of their role in making me the person I am today. (Tammet, 2006, pp. 27–28)

WWW

For a full suite of assignments and additional learning activities, use the access code located in the front of your book to visit this exclusive website: http://go.jblearning.com/dechesnay. If you do not have an access code, you can obtain one at the site.

REFERENCES

American Psychiatric Association. (2000). *Diagnostic and statistical manual for mental disorders* (4th ed.). Washington, DC: American Psychiatric Publishing.

Beatson, J. E. (2008). Walk a mile in their shoes: Implementing family-centered care in serving children and families affected by autism spectrum disorder. *Topics in Language Disorders*, *28*(4), 309–322.

Cameron, C., Ungar, M., & Liebenberg, L. (2007). Cultural understandings of resilience: Roots for wings in the development of affective resources for resilience. *Child and Adolescent Psychiatric Clinics of North America, 16*, 285–301.

Carbine, P., Behl, D., Azor, V., & Murphy, N. (2010). The medical home for children with autism spectrum disorders: Parent and pediatric perspectives. *Journal of Autism and Developmental Disorders, 40*, 317–324.

Carr, E. G., & Owen-DeSchryver, R. (2007). Physical illness, pain, and problem behavior in minimally verbal people with developmental disabilities. *Journal of Autism and Developmental Disorders, 37*, 413–424.

Di Martino, A., Melis, G., Cianchetti, C., & Zuddas, A. (2004). Methylphenidate for pervasive developmental disorders: Safety and efficacy of acute single dose test and ongoing therapy. *Journal of Child and Adolescent Psychopharmacology, 14*(2), 201–218.

Elder, J., & D'Alessandro, T. (2009). Supporting families with autism spectrum disorders: Questions parents ask and what nurses need to know. *Pediatric Nursing, 35*(4), 240–253.

Fombonne, E. (2005). Epidemiological studies of pervasive developmental disorder. In F. R. Volkmar, A. Kiln, R. Paul, & D. Cohen (Eds.), *Handbook of autism and pervasive developmental disorders*, (3rd ed. pp. 42–69). Hoboken, NJ: John Wiley & Sons.

Greenspan, S. L., & Brazelton, T. B. (2008).Guidelines for identification, screening, and clinical management of children with autism spectrum disorders. *Pediatrics, 121*, 828–830.

Howlin, P. (2005). Outcomes in autism spectrum disorders. In F. R. Volkmar, R. Paul, A. Klin, & D. Cohen (Eds.), *Handbook of autism and pervasive developmental disorders* (3rd ed., Vol. II, pp. 201–209). Hoboken, NJ: John Wiley & Sons.

Kanne, S., Christ, S., & Reisersen, A. (2009). Psychiatric symptoms and psychosocial difficulties in young adults with autistic traits. *Journal of Autism and Developmental Disorders, 39*, 827–833.

King, B., & Bostic, J. (2006). An update on pharmacologic treatments for autism spectrum disorders. *Child and Adolescent Psychiatric Clinics of North America, 12*(11), 161–175.

Lord, C., & McGee, J. (Eds.), &Commission on Educational Interventions for Children with Autism. (2001). *Educating children with autism*. Washington, DC: National Academies Press.

Mandell, D., Maytali, M., & Zubritsky, C. (2005). Factors associated with age of diagnosis among children with autism spectrum disorder. *Pediatrics, 116*(6), 1480–1486.

Martinez-Pederast, F., & Carter, A. (2009). Autism spectrum disorders in young children. *Child and Adolescent Psychiatric Clinics of North America, 18*, 645–663.

Myers, S., Johnson, C., & American Academy of Pediatrics Council on Children with Disabilities (2007). Management of children with autism spectrum disorders. American Academy of Pediatrics. *Pediatrics, 120*(5), 1162–1182.

Seltzer, M., Kraus, M., Osmond, G., & Vestal, C. (2000). Families of adolescents and adults with autism: Uncharted territory. In L. Chidden (Ed.), *International review of research in mental retardation: Autism* (Vol. 23, pp. 267–294). San Diego, CA: Academy Press.

Seltzer, M., Shattuck, P, Abbeduto, L., & Greenberg, J. (2004). Trajectory of development in adolescents and adults with autism. *Mental Retardation and Developmental Disabilities Research Review, 10*, 234–247.

Tammet, D. (2006). *Born on a blue day*. New York, NY: Free Press.

Tsakanikos, E., Costello, H., & Holt, G. (2006). Psychopathology in adults with autism and intellectual disability. *Journal of Autism and Developmental Disorders, 36*, 1123–1129.

Witwer, A., & Lecavalier, L., (2005). Treatment incidence and patterns in children with autism spectrum disorders. *Journal of Child and Adolescent Psychopharmacology, 15*, 671–681.

CHAPTER 30

Developing a Nurse Practitioner–Run Center for Residents in Rural Appalachia

Joyce M. Knestrick and Mona M. Counts

Objectives

At the end of this chapter, the reader will be able to

1. Create a problem statement for a nurse-run clinic to serve a vulnerable population.
2. Describe how the community might be involved in creating a new nurse-managed clinic.
3. Discuss staffing needs for a clinic to be operated by nurses in conjunction with other health professionals.

In rural Appalachia, the population experiences barriers to primary care, a higher risk of acute and chronic illness, inconsistency in healthcare services, and geographic separation from healthcare services that make this population vulnerable. The barriers faced by this population affect their quality of life physically, socially, and spiritually. The provision of healthcare services for the residents in rural Appalachia by providers who consider the culture of residents while providing evidence-based health care is the major focus of the nurse practitioner–run primary care practice described here.

The purpose of this chapter is to describe the vulnerable population in the rural Appalachian region of southwestern Pennsylvania; to describe the planning, implementation, and sustainability of a nurse practitioner–run primary care practice; to present selected outcome data; and to suggest future projects to serve the area.

FOCUS OF THE CENTER

Problem Statement

In a rural Appalachian area in southwestern Pennsylvania, a need was identified to develop and maintain a nurse practitioner–run primary care center to serve the primary healthcare needs of the community. Development and especially sustainability of the center were considered paramount to providing culturally competent care to this population.

Values

The authors of this chapter are both residents of rural Appalachia. Several core values of the rural Appalachian population drive the purpose and the operations of the center, and several characteristics drive the healthcare behaviors and healthcare-seeking behaviors of the community. The concepts of family, hardiness, acceptance, spirituality, and continuity are highly valued by the culture (Counts, 1992; Huttlinger & Purnell, 2008). It is essential to understand the concepts of structure, organization, and sustainability from the point of view of the community to develop effective interventions for this population.

Mission

The mission of the nurse practitioner–run primary care center is to provide culturally competent, patient-centered, and comprehensive healthcare services to the community. The primary care center is the patient's healthcare home.

CENTER DEVELOPMENT PROCESS

Center Development

In the 1980s, healthcare services in this area of Appalachia were limited. Barriers to access to health care included the need for travel to a tertiary care center in a neighboring state or to a tertiary care center located 60 miles from the community. The establishment of foreign-born physicians' private practices and clinics provided inconsistent providers and care as well as limited access for individuals and families without healthcare insurance. A nurse practitioner (NP) living in the community was bombarded by community members seeking health care on her porch. The community reached out to her to start a center to provide healthcare services to the area. In response, the NP did an ethnographic analysis of the community, which led to the development of a nurse practitioner–run center in a local town.

As individuals, families, and other community members began to express their healthcare concerns and needs to the providers in the primary care center, the need for more data on the population surfaced. The Appalachian Patterns General Ethnographic Nursing Evaluation Studies in the State III (Counts, 1992; Russell, Gregory, Wotton, Mordoch, & Counts, 1996) were conducted in the county to further assess the healthcare concerns and health needs of the community. The study revealed the need for culturally competent healthcare services. A commitment to the community and integration of the primary care center with the community were essential elements identified in the study. In addition, the characteristics of this particular Appalachian community were further defined.

Stakeholders

The primary care center practice was started and run by a corporation of nurse practitioners. To include and increase community participation and to develop more intense community involvement, the structure was eventually changed to that of a 501C3 nonprofit organization. These changes led to improved access to additional funding sources. The community residents became the owners of the practice and had a vested interest in sustainability of the center. In addition to the community at large, stakeholders included the township supervisors, the state representative, local businesses, churches, and senior organizations. From the group of concerned citizens, a board was established to oversee the operations and sustainability of the center. The establishment of community ownership of the nonprofit organization led to the application to become a federally qualified health center look-alike (FQHC-LA), which is the clinic's current status.

Characteristics of the Population

This community exhibits many of the traits found in the literature regarding Appalachian populations (Huttlinger & Purnell, 2008). When the community describes its members, "being hardy" is a common descriptor. They have lived in this mountainous area for a long period of time, have survived economic losses, and have limited employment opportunities, yet they continue to carry on with their lives and their culture.

Family ties are strong in the community. In this area, family is defined as more than one's blood relatives; it also includes individuals who have married into the family, and individuals or families who have been adopted into the family (formally or informally). Family is stronger than an individual; therefore, a member of the community may refer to the family when speaking—for example, "We want a healthcare center that is going to stay here" or "We only want to see the nurse provider." The families take pride in "doing for each other." Most of the families have extended family members who live nearby, so that the entire family may become involved in an issue that some other cultures might consider personal. For example, if a teenager is pregnant, the family may get together to offer advice and decide how to handle the teen and her pregnancy. Elders are respected and often live with family members. These elders often are the main providers of child care and also provide care for other less healthy elders in the extended family. The family ties are so strong that the obligations to family may outweigh other obligations such as school, work, or healthcare appointments.

To gain acceptance in the community, continuity of care has to be established. The long-held distrust of outsiders is reinforced when services are started and then are moved or closed. Previously, centers were started in the area that employed foreign physicians, but the language barriers created additional trust issues. The gathering of research data from the community by faculty in universities and medical schools left a "bad taste" for outsiders offering healthcare services because there was no plan for follow-up on the research findings.

The process of acceptance by the community is ongoing. The NP has to demonstrate respect for the individual and the family. When one of the authors first came to the center, a grandmother stated, "You can see my granddaughter but I will not see you; you are a northerner." When the NP (who lives less than 30 miles away in the same Appalachian region) turned to acknowledge the grandmother and offered to make an appointment with the other NP, the grandmother noticed the NP had "Elvis" on her shirt. The grandmother remarked, "You did a good job with my grandbaby, and you like Elvis, so you are okay by me. I will see you now." Those encounters set up the acceptance of the provider.

Spirituality in this community is deep rooted in a belief in God and Christ. Some members of the population have strong ties to their churches. The church often provides a means of support and a mechanism for socialization. Doing good deeds and living right on earth are often perceiving as a way to gain rewards in heaven; thus one cannot change the future, and certain circumstances are seen as something that has to be endured on this earth.

Appalachian Outcomes

An essential concept in this community is "neighboring," which is described as neighbors taking care of one another when a need arises. If a person is sick, the neighbors will do what they can to take care of him or her. If the person is laid off from work, the neighbors will help with food and other services such as babysitting while the individual searches for a job. As a neighbor, the person receiving the services will help another neighbor in turn.

For the population served by the center, health is defined as "the ability to function." Members of the community will ignore health problems until they are not able to go to work, cannot attend to their farm or household chores, or experience complete incapacity. For this population, as long as people are able to continue to work, they are perceived as healthy. Health is intertwined with the mind, body, and spirit (Counts, 1992). Although health care is focused within the family, a sense of individual responsibility for self-care exists. As part of the self-care practices, the family may prescribe folk medicines and treatments before they seek traditional health care services. Mental health problems are generally accepted by the community as "fate."

In the Appalachian community served by the center, the population is aging in place. The elderly population is increasing. As with the elder population in bordering West Virginia, the elders are less educated, are often unemployed, and are uninsured or underinsured (Counts, 1992). More than 13% of the patients at the primary care center are older than the age of 65—a percentage consistent with the 15% proportion of the U.S. population that is elderly and the 15% proportion in Pennsylvania (U.S. Census Bureau, 2010).

The general population of this area has limited economic resources. Many are underinsured or uninsured. Many also leave the area to gain employment and then return to care for family. The general population of the county reported a $20,125 annual per capita income, with 17.5% of the community being below the poverty level. The percentage of families below the poverty level in the county is 13.5% versus the national average of 9.6% (U.S. Census Bureau, 2010). The patients at the primary care center have incomes below the county averages.

Community Outreach

The goals of the primary care center are not only to provide healthcare services but also to partner with the community to make improvements in the lives of residents. The area historically has had several extraction industries. Coal mining continues to be an integral activity in the area. In addition, strip mining and gas drilling are becoming more prevalent. Workers often come from other areas to work in these industries. Recreational activities related to the beautiful mountains, lakes, and streams are also owned or managed by outside agents. Therefore, to help the community economically, the goal has been to hire staff from within the community and train the staff to become successful so that they can give back to the community. The primary care center employs an office manager, a receptionist, a billing clerk, and a medical assistant, all of whom were trained on site. Office staff have gone school to become licensed practical nurses, registered nurses, and nurse practitioners.

THE OPERATIONAL PLAN

A plan was developed with the input of the community to establish a center that would be community owned, staffed by local residents and caring providers, and culturally sensitive. The primary care center was started by the nurse practitioners, but support was then obtained from the community and grants were written to allow the clinic to become a FQHC-LA. The center was established with four NPs (total of 1.2 full-time equivalents) and seven other personnel, including a registered nurse, a medical assistant, a receptionist, and a billing clerk.

Seeking Funding

The community identified a board of directors to establish community oversight of the center. Grants were written to fund the primary care center. Local state representatives were enlisted to help at the state level. In addition, the federal representative and a state senator were contacted to help fund the center.

Need for Social Services

Early in the development of the primary care center, a need for social services became apparent. This area of Appalachia has high poverty levels and limited access to mental health services, leaving the community vulnerable in case of injuries related to violent acts, and issues related to substance abuse. Mental health problems tend to be accepted by the families, and treatment is not sought unless the person is not able to function in the family.

The need for addition of a social worker to the primary care center was carefully assessed and initially funded by a grant from Stuanton Farm Foundation. The person had to be culturally competent, accepted by the community, and perceived by the community as providing different services than a traditional social worker. Many of the residents expressed concerns related to prior bad experiences with social workers, such as "They came and took my cousin's kids away" and "That social worker put my mother in a home." The social worker was charged with providing mental health screenings and assessments, delivering counseling services, and maintaining links with area mental health providers. In addition, the social worker was expected to play a role in assisting with acquiring services to help keep the elderly and disabled patients in their homes.

Sources of Funding

The primary care center is funded by private insurers, Medicare, Medicaid, and cash payments via a sliding scale, so some patients do not pay for their services. It is important to note that some private insurers recognize the NPs as primary care providers while others do not. Another caveat with a few of the private insurers is that the NPs may not be recognized as primary care providers, but are listed as specialists. The primary care center also is funded by donations, program grants, and contracts with companies for wellness and drug screening services.

OUTCOMES

For the past 10 years, the center has been acknowledged by a state Medicaid-managed care insurer for providing excellent, highest-quality standards of care. This designation is evidenced by accessibility to the company's subscribers, prevention of illness via immunizations, screening for potential illnesses, and efforts to minimize the impact of nonpreventable illness. The center has partnered with various agencies to provide preventive services such as cervical cancer screening, breast examinations, and mammogram services to women in the community.

During the past five years, more than 90% of the adult patients have had cholesterol screening, with follow-up education on diet and lifestyle changes and medications as necessary. In a sample of patients with type 2 diabetes (n = 40), 84% had their previously elevated glycohemoglobin A_{1c} levels decreased to 6.5 or another goal. A protocol change that increased patient diabetic education and aggressive treatment strategies was implemented to decrease the complications of diabetes. Programs were initiated to help with smoking cessation.

Although the population believes that what one eats can lead to better health, food choices are often limited due to limited budgets or lack of money to buy nutritious foods. The laid-back lifestyle of the population and the poor diet often leads to obesity, which is becoming more prevalent in the population. Programs emphasizing lifestyle changes, diet education, and exercise have been initiated with the help of community partners to assist with recreational activities. The overreaching goal of the center is to improve the overall quality of life for the community.

In 2008, a mobile unit was funded by the Pennsylvania Department of Health and established to provide county-wide health care and health promotion and prevention services. In collaboration with a large university and with smaller universities in the area, the mobile unit is staffed with NPs, volunteer registered nurses (RNs), nursing faculty, and students. The mobile unit visits senior centers, community centers, and schools throughout the county. Blood pressure, cholesterol, and height and weight screenings are provided. County residents who do not have a healthcare provider are offered appointments and follow-up care services. Recently, funding was received from the Pennsylvania Department of Health to retrofit the mobile unit to provide dental services.

BARRIERS TO CONTINUING CARE

Access to healthcare services is becoming an increasingly complex problem that functions as a barrier to good health in the current tough economic times. In poor rural areas, money for food typically takes precedence over gasoline to drive to the primary care center for care. Severe weather conditions such as extreme heat, rain, or cold also influence access to care, as many patients need to walk to the center.

Other access issues affect care at the provider level. Barriers to full-scope practice for NPs persist in the state. Although most local hospitals now accept the NPs' orders for diagnostic testing, some do not. Differences in implementation of prescriptive authority also complicate the NPs' ability to work smoothly in an integrated healthcare environment.

Problems with billing and reimbursement occur frequently. Although the primary care center accepts insurance from many sources and is listed on provider panels for multiple insurers, the majority of the patients are covered by Medicaid (31%), Medicare (17%), or other third-party payers (22%) or are self-pay clients (30%). Due to the FQHC-LA status of the center, 48% of the visits are paid at a base level. Finally, funding to run the center often depends on payment from insurers that are notorious for not providing reimbursement in a timely manner.

OPPORTUNITIES

Continued community support, growth in the number of patients, and continued stakeholder support provide opportunities for further growth of the primary care center. The need to provide services to the Appalachian population continues to increase. In addition, healthcare reform legislation has called for more effective ways to deliver primary healthcare services. An opportunity exists to demonstrate how the nurse practitioner model of primary care can effectively reduce healthcare costs while providing high-quality and culturally sensitive primary care services.

CURRENT STATUS

With changes in the healthcare system, the nurse practitioner–run primary care center is in the process of becoming part of a larger health system in the county. This federally qualified community health center, which began operations in 1977, was also established by a group of citizens. Community volunteers helped to build and design this system, which now offers a full range of primary care, preventive care, and dental and mental health services.

This partnership is a logical step to sustain culturally competent care to this vulnerable population for several reasons. First, the evolution of this system and that of the primary care center are similar. Second, the types of populations served are similar for both systems. Third, both systems were begun as NP-managed practices and expanded to include services by other professionals.

SUMMARY

This chapter has described the implementation of a nurse-managed center to provide primary healthcare services to an area in rural Appalachia. Because they already lived in this region, the NPs who started the center began with a good grasp of the healthcare needs of the community. Nurse practitioners and other advanced practice nurses have the skills to provide high-quality, cost-effective, culturally sensitive care to this vulnerable population. The NPs have worked to empower their patients in this rural Appalachian community to improve their quality of life and limit the effects of chronic disease by providing health care, prevention, education, social services, and screening. The outcomes indicate that attention to the community priorities and the cultural needs of the patients can enable NPs to provide culturally competent primary health care to a vulnerable population.

For a full suite of assignments and additional learning activities, use the access code located in the front of your book to visit this exclusive website: http://go.jblearning.com/dechesnay. If you do not have an access code, you can obtain one at the site.

REFERENCES

Counts, M. (1992). *GENESIS III: General Ethnographic Nursing Evaluation Studies in the State, 1985–2002.* Unpublished manuscript, Department of Nursing, West Virginia University, Morgantown, WV.

Huttlinger, K. W., & Purnell, L. D. (2008). People of Appalachian heritage: In L. D. Purnell & B. J. Paulanka (Eds.), *Transcultural health care: A culturally competent approach* (3rd ed., pp. 95–112). Philadelphia, PA: F. A. Davis.

Russell, C., Gregory, D., Wotton, D., Mordoch, E., & Counts, M. (1996). ACTION: Application and extension of the GENESIS community analysis model. *Public Health Nursing, 13*(3), 187–194.

U.S. Census Bureau. (2010). Retrieved September 30, 2010, from http://factfinder.census.gov/servlet/ACSSAFFFacts?_event=ChangeGeoContext&geo_id=05000US42059&_geoContext=&_street=&_county=Greene+County&_cityTown=&_state=&_zip=&_lang=en&_sse=on&ActiveGeoDiv=&_useEV=&pctxt=fph&pgsl=010&_submenuId=factsheet_1&ds_name=ACS_2008_3YR_SAFF&_ci_nbr=null&qr_name=null&reg=null%3Anull&_keyword=&_industry=

Strategies for Working with Individuals with Fetal Alcohol Spectrum Disorder: Lessons Learned in Alaska

Marilyn Pierce-Bulger

Objectives

At the end of this chapter, the reader will be able to

1. Describe Fetal Alcohol Spectrum disorders.
2. Explain the dangers and disabilities that can result from Fetal Alcohol Spectrum disorders.
3. Explain the extent to which Alaska's program can be used in other states.

WWW

INTRODUCTION

Caring for vulnerable individuals characterizes the history of nursing. To be vulnerable has explicit and implicit meanings that encompass lack of protection from physical or emotional harm; being easily persuadable; inability to resist illness; debility or failure; and openness to attack. An individual who has had prenatal exposure to alcohol is at risk for all of these vulnerabilities. Most often, these individuals have a hidden disability that is not easily identified by outward physical signs. This chapter discusses fetal alcohol spectrum disorders (FASD), nursing strategies for working with someone suspected of having FASD, and suggestions for advocacy on behalf of these vulnerable individuals.

FETAL ALCOHOL SPECTRUM DISORDERS

Fetal alcohol syndrome (FAS) was first identified in a descriptive analysis done by Dr. Paul Lemoine in France in 1968. The breakthrough in understanding FAS occurred in 1973 at the University of Washington when Drs. Kenneth Lyons Jones and David Smith followed a group of children whose mothers had consumed high levels of alcohol during their pregnancies. These children exhibited a similar pattern of facial features (Jones & Smith, 1973). The cardinal facial features associated with this syndrome are phenotypical to FAS; that is, no other agent causes this *combination* of shortened palpebral fissure length (small eye openings), smooth philthrum (vertical groove under the nose to upper lip), and thin vermillion border of the upper lip. FAS has other associated features including epicanthal folds, low-set ears, flat midface, short nose, and a low nasal bridge. To meet the medical definition of FAS, an individual must have the aforementioned facial features, small stature (under the 10th percentile), and central nervous system disabilities (Astley, 2004; Bertrand et al., 2004).

These facial features develop during the third week of gestation, when many women are unaware or have just learned that they are pregnant. Public education efforts since the first U.S. Surgeon General's public (1981) health advisory have increased awareness about the potential harm to the fetus when the mother consumes alcohol during pregnancy. Most women, if they are not addicted to alcohol, stop alcohol use when they learn they are pregnant. Despite increasingly numerous safe and highly effective options for contraception today, nearly half (49%) of American women still have a mistimed or unintended pregnancy. Many of these women are consuming alcohol at the time of conception (Centers for Disease Control and Prevention [CDC], 2010).

Any reproductive-age woman who is drinking alcohol and having intercourse without effective contraception may unintentionally harm her fetus. The latest U.S. Surgeon General's public health advisory states that a pregnant woman should not drink any amount of alcohol during pregnancy. If she has already consumed alcohol during her pregnancy, she should stop to minimize further risk. Any woman who is contemplating pregnancy should abstain from alcohol (Office of the Surgeon General, 2005).

Because the window for the development of the facial features is so small, many children who have had prenatal alcohol exposure do not demonstrate physical signs of their disability. These individuals may experience a myriad of physical, mental, behavioral, and learning disabilities that are collectively referred to as fetal alcohol spectrum disorders. These diagnoses include static encephalopathy (SE) and alcohol-related neurobehavioral disorder (ARNBD.) An older term, fetal alcohol effect (FAE), is no longer used (Bertrand et al., 2004).

Alcohol use during pregnancy is the leading preventable cause of mental retardation and birth defects in the United States. The scope of this disability is challenging to identify, because women may not always disclose their alcohol use and healthcare providers may not screen them for alcohol use. The CDC reports FAS prevalence rates ranging from 0.2 to 1.5 cases per 1000 births across various population groups in the United States (CDC, 2002; May & Gossage, 2010). These rates are comparable to or greater than the rates for other common developmental disabilities such as Down syndrome and spina bifida. Disadvantaged groups such as American Indians/Alaska Natives and other minorities have documented prevalence rates as high as 3 to 5 cases per 1000 births (May & Gossage, 2010). Research at the University of Washington (UW) identified a prevalence rate of 10 to 15 cases per 1000 children in the foster care system in the state of Washington (Astley, Stachowiak, Clarren, & Clausen, 2002).

IMPACT OF ALCOHOL

Contrary to popular belief, fetal alcohol exposure is worse than fetal exposure to many illicit substances and medications. Because of alcohol's ubiquitous nature in U.S. culture and its status as a legal substance, the public is often unclear about the potential severity of its impact on the developing fetus. More than half of all women of childbearing age (ages 18–44) report some alcohol use, and one in eight reports drinking while pregnant (CDC, 2010). Moreover, both binge-pattern drinking and the reported amounts of alcohol consumed are on the rise. These trends are concerning because binge doses of alcohol are found to have greater detrimental impact on the fetus than lower levels at the same point in time. In addition, initial alcohol use is occurring at younger ages and is a key predictor of adult alcohol abuse and dependency (National Institute on Alcohol Abuse and Alcoholism [NIAAA], 2000). There are no known safe amounts or types of alcohol that may be consumed during pregnancy.

Alcohol, as a teratogen causing developmental malformations, has a direct toxic effect on fetal cells. It exerts its impact on the nervous system in many ways, including interfering with normal proliferation of nerve cells; increasing the formation of free radicals; altering the cell's ability to produce or regulate growth, division, and survival impairing cell migration; and interfering with normal adhesion of cells. It also alters formation of axons, cell membranes, biochemical pathways and electrical signals, cellular calcium regulation, and the expression of certain genes (NIAAA, 2000).

Alcohol exposure during the first trimester of pregnancy can result in fetal malformations, such as the cardinal facial features associated with FAS. Individuals with FAS may also experience other central developmental defects, such as visual, auditory, palate, dental, or sinus abnormalities. Orthopedic, cardiac, and other anomalies have also been reported. For further information on key embryological developmental impacts associated with weeks of gestation, visit the National Organization on Fetal Alcohol Syndrome website: http://www.nofas.org/healthcare/QIP%20Materials/Patient%20Education%20Materials/Fetal%20Development%20Chart%20Outline.pdf.

Although the fetal brain can be affected by maternal alcohol consumption during the entire nine months of pregnancy, some parts of the fetal brain appear to be especially sensitive to the detrimental effects of alcohol. The corpus callosum passes information between the right and left hemispheres; in some cases, it has been shown to be reduced in size or absent in individuals with FASD. This defect may result in attention problems and difficulties with reading, verbal memory, and executive and psychosocial functioning (U.S. Department of Health and Human Services [USHHS], 2010a).

The basal ganglia are involved with the ability to detect the progress of movement, spatial memory, and the ability to perceive time. The caudate plays a role in inhibiting inappropriate behaviors. Extensive connections from this area of the brain to the frontal lobes may be altered in FAS, interfering with the ability to plan, sequence, and shift from one task to the next. The hippocampus, a part of the limbic system, is involved with emotional aspects of survival and plays a role in memory. The cerebellum appears to be most impacted by maternal alcohol consumption during the third trimester. Functional and magnetic resonance imaging (MRI) data support the findings of altered cellular functioning and evidence of cerebellar hypoplasia in children affected by FAS (Astley et al., 2006).

The end result of these central nervous system impacts is that individuals with FASD may be missing or have disordered cellular connections in their brains, resulting in dysfunctional or absent neural pathway communication and prolonged processing speed. For example, individuals with FASD may be able to "talk the talk," because they may be good mimics, but that may not be able to "walk the walk"—that is, carry through with what they just promised to do. They may have organic brain damage from prenatal alcohol exposure. Stopping alcohol use during any stage of the pregnancy is helpful in improving fetal outcome.

FASD MYTHS

Many myths about fetal alcohol syndrome exist. For instance, one myth is that the child will outgrow this disability. In reality, an affected individual does not outgrow this disability, nor is it a genetic condition. While genetics does play a role in alcohol processing, individuals experience FASD because of prenatal exposure and alcoholism patterns across multiple generations in a family.

Another myth is that FAS is a "more severe" form of FASD. Actually, FAS accounts for only 10% of those affected by prenatal alcohol exposure. Indeed, the outward physical signs of FAS, such as the characteristic facial features, may allow for identification so that affected individuals receive help. The remaining 90% of individuals experience a hidden disability. They often do not get services or the accommodations needed, and their adverse behaviors due to FASD may be interpreted as willful. Behavioral problems may be attributed to poor parenting. Some individuals with FASD have an intelligence quotient (IQ) in the mental retardation range, but many do not.

FASD is not specific to certain ethnic or racial groups. The Alaska Native community is an example of a community that is stereotyped in this regard. Some groups, such as Alaska Natives, have greater awareness of the problem and have acknowledged the problematic nature of alcohol abuse in their communities. This issue is discussed in more depth in the Alaska-specific section of this chapter.

PRIMARY DISABILITIES

A primary disability is an effect or direct result of the prenatal alcohol exposure. Primary disabilities associated with FASD include expressive and receptive language problems, poor memory and judgment, challenges with abstract reasoning and predicting outcomes, over- or under-sensitivity to environmental stimuli, dysmaturity (socially younger age than the individual's chronological age), slow response time, poor time management skills, and problems with cognition and learning. Nurses may see these effects manifested differently depending on the age of the client.

Early Childhood

Infants and toddlers with prenatal alcohol exposure may present as small for gestational age with a small head circumference. They may experience seizure disorders, exhibit feeding problems, or have delays in motor and speech development. Infant learning and early intervention programs are excellent services for these at-risk children. During early childhood, affected individuals may also experience sensory integration issues that result in hyperactivity, attention deficits, anger outbursts, and expulsion from preschool programs. Evaluation by occupational and physical therapists may help discern an individual child's sensory challenges and lead to recommendations for environmental changes helpful for both the child and caregivers (Coles, Smith, Fernhoff, & Falek, 1985; Mitchell, 2002; O'Connor, Shah, Whaley, Croni, Gunderson, & Graham, 2002; USHHS, 2010b).

Early School Age

By the time they reach school age, children with prenatal alcohol exposure may present with increasingly challenging behaviors in the classroom setting, have difficulties making friends, or begin to have difficulties with math or reading. Their organic brain damage interferes with the ability to meet the increasingly complex daily expectations of children in this age group. Affected children may behave impulsively, as they cannot inhibit inappropriate behaviors. Their inability to read social cues may make them the class outcast. Their inability to modulate incoming sensory messages may prove overwhelming for them, such that they demonstrate anger and emotional outbursts. Their attention-deficit behavior may be noted by pediatric primary care providers, parents, or teachers. All of these characteristics render the child more vulnerable to early manifestations of mood disorders (Bertrand et al., 2004; Kable & Coles, 2004).

Middle School Age

The onset of puberty adds a new complexity to the mix, because reproductive hormones share the same pathways in the brain as the neurotransmitters that modulate behavior and mood. Adolescents with FASD may begin to act out sexually because they are impulsive and cannot easily inhibit their sexual urges. Moreover, their social dysmaturity may result in acting out sexually with younger-age children.

The complex demands of a middle school setting require students to interact with multiple teachers in several classrooms and to demonstrate organizational skills related to homework and time keeping. Adolescents with FASD are often unable to meet these demands, and their lives may become increasingly miserable. If they cannot read important social cues and interpret language correctly due to expressive or receptive language problems, they are likely to be ostracized at a critical developmental period. They may continue to experience failures on many functional fronts and become increasingly vulnerable to others who may prey on them. A desire to "fit in" has led many individuals with FASD to follow through with detrimental behaviors in an attempt to please their peers, leading to trouble with the law or in school.

If they have not been identified for supportive services by now, adolescents with FASD may be experiencing increasing mental health problems, such as depression or experimentation with alcohol or drugs. They may also have numerous diagnoses (e.g., attention-deficit/hyperactive disorder, oppositional defiant disorder, or conduct disorder) that reflect the symptoms *but not the etiology* of their underlying brain damage. They may be at higher risk for suicide because of their inability to understand cause and effect, impulsivity, poor acceptance within their peer community, and patterns of recurrent failure in school and social settings (O'Malley & Huggins, 2005).

Missing the underlying diagnosis can lead to delayed or inadequate treatment and medication, a rising sense of failure, and a sense of hopelessness. Conversely, correctly identifying the underlying organic brain damage can lead to appropriate treatment and accommodations for these children. If their family, school, healthcare providers, and community understand the root cause of their problems—that is, prenatal exposure to alcohol—there is a much better chance that they will receive services.

Young Adults and Adults

An individual with FASD comes into adulthood with organic brain damage. These persons are very likely over-represented in the prison population because they cannot link cause and effect, are vulnerable to suggestion by predatory adults and peers, are more vulnerable to the effects of alcohol and substances, and have social dysmaturity that may link them romantically with under-age partners (Streissguth, Barr, Kogan, & Bookstein, 1996; Streissguth, Bookstein, Barr, Sampson, O'Malley, & Young, 2004). They are challenged by the organizational requirements of an increasingly complex educational system and likely cannot complete school without significant assistance.

Their brain damage makes parenting and caregiving a significant challenge, although they are often loving, caring parents when they have children. Older persons with FASD may experience recurring job failures due to a poor match with job requirements and their lack of executive functioning skills. They may be denied family support services because they cannot complete paperwork, case plans, or required training, or keep appointments without support. Children and adults with FASD can lead successful, meaningful lives, but they require significant accommodations and may need lifelong supportive services.

SECONDARY DISABILITIES

Secondary disabilities are those that occur because the primary disability has not been recognized or addressed effectively. Those persons with FASD who are not identified at an early age are more likely to develop secondary disabilities, such as trouble with the law and incarceration, mental health issues, alcohol or drug problems, disrupted school experiences, or inappropriate sexual behaviors. Correct diagnosis by age 6, a stable living situation, not being a victim of violence, and documented eligibility for developmental disability services have all been shown to be protective against secondary disabilities (Streissguth et al., 1996; Streissguth et al., 2004).

THE EXPERIENCE IN ALASKA

The state of Alaska began to work with FASD in the 1980s when the Indian Health Service (IHS) created a network of FAS coordinators/educators at its service unit hospitals. These

Box 31-1 Case Study: Dena a Coy: Substance and Mental Health Services

- Dena a Coy provides substance and mental health treatment services for affected women in a setting with their young children. The women receive services during the pregnancy and for several weeks postpartum. Discharge planning is a continuous process, so that mothers are assisted to obtain the community supports they need to maintain a clean and sober lifestyle following their treatment.
- An adjunct program to the services of Dena a Coy is the Alaska Women's Recovery Project. This project provides ongoing peer-driven and peer-led community-based activities (see http://www.southcentralfoundation.com/services/denaAcoy.ak and http://www.southcentralfoundation.com/services/AWRP.ak).

healthcare providers interviewed women when they presented for prenatal care, assessed their alcohol and substance use, and offered education and assistance with entry into treatment if indicated. During the 1990s, when the Alaska Native Tribal Health Consortium and tribal entities assumed control of their healthcare systems, some of these IHS programs continued. The Alaska Native sobriety movement and a residential treatment facility for pregnant women (such as the Southcentral Foundation's Dena a Coy; see **Box 31-1**) are examples of programs that continue to provide assessment, support, intervention, and treatment options for women who experience alcohol and substance use issues.

In 2000, the state of Alaska received a $29 million, five-year grant from the Substance Abuse and Mental Health Services Administration (SAMHSA) to fund the following programs:

- Public and professional knowledge, attitude, and beliefs surveys about FAS
- Public and professional awareness and education campaigns
- A network of FASD diagnostic teams around the state
- FAS tracking and reporting in the Alaska Birth Defects Registry (ABDR)
- Integrated FASD training and education into health, education, criminal justice, social service, and other support systems

The FASD diagnostic teams funded by the state of Alaska use the *Diagnostic Guide for Fetal Alcohol Spectrum Disorders: The 4 Digit Diagnostic Code*, third edition, 2004 (Astley, 2004), as a guide for the multidisciplinary healthcare team making the diagnosis. The process of diagnosis involves evaluation of the individual's facial features, growth, and central nervous system function, and an assessment of the alcohol exposure. The multidisciplinary teams typically include a physician or nurse practitioner, psychologist, occupational and/or physical therapist, and speech language pathologist. In Alaska, parent navigators are also key team members and have the expertise that comes from having a child with FAS, FASD, or another disability. Their voices of experience provide valuable support and advocacy for the family and/or individual going through the diagnostic process and attempting to follow recommendations. In the absence of an alcohol history (such as in a case of a foreign-born adopted child), an FAS diagnosis can still be made if a child has the full facial features associated with this syndrome. Many of the Alaska teams use the University of Washington's FAS Facial Photographic Screening Tool, which analyzes digital photos of the child's face to determine whether a diagnosis is warranted. This FAS screening tool, which is used in the foster care population in Washington, is highly sensitive (Astley et al., 2002).

Sustainable funding streams throughout Alaska (except for the northwestern region) ensure access to FASD diagnostic services. The ABDR reporting system continues to feature FASD issues and collaborates with other epidemiologic partners such as the Pregnancy Risk Assessment Monitoring (PRAMS) data system to ascertain trends in the behaviors of pregnant and postpartum women. Community readiness for FASD prevention and intervention efforts can be quite variable, and valuable lessons about creating diagnostic teams and managing system-related have been learned over the 10 years of the program's existence. To be sustainable, program efforts require active community leader engagement, creativity in securing team members, and efficient coordination of the multidisciplinary teams. Some diagnostic teams, for example, are tracking clients after diagnosis to determine whether clients are able to secure needed accommodations and services. Vocal parent and community advocacy groups have played a key role in making needed changes. As an example, Alaska state Medicaid regulations prohibited psychologists who were not affiliated with a mental health center from providing evaluation services, which created a significant barrier to diagnosis for those patients in rural settings. Recognizing the detrimental effect of this regulation, the state eventually removed that barrier. Other service innovations include the creation of a respite program for families who have a child with FASD (Family Camps) and a Medicaid waiver program that provides comprehensive services for youth with a serious emotional disturbance (SED) who are suspected or diagnosed with an FASD.

Box 31-2 Case Study: Southcentral Foundation Nutaqsiivik Home Visitation Service

The Southcentral Foundation's Nutaqsiivik home visitation service (http://www.southcentralfoundation.com/services/nutaqsiivik.ak) was originally intended to assist socially high-risk Alaska Native and American Indian women who gave birth in Anchorage. In the 1990s, monitoring data indicated that a significant percentage (28%) of these women had FASD (Pierce-Bulger & Nighswander, 2001). The original aim was to reduce post-neonatal infant mortality; the program demonstrated a 50% mortality reduction in this regard. The clear efficacy of the program led to continued institutional support for it.

The Nutaqsiivik program provides public health nursing services, care coordination, and family intervention. Women and their infants benefit from prenatal, lactation, infant health, immunization, and contraceptive services as well as community referrals and support as needed. The program is now available for all women, not just those at highest risk. It was recently awarded additional home visitation funds earmarked for tribal groups as part of national healthcare reform legislation (USHHS, 2010c).

Recent ABDR data collected on Alaskan children born between 1996 and 2002 have demonstrated an overall 32% reduction in the prevalence of FAS in Alaska. Of note, the FAS rate among Alaska Natives decreased by 49%, while the rate for non-Natives *increased* by 64% (State of Alaska, 2010). The greater awareness and historical focus on the topic of FAS in the Native Alaska community is likely in part to be responsible for the reduction. There has been no specific FASD prevention focus among the non-Native community, so providers and community members are less likely to consider it a problem in this group. Healthcare providers, for example, may (erroneously) make the assumption that non-Native women do not drink when pregnant.

While much more work remains to be done, there is also much to applaud. An example of a sustainable program is the Nutaqsiivik program (**Box 31-2**).

Alaska is truly committed to the ongoing prevention of FAS and the creation of systems of care that are responsive to those with an FASD.

CARING FOR INDIVIDUALS WHO MAY HAVE FASD

Nurses need to be aware that unusual behavior may indicate the presence of FASD and that behavior change applications are not effective because these behaviors are the result of organic brain damage. Instead, interventions must focus on changing the environment. Given that alcohol exposure is variable in dose and timing, individuals with prenatal alcohol exposure are likely to demonstrate different manifestations of organic dysfunction, and interventions must be tailored to their unique circumstances. Nevertheless, some general strategies may be helpful for working with affected individuals.

It is important to be nonjudgmental with clients, as their aberrant behaviors are likely to be unintentional. The client who always misses her appointments or does not follow through on recommendations, for example, may have FASD. Developmental age may be markedly different from the chronological age. Helping family and community members who interact with the client to understand this fact may help them to be more empathetic. In addition, because the person with FASD may be overly sensitive to criticism, it is important to be careful with body language and verbal feedback that may be perceived as negative.

Repetition of directions, instructions, and concepts is very important. Making a new memory is challenging for a person with FASD. The repetition helps to get the information stored in the hippocampus—that is, the "habit area of the brain." Multimode cues, such as visual lists, simple action pictures, and graphics, can help with this type of memory storage. Return demonstration is essential to reinforce information, although affected persons may repeat information back yet not fully understand it. Assess for understanding and follow through as needed. Saying "Do you understand?" is not enough. The person may willingly agree but have no comprehension. Have the client repeat, model, and tell you what he or she knows.

Routines can help the person with FASD to expect consistency and to function more effectively. When a routine must be interrupted, advance multimode warnings repeated many times may help with required transitions.

One strategy is to act out or role-model behaviors to help clients with FASD in interaction with others and in controlling impulsive behaviors. In particular, clients need to learn how to control voice tone and volume, recognize personal space, and understand limits for alcohol and substances.

Individuals with FASD are prone to sensory overload, which may be manifested as frustration, anger, or emotional outbursts. Finding a safe, quiet, less stimulating environment of their choice will help them to calm down. In a busy clinic or emergency room (ER) setting, this practice may mean taking clients to a more gently lighted or quieter office space to interact. Remove distractions and clutter, and create clear boundaries. Think about odors, lights, colors, touch, textures, and sound—clients may react to any or all of these stimuli.

Learning new skills and retaining the information are achieved in small steps. Teach clients with FASD slowly, repeating the information often. If they are sent home with complicated discharge instructions, arrange for them to have a home-visiting nurse or rapid follow-up for reassessment. They may need to move around physically while learning. Give them extra time to complete a task, and remember that processing speed is likely to be slower than normal.

Time concepts are challenging for persons with FASD. External cues such as smart phone and watch alarms for appointments, calendars, and phone call reminders for appointments are helpful tools in time management. Money concepts are abstract and, therefore, challenging to individuals with FASD, so automatic bill pay accounts can help them manage their financial affairs; some may need a financial custodian, however. A trusted friend or family member may need to come with them to appointments to assist with interpreting and remembering information. Identifying strengths and ways to compensate for these challenges is an important contribution of the nurse working with a FASD-affected person.

ADVOCACY AND ACTIONS

A woman with a severe alcohol problem may not seek care or request help. Some signs of severe alcohol abuse include poor nutritional status, anemia, and inadequate weight gain during pregnancy. It is critical that the nurse takes every opportunity to screen reproductive-age women for at-risk alcohol consumption and effective contraception (Savage, 2008). Assessment of last menstrual period and inquiry about contraceptive use should be included at every encounter for reproductive-age women, whether they are presenting for a women's health-related issue or not. An inquiry about last alcohol use and the amount consumed offers a glimpse into the drinking pattern and provides an opportunity for brief intervention (Floyd, Ebrahim, Tsai, O'Connor, & Sokol, 2006; Ingersoll, Floyd, Sobell, & Velasquez, 2003). Research has shown that screening and brief intervention can be effective in reducing the risk of alcohol-exposed pregnancies. Several screening tools have been shown to be very effective with pregnant and reproductive-age women, including the CAGE, TWEAK, and T-ACE instruments (Chang, 2010; "Drinking and Reproductive Health," 2010).

Prenatal healthcare providers do not always give clear and factual information about alcohol use and its possible effects on the fetus during pregnancy. They may not want the woman to worry and they may perceive that they cannot control what has already occurred. One way to deliver a clear message about alcohol impact is to show the woman fetal developmental dates on a gestational wheel. Conception occurs at roughly 10 to 17 days after the onset of her last menstrual period. Implantation occurs about a week later. Any alcohol she consumed after this week has reached her fetus. If she has a binge pattern of drinking, the risk to the fetus is even higher. Although there is no way to detect FASD in utero, the pregnant woman can be encouraged to make healthy choices, learn about early signs of FASD, and seek assistance if she is concerned about the child's development.

Maternal alcohol history often does not get transferred to the baby's medical record at the time of birth. The birth mother may not be involved with the diagnostic process, and her records cannot be accessed without her consent. These factors increase the complexity for FASD diagnostic teams trying to establish the maternal alcohol history for a child. The nurse can help to ensure correct diagnosis for the baby by documenting the timing and amount of reported maternal alcohol consumption.

CONCLUSION

There is no safe amount of alcohol use in pregnancy. Maternal alcohol consumption can cause damage to the fetus at all stages of pregnancy, and stopping at any time is helpful to the fetus's development. FASD is a phenomenon that occurs in all races and communities. While some communities are addressing this problem, most in the United States are not. Indeed, the people with the greatest difficulties may be the ones least recognized.

The nurse can be an interpreter for persons with FASD, as such individuals speak a different cognitive language and experience social cues differently than those unaffected by FASD. Their behaviors may be challenging—but there is a reason behind the behaviors. Partnering with these highly vulnerable persons can increase their abilities to negotiate a difficult and often incomprehensible world.

For a full suite of assignments and additional learning activities, use the access code located in the front of your book to visit this exclusive website: http://go.jblearning.com/dechesnay. If you do not have an access code, you can obtain one at the site.

REFERENCES

Astley, S. (2004). *Diagnostic guide for fetal alcohol spectrum disorders: The 4-digit diagnostic code* (3rd ed.). Seattle, WA: University of Washington.

Astley, S., Aylward, E., Brooks, A., Carmichael-Olson, H., Coggins, T., & Davies, S. (2006). Association between brain structure, chemistry, and function as assessed by MRI, MRS, FMRI and neuropsychological testing among children with fetal alcohol spectrum disorders (FASD). *Alcoholism: Clinical & Experimental Research, 30*(6), 229A.

Astley, S., Stachowiak, J., Clarren, S., & Clausen, C., (2002). Application of the fetal alcohol syndrome facial photographic screening tool in a foster care population. *Journal of Pediatrics, 141*, 712–717.

Bertrand, J., Floyd, R., Weber, M., O'Connor, M., Riley, E., & Johnson, K. (2004). *Fetal alcohol syndrome: Guidelines for referral and diagnosis.* Atlanta, GA: Centers for Disease Control and Prevention.

Centers for Disease Control and Prevention (CDC). (2002). Fetal alcohol syndrome—Alaska, Arizona, Colorado, and New York, 1995–1997. *Morbidity and Mortality Weekly Report, 51*(20), 433–435. Retrieved October 9, 2010, from http://www.cdc.gov/mmwr/preview/mmwrhtml/mm5120a2.htm

Centers for Disease Control and Prevention (CDC). (2010). Centers for Disease Control features drinking while pregnant still a problem. Retrieved October 9, 2010, from http://www.cdc.gov/Features/dsAlcoholChildbearingAgeWomen/

Chang, G. (2010). Alcohol-screening instruments for pregnant women. *NIAAA Publications*, Retrieved October 10, 2010, from http://pubs.niaaa.nih.gov/publications/arh25-3/204-209.htm

Coles, C., Smith, I., Fernhoff, P., & Falek, A. (1985). Neonatal neurobehavioral characteristics as correlates of maternal alcohol use during gestation. *Alcoholism: Clinical & Experimental Research, 9*(5), 454–460.

Drinking and reproductive health: A fetal alcohol spectrum disorders tool kit. (2010). American College of Obstetrics and Gynecology and Centers for Disease Control and Prevention. Retrieved October 10, 2010, from http://www.acog.org/departments/HealthIssues/FASDToolKit.pdf

Floyd, R., Ebrahim, S., Tsai, J., O'Connor, M., & Sokol, R. (2006). Strategies to reduce alcohol-exposed pregnancies. *Maternal Child Health Journal, 10*, S149–S151.

Ingersoll, K., Floyd, R., Sobell, M., & Velasquez, M. (2003). Project CHOICES Intervention Research Group: Reducing the risk of alcohol-exposed pregnancies—a study of motivational intervention in community settings. *Pediatrics, 111*, 1131–1135.

Jones, K., & Smith, D. (1973). Recognition of the fetal alcohol syndrome in early infancy. *Lancet, 2*, 999–1001.

Kable, J., & Coles, D. (2004). Teratology of alcohol: Implications for school settings. In R. T. Brown (Ed.), *Handbook of pediatric psychology in school settings* (pp. 379–404). Mahwah, NJ: Lawrence Erlbaum Associates.

May, P., & Gossage, J. (2010). Estimating the prevalence of fetal alcohol syndrome: A summary. Retrieved October 9, 2010, from http://pubs.niaaa.nih.gov/publications/arh25-3/159-167.htm

Mitchell, K. (2002). *Fetal alcohol syndrome: Practical suggestions and support for families and caregivers.* Washington, DC: National Organization on Fetal Alcohol Syndrome.

National Institute on Alcohol Abuse and Alcoholism (NIAAA). (2000). *10th special report to the U.S. Congress on alcohol and health.* NIH Pub No. 00-1583. Washington, DC: U.S. Department of Health and Human Services.

O'Connor, M., Shah, B., Whaley, S., Croni, P., Gunderson, B., & Graham, J. (2002). Psychiatric illness in a clinical sample of children with prenatal alcohol exposure. *American Journal of Drug & Alcohol Abuse, 28*(4), 743–754.

Office of the Surgeon General. (2005). *Advisory on alcohol use in pregnancy.* Washington, DC: U.S. Department of Health and Human Services.

O'Malley, K., & Huggins, J. (2005). Suicidality in adolescents and adults with fetal alcohol spectrum disorders. *Canadian Journal of Psychiatry—Revue Canadienne de Psychiatrie, 50*(2),125.

Pierce-Bulger, M., & Nighswander, T. (2001). Nutaqsiivik: An approach to reducing infant mortality using quality improvement principles. *Quality Management in Health Care, 9*(3), 40–46.

Savage, C. (2008). How to screen patients for alcohol use disorders. *American Nurse Today, 3*(12). Retrieved October 10, 2010, from http://www.americannursetoday.com/article.aspx?id=4124&fid=4104#

State of Alaska. (2010, February 17). Decline in the birth prevalence of fetal alcohol syndrome in Alaska. *Epidemiology Bulletin No. 3.* Retrieved October 9, 2010, from http://www.epi.alaska.gov/bulletins/docs/b2010_03.pdf

Streissguth, A., Barr, H., Kogan, J., & Bookstein, F. (1996). *Understanding the occurrence of secondary disabilities in clients with fetal alcohol syndrome (FAS) and fetal alcohol effects (FAE): Final Report to the Centers for Disease Control and Prevention (CDC).* Report No. 96-06. Seattle, WA: University of Washington, Fetal Alcohol & Drug Unit. Technical.

Streissguth, A., Bookstein, F., Barr, H., Sampson, P., O'Malley, K., & Young, J. (2004). Risk factors for adverse life outcomes in fetal alcohol syndrome and fetal alcohol effects. *Journal of Developmental & Behavioral Pediatrics, 25*(4), 228–238.

U.S. Department of Health and Human Services (USHHS), Centers for Disease Control and Prevention (CDC), National Center on Birth Defects and Developmental Disabilities, FASD Regional Training Centers, and National Organization on Fetal Alcohol Syndrome (NOFAS). (2010a). Fetal alcohol spectrum disorders competency-based curriculum development guide for medical and allied health education and practice—Competency IV: Biological effects of alcohol on fetus. Retrieved October 9, 2010, from http://www.cdc.gov/ncbddd/fasd/curriculum/FASDguide_web.pdf

U.S. Department of Health and Human Services (USHHS), Centers for Disease Control and Prevention (CDC), National Center on Birth Defects and Developmental Disabilities, FASD Regional Training Centers, and National Organization on Fetal Alcohol Syndrome (NOFAS). (2010b). Fetal alcohol spectrum disorders competency-based curriculum development guide for medical and allied health education and practice—Competency VI: Treatment across the life span for persons with fetal alcohol spectrum disorders. Retrieved October 9, 2010, from http://www.cdc.gov/ncbddd/fasd/curriculum/FASDguide_web.pdf

U.S. Department of Health and Human Services (USHHS). (2010c). News release: Pregnancy assistance fund and tribal home visiting grants to states. Retrieved October 10, 2010, from http://www.hhs.gov/news/press/2010pres/09f/state_charts2.html

U.S. Surgeon General. (1981). Surgeon General's advisory on alcohol and pregnancy. *FDA Drug Bulletin, 11*, 9–10.

UNIT VI

Teaching–Learning

Teaching should be full of ideas instead of stuffed with facts.
—Source Unknown

CHAPTER 32

Teaching Nurses About Vulnerable Populations

Mary de Chesnay

Objectives

At the end of this chapter, the reader will be able to

1. Discuss ways in which students can be helped to understand their own ethnocentrism.
2. Discuss specific things about other cultures that students need to learn.
3. For each model described, identify sources of commonality that can be used in other settings.

The American Academy of Nursing (AAN) and the American Association of Colleges of Nursing (AACN) have devoted much attention to teaching students to be culturally competent. The AAN has an expert panel assigned to the topic (AAN, 2011; Giger, Davidhizer, Purnell, Harden, Phillips, & Strickland, 2007), and the AACN has mandated cultural competence as an outcome of baccalaureate education. The *BSN Essentials* document lists five competencies that baccalaureate students are expected to demonstrate by graduation. A toolkit for graduate students is available on the website, along with competencies for graduate students (AACN, 2010). Much attention in the literature is devoted to teaching people how to be culturally competent; in fact, a book on this issue won a well-deserved *American Journal of Nursing* "Book of the Year" award (Jeffreys, 2010). Moreover, a cottage industry of cultural trainers has sprung up and consultants are easily found who stand ready to teach courses on cultural sensitivity, competence, or awareness.

It would seem that cultural competence is a good thing to know and, therefore, must be taught. As with any bandwagon, however, it is essential to critically examine the nature of the concept and determine what it means to teach students to be culturally competent. Dreher and MacNaughton (2002) caution that we should pay attention to the fact that individuals and their cultures do not represent a settled, static relationship; in addition, culture evolves over time, making it difficult for clinicians to keep up. These authors assert that, in public health, which focuses on populations instead of individuals, it is useful to understand as many cultural factors as possible about the group, although such understanding might be difficult to achieve in acute care settings. They caution against the danger of attributing poor communication to "cultural differences" instead of to poor interpersonal skills on the part of the nurse. In short, their contention is that cultural competence is simply nursing competence.

Having said that, there still seems to be an important place in nursing education for teaching students to be competent communicators with people who are different from themselves. This chapter provides some ideas on this subject for faculty and students.

There are many ways to teach nursing students how to work with vulnerable people, and there are numerous activities students can undertake to gain practice in providing culturally competent care. This chapter presents some ideas for faculty with regard to the use of these strategies and seeks to inspire them to devise similar learning activities for their own students. For students who read this chapter, it is hoped that they find some of the experiences presented here inspirational with regard to their own fieldwork.

For any activity designed to prepare nurses to provide culturally competent care, it is critical to emphasize two key points: know yourself and show respect for others. First, the best way that nurses can prepare for working with vulnerable people is to know themselves. The more a person knows and acknowledges his or her own biases, the more easily the nurse can put these prejudices aside and concentrate on the patient as a person instead of a stereotype. *Ethnocentric bias* is a term derived from anthropology that refers to the notion that one's own cultural beliefs, practices, folkways, values, and norms are the right ones. Ethnocentric biases develop from our experience of living within our own cultures: growing up in families, attending educational institutions with certain emphases, and interacting with people we like or do not like. Ethnocentrism is neither good nor bad—it just is. To acknowledge that we all have biases simply indicates that we are human. People tend to get in trouble, however, when they act toward others as if their own way is the only right way or when they confuse bias with truth.

How do we learn to deal with ethnocentric bias? It is essential to recognize a particular feeling or attitude as bias and then to critically examine all of our own values and beliefs, particularly in terms of how we see others who are different from ourselves. This principle of self-examination relates to everyone, not just to members of majority groups. It might be helpful to apply the general system theory concept of multi-finality, which holds that there are many ways to reach the same end. Appreciating that other ways of achieving the goal might be equally effective and valid is a key component of self-awareness.

The second way that nurses can prepare for working with vulnerable people is to learn to show respect. Novices tend to expend large amounts of time and energy trying to learn cultural material quickly so that they can interact "appropriately" in terms of superficial gestures, such as making eye contact or not, shaking hands or not, or touching arms. Yet, despite the best of intentions, these actions can sometimes be interpreted as mocking the group. Being yourself, yet doing your best in terms of showing the most respect according to your own cultural standards, is more likely to be understood by the patient as respectful than is adopting gestures or expressions that are obviously not your own. In this regard, cultural competence is a misleading concept because it implies that one is competent to practice another group's cultural behaviors. A more useful view of cultural competence is that it entails being comfortable while interacting with diverse people who behave in ways and hold values that are different from one's own without judging the other group by one's own standards.

Another key point in providing culturally competent care is to reframe compliance or adherence in light of the patient's or group's cultural norms, values, and folkways. For example, students might not understand food taboos and offer pork to a Muslim or Jewish patient, then wrongly interpret the patient's rejection of pork as loss of appetite. Many Arabs and Jews do not observe the dietary laws—but many do, so it is important to ask about this issue.

The patient and family are always the best teachers of their culture. The salient point for the culturally competent provider is to ask and not to assume. Think of your patients and their families as your best teachers about their culture.

WHY TEACH NURSING STUDENTS ABOUT VULNERABLE POPULATIONS?

Global demographics are changing as populations evolve into ever more complex societies. Demographics of individual countries are also changing rapidly as people move within their countries or from one country to another to find food, jobs, or simply better lives for their families. As the costs of living and health care spiral higher, the most vulnerable members of the population become even more entrenched in the daily ordeal of living. The nursing profession cannot afford for its practitioners to be isolationistic in the way they treat patients and families, nor can it afford to ignore communities. Community-based care and focus on populations are aspects of nursing that students need to learn to provide cost-effective, culturally competent care.

The kinds of experiences students have in their basic educational programs can improve their confidence. This chapter presents three models from different universities. Although two of these universities happen to be private, the strategies and activities are universal and can be adapted by anyone interested in helping students develop or improve cross-cultural interpersonal relations. Many schools have implemented similar programs on behalf of the vulnerable populations of their own or international communities. Websites for the schools are a good source of information.

WHAT SHOULD STUDENTS LEARN?

Nurses need experiences that teach them to be comfortable with people different from themselves, which in turn requires interaction with many kinds of people. It is not sufficient to simply review the literature and write papers on vulnerable populations. Although writing papers is useful, it can be an empty intellectual exercise if not combined with developing competence at talking with people. Fieldwork is an excellent way to develop interaction skills; immersion programs such as study-abroad programs in which students live with local families are even better.

Students need to develop an understanding of culture and become aware of their own ethnocentric biases. In doing so, they need a safe context for their own experimentation in which they will not be criticized by their faculty for attitudes they hold but rather coached to develop new ideas or views about the vulnerable. For example, it is not useful to berate students who believe that all homeless people should take menial jobs so they can get off the street. Instead, they should be guided to understand the complexities of homelessness and the reasons why even menial jobs are not an option for many people.

Even though the statistical information on vulnerable populations often becomes obsolete before it is printed because the health disparities tend to increase with population increases, students still need to know who the vulnerable are and recognize the health disparities associated with the vulnerable populations in their own communities. Students should be encouraged to review the literature critically for applicability to vulnerable populations and to formulate practices that better serve the vulnerable.

Finally, students should learn how to reverse vulnerability. Nursing means not only curing and preventing illness, but also strengthening the patient's resources so that the patient becomes less vulnerable. Once trendy, the term "empowerment" has fallen out of favor because it has a patriarchal connotation, yet the notion that people can be helped to attain autonomy is still useful in teaching students to care for the vulnerable. Perhaps a more appropriate intervention is helping the patient develop or increase resilience. Everyone has strengths, and focusing on strength rather than weakness is a good therapeutic technique. Several chapters in this book, for instance, emphasize the nature of resilience.

MODELS OF EXPERIENTIAL LEARNING

Duquesne Model

Duquesne University is a small liberal arts institution founded in 1878 and operated by the Spiritans, an order of priests with strong service ties to developing countries in Africa and South America. Through its school of nursing, Duquesne confers undergraduate and graduate degrees, including a PhD, and it offers a variety of certificate and continuing education programs. During the author's tenure as dean of the school from 1994 to 2002, the faculty created a variety of programs and experiences for students and faculty so as to operationalize the service mission of the university. Two major outreach programs (local and international) are particularly relevant to the education of nursing students in caring for people from vulnerable populations, and these programs involve students at all levels: baccalaureate, master's, and doctoral.

Nurse-Managed Wellness Centers

The first outreach program was initially funded by the school of nursing and later by a grant from the U.S. Department of Housing and Urban Development (HUD). The faculty member who coordinated the gerontological clinical nurse specialist track in the master of science in nursing (MSN) program created a model for outreach into the community by starting a wellness clinic in a high-rise apartment building designated for senior citizens (Taylor, Resick, D'Antonio, &

Carroll, 1997). Students and faculty conducted many health screening and health promotion activities. The model was evaluated as successful by residents, staff, faculty, and students, with the result that the clinic was replicated later in a federally funded project to expand services to African Americans in the poor neighborhoods near the university.

With the success of the prototype center, two additional centers were opened in the African American communities called the Hill District and East Liberty (Resick, Taylor, & Leonardo, 1999). Later, the Visiting Nurse Association in Butler County, Pennsylvania, adopted the model for a rural community north of the city. To prepare for the expansion of the clinic, the faculty used ethnographic methods to gain access to the community, to establish rapport with civic leaders and community residents, and to identify unmet needs that the school of nursing could fulfill (Resick, Taylor, Carroll, D'Antonio, & de Chesnay, 1997). The community members initially had reservations about the proposed clinic because they perceived previous experiences, when outsiders had come into the community for various research projects, as disrespectful to them. However, by using the principles of ethnographic research and the methods of participant observation and interviewing, the faculty found ways to involve the community in planning so that when the second clinic opened, the community members reported that they felt a sense of ownership.

As of this writing, the original clinic and the Hill District clinic are thriving and provide a continuous educational experience for students and a practice setting for the nurse practitioner faculty. Faculty and students conduct health assessments, medication evaluations, teaching presentations, exercise classes in the form of dance therapy, and other health promotion activities. One of the projects at the clinics involved creating a chart audit system for measuring outcomes. This experience provided graduate students with the opportunity to apply theory to the practice of nursing in a functioning practice setting and allowed them to test the validity and reliability of the audit tool in a real setting in a way that would be used by the staff (Resick, 1999).

When necessary, staff refer residents to their primary care providers and, in some cases, directly to the emergency room. Students who rotate through the clinics obtain a sophisticated understanding of the healthcare issues of the elderly in the two independent-living high rises, one of which has a predominantly white population and the other a predominantly African American population. Through the clinics, students learn firsthand about the issues of the elderly as a vulnerable population.

Other activities in the local communities were initiated at the request of the community leaders, who had identified problems. One highly successful program taught cardiopulmonary resuscitation (CPR) to residents of all ages. A research project was conducted by faculty to examine community knowledge about CPR, and the results were helpful in developing the CPR programs (Winter, 2001). Classes were conducted by certified faculty in the community centers, and people of all ages completed the course.

Center for International Nursing

The Center for International Nursing was created in 1992 (Carty & White, 1993; White & Smith, 1997) to provide an administrative structure within which students and faculty could conduct educational programs, service projects, and research abroad. Initially, the Center's focus was Nicaragua, but later the Center expanded to South America, Africa, and Europe to complete specific initiatives. From 1994 to 2002, more than 130 students at all levels completed international projects, and each year 6 to 10 undergraduate students completed part of their community health nursing clinical requirement in a barrio in Managua in conjunction with Duquesne faculty and faculty in Duquesne's sister school, Universidad Politecnica de Nicaragua (UPOLI) (L. Cunningham & S. Colvin, personal communication, August 2000). The students conducted community assessments, performed health assessments, intervened in referrals to the community health clinics, and conducted health fairs to teach the community residents a variety of health promotion techniques. In another project, one of the critical care faculty taught part of the trauma content to students in a hospital in Managua (C. Ross, personal communication, September 1999).

Due largely to the publicity about the activities of the Center, the nursing school was approached by the Pittsburgh Rotary Club, whose members wanted to begin an international health project. They built a clinic in partnership with the Rotary Clubs of Managua and Jinotega in a northern community of Nicaragua near the city of Jinotega. When the community residents were asked what they wanted to name their clinic, they indicated that they wanted it named for the late member of the Pittsburgh Pirates baseball team—La Clinica de Roberto Clemente. Clemente died in a plane crash while trying to deliver medical supplies after the Managua earthquake of 1972 and is still revered in Nicaragua. This clinic is used by nurse practitioner faculty as a clinical site for training graduate students, and the community was the site of an ethnographic study on men's health conducted as dissertation research by a doctoral student, as described in Chapter 34 of the first edition of this book (Ross, 2000).

A second international study was conducted as action research by a doctoral student who worked in Peru on the clean water project run by the Sisters of Mercy (Zolkoski, 2000). Other doctoral students have conducted independent studies in Nicaragua and served as teaching faculty for some of the programs offered to the local nurses and physicians.

Faculty made a commitment to the sister school (UPOLI), and many other projects were conducted with the poor of Nicaragua. The emphasis on the "train the trainer" approach meant that the faculty tried to work with the local nurses as much as possible; many projects were accomplished with the support of the sister school faculty. The study by Colvin, de Chesnay, Mercado, & Benavides (2005) described in Chapter 17 of the first edition of the book, "Child Health in a Barrio of Managua," was an outcome of the work conducted under the auspices of the *hermanamiento* (sister school relationship). Many other projects and programs have been conducted as well—too many to mention all of them here.

Online Doctoral Program

Concurrent with the increasing international visibility of the Duquesne University School of Nursing, the faculty became aware of the desire of nurses in developing countries to improve nursing education for their people. Dr. John Murray, the university president, challenged the deans to experiment with distance learning strategies, and the faculty chose to meet his challenge by creating opportunities for nurses in developing countries to earn Duquesne's PhD in nursing through synchronous Web-based courses, coupled with residency on campus during the summers. The first course was taught by Dr. Jeri Milstead in the summer of 1997 (Milstead, 1998). Although some international nurses applied to the program, Duquesne's faculty were surprised at the popularity of the program among nurses who lived within driving distance of the university. Many lived in medically underserved areas where they needed to continue working because there was no one to replace them or because they still had children at home, but they were highly motivated, and the program became extremely competitive.

Seattle University Model

The Seattle University College of Nursing has a long tradition of furthering the mission of the university to promote social justice by serving the poor. In response to changes in health care during the 1980s, faculty revised the master's degree program to teach advanced practice nurses to work with vulnerable populations (Vezeau, Peterson, Nakao, & Ersek, 1998). Originally developed as a clinical specialist program, the faculty recognized the need for a corresponding program for nurse practitioners and added a family nurse practitioner track. More recently, the Seattle nursing school has developed an innovative second-degree immersion track for people with college degrees in other disciplines who wish to be nurses.

Many experiences in other courses (for example, the clinical courses and the thesis/scholarly project) enable the students to develop comfort and skill in working with diverse patients, families, and communities. For their thesis or other scholarly project, the students are expected to develop projects significant to their own future roles as advanced practice nurses and to vulnerable populations. Chapters 19 (Grandmason) 23 (Pasumansky), and 24 (Cogen) are reports of research with implications for vulnerable populations in Africa and the United States.

In the BSN program, students work in the poor neighborhoods, called garden communities, located near the university. Garden communities are scattered around the city and students spend a good bit of clinical time there. Faculty are assigned to each community and provide clinical supervision and support. The undergraduate course on vulnerable populations is a two-credit required course in which the students conduct fieldwork by interviewing persons different from themselves so as to develop comfort with and competence at interacting with culturally diverse people and groups. Students discuss their fieldwork in a variety of settings in the United States and Belize.

Kennesaw State University Model

Located just north of Atlanta, Kennesaw State University emphasizes global learning in a way that has moved the university onto the world stage in several disciplines, and its School of Nursing is a leader in this effort. For many years, the WellStar School of Nursing has sent students to Oaxaca, Mexico, to live with families, study Spanish, and learn in the local hospitals and community agencies. Students report that their experiences there are life-changing. Even though many may not travel abroad again, they express an appreciation for the Mexican culture of clients they serve in this country. A second Mexican initiative for Kennesaw State graduate students in the nurse practitioner track is described in Chapter 35 in this book on graduate fieldwork.

For a course on "vulnerable populations," the author of this chapter assigned undergraduate students to conduct fieldwork with populations different from their own. The groups might be of different races or ethnicity or simply be members of a population that is medically underserved or disadvantaged such as homeless people. Students interviewed a variety of service providers and group members and presented what they learned to the class. One group of students interviewed affluent adolescents for a research project the author conducted; their work is reported in Chapter 18 on life history research.

Finally, Kennesaw State University's nurse-managed clinic serves as a primary teaching site for its students. Run by a nurse practitioner faculty member, Donna Chambers, the clinic staff have an average of 3000 patient visits per year. Now that a formal agreement has placed the clinic under the auspices of Kennesaw State University, plans are to rotate all nursing students (as well as social work and health promotion and sports management students) through the clinic at some point in their studies.

KEY COMPONENTS OF EDUCATIONAL EXPERIENCE

A plan for teaching nursing students how to care for vulnerable populations might include the following components:

- Identify the vulnerable populations within the community. If international nursing is an interest of the school, then faculty might capitalize on their own international research or service experiences. Sister school relationships such as the Duquesne hermanamiento could provide wonderful opportunities for faculty and student exchanges, service learning projects, or collaborative research with nursing faculty in other countries.
- Develop a set of guidelines for students to follow for their fieldwork with the expected outcomes clearly stated. (The *Instructor Guide* for this book contains sample syllabi and detailed guidelines.) Outcomes should include an expectation for improved self-awareness.
- Designate key faculty to coordinate or guide the process. Not every faculty member will want to be involved, but it is essential to have at least one faculty champion for each project.
- Establish the need for specific projects in concert with stakeholders who are key members of the population.
- Decide whether service learning projects will be part of the curriculum and conducted within specific courses or whether they will be free-standing efforts that are initiated as people express interest in them. One way to focus on vulnerable populations without undertaking major curriculum changes is to allow students to use independent study courses for fieldwork.
- Design and implement a small-scale project that can be funded through existing resources. Later, after individual faculty have established a track record, more sophisticated projects can be funded through grants and contracts.

- Evaluate the projects not only in terms of student satisfaction and learning, but also in terms of benefits to the population.
- Consider evaluation data carefully before designing subsequent projects.

SUMMARY

The models presented here have several characteristics in common that contributed to their effectiveness in meeting the objectives of the courses and programs. Successful experiences for students include opportunities for developing self-awareness, fieldwork that enables them to develop communication skills and interact with people different from themselves, and review of available literature on the population of interest. Although these experiences are challenging, the students generally rate them as positive. In many cases in which students have traveled to other areas to become immersed in another culture, they indicate that their experiences were life-changing. The success of these service learning programs demonstrates that providing such opportunities at undergraduate and graduate levels is a crucial aspect of nursing education with regard to vulnerable populations.

For a full suite of assignments and additional learning activities, use the access code located in the front of your book to visit this exclusive website: http://go.jblearning.com/dechesnay. If you do not have an access code, you can obtain one at the site.

REFERENCES

American Academy of Nursing (AAN). (2011). Cultural competence: Expert panel report. Retrieved January 4, 2011, from www.aannet.org/i4a/pages/Index.cfm?pageID=3555

American Association of Colleges of Nursing (AACN). (2010). Cultural competence in nursing education. Retrieved October 18, 2010, from www.aacn.nche.edu/Education/cultural.htm

Carty, R., & White J. (1993). *Nicaraguan–American nursing collaborating project.* Washington, DC: American Association of Colleges of Nursing, pp. 37–38.

Colvin, S., de Chesnay, M., Mercado, T. & Benavides, C. (2005). Child health in a barrio of Managua. In M. de Chesnay (Ed.) *Caring for the vulnerable: Perspectives in nursing practice, theory and research.* Sudbury, MA: Jones and Bartlett.

Dreher, M., & MacNaughton, N. (2002). Cultural competence in nursing: Foundation or fallacy? *Nursing Outlook, 50,* 181–186. doi: 10.1067/mno.2002.125800

Giger, J., Davidhizer, R., Purnell, L., Harden, J. T., Phillips, J., & Strickland, O. (2007). American Academy of Nursing Expert Panel report: Developing cultural competence to eliminate health disparities in ethnic minorities and other vulnerable populations. *Journal of Transcultural Nursing, 18*(2), 95–102. doi: 10.1177/1043659606298618

Jeffreys, M. (2010). *Teaching cultural competence in nursing and health care* (2nd ed.). New York, NY: Springer.

Milstead, J. (1998). Preparation for an online asynchronous university doctoral course: Lessons learned. *Computers in Nursing, 16*(5), 247–258.

Resick, L. (1999). Challenges in measuring outcomes in two community-based nurse-managed wellness clinics: The development of a chart auditing tool. *Home Health Care Management and Practice, 11*(4), 52–59.

Resick, L., Taylor, C., Carroll, T., D'Antonio, J., & de Chesnay, M. (1997). Establishing a nurse-managed wellness clinic in a predominantly older African American inner-city high rise: An advanced practice nursing project. *Nursing Administration Quarterly, 21*(4), 47–54.

Resick, L., Taylor, C., & Leonardo, M. (1999). The Nurse-Managed Wellness Clinic Model developed by Duquesne University School of Nursing. *Home Health Care Management and Practice, 11*(6), 26–35.

Ross, C. (2000). *Caminando mas cerca con Dios [A closer walk with Thee]: An ethnography of health and well-being of rural Nicaraguan men.* Unpublished doctoral dissertation, Duquesne University, Pittsburgh, PA.

Taylor, C., Resick, L., D'Antonio, J., & Carroll, T. (1997). The advanced practice nurse role in implementing and evaluating two nurse-managed wellness clinics: Lessons learned about structure, process and outcomes. *Advanced Practice Nursing Quarterly, 3*(2), 36–45.

Vezeau, T., Peterson, J., Nakao, C., & Ersek, M. (1998). Education of advanced practice nurses serving vulnerable populations. *Nursing and Health Care Perspectives, 19*(1), 124–131.

White, J., & Smith, C. (1997). Developing an international nursing partnership with Nicaragua. *International Nursing Review, 44*(1), 13–18.

Winter, K. (2001). Bystander CPR in two Pittsburgh communities. *Cultura de los Cuidados, 5*(9), 82–89.

Zolkoski, R. (2000). *Clean water for Chimbote, Peru: Transcultural nursing in participatory action research.* Unpublished doctoral dissertation, Duquesne University, Pittsburgh, PA.

CHAPTER 33

Healthy Communities and Vulnerability: Enhancing Curricula for Teaching Population-Based Nursing

Barbara A. Anderson

Objectives

At the end of this chapter, the reader will be able to

1. Describe a healthy community in terms of the vulnerable populations it contains.
2. Identify areas for improvement in nursing curricula that adequately address the needs of the whole community.
3. Discuss ways in which resilience of populations can be addressed.

INTRODUCTION

Vulnerability, as a concept applicable to either individuals or populations, can be interpreted as a pejorative term. Vulnerable populations are often characterized as helpless, susceptible, at risk, or marginalized; rarely do depictions of such groups refer to their resilience and strengths. Individuals within a specified group, however, may not feel vulnerable, resisting this categorization as prejudicial or deflecting attention from their strengths (de Chesnay, 2005)

Vulnerable populations, which frequently encompass strong people facing difficult circumstances, have the potential for resilience when their strengths are mobilized. Resilience—"the process of adapting well in the face of adversity, trauma, tragedy, or even significant sources of stress" (Newman, 2003, p 42)—is characterized by hope, positive action, and movement toward wholeness (de Chesnay, 2005). Certainly, these chararacteristics of hope and positive action were central points of discussion in the 2008 U.S. presidential campaign, reflecting a perceived national sense of hopelessness about a vulnerable system.

Powerful factors influence whether an individual, an aggregate, or even a nation feels vulnerable or resilient in the face of adversity. Factors affecting a sense of vulnerability include family support, religious systems, cultural norms, and individual characteristics (Greeff &

Human, 2004). The influence of the larger community on the sense of vulnerability is a factor that is rarely addressed as a variable. Does a community that is *healthy* make vulnerable populations less vulnerable, more hopeful, and more resilient? What is a *healthy community* and how is it characterized? What does an *unhealthy community* look like, and does it lessen resiliency or increase susceptibility to adverse outcomes among vulnerable populations? These questions are rarely addressed in population-based nursing education curricula.

Other factors that are minimized in the curricula include the influence of vulnerable populations on the health of a community and the response of the community to vulnerable populations. Do vulnerable populations bring strength, resilience, and different paradigms to the community, or do they create uncomfortable questions, economic instability, and social disruption? In the general population, lip service is often paid to various beliefs about vulnerable groups—for example, they contribute to building of healthy communities, they undermine prevailing values, they erode the health of community, or they threaten the economic order. As recent events in the United States demonstrate, immigrants, as an example of a vulnerable group, are frequently marginalized, considered to be freeloaders, characterized as dangerous, and made to feel unwelcome. They may be targeted as the root cause of community problems by contributing to economic instability and absorbing desirable jobs, despite the fact that they frequently work in the lowest and least visible sectors of the informal economy. Moreover, they may be labeled as creating unhealthy communities, endangering the health of the public.

This detrimental community response to vulnerable populations has been seen historically in periods of economic downturn (Friedman, 2005; Sen, 2006). It is frequently expressed in highly salient social messages that imply intentional threat from vulnerable groups (Anderson & Anderson, in press; Sen, 2006). This labeling of the vulnerable in times of community stress is the hallmark of an unhealthy community (Anderson & Anderson, in press). The threads of such messages, as they influence resilience among the most vulnerable, are rarely systematically factored into the curricula of population-based nursing education. Beyond this curricular oversight is the larger issue of stagnated approaches to nursing education in general.

GONE MISSING: NURSING FACULTY

There is a huge need for renovation of, and innovation in, nursing curricula. While valiant efforts are being made to close the gap in nursing leadership, these efforts are hampered by the severe lack of nursing faculty in the United States. Admission of nursing students, at all levels, is dampened by the shortage of faculty (Aiken, 2007; Allen, 2008; American Academy of Nursing, 2006; American Association of Colleges of Nursing [AACN], 2008a, 2008b; Buerhaus, Staiger, & Auerbach, 2008; International Council of Nurses [ICN], 2006; The Joint Commission, 2008; Potempa, Redman, & Landstrom, 2009; Proto & Dzurec, 2009; Ross, Polsky, & Sochalski, 2003; Yordy, 2006). This national faculty shortage is affecting the development of innovative nursing curricula at all levels of nursing education. Even so, highly original and creative ideas and programs are being generated to increase graduates' understanding of population-based health as foundational to improving the health of the nation. Basic premises include understanding the hallmarks of a healthy community and promoting models of resilience among communities and vulnerable populations.

THE PREVAILING CURRICULAR PARADIGM

The historical paradigm in population-based nursing curricula has been that vulnerable populations bring problems and that the community, as a reservoir of programs, can solve these problems. This paradigm assumes a problem-based assessment, active interventions for solutions to problems with or without the input of those affected, and outcome evaluation for programs addressing identified problems. Curricular approaches use this paradigm to craft problem-based learning, beginning with the word "problem." Nursing students, at both undergraduate and graduate levels, quickly adapt to this problem-oriented approach. As a consequence, they often fail to assess for individual or aggregate resiliency, the state of dynamism and health of the community in which the vulnerable must navigate, the perceived and actual effects that the vulnerable have upon a community, and the community's attitude toward specific vulnerable populations.

This approach of problem orientation is antithetical to the way that students of nursing learn pathophysiology. First, they learn normal anatomy and physiology, fundamentals of health, and conduct of a normal health assessment. Likewise, they study psychology before engaging in psychiatric nursing. Learning to recognize health is foundational to understanding pathology. Only then, after establishing a basis for recognizing health, do nursing students move to learning about deviations from health. Thus population-based nursing curricula, in using the problem-oriented approach without first examining resiliency, fail to lay a foundation for normalcy before moving into pathology.

ENVISIONING A RESILIENCY MODEL FOR POPULATION-BASED NURSING CURRICULA

Vulnerable populations can optimally mobilize their strengths in facing difficult circumstances if they are supported by a healthy community. Likewise, communities can become healthier and more whole as they learn from and incorporate the resiliency and knowledge of vulnerable populations in their approach to overall health. The nation's blueprint for health, *Healthy People 2010: Understanding and Improving Health* (U.S. Department of Health and Human Services [USDHHS], 2000) is now updated in the *Healthy People 2020* version (Healthy People 2020, n.d.) The 2010 version has brought much greater understanding about the integration of individual and community health as a comprehensive framework for understanding the determinants of the nation's health (Institute of Medicine [IOM], 2003a, 2003b). The social ecological model (Skokols, 1996) and the ecological model of health (IOM, 2003b) have furthered understanding that both individual and aggregate health are determined by daily and lifetime interactions within the community. Thus linking biological, sociocultural, and environmental determinants of health is now mainstream thinking.

Although the ecological model of health remains a potent framework for linking vulnerability and community, a directional change in nursing curricula is essential to move toward a resiliency model. Nursing educators need to design curricula that help students seek out strengths before problems, indicators of healthy functioning of a community, and evidence of interactions between vulnerable populations and their community that promote mutual resiliency.

DESIGNING A RESILIENCY MODEL POPULATION-BASED NURSING CURRICULA

The movement of population-based nursing curricula from a problem-based model to a resiliency model assumes that both the community and the vulnerable populations residing in the community can learn from and teach one another. The curricula need to reflect this overarching assumption, which incorporates a readiness to collaborate in mutual planning, mutual respect for vulnerable individuals and the community in which they live, and a spirit of service on both sides. The community serves, is served by, and learns from vulnerable populations. Vulnerable populations, likewise, have a responsibility to serve and take a recognized place within the community. These are major assumptions, calling on a community to demonstrate good health and vulnerable populations to muster inner resources of resiliency.

Identifying the Hallmarks of a Healthy Community

How is a healthy community characterized? What does an unhealthy community look like? Does a healthy community foster resilience or decrease susceptibility to adverse outcomes among vulnerable populations? These are critical questions that need to be incorporated into population-based nursing curricula utilizing a resiliency model.

The ecological model of health, as defined by the Institute of Medicine (2003b), remains an excellent framework for studying the interface of vulnerability and community. The community can be a healthy environment for its citizens, including those most vulnerable, or it can be a place that destroys the health and spirit of its denizens. An urban environment with sprawl, poor hygiene, and inadequate planning creates conditions that encourage a sedentary lifestyle, development of illnesses linked to environmental pollutants, and conditions of mental stress, social division, and alienation (Franklin, Frank, & Jackson, 2004). In contrast, a community characterized by citizen empowerment, inclusive of those who are most vulnerable, possesses hallmarks of a healthy community (Diers, 2004).

Which components should be built into curricula for the assessment of a healthy community? The Healthy Cities initiative, designed by the World Health Organization (WHO), sets a standard for health promotion and citizen participation, including those who are most vulnerable. In October 2003, political leaders throughout Europe convened in Belfast, Ireland, to draft a strategic plan and call for action. "The Belfast Declaration for Healthy Cities: The Power of Local Action" is a blueprint that has been widely accepted as definitive of the "healthy city." According to the Belfast Declaration, a healthy city is an urban environment that promotes human health in the following ways:

- Reducing inequalities and addressing poverty
- Building strategic partnerships for human health

- Considering health impacts in urban planning
- Including citizens in planning and policy decision making
- Working toward the United Nations Millennium Development Goals
- Strengthening linkages with other cities nationally and globally
- Sharing resources and lessons learned with other cities (WHO, 2003)

A hallmark of a healthy city is that it promotes the health of the population, including those most vulnerable (**Table 33–1**).

Community initiatives to promote resiliency in rural areas also have a profound effect on the health of vulnerable populations. For instance, the Andean Rural Health Care project in Bolivia, South America, demonstrated the effectiveness of local community partnerships with private nongovernmental organizations. This project, which was built on principles from the ecological model, used local resiliency and initiative to provide vulnerable populations with accessible primary health care (Perry et al., 1991).

Population-based nursing curricula need to use such examples in demonstrating policy initiatives and program implementation. Through curricula built on a model of resiliency, students can learn to identify how a community contributes to resiliency, vulnerability, or perhaps both simultaneously. They can examine how the community responds to those persons who are vulnerable and how members of vulnerable populations within the community initiate community action. Students can also look at highly salient social messages about vulnerability. For example, in an economically depressed community, what is the response to persons affected by unemployment and homelessness? What does the community have to say about the role of

Table 33–1 Indicators of a Healthy Urban Environment

Adequate space for exercise, active lifestyle, and cultural events
Promotion of social networks
Affordable, high-quality housing
Equity and programs for poverty reduction
Opportunities for local food production and healthy food outlets
Diverse employment opportunities
Accessible, ecological, safe transport systems
Reduction in emissions that threaten climate stability
Acceptable noise levels
Good air and water quality
Good sanitation and waste disposal
Adequate planning for community safety and disaster management

Source: WHO, 2005.

vulnerable populations in such an economic climate? Does the community perceive that vulnerable populations undermine cultural norms and values? Pose public health or economic threats? Make substantial contributions to the well-being of the community? Do vulnerable populations in the community feel they are using their strengths? Do they believe that they are contributing to the community? Do they feel welcomed and respected?

Curricular methods used to assess resiliency include direct observation, engaged, immersed participation, and deep introspection (Scott, Harrison, Baker, & Wills, 2005; Tanner, 2006). Such curricula support the learning of emotional intelligence (Leonard & Swap, 2004).

In the author's experience, nursing students engaged in population-based coursework have limited exposure to community assessment from a resiliency perspective. They do not know how to identify the signs of resiliency within a community, the strengths of a population experiencing vulnerability, or the hallmarks of healthy interface between community and vulnerability. Rather, they initially focus on the problems; seeing the problems and the shadows, they may never see the hallmarks of health.

Broadening the Definitions of Community Experience

A resiliency model of population-based nursing curricula needs to embrace an interdisciplinary approach to learning (**Table 33–2**). This concept receives much lip service from the profession of nursing, yet nursing remains one of the most enclaved of professions—a characteristic that is reflected in its teaching–learning environment.

A resiliency model of curricula needs to deliberatively seek specific learning opportunities (not teaching opportunities) from community-based organizations and a wide variety of disciplines, including myriad health professions and other professions. To understand how a community functions and its state of health, the student needs exposure and opportunities to learn from the multiple dimensions of community organization: electoral offices, community services, law enforcement, education at all levels, and outreach services, to mention a few.

Table 33–2 Resiliency: Curricular Concepts

Question	Suggested Learning Resource
What does a healthy community look like?	"Healthy Cities" indicators
Is this a healthy community?	The ecological model of health
What is vulnerability?	Examine the community context and definitions of vulnerability within the community
Which variables contribute to vulnerability?	Examine the community context and salient social messages
Does the community decrease or exacerbate vulnerability?	Examine the role and the power of vulnerable populations in community action

A paradigm of resiliency in a healthy community is the platform for the learning (Gormley, Frerick, & Dean, 2009; Potempa et al., 2009; Proto & Dzurec, 2009). This paradigm (learning how a healthy system works) is counter-intuitive to the problem-oriented paradigm (learning to see shadows everywhere). Yet, it is not all that different from teaching fundamentals of health before moving to pathology. The paradigm of resiliency requires careful reflection, building on the experiences of students deeply immersed in the community. It is "the process by which the learner reflects on his or her experience and draws significance and meaning from such reflection" (Strauss et al., 2003).

WHAT IF?

What if population-based nursing curricula were directed away from looking initially at the "problems of vulnerable populations" and toward the identification of signature strengths and evidences of resiliency in both communities and vulnerable populations? What if the word "problem" was never introduced, or at least was introduced only after an assessment for resiliency? What if students were encouraged to participate in community organization and development from the rubric of how vulnerable populations strengthen the community and how communities become healthier as a result of working with vulnerable populations? Would this approach take the "problem" out of problem-based learning and substitute an ecological model of learning that acknowledges multiple levels of health determinants and the dynamic interface between communities and vulnerable populations? This paradigm for population-based nursing education proposes that curricula guide students to first examine how healthy communities make vulnerable populations more resilient and how vulnerable populations' strengths can be used to build healthy communities, looking for wellness before ascribing pathology.

For a full suite of assignments and additional learning activities, use the access code located in the front of your book to visit this exclusive website: http://go.jblearning.com/dechesnay. If you do not have an access code, you can obtain one at the site.

REFERENCES

Aiken, L. (2007). U.S. nurse labor market dynamics are key to global nurse sufficiency. *Health Services Research*, 42, 1299–1320.

Allen, L. (2008). The nursing shortage continues as faculty shortage grows. *Nursing Economics*, 26, 35–40.

American Academy of Nursing, Expert Panel on Global Nursing and Health. (2006). White paper on global nursing and health: A brief. *Nursing Outlook*, 32, 111–113.

American Association of Colleges of Nursing (AACN). (2008a, September). *Addressing the nursing shortage: A focus on nurse faculty*. Washington, DC: Author.

American Association of Colleges of Nursing (AACN). (2008b, September). *Nursing faculty shortage fact sheet.* Washington, DC: AACN.

Anderson, G., & Anderson, B. *Genocide. A comparative study of epidemiology.* New York: The Edwin Mellen Press, (In press).

Buerhaus, P., Staiger, D., & Auerbach, D. (2008). *The future of the nursing workforce in the United States: Data, trends and implications.* Sudbury, MA: Jones & Bartlett.

de Chesnay, M. (Ed.). (2005). *Caring for the vulnerable.* Sudbury, MA: Jones and Bartlett.

Diers, J. (2004). *Neighbor power: Building community the Seattle way.* Seattle: University of Washington Press.

Franklin, H., Frank, L., & Jackson, R. (2004). *Urban sprawl and public health: Designing, planning and building for healthy communities.* Washington, DC: Island Press.

Friedman, B. (2005). *The moral consequences of economic growth.* New York, NY: Knopf.

Gormley, D., Frerick, J., & Dean, A. (2009). Pathways to nursing: An innovative program to encourage high school students to enter nursing. *Kentucky Nurse, 57*(4), 7–8.

Greeff, A. & Human, B., (2004). Resilence in families in which a parent has died. *American Journal of Family Therapy, 37*(1), 27–42.

Healthy People 2020—Improving the health of Americans (n.d.) Retrieved from http://www.healthypeople.gov

Institute of Medicine (IOM). (2003a). *The future of the public health in the 21st century.* Washington, DC: National Academic Press.

Institute of Medicine (IOM). (2003b). *Who will keep the public healthy?: Education public health professionals for the 21st century.* Washington, DC: National Academic Press.

International Council of Nurses (ICN). (2006). *The global nursing shortage: Priority areas for intervention.* Geneva, Switzerland: Author.

The Joint Commission. (2008). Health care at the crossroads: Guiding principles for the development of the hospital of the future. Retrieved December 10, 2008, from http:www.aramarkhealthcare.com

Leonard, D., & Swap, W. (2004). Deep smarts. *Harvard Business Review, 82*(9), 88–97, 137.

Newman, R. (2003). Providing direction on the road to resilience. *Behavioral Health Management, 23*(4), 42–43.

Perry, H., Robison, N., Chavez, D., Taja, O., Hilari, C., Shanklin, D., & Wyon, J. (1991). Attaining health for all through community partnerships: Principles of the census-based, impact-oriented (CBIO) approach to primary health care developed in Bolivia, South America. *Social Science Medicine, 48*(8), 1053–1067.

Potempa, K., Redman, R., & Landstrom, G. (2009). Human resources in nursing education: A worldwide crisis. *Collegian, 16*(1), 19–23.

Proto, M., & Dzurec, L. (2009). Strategies for successful management and oversight of nurse faculty workforce initiatives: Lessons from the field. *Journal of Professional Nursing, 25*(2), 87–92.

Ross, S., Polsky, D., & Sochalski, J. (2003). Nursing shortages and international nurse immigration. *International Nursing Review*, 32, 231–262.

Scott, S. B., Harrison, A. D., Baker, T., & Wills, J. D. (2005). An interdisciplinary community partnership for health professional students: A service-learning approach. *Journal of Allied Health, 34*(1), 31–35.

Sen, A. (2006). *Identity and violence.* New York, NY: W. W. Norton.

Skokols, D. (1996). Translating social ecological theory into guidelines for community health promotion. *American Journal of Health Promotion, 10*, 282–298.

Strauss, R., Mofidi, M., Sandler, E. S., Williamson, R. III, McMurtry, B. A., Carl, L. S., & Neal, E. M. (2003). Reflective learning in community-based dental education. *Journal of Dental Education, 67*(11), 1234–1242.

Tanner, C. (2006). The next transformation: Clinical education. *Journal of Nursing Education, 45*(4), 99–100.

U.S. Department of Health and Human Services (USHHS). (2000). *Healthy people 2010: Understanding and improving health* (2nd ed.). Washington, DC: U.S. Government Printing Office.

World Health Organization (WHO). (2003). Belfast declaration for healthy cities: The power of local action. Retrieved November 21, 2006, from http://www.who.dk/healthy-cities

World Health Organization (WHO). (2005). Designing healthier and safer cities: The challenge of urban planning. Retrieved November 21, 2006, from http://www.who.dk/healthy-cities

Yordy, K. (2006). *The nursing faculty shortage: A crisis for health care.* Princeton, NJ: Robert Wood Johnson Foundation.

CHAPTER 34

Preparing Nursing Professionals to Be Advocates: Service Learning

Lynda P. Nauright and Astrid Wilson

Objectives

At the end of this chapter, the reader will be able to

1. Describe how advocacy came to be a key concept in nursing.
2. Describe how service learning has improved nursing education.
3. Develop a service learning project for the community in which you expect to practice.

THE EVOLVEMENT OF ADVOCACY AS A NURSING ETHIC

Paralleling the women's movement, nursing in the 1960s and 1970s was evolving from the ethic of loyalty to the physician and hospital to a new ethic of patient advocacy. Modern nursing, which began on the battlefield of the Crimea, had long adhered to a military metaphor: Nurses wore uniforms, caps, and cloaks; different schools had unique insignia; and stripes were added as the student progressed up the ranks (Winslow, 1984).

Consistent with the military theme, loyalty to the commanding officer and strict obedience to his orders were a major part of the nursing ethic. The Nightingale pledge, written in 1893, states, "with loyalty, I will endeavor to aid the physician in his work" (Davis & Aroskar, 1978, pp. 12–13). Charlotte Aikens' classic text on nursing ethics, published in 1916, reiterates this theme:

> Loyalty to the physician is one of the duties demanded of every nurse, not solely because the physician is her superior officer, but chiefly because the confidence of the patient in his physician is one of the important elements in the management of his illness, and nothing should be said or done that would weaken this faith or create doubts as to the character or ability or methods of the physician. (p. 44)

The moral power of this reasoning was compelling. Nurses were concerned about their patients' well-being and were taught repeatedly that the "faith" that people have in a physician is as much a healing element as is any medicinal treatment. Thus, even if the physician blundered, the patient's confidence was to be maintained at all costs. Parsons' (1916) text states:

> If a mistake has been made in treating a patient, the patient is not the person who should know it if it can be kept from him, because the anxiety and lack of confidence that he would naturally feel might be injurious to him and retard his recovery. (p. 32)

Beginning in the twentieth century, however, some thoughtful nurses questioned and debated among themselves where such loyalty should end ("Where Does Loyalty to the Physician End?", 1910). Indeed, as early as 1932, Annie Goodrich spoke of modifying, if not abolishing, nursing's militarism. Nevertheless, the *Code for Nurses*, accepted by the American Nurses Association (ANA) in 1950, and a similar code accepted by the International Congress of Nursing (ICN) in 1953, called for nurses to verify and sustain physicians' orders, sustain confidence in the physician, and report incompetence or unethical conduct "only to the proper authority" (ANA, 1950, p. 196; ICN, 1953).

In the turbulent 1960s and 1970s, challenges were issued to all institutions that demanded unquestioned loyalty of its authority—and the medical profession was no exception. A diminishing confidence in physicians was coupled with rising consumerism and an emerging feminism. Collectively, these forces brought about changes in perspective on the part of both nurses and patients. Leaders of the patients' rights movement turned to nurses for assistance in securing the fundamental rights of patients for informed consent, the right to refuse treatment, and the right to have full information about diagnosis and prognosis.

George Annas, an attorney, first defined patient rights and urged nurses to be patient advocates (1974). Later in *The Rights of Hospital Patients* (1975), he explicitly attacked the military metaphor and again called for nurses to accept the new responsibility of patient advocacy. He was not disappointed. Nurses enthusiastically embraced their role as patient advocates. The nursing literature of the 1970s and 1980s is replete with discussions of advocacy as an essential role of the nurse, and use of the concept of advocacy as an appropriate philosophical base for nursing.

Nursing codes of ethics were revised as well. In 1973, ICN dropped all mention of loyal obedience to the physician's orders, instead stating that "The nurse's primary responsibility is to those people who require nursing care" (Davis & Aroskar, 1978, pp. 13–14). The 1976 revision of the ANA' *Code for Nurses* specifically required nurses to protect the "client" from the "incompetent, unethical or illegal practice of any person" (ANA, 1976, p. 8). Gone from the revised *Code* were rules obliging the nurse to maintain confidence in physicians or obey their orders. In fact, the word "physician" did not even appear in the revised *Code for Nurses.*

Given that patient advocacy is a nursing value, how, then, do we prepare students to be patient advocates, to care about advocacy, and to exercise social responsibility? One method is through learning strategies such as experiential and service learning. Service learning is defined as educational experiences in which students participate in an activity that provides needed assistance. Service learning can be thought of as a holistic model of education that emphasizes student active learning while providing a needed community service encouraging social responsibility (Wittmann-Price, Anselmi, & Espinal, 2010).

Service learning connects thought and feeling in a deliberate way, creating a context in which students can explore how they feel about what they are thinking and what they think about how they are feeling. A variety of service learning opportunities, in which students are able to use their skills and knowledge to help the community while furthering their learning, can serve as powerful tools for teaching students to be advocates.

The concept of service learning is based on Kolb's (1984) theory of experiential learning. Kolb's model outlines four components. First, there is (1) an immediate concrete experience during and after which a person makes observations and reflections. Out of these reflections comes (2) an abstract theory of why things are as they are, which leads to (3) ideas on how to address the situation experienced. This, in turn, leads to (4) active experiments and, therefore, learning.

Several other educational theories and principles support the teaching/learning strategy of service learning. Early learning theorist and researchers observed that rewarded or reinforced behaviors are more likely to occur in the future. Furthermore, what is learned is more likely to be retained if it is learned in a situation similar to that in which it is to be used. In his adult learning theory, Malcolm Knowles (1984) proposed that adults are motivated to learn when they experience a need to know something so as to deal with a particular situation or problem.

Another theory related to service learning is social learning theory. Bandura (1977, 1986, 2001) outlined the behaviorist, cognitive, and social cognition dimensions of this theory. Components of social learning theory include role modeling, reflection, observation, and reproduction of role-modeled activities (Bastable, 2003). Other concepts are reciprocal learning, developing citizenship skills, achieving social change, addressing community-identified needs, and the integral involvement of community partners (Bradshaw & Lowenstein, 2007).

Service learning differs from classroom strategies in that professors are more likely to serve as facilitators, encourage active participation, share responsibility for learning, encourage reflection, and look at long-term goals (Billings & Halstead, 2009). Thus, in this approach, professors move from being the "sage on the stage" to acting as the "guide on the side."

BENEFITS OF SERVICE LEARNING

One obvious benefit of service learning is that it meets actual community needs. This benefit is not the only one, however. Service learning fosters caring for others, allows students to experience firsthand how vulnerable populations are affected by public policy, and helps them develop empathy with diverse individuals. Reflection about the experience is a critical component of service learning. In the meantime, this practice fosters moral development, while simultaneously enhancing moral decision making.

This direct participation with vulnerable populations often causes students to develop a better understanding of themselves, including a greater appreciation of their own strengths and weaknesses. In addition, they may develop skills in problem solving, critical thinking, leadership, and ethical decision making through a program. An increased sense of civic responsibility, increased political/global awareness, and the development of cultural competence may also be outcomes (Mueller & Norton, 1998).

Benefits also accrue to the institutions that engage in service learning. The foundation of an effective service learning program is a balanced long-term partnership between communities and institutions of higher education. This "hands-on" community involvement enhances institutional visibility. It may also appeal to potential donors, while helping to minimize the traditional separation between "town and gown" (Pellietier, 1995).

EXPERIENTIAL AND SERVICE LEARNING: STRATEGIES

Study Abroad Program: Oaxaca, Mexico Practicum

The WellStar School of Nursing at Kennesaw State University (KSU) is a leader in preparing undergraduate and advanced practice nurses to meet the needs of the citizens of Georgia and throughout the world. KSU has a strong commitment to global learning, with diverse study-abroad courses being offered in which students have the opportunity to broaden their understanding of different cultures and participate in service learning. Service learning and advocacy are concepts threaded through university curricula. The literature provides strong documentation of the effectiveness of service learning in such study-abroad programs and international experiences (Amerson, 2010; Johanson, 2009; Larson, Ott, & Miles, 2010; Lindsey, 2009; Pechak & Thompson, 2009; Wong, 2009; Yeh, Rong, Chen, Chang, & Chung, 2009).

One such study-abroad course in nursing is the Nursing Practicum in Oaxaca, Mexico (developed by Dr. Carol Holtz more than 15 years ago), which provides an immersion experience in Mexican culture. Students live with a Oaxacan family for two weeks, practice nursing in a general hospital in the city and a children's hospital outside the city, study Spanish, have cultural excursions, and interact with the local people. These experiences help form the learning foundation for advocacy through service.

One of the authors of this chapter joined Holtz in her over the last three years and has the primary responsibility of supervising students at the Hospital de la Ninez Oaxaquena in San Bartolo Coyotepec, south of the city of Oaxaca. Students share their interests with faculty and are then assigned to different nursing units such as the emergency room, neonatal intensive care, hematology/oncology, or medical–surgical service. A prevailing issue in all of the units is children's responses to hospitalization. One approach that allows nurses and students to partially address the anxiety and stress of hospitalization and become the child's advocate is *play*.

Child's play in a hospital is a term that can conjure up the idea that such activities have little importance. In reality, *the work of the child is play*, and play is very significant for successful growth and development. Play need not stop when a child enters a hospital, because play is the language of all children. Play can be a powerful tool in communicating, teaching, and bringing comfort to hospitalized children. Children can express their thoughts and feelings through play and be better able to understand why they are where they are.

A former nursing student provided finger puppets from Peru to be used in the Oaxaca Practicum. After faculty role-modeling, the students became very proficient with interacting with patients and their family members using finger puppets as a means of eliciting communication. The students were most impressed with how the children responded when they were given the puppets. Some frowns changed to smiles, some children who were silent began talking, and others played with other patients. Parents' faces also lit up when asked if their child could have a puppet. One student was delighted when she returned from a break and found a mother wearing the finger puppet and interacting with her young child.

The coordinator of education at the hospital was so pleased with the children's responses to the finger puppets that she requested the nursing students distribute more puppets in other units than the ones to which they were assigned. The resources at the hospital included a well-stocked school room, a play room, and a rehabilitation room, but individual toys were limited. The nursing students became advocates for many of these children, increasing their play experience.

Other advocacy opportunities that flowed from the Oaxaca Practicum occurred at the Hospital Civil in Oaxaca. Nursing students were able to assist in the labor and delivery process, assess and report patients' conditions, and provide food for indigent Indians outside the hospital. Developing a new understanding of the Mexican culture from this study-abroad program will enable the students to be better advocates for Mexican patients whom they encounter in the United States.

Fuld Fellowship Program

Funded through the Helene Fuld Health Trust, the Fuld Fellowship program is an award extended to second-career nursing students committed to improving care for vulnerable populations. Fellows are enrolled through a degree option for non-nurses with degrees in other fields. One of the unique strengths of the Fuld program is its blending of academics and leadership training during hands-on provision of health care to the poor and disenfranchised ranging from inner-city residents to rural migrant workers.

One example of its services is Café 458, a restaurant for the homeless in downtown Atlanta, Georgia. Guests order from a menu, sit at small tables with student volunteers, and receive counseling, social services, and legal services. The innovative café, which provides not only delicious food but also dignity to its patrons, was founded by A. B. Short and his wife, Ann Connor.

Other community outreach activities available in the metro Atlanta area include MedShare International, which collects and recycles surplus medical supplies and equipment for distribution to other countries; Joe's Place, a foot care clinic for the homeless; Project Open Hand, which provides meals and nutrition services to people with symptomatic HIV/AIDS, homebound elderly persons, and others with critical illnesses or disabilities; and the International Rescue Committee (IRC), a refugee resettlement agency. "Through the IRC, I was introduced to a newly arrived family from Kabul, Afghanistan, and have developed a strong relationship with the parents and their children," said Jordan, a senior who intends to work in international health. "I witnessed the birth of the fifth child and felt thankful to share that precious moment with them" (Loftus, 2005).

Farm Worker Family Health Project

Georgia's migrant farm workers travel across the country, working as many as 18 hours per day harvesting tobacco, fruits, and vegetables and working at packing houses. They have no primary physician or health insurance, and virtually no time or resources to attend to their health needs or those of their children. According to Judith Wold, who has directed the volunteer Farm Worker Family Health Program since 2002, "Agriculture is one of the most dangerous occupations in the United States and the migrant farm workers are terribly at risk" (Comeau, 2006).

The Farm Worker Family Health Program, based in rural Moultrie, Georgia, has engaged in a two-week intensive health service delivery initiative each June to care for more than 1000 migrant farm workers and their families. The most common conditions treated are muscle strains, back problems, foot fungus, urinary tract infections, parasitic infections, skin rashes, eye and ear infections, anemia, hypertension, and diabetes (Comeau, 2006). As part of this program, family nurse practitioner, adult nurse practitioner, family nurse midwife, and women's health nurse practitioner students provide screening, educational, and counseling services.

Nursing students begin their long day at elementary schools, where they offer a variety of preventive and assessment services. The children are given health, developmental, and psychological evaluations. If needed, nurse practitioner students refer the children to local healthcare facilities. Dental hygiene students apply sealants and provide fluoride treatments, referring those needing additional intervention to the evening clinic. In the process, each child's school health record is updated on a database created by a student majoring in nursing leadership and administration. In the afternoons, students attend seminars on topics related to migrant health. As these nurses visit their family caseload, they are sometimes accompanied by county outreach workers. Some students have to battle the southern Georgia heat and humidity to observe the workers as they do their own jobs. A few actually tried their hand at harvesting alongside the workers—but did not last long!

In the evening, the students and faculty set up tables and supplies in the front yard of a church or whatever space is willing to donate access to electricity. Much of the in-depth physical assessments are conducted in the Nightingale van, a mobile clinic borrowed from South Georgia College. At sunset, about 9:00 P.M., workers come in from the fields to be seen, along with children referred earlier in the day from the school screening. Nursing students check in and screen farm workers and family members. Faculty members then conduct more extensive evaluations in the van for those who need them. Separate tents offer physical therapy and dental care, with volunteer dentists providing tooth extractions and other dental services. Volunteers from the community assist with setup and serve as interpreters.

Caring for these families has a profound effect upon students. "Before the trip, I was scared to death," confessed Rebecca, a third-year MSN candidate. "I was afraid I would be so lost, but I wasn't. I was hoping to come away with a little more knowledge. I came away with the world" (Loftus, 2005, p.2).

Beads for Books Campaign

Hurricane Katrina devastated the low-lying city of New Orleans, not only with wind damage but also with flooding when many of the levies were breached. One of this chapter's authors, who attended nursing school at Louisiana State University (LSU) in New Orleans, was the initiator of the Beads for Books campaign, which sought to assist nursing students in the wake of the 2005 disaster. She had visited the city a month before Katrina ravaged the area, meeting with the Dean of Dillard's School of Nursing to ask her to encourage the school's baccalaureate graduates to seek a master's degree in leadership from her program in the metro Atlanta area.

When Katrina came ashore, the Dillard University campus was flooded with approximately six feet of water for three weeks. Almost all buildings had to be gutted for repairs. All library books were lost, including the personal libraries of many of the faculty, who lived close by. The author received permission from Dillard's nursing school dean to initiate a book drive. A doctoral student research conference was eminent, so the author solicited nursing textbooks from faculty and students attending the conference.

After learning of the project, Carol Buisson, a New Orleans native and businesswoman and also a nurse and a friend of one of the authors, volunteered to contribute Mardi Gras beads to thank book donors. Thus the Beads for Books campaign was born. Nursing students (not only doctoral candidates, but also master's and undergraduate students) enthusiastically embraced the project, donating more than 300 expensive nursing textbooks, and driving twice to New Orleans to deliver them.

The book drive received national publicity and donations flooded (in a positive way) in. In all, 34 boxes of books were delivered by Nauright's campaign, approximately half of which were new. Many more were contributed by sorority groups. The campaign was stopped only when the Dean said, "We have no more room." (Nauright, unpublished manuscript).

IN THEIR OWN WORDS: IMPACT OF SERVICE LEARNING ON STUDENTS

For several years, one of the authors (Nauright, unpublished manuscript) taught an undergraduate policy course that had a service learning component. Students were allowed to choose a vulnerable population, interact with the population for at least 40 hours, identify a political or policy issue that affected their group, and advocate with state or federal legislators on behalf of their population. Just the simple act of interacting with at-risk populations and becoming personally involved in actions on their behalf proved to be a life-altering event for them. Students were encouraged to reflect on their experiences and to record their reflections in a journal. Their journal reflections, cited with their written permission, on the impact of service learning make the case far better than any narrative written by faculty.

After participating in a course using service learning, one student wrote:

> Before taking this class, I did not have any idea of the importance of personal involvement. Having graduated 20 years ago, I was "trained" to do tasks, not think too much, and be a good girl. Thank God times have changed.

> I have been helping myself as well as others by volunteering. The time that I have spent at [a homeless shelter] has given me a broader understanding of the word "care."

Students interacted with susceptible populations in a variety of ways, volunteering with such organizations as the American Red Cross, the State Council on Maternal and Infant Health, the State Nurses' Association School Health Task Force, children's shelters, food banks, Planned Parenthood, the Salvation Army, refugee programs, the State Council on Aging, AIDS outreach programs, and various agencies serving the homeless with shelters, health clinics, treatment centers for addiction, and educational programs. Volunteer activities were both challenging and rewarding. One student reported on her day building a house with Habitat for Humanity volunteers:

> We had to dance around large families of baby mice. We made walls until all the prepared materials were gone. This was inside an unheated warehouse but we kept on swinging those hammers . . . We got pretty good! My family all want to come another time and try it.

After coaching a blind young woman about interviewing for jobs over the phone, a student reported, "By the fourth call, she was amazing! She had poise and confidence that surprised both of us. Needless to say, she made several appointments for job interviews. It made me feel incredibly good to have made such a difference in this young lady's job search."

Another student who worked in a mobile clinic that visits shelters and places where homeless people congregate to provide healthcare services, observed: "I've begun to recruit my friends into volunteering with the Task Force [for the Homeless]. I laugh to myself at the crusader I've become."

Some activities led students to move out of their comfort level. A female student who volunteered at the Atlanta Union Mission, which serves the homeless, wrote,: "When I walked into that building I felt so AFRAID. I can't imagine what the people feel like who have to live out there on the streets." One of the biggest eye openers was the plight of the homeless. "Last year I began working in the homeless clinic to meet a class requirement. This was my first introduction to the homeless. I began to realize that these men and women were individuals much like myself." Another student wrote: "How can this situation we call homelessness but includes joblessness, hopelessness, nutritionessless [sic] and respectlessness [sic] be happening in what is supposed to be the greatest country in the world? It is mind-boggling and heart-wrenching and irrational."

Students welcome the opportunity to be advocates. Using service learning, especially with at-risk populations, is an effective way to teach advocacy and to expose students to experiences that will affect the way they look at vulnerable clients and the way they practice nursing. An additional benefit is the recognition by students that political awareness and activism are critical components of the nurse advocacy role.

For a full suite of assignments and additional learning activities, use the access code located in the front of your book to visit this exclusive website: http://go.jblearning.com/dechesnay. If you do not have an access code, you can obtain one at the site.

REFERENCES

Aikens C. A. (1916). *Studies in ethics for nurses.* Philadelphia, PA: Saunders.

American Nurses Association (ANA). (1950). A code for nurses. *American Journal of Nursing, 50*(4), 196.

American Nurses Association (ANA). (1976). *Code for nurses with interpretive statements.* Kansas City, MO: Author.

Amerson, R. (2010). The impact of service-learning on cultural competence. *Nursing Education Perspectives, 31*(1), 18–22.

Annas, G. (1975). *The rights of hospital patients: The basic ACLU guide to a hospital patient's rights.* New York, NY: Discus.

Bandura, A. (1977). *Social learning theory.* Englewood Cliffs, NJ: Prentice-Hall.

Bandura, A. (1986). *Foundations of thought and action: A social-cognitive theory.* Englewood Cliffs, NJ: Prentice-Hall.

Bandura, A. (2001). Social cognitive theory: An agenic perspective. *Annual Review of Psychology, 52,* 1–26.

Bastable, S. (2003). *Nurse as educator* (2nd ed.). Sudbury, MA: Jones and Bartlett.

Billings, D. M., & Halstead, J. A. (2009). *Teaching in nursing: A guide for faculty* (3rd ed.). St. Louis, MO: Saunders.

Bradshaw, M. J., & Lowenstein, A. J. (2007). *Innovative teaching strategies in nursing* (4th ed.). Sudbury, MA: Jones and Bartlett.

Comeau, A. (2006, May 30). *Emory nursing students provide care for migrant workers and their families* [Press release]. Atlanta, GA: Emory University.

Davis, A. J., & Aroskar, M. A. (1978). *Ethical dilemmas and nursing practice.* New York, NY: Appleton-Century-Crofts.

Goodrich, A. W. (1932). *The social significance of nursing.* New York, NY: Macmillan.

International Congress of Nursing (ICN). (1953). International code of nursing ethics. *American Journal of Nursing, 53*(9), 1070.

Johanson, L. S. (2009. Service-learning: The deepening students' commitment to serve. *JCN, 26*(2), 95–98.

Knowles, M. (1984). *The adult learner: A neglected species.* Houston, TX: Gulf Publishing.

Kolb, D. A. (1984). *Experiential learning: Experience as the source of learning and development.* Englewood Cliffs, NJ: Prentice-Hall.

Larson, K. L., Ott, M., & Miles, J. M. (2010). International cultural immersion: En vivo reflections in cultural competence. *Journal of Cultural Diversity, 17*(2), 44–50.

Lindsey, L. (2009, July–September). Belize service learning project for WKU nursing students. *Kentucky Nurse,* 12.

Loftus, M (2005, Winter). Making bigger beds. *Emory Nursing.* Atlanta, GA: Emory University.

Mueller, C. & Norton, B. (1998). Service Learning: Developing values and social responsibility. In M. Billings & J. Halstead (Eds.), *Teaching in nursing education.* Philadelphia, PA: Saunders.

Nauright, L. (n.d.). Unpublished manuscript.

Parsons, S. E. (1916). *Nursing problems and obligations*. Boston, MA: Whitcomb & Barrows.

Pechak, C. M., & Thompson, M. (2009). A conceptual model of optimal international service-learning and its application to global health initiatives in rehabilitation. *Physical Therapy, 89*(11), 1192–1204.

Pellietier, S. (1995). The quiet power of service learning: Report from the National Institute on Learning and Service. *The Independent, 95*(2), 6.

Where does loyalty to the physician end? [Letter]. (1910), *American Journal of Nursing, 10*(1), 274–276.

Winslow, G. R. (1984). From loyalty to advocacy: A new metaphor for nursing. In *The Hastings Center report* (pp. 32–40). Hastings on Hudson, NY: Hastings Center.

Wittmann-Price, K. A., Anselmi, K. K., & Espinal, F. (2010). Creating opportunities for successful international student service-learning experiences. *Holistic Nursing Practice, 24*(2), 89–98.

Wong, J. (2009, Fall). Africa: My mission, my passion, one day at a time a nurse's perspective. *Stanford Nurse*, 18–19.

Yeh, M., Rong, J., Chen, M., Chang, S., & Chung, U. (2009). Development of a new prototype for an educational partnership in nursing. *Journal of Nursing Education, 48*(1), 5–10.

CHAPTER 35

Working with Graduate Students to Develop Cultural Competence

Mary de Chesnay, Genie Dorman, and David Bennett

Objectives

WWW

At the end of this chapter, the reader will be able to

1. Compare and contrast models of fieldwork for graduate and undergraduate students.
2. Describe how nurse practitioner students can be involved in international clinical experiences despite their heavy clinical schedules.
3. Provide a case for service learning at the graduate level.

INTRODUCTION

This chapter reflects two approaches to graduate education that emphasize fieldwork with vulnerable populations as a way to develop cultural competence. One approach is clinical instruction of nurse practitioner students. The other is traditional fieldwork, in which students spend time immersed in the culture and complete a project with outcomes that might be useful to the community. The ideas for the fieldwork presented here were generated in nursing, but could easily be transferred to other disciplines.

Fieldwork is a useful way of teaching students to work with people who are different from themselves. It enables students to confront their ethnocentric biases, learn to tolerate ambiguity, and handle conflict, by having students conduct real projects that benefit the communities in which they are working. Similar to participatory action research, fieldwork projects such as those described in this book enable students to design, implement, and evaluate work that can be used by the community when they leave. This chapter includes a rich description of how nurse practitioner students can fit a study-abroad experience into their highly structured curriculum. Following this chapter are two chapters that describe fieldwork conducted by doctoral students of the first author as a course requirement for a doctoral elective in working with vulnerable populations.

MASTER'S-LEVEL FIELDWORK

Previous editions of this book have highlighted how some creative graduate faculty prepare their students to work with vulnerable populations. In the first edition, Phillips and Peterson (2005) described projects their students completed for a master's-level course in vulnerable populations. In the second edition, Peterson and colleagues (2008) discussed the process of mentoring master's degree students as they sought to develop innovative practice models for vulnerable populations. These projects generated a vulnerability assessment model, a way to help students understand the complexity of vulnerability by using a game (Jenga) and a form of play with visual symbols as a way of modeling (a bicycle and barbells).

The course taught by Phillips and Peterson used Aday's (2001) classic book as a text, but it was found to be too statistical and not clinically focused for nurses. This book was written to fill that specific need—for an undergraduate and graduate text that can be used in courses designed to teach both undergraduate and graduate nursing students to care for the vulnerable.

One of the most exciting ways in which to capture students' imagination for creative solutions to social problems is to encourage them to develop projects that address the needs of special populations in which they have a particular interest. For example, a student who works in pediatrics might examine the needs of children in a culture with which the student is unfamiliar. A student who has a passion for helping the medically underserved might volunteer his or her clinical services to a free clinic as a quid pro quo for conducting a research project there as a master's degree requirement.

Other projects to help graduate students learn cultural competence might focus on creating a business plan for a free clinic, interviewing stakeholders for an evaluation study of services provided by a homeless shelter, writing a grant to fund a mobile clinic, and developing a resource guide for teenagers to help them learn how to prevent communicable diseases. These projects would require students to spend time in the company of stakeholders, assess needs, talk with staff who serve the populations, identify resources available for the populations, and evaluate existing services.

An example of how effective graduate fieldwork can benefit the population is Brown's work on behalf of homeless adolescents in Seattle. At Seattle University, graduate students may choose either a thesis or a project that serves the vulnerable. Brown, a nurse practitioner student, was concerned about the spread of hepatitis B among the homeless adolescents of the city—an issue that inspired her to develop a short video as a teaching guide for preventing hepatitis B. She wrote a script, pilot tested it with her friends and family members acting as homeless adolescents, incorporated their critiques, and distributed edited copies to agencies that serve homeless children, who are mostly runaways (Brown, de Chesnay, & Phillips, 2005).

DOCTORAL FIELDWORK

The two chapters that follow this one—Chapter 36 by Jackson and Chapter 37 by Green—were completed as course requirements for a doctoral elective in working with vulnerable populations. The course provides students with an opportunity to explore in-depth special issues related to nursing in today's increasingly complex healthcare climate. Students select topics to explore, make a seminar presentation to the group on their topics, complete a fieldwork assignment related to the topic, and develop a publishable paper as the final outcome.

The objectives of the course were as follows:

- Analyze the literature on a special topic related to vulnerable populations.
- Complete fieldwork that improves the student's own cultural competence with a specific population.
- Prepare a teaching plan for undergraduate or graduate students or a project for practicing nurses that promotes cultural competence with a specific population.

The fieldwork project accounted for 30% of the students' grades. Instructions were to review the literature on the topic; complete a project that addressed a vulnerable population in terms of health-related issues; develop a goal statement and objectives to demonstrate how the student planned to achieve his or her objectives; and provide a timetable of activities designed to accomplish the goal and objectives for the project. The final paper was required to include a plan for teaching the content to either undergraduate or graduate students. The final project report was the graded outcome.

The students chose topics of great relevance to their current work. Green developed a cultural competence training program for school nurses in the south Georgia community in which she works and lives. Jackson is a nurse educator who has long been concerned with the issues of the homeless in her community south of Atlanta. Her assessment opened her eyes to the local community, and she has new experiences to share with her students as a result. These authors' rich descriptions of their work follow this chapter.

CLINICAL PRACTICE FOR NURSE PRACTITIONER STUDENTS

Another dimension of graduate student education is clinical experiences for nurse practitioner students. Two of this chapter's authors (Dorman and Bennett) are faculty who take family nurse practitioner students to Xalapa, Mexico, for their women's health clinical practicum. These experiences provide students with an outstanding immersion experience that is not often available in high-pressure nurse practitioner programs. Immersion experiences for undergraduates (Ailinger, Molloy, & Sacasa, 2009; Christoffersen, 2008; Stevens, 1998) are quite common, but nurse practitioner programs tend to be so structured that they usually do not allow for cross-cultural education. Yet, the co-authors of this chapter have made a commitment to provide intensive precepted clinical work in women's health in Mexico. Their students have intensive language, lifestyle, cultural, and clinical experiences with locals similar to those provided by undergraduate study-abroad courses.

Although the literature rarely describes the provision of such experiences for graduate students in nurse practitioner programs, some faculty have published details of how they accomplish cross-cultural clinical experiences for their students. When one of this chapter's authors (de Chesnay) was dean of a school with graduate programs, she arranged for immersion experiences for students at all levels—baccalaureate, master's, and doctoral. This school of nursing had started a clinic in northern Nicaragua, and one of its faculty took nurse practitioner students there every year for intensive immersion. He also was a primary faculty member in the undergraduate immersion work in a barrio of Managua (Ross, 1999).

Also in Nicaragua, Rita Ailinger, of George Mason University, has worked for years with undergraduates in community health nursing and, more recently, with graduate students. She has described an intensive two-week experience in which students collaborate with students and faculty at a Nicaraguan university not only to learn the culture but also to manage clinical problems in an area not known for its bountiful resources for patients (Ailinger, Zamora, Molloy, & Benavides, 2000).

Yale University nurse practitioner students and faculty provided health care to children in a poor neighborhood of Managua in an intensive four-day period each year for a five-year project. Students completed annual health histories for the children, created comprehensive medical records in Spanish and English for each child, treated existing conditions and developed follow-up plans, trained teachers, and built relationships with local providers to ensure continuity of care (Allen, Meadows-Oliver, & Ryan-Krause, 2008).

GRADUATE CLINICAL COURSE: A CULTURE-FOCUSED WOMEN'S HEALTH FAMILY NURSE PRACTITIONER (FNP) PRACTICUM IN XALAPA, MEXICO

Like many other areas of the United States, greater metropolitan Atlanta, Georgia, has experienced an explosive growth in its Latino population in recent years, with a documented 300% increase in this group in the past decade. The Latino population (most of whom are Mexican) of the city of Atlanta and surrounding counties now numbers approximately 500,000. Most of these individuals are undocumented, lack knowledge of the healthcare system, and have little or no access to health care other than emergency services.

The Xalapa Project

The faculty of the WellStar Primary Care Nurse Practitioner Program believe that for their graduates to be effective providers of care for their Latino clients, they must possess knowledge and sensitivity regarding the clients' culture and health beliefs, and many of their students have expressed their desire to learn more about the values and expectations related to health care held by this population. As actual experience with persons of another culture is necessary to develop cultural sensitivity, the faculty of the WellStar Primary Care Nurse Practitioner Program, in collaboration with the School for Foreign Students (*la Escuela para Estudantes Extranjeros*) of the University of Veracruz (*Universidad Veracruzana*) in Xalapa, Mexico, developed a women's health practicum experience focusing on cultural and health beliefs.

Xalapa, Mexico, is the cultural, academic, and political capital of the state of Veracruz, and it affords nurse practitioner students a unique opportunity to explore the function and structure of women's health care in a cultural setting that is assuming an increasingly significant position within the cultural context of the United States. The healthcare system of Xalapa comprises private-pay clinics and hospitals, government-sponsored clinics and hospitals, and traditional medicine practices provided by *curanderos.*

This practicum, which is based in the government-sponsored *Universidad Hospital de Maternidad,* emphasizes experiences within the Xalapan public healthcare system including both hospital-based and community clinic-based experiences. Services offered by the hospital and clinics include gynecological care (Pap smears), family planning and birth control, prenatal care, labor and delivery, postpartum care, and pediatric care to infants and children. In these settings, the students are paired with local physicians and nurses to provide care to mothers, infants, and children who lack any other means of obtaining that care. The students complete prenatal admission assessments, support laboring mothers, assist in both vaginal births and cesarean sections, complete gynecological examinations, and provide patient education.

Cultural immersion is another important aspect of this experience. Students are housed with local families and attend daily Spanish language, culture, and nutrition classes as well as local cultural events. The culture and language immersion encourages each student to pursue an in-depth exploration of the values, beliefs, customs, and practices that affect the healthcare status of this community.

Since its inception in fall 2000, five groups (a total of 60 family nurse practitioner students) have completed the practicum. A sixth group, consisting of 10 students, was scheduled to participate in the practicum in fall 2010. In Fall, 2009, there were 7 participants. The most recent group to complete the practicum in Fall, 2010 consisted of 9 participants. Similar to the situation with the participants in 2000, 2004, 2007, and 2008, data collected from these students regarding the practicum experience revealed extremely positive outcomes for both the students and the Latino clients whom they served. These outcomes included plans to actively seek positions caring for Latino clients, ongoing Spanish language study, and continued participation in Latino cultural events.

Selected Student Notes on the Xalapan Experience

Student 1

As a participant in the week-long study abroad program to Xalapa, Mexico, I feel like my perspective on Mexicans has changed completely. Even though I was raised in Houston, Texas, with many Hispanic friends and influences, I realize now that I have been ignorant in my view of Mexicans. As unbelievable as it is for me to begin to understand why I would think otherwise, I now truly understand that they share a lot of similar life experiences. They can be farmers and from the country, or they can be blonde and metropolitan—just like you would see in the United States. They may accomplish things differently than the United States, but they deal with many of the same issues and obstacles as people in the United States, and they ultimately generally share the desire to do better and achieve more for themselves and their families.

This seems like it would be obvious or just assumed, but this trip has really helped me to know and understand that internally. As open minded and nonjudgmental as I believed myself to be, this trip basically exposed within myself my own shortcomings. I think that this is going to have a significant implication in my practice as a nurse practitioner. Not only will I have a better understanding of specific cultural beliefs and practices in the Mexican culture, but more importantly, this experience will always remind me of my own potential to have misconceptions about people from any other groups or walks of life.

Student 2

There were really two aspects of this trip that were extremely valuable to me as a clinician. The first was the time that I spent with the female doctor who was doing [Pap smears]. She was very knowledgeable and very much tuned into her patient population. I admired her ability to really communicate with her patient, and she seemed to really care about what she was doing. The patients seemed to feel at ease with her, and she had a good balance of professionalism and friendliness. She was also very aware of her patient population and the resources they have available in terms of their finances for health care. She was very happy to have us with her and was excited to teach us about what she knew and the population.

The second aspect that [was valuable was] cultural. I went into this experience with the philosophy that I would truly make my best effort to completely embrace the culture and people of Mexico, and I feel like I really did that. My home-stay mom was amazing and really treated us like we were her own daughters. I enjoyed walking around the city and really experiencing the people, the food, and the culture of the city.

Student 3

The trip to Xalapa, Mexico, was an exceptional learning experience for a number of reasons. The clinical portion of the experience brought me greater understanding of the scope of care for the very poor in Mexico. Although the technology was very limited and basic, the healthcare team did the best with what they had, and I did feel the team members cared deeply for their patients.

I loved the cultural part of Xalapa, and being totally immersed in the culture. Although living with a family that one does not know was a bit uncomfortable, they were extremely gracious and welcoming. The mother was very proud of her culture and did her best to impress us with certain aspects, such as the upcoming "Day of the Dead." She encouraged us to speak Spanish, and helped us understand when possible.

The most important thing I learned was how it feels to be in a foreign land, surrounded by people who are very similar, yet very different. When the Xalapan natives realized that I did not speak Spanish well, they went out of their way to be helpful and welcoming. I note the contrast in the United States, in which many U.S. citizens often look on those from other countries with disdain, and even speak harshly to them, [telling them] to "learn the language!"

Student 4

I have a new appreciation for the work that I do presently in public health. I see women daily who have little means and overwhelming problems, and sometimes I get weary. This experience has opened my eyes in many ways. I am indeed spoiled and take many things for granted. I have new eyes with which to see all my patients, and especially those who speak a different language. Honestly, I have never "felt" the need to learn Spanish. Because of this experience I am becoming a student of Spanish and look forward to offering my Hispanic patients more compassionate care and understanding.

IMPLICATIONS FOR WORKING WITH VULNERABLE POPULATIONS

As a result of the clinical practice and fieldwork conducted in these courses, students learned several important lessons about working with vulnerable populations and about teaching nursing students to do the same. Perhaps the most important lesson is the necessity of confronting one's own ethnocentrism and developing the ability to appreciate cultural differences. Seeing how nurses in other cultures handle problems can help us to think creatively about our own healthcare problems and devise new solutions based on patients' needs rather than a paternalistic approach of determining what is right for them. An example might be framing recommendations about controlling diabetes through diet by taking the time to understand which kinds of foods are not only culturally specific, but also available to the family. There is no substitute for developing an understanding of why young children in rural areas of less-developed countries experience a high rate of burns by visiting their homes and seeing the open cooking fires in the middle of cinder-block shacks.

While some characteristics, values, and beliefs may be common to members of a cultural group, it is essential to recognize that patients and their families are also individuals who fit into their own communities in unique ways that may or may not be representative of their culture. Demonstrating respect for differences by not stereotyping is a skill that is more easily learned by interacting with people in their own settings than by reading about them as a cultural group. The individuality of health beliefs, problem-solving approaches, application of spirituality, and decision-making capacity varies widely within a culture.

It might seem paradoxical to appreciate cultural differences without stereotyping. At what point does practicing cultural competence cross the line into stereotyping? At what point is "being yourself" inadequate when interacting with members of other cultural groups? Nurses who work with people different from themselves, whether vulnerable or not, need to answer these questions for themselves.

What is clear, however, is that immersion programs can be a powerful teaching technique to help students sort out their biases and learn to appreciate cultural differences. Vulnerability is related to risk factors at a given point in time; it is not always related to poverty or minority status. Anyone can be vulnerable to a variety of stressors. Facilitating clinical experiences with culturally diverse groups enables nursing students to understand vulnerability at a deeper level than reading the literature can provide.

For a full suite of assignments and additional learning activities, use the access code located in the front of your book to visit this exclusive website: http://go.jblearning.com/dechesnay. If you do not have an access code, you can obtain one at the site.

REFERENCES

Aday, L. A. (2001). *At risk in America: The health and health care needs of vulnerable populations in the United States* (2nd ed.). San Francisco, CA: Jossey-Bass.

Ailinger, R., Molloy, S., & Sacasa, E. (2009). Community health nursing student experience in Nicaragua. *Journal of Community Health Nursing, 26*, 47–53.

Ailinger, R., Zamora, L., Molloy, S., & Benavides, C. (2000). Nurse practitioner students in Nicaragua. *Clinical Excellence for Nurse Practitioners, 4*(4), 240–244.

Allen, P., Meadows-Oliver, M., & Ryan-Krause, P. (2008). Establishing a school-based clinic in Managua, Nicaragua. *Pediatric Nursing, 34*(3), 262–266.

Brown, D., de Chesnay, M., & Phillips, D. (2005). Hepatitis B and homeless adolescents: Creating educational opportunities. In M. de Chesnay (Ed.), *Caring for the vulnerable* (pp. 289–294). Sudbury, MA: Jones and Bartlett.

Christoffersen, J. (2008). Leading a study-abroad group of nursing students in Nicaragua: A first-timer's account. *Nursing Forum, 43*(4), 238–246.

Peterson, J., Andersen, H., Mercado, J., Shellhorn, J., Speyer, J., & Thiagarag, L. (2008). Designing a model for predicting or working with vulnerable populations based on graduate fieldwork. In M. de Chesnay & B. Anderson (Eds.), *Caring for the vulnerable* (pp. 483–496.) Sudbury, MA: Jones & Bartlett.

Phillips, D., & Peterson, J. (2005). Graduate studies approach to vulnerability. In M. de Chesnay (Ed.), *Caring for the vulnerable* (pp. 385–394). Sudbury, MA: Jones and Bartlett.

Ross, C. (1999). Preparing American and Nicaraguan nurses to practice home health nursing in a transcultural experience. *Home Health Care Management and Practice, 11*(1), 66–70.

Stevens, G. (1998). Experience the culture. *Journal of Nursing Education, 37*(1), 30–33.

CHAPTER 36

Assessing the Needs of the Homeless in Townsville, USA

Annette Jackson

Objectives

At the end of this chapter, the reader will be able to

1. Describe the extent of the problem of homelessness in the United States.
2. Discuss the health issues related to homelessness.
3. Describe the role of nurses in assisting the homeless.

INTRODUCTION

Approximately 3 million Americans experience homelessness each year. It is estimated this number will increase over 2009 and 2010 by 1.5 million (National Coalition for the Homeless, 2010). Nearly 200,000 people in the United States have been homeless for more than a year (Drury, 2008). Due to multiple factors, the homeless are difficult to number, and estimates are likely to reflect an undercount of the true numbers of homeless individuals (de Chesnay, 2008).

Causes of homelessness vary greatly, and are often associated with the economy, federal laws and regulations, and personal choices of homeless persons (National Coalition for the Homeless, 2010). Inability to pay rent or mortgage payments, mental illness, domestic violence, and unaffordable health care are general reasons for lack of a permanent residence reported by the majority of homeless individuals (National Coalition for the Homeless, 2010). Regardless of the cause, many homelessness individuals find themselves unable to meet basic needs of food and shelter, much less navigate the healthcare system. Communities have a responsibility to provide services to members of vulnerable populations to improve health of both the individual and the community. Assessment of community resources is a first step in determining unmet needs and planning future interventions.

This chapter describes a needs assessment of the homeless carried out in a small city in the southern United States. Assessment of this city's provision of food, shelter, and health care are discussed. Other issues of importance to the homeless, such as permanent, affordable housing were not included in this assessment, due to time constraints. Also discussed are several recommendations for the future care of the homeless in this city.

EXTENT OF THE PROBLEM

The recent economic downturn in the United States has left more people unable to afford sufficient food and housing for themselves and their families. A survey conducted by the U.S. Conference of Mayors (National Coalition for the Homeless, 2009) found that 82% of surveyed cities reported an increased demand for shelter over a one-year period of time, and 25% of requests for emergency food assistance went unmet in 2009. Most U.S. cities are unable to meet this increased demand for food and shelter (National Coalition for the Homeless, 2010).

Food and shelter are basic human needs necessary for survival. Scarcity of food is associated with impaired access to medical and mental health care and prescription medications (Baggett, O'Connell, Singer, & Rigotti, 2010). Often basic needs of food and shelter take priority over permanent housing and other needs (Drury, 2008). The right to food is a well-recognized and -documented human right explicitly addressed in the domestic constitutions of 22 nations (Food and Agriculture Organization of the United States, 2010).

Many U.S. cities have in place adequate responses for the provision of food to the homeless. Churches and community and civic organizations are the primary means by which food is distributed through food pantries, soup kitchens, and shelters. Unfortunately, some U.S. cities choose to place restrictions on what is called food sharing. These restrictions prohibit individuals and organizations from sharing food with homeless people in public settings. City governments struggle to move the homeless out of sight, largely for economic reasons and because of the "not in my backyard" attitude of many citizens (National Coalition for the Homeless, 2010). It has long been a myth that feeding the homeless enables them to remain homeless.

HEALTH ISSUES

Homeless people carry multiple burdens that potentiate vulnerability. Many suffer from chronic and acute illnesses, such as hypertension, diabetes, asthma, HIV/AIDS, and tuberculosis. Mental illness, substance abuse, poor dental hygiene, and visual impairment are common in the homeless population (Baggett et al., 2010). The homeless experience poor access to health care, often delay seeking treatment, tend to utilize emergency rooms for primary care, are hospitalized at higher rates, and have higher incidence of morbidity and mortality than the general population (Gelberg, Andersen, & Leake, 2000; Savage, Lindsell, Gillespie, Dempsey, Lee, & Corbin, 2006; Schanzer, Dominguez, Shrout, & Caton, 2007; Zlotnick & Zerger, 2008). The health issues of the homeless negatively affect their ability to function socially to secure employment, housing, and health care. Health problems for the homeless population are primarily chronic in nature, and require multiple interventions (Bottomley, Bissonnette, & Snekvik, 2001; Savage et al., 2006).

A review of the literature reveals that, contrary to popular thought, the homeless are willing to seek health care when they perceive a condition is serious, even in light of mental illness, substance abuse, and lack of housing (Gelberg et al., 2000). Over-arching themes in the research of the homeless and their health-seeking behaviors include a lack of available resources (Martins, 2008; Nickash & Marnocha, 2009), lack of compassionate care (Hudson, Nyamathi, & Sweat, 2008; Macnee & McCabe, 2004; Martins, 2008; Nickash & Marnocha, 2009), labeling and stigma (Darbyshire, Muir-Cochrane, Fereday, Jureidini, & Drummond, 2006; Diaski, 2007), putting off health care until an emergency occurs (Martins, 2008; National Coalition for the Homeless, 2010), feeling unwelcome and out-of-place (Wen, Hudak, & Hwang, 2007), and the experience of barriers to care related to communication. Communication-related barriers include authoritative and one-way communication as well as lack of communication skill on the part of healthcare providers (Hatton, 2001; Hatton, Kleffel, Bennett, & Gaffrey, 2001).

A comprehensive community assessment is critical for city governments and other agencies to understand unmet need and determine the direction of future policies and practices in caring for the homeless. Needs assessment allows for delivery of the most effective care to those in greatest need, permits application of the principles of social justice and equity, and ensures that scarce resources are responsibly allocated. Considered to be the most effective approach to prevent and reduce homelessness, the Homeless Continuum of Care model (U.S. Department of Housing and Urban Development [HUD], 2010) is a planning model designed to assist the homeless at every level of need to move them to permanent housing. The continuum addresses the underlying causes of homelessness, such as mental illness, domestic violence, and substance abuse (HUD, 2010). The Continuum of Care model is composed of six components: prevention, outreach and assessment, emergency shelter, transitional housing, supportive housing, and supportive services. This model served as a guide for the assessment of a city in the southern United States, hereafter referred to as "Townville."

ASSESSMENT OF HOMELESSNESS IN TOWNVILLE

The city of Townville is approximately 52% female and 48% male. The racial make-up of the population is nearly 67% white, approximately 31% black, and 2% "other" races. The median home value in Townville is $25,000 less than the state median home value. Per capita income is 20% less than the state average, and nearly 16% of the residents live below the poverty level. More than 5000 people in Townville are uninsured (hopehealthclinic.com, 2010).

The continuum component "prevention" was not assessed in Townville. This component involves community efforts to prevent homelessness. The continuum component "outreach and assessment" was loosely analyzed. No efforts to assess the homeless and available resources or efforts to reach out to the homeless to inform and engage them in available services were observed.

The component "emergency shelter" proved to be a central element of the Townville assessment. The shelter in Townville is the sole emergency shelter for the county. It can house 32 people for two- to four-week stays, and accepts men, women, and children. This shelter meets a tremendous need in the community, and is at risk of imminent closure due to lack of funding.

Sheltered individuals receive a hot breakfast every day, but are required to leave the property afterward until the shelter reopens in the late afternoon, when a hot evening meal is served. During the day, sheltered and unsheltered homeless persons can be found congregating underneath two bridges in Townville.

The component "transitional housing" describes a type of supportive housing that facilitates the movement from emergency shelter to permanent housing. Transitional housing was assessed as lacking in Townville. One transitional home for men is operated by a local church and houses a maximum of 15 men. One center for women will accept women who are homeless for any reason; however, the primary mission of this center is to serve women who are victims of domestic violence. Women experiencing domestic violence are accepted before women who are homeless for other reasons. Transitional housing is offered to a small number of homeless who enroll in substance abuse treatment at a local recovery organization. The component "supportive and permanent affordable housing" was not assessed in Townville.

The component "supportive services" includes case management; employment, training, and education; health care; substance abuse treatment; mental health; and child care. Case management for the homeless in Townville is situated within the services accessed by this population. There is not a universal case management effort in Townville. Health care, substance abuse treatment, mental health services and food resources were the primary focus of the assessment in Townville.

Health care is provided to the homeless in Townville by a local community clinic, a free clinic located within the county health department, and the local hospital emergency room. The local community clinic is heavily utilized by the working poor and uninsured in Townville. Providers at this clinic see, on average, 60 patients per day. Patients are seen by appointment only, which serves as a huge barrier to care for the homeless. This clinic is conveniently located next door to the local food kitchen. The free clinic located in the health department will see patients on a walk-in basis, but it is located approximately four miles from the shelter, and is situated on a busy four-lane highway with no sidewalk access. No public transportation is available in Townville. The community clinic focuses on chronic care, and the free clinic provides acute care. Plans are in motion to merge the community clinic and free clinic into one site, to be located next to the current community clinic, which is located next to the weekly food pantry. This new clinic will see patients with acute and chronic conditions on both walk-in and appointment bases. The merger is expected to provide the clinic with greater funding opportunities while decreasing operating costs.

Currently, the barriers to access to each facility promote use by the homeless of the local emergency room for health care. The nurse manager of the emergency room and several staff nurses agreed that this emergency room is utilized by the homeless at a high rate, but this utilization did not overly stress the department.

A dental clinic is located within the free health department clinic, and will be located in the new merged health clinic. In addition, a local dentist schedules one Saturday per month to perform extractions for the homeless at no cost.

Mental health services are provided free of charge for the homeless through a regional community services organization. Homeless patients are provided with counseling and medications if necessary. This organization also assists with job placement and other services. Substance abuse treatment is delivered through a local organization that can house people in recovery, on both short-term and long-term bases.

Two soup kitchens are in operation in Townville; one serves a hot lunch Monday through Thursday and a sack lunch on Friday, and the other functions as a weekend soup kitchen that provides a hot meal for lunch Saturday and Sunday. The weekly soup kitchen is thriving. As many as 100 people are served daily. The director reports an overabundance of volunteers, some of whom are occasionally turned away due to lack of work. The weekend soup kitchen is new, and is expected to do well in this community. A clothes closet is located in the weekend soup kitchen, and other clothes closets are located within several local churches.

Over the course of the community assessment, the author of this chapter communicated extensively with key stakeholders on primarily a face-to-face basis, but also by phone and e-mail. These stakeholders included the director of the food pantry and community clinic, the soup kitchen directors and workers, staff nurses, nurse practitioners, the county nurse manager, ministers, police, the county coroner, restaurant and grocery store managers, directors of transitional homes, the director of the emergency shelter, and, most importantly, the homeless themselves. Homeless persons were interviewed in a variety of venues to get their thoughts and opinions of the services they were or were not able to access in Townville.

Five homeless persons were asked general, informal questions regarding their health and life in the shelter (no unsheltered homeless were available for discussion). All but one of these homeless people were younger than 40 years of age, and all but one were male. These observations were supported by the work of Lafuente and Lane (1995), who reported that homeless men remain the most visible segment of the population, and that currently homeless people are younger, with a mean age of 31 to 38 years old. One man represented a family of five—his wife and three children younger than the age of 5 were staying together in the shelter. One man was a victim of assault by a roommate and was nursing a knife wound to the abdomen. He reported his incision was healing well, and that he had been given adequate supplies to care for his wounds. When asked what he needed most right now, he began to weep and responded, "A job!" Another man was a convicted felon who had completed his prison sentence and was released to the street. He also began to weep as he described how his life had taken "a bad turn," but he was optimistic about his current situation and hopeful regarding an upcoming job interview.

One young man expressed no needs except a job. A pregnant young woman spoke at length about her pregnancy and the baby's father—another shelter resident. She spoke freely and honestly about her to efforts to "get back on her feet." She stated that she could hardly wait to get her own place so she could decorate a nursery for the baby. This woman also spoke of her struggles to locate an obstetrician willing to care for her and her baby. As Swanson, Andersen, and Gelberg (2003) reported, services for the homeless are usually not organized to care for the needs of pregnant women.

All of the homeless persons interviewed spoke positively regarding the shelter, although most reported they did not like having rules and being "kicked out" in the mornings. Each felt shelter staff truly cared for them.

Regarding healthcare access in Townville, most had only negative comments. One man stated, "It's too far to walk to the health department, and you can't get an appointment at the clinic . . . so I just don't go." The father of three recalled a recent struggle to get his infant son seen for what turned out to be bronchitis. Swanson et al. (2003) found that having children negatively and significantly affected healthcare quality and access satisfaction. At least two homeless persons reported they did not get sick and had not needed health care—evidence that preventive health care may not be a priority for the homeless.

As described by Markos and Allen (2001) and Schanzer et al. (2007), the homeless frequently seek medical treatment in hospital emergency rooms due to lack of access to basic health care. All five homeless people from Townville stated their first choice for health care would be the local emergency room and cited reasons supported by Carter, Green, Green, and Dufour (1994): accessibility, transportation, present-time orientation, and limited resources. Savage et al. (2006) suggest reduction in use of emergency departments by the homeless can be achieved by adding community-based approaches that provide cost-effective care and enable the homeless to better care for themselves. O'Toole et al. (2007) underscore the importance to the homeless of treatment on demand. The merger of the two health clinics in Townville may very well accomplish this task.

Each homeless person reported feeling stigmatized and disrespected by healthcare providers and the community in general. One young man stated, "You walk all over this city for hours putting in applications, and as soon as they know you're homeless or you use the shelter address, they're not interested." As found in a study by Carter et al. (1994), regarding life in general, each homeless person voiced dissatisfaction with his or her current situation.

CONCLUSIONS AND RECOMMENDATIONS ABOUT HELP FOR THE HOMELESS IN TOWNVILLE

Overall, it appears that Townville takes good care of the homeless. Several needs were identified by this student and key stakeholders for the homeless in this community, including transportation, increased funding for the emergency shelter, more shelters and transitional homes, a day center, and greater accessibility to health care. Other needs identified include job training and a universal case management system for the homeless in Townville.

Recommendations for the future include an in-depth, formal study of Townville's homeless population, their health, and their healthcare-seeking behaviors. Valuable data could be collected through replication of a study by Gelberg, Andersen, and Leake (2000) that investigated the health and use of healthcare services by the homeless using the framework of the Behavioral Model for Vulnerable Populations. This health services utilization model considers predisposing, enabling, and need components as predictors of healthcare services utilization. Findings from this study could then be integrated into the assessment aspect of the three core functions of public health, the other two being policy development and assurance (Hatton et al., 2001). Assessment includes all activities involved in community diagnosis, such as needs assessment and appraisal of the health of the homeless, health screenings, case finding, and monitoring (Hatton et al., 2001). It is this crucial assessment piece that guides policy development and provides assurance that necessary services are provided and goals are met.

Alternatively, Townville could engage in the U.S. Federal Strategic Plan to Prevent and End Homelessness (U.S. Interagency Council on Homelessness, 2010). This strategic plan has four goals:

- Finish the job of ending chronic homelessness in 5 years
- Prevent and end homelessness for families, youth, and children in 10 years
- Prevent and end homelessness among veterans in 5 years
- Set a path to ending all types of homelessness.

Built into this federal strategic plan are 10 objectives, of which objectives 7, 8, and 9 address the health of the homeless. This comprehensive plan seeks to integrate health care and housing so as to provide the homeless with greater stability as they transition from homeless to housed.

Townville is doing many things right. The homeless in this community are well fed, well dressed, and, for the most part, well sheltered. The merger of the clinics is anticipated to greatly improve access to health care and dental care by the homeless in Townville.

The experience of speaking to the homeless was extremely valuable. Preconceived notions were shattered, as these people were pleasant, friendly, and interested in telling their stories. Their physical appearance did not fit the stereotypical homeless person. This student would never have guessed these people were homeless based solely on their appearance. As a heterogeneous group, the homeless cannot be characterized by long-held stereotypes. This assignment proved enlightening and moving, and will be long remembered, as new networks and contacts were formed, and several volunteer opportunities opened to this student.

For a full suite of assignments and additional learning activities, use the access code located in the front of your book to visit this exclusive website: http://go.jblearning.com/dechesnay. If you do not have an access code, you can obtain one at the site.

REFERENCES

Baggett, T., O'Connell, J., Singer, D., & Rigotti, N. (2010). The unmet health care needs of homeless adults: A national study. *American Journal of Public Health, 100*(7), 1326–1331.

Bottomley, J., Bissonnette, A., & Snekvik, V. (2001). The lives of homeless older adults: Please, tell them who I am. *Topics in Geriatric Rehabilitation, 16*(4), 50–64.

Carter, K., Green, R., Green, L., & Dufour, L. (1994). Health needs of homeless clients accessing nursing care at a free clinic. *Journal of Community Health Nursing, 11*(3), 139–147.

Darbyshire, P., Muir-Cochrane, E., Fereday, J., Jureidini, J., & Drummond, A. (2006). Engagement with health and social care services: Perceptions of homeless young people with mental health problems. *Health and Social Care in the Community, 14*(6), 553–562. doi: 10.1111/j.1365-2524.2006.00643.x

de Chesnay, M. (2008). Vulnerable populations: Vulnerable people. In M. de Chesnay & B. Anderson (Eds.), *Caring for the vulnerable: Perspectives in nursing theory, practice, and research* (2nd ed., pp. 3–14). Sudbury, MA: Jones & Bartlett.

Diaski, I. (2007). Perspectives of homeless people on their health and health needs priorities. *Journal of Advanced Nursing, 58*(3), 273–281. doi: 10.1111/j1365-2648.2007.04234.x

Drury, L. (2008). From homeless to housed: Caring for people in transition. *Journal of Community Health Nursing, 25*, 91–105. doi: 10.1080/07370010802017109

Food and Agriculture Organization of the United States. (2010). Retrieved from http://www.fao.org/WorldFoodSummit/english/fsheets/food.pdf

Gelberg, L., Andersen, R., & Leake, B. (2000). The behavioral model for vulnerable populations: Application to medical care use and outcomes for homeless people. *Health Services Research, 34*(6), 1273–1302.

Hatton, D. (2001). Homeless women's access to health services: A study of social networks and managed care in the U.S. *Women and Health, 33*(3/4), 167–181.

Hatton, D., Kleffel, D., Bennett, S., & Gaffrey, E. (2001). Homeless women and children's access to health care: A paradox. *Journal of Community Health Nursing, 18*(1), 25–34.

hopehealthclinic.com. (2010). Retrieved from http://www.hopehealthclinic.com

Hudson, A., Nyamathi, A., & Sweat, J. (2008). Homeless youth's interpersonal perspectives of health care providers. *Issues in Mental Health Nursing, 29*, 1277–1289. doi: 10.1080/01612840802498235

Lafuente, C., & Lane, P. (1995). The lived experience of homeless men. *Journal of Community Health Nursing, 12*(4), 211–219.

Macnee, C., & McCabe, S. (2004). Satisfaction with care among homeless patients: Development and testing of a measure. *Journal of Community Health Nursing, 12*(3), 167–178.

Markos, P., & Allen, D. (2001). A model of primary healthcare service delivery for individuals who are homeless. *Guidance and Counseling, 16*(4), 127.

Martins, D. (2008). Experiences of homeless people in the health care delivery system: A descriptive phenomenological study. *Public Health Nursing, 25*(5), 420–430. doi: 10.1111/j.1525–1446.2008.00726.x

National Coalition for the Homeless. (2010). Retrieved from http://www.nationalhomeless.org

Nickash, B., & Marnocha, S. (2009). Healthcare experiences of the homeless. *Journal of the American Academy of Nurse Practitioners, 21*, 39–46. doi: 10.1111/j1745-7599.200800371.x

O'Toole, T., Conde-Martel, A., Gibbon J., Hanusa, B., Freyder, P., & Jine, M. (2007). Where do people go when they first become homeless? A survey of homeless adults in the USA. *Health and Social Care in the Community, 15*(5), 446–453. doi: 10.1111/j.1365-2524.2007.00703.x

Savage, C., Lindsell, C., Gillespie, G., Dempsey, A., Lee, R., & Corbin, A. (2006). Health care needs of homeless adults at a nurse-managed clinic. *Journal of Community Health Nursing, 23*(4), 225–234.

Schanzer, B., Dominguez, B., Shrout, P., & Caton, C. (2007). Homelessness, health status, and health care use. *American Journal of Public Health, 97*(3), 464–469.

Swanson, K., Andersen, R. & Gelberg, L. (2003). Patient satisfaction for homeless women. *Journal of Women's Health, 12*(7), 675–687.

U.S. Department of Housing and Urban Development (HUD). (2010). Retrieved from http://www.hudhre.info

U.S. Interagency Council on Homelessness. (2010). Retrieved from: http://www.usich.gov

Wen, C., Hudak, P., & Hwang, S. (2007). Homeless people's perceptions of welcomeness and unwelcomeness in healthcare encounters. *Journal of General Internal Medicine, 22*, 1011–1017. doi: 10.1007/s11606-007-0183-7

Zlotnick, C., & Zerger, S. (2008). Survey findings on characteristics and health status of clients treated by the federally funded (US) Healthcare for the Homeless programs. *Health and Social Care in the Community, 17*(1), 18–26. doi: 10.1111/j.1365-2524.2008.00793.x

Designing and Implementing a Cultural Competence Education Model of School Nurses: Working with African American Children and Families

Rebecca Green

Objectives

WWW

At the end of this chapter, the reader will be able to

1. Describe the cultural factors of South Georgia that necessitate a cultural competence approach to school nursing.
2. Describe an intervention that school nurses can use to provide health care for African American children.
3. Describe the outcomes that would be expected from the intervention and how to measure them.

The doctor of nursing science program at a mid-size metropolitan university in Georgia offers a "Special Topics: Vulnerable Populations" course, which provides an opportunity for doctoral-level nursing students to explore in-depth special issues related to nursing education in an increasingly complex healthcare climate. The course requirements include a literature analysis on a special topic of the student's choice related to vulnerable populations; completion of fieldwork designed to improve the student's cultural competence with a specific population; and preparation of a teaching plan for undergraduate or graduate students, or a project for practicing nurses, to promote cultural competence with a specific population.

One student, a practicing school nurse in a metropolitan school district in south Georgia, elected to complete an analysis of available literature related to her primary population of service, African Americans, with particular attention to African American culture as it relates to health care, health disparities, and health issues of African Americans. A survey of cultural competence educational tools and curriculum was included in the review as well. She used information acquired during the review of literature to improve her own cultural competence, and to design and implement an educational module for the school nurses in her system to promote cultural competence in working with African American children and families. The literature analysis was begun in late August and continued through September; design of the education module was completed in October; and implementation, consisting of a two-hour in-service program held in the school district's central office, took place in early November. A report of the completed project was delivered in the final "Special Topics: Vulnerable Populations" class meeting, and the culminating paper was completed by the end of the semester, in early December.

DESCRIPTION OF SCHOOL SYSTEM, POPULATION, AND SCHOOL NURSES IN SOUTH GEORGIA

The small city school system in south Georgia serves approximately 7500 students, approximately 77% of whom are African American. The area has long struggled with racial disparities that exist between two school systems. The city school system serves primarily minority families, whereas the county system serves primarily white families. All of the schools in the city system are Title I schools, which indicates that at least 40% of the students in the school qualify for free or reduced-price lunch. Title I status is a federal educational funding program for school systems that enroll a high proportion of students at risk for failure and living at or near the poverty level (U.S. Department of Education, 2010).

Both the county and city school systems have long benefited from progressive school nurse programs and policies. Even before the Tobacco Master Settlement of 1998 created a start-up funding source for school nurse programming in Georgia (Master Settlement Agreement, 2002), the regional district health director had established a school nurse program for the whole health district, using public health funds. Over the years, that initiative morphed into a local school nursing program that currently is funded primarily through local school board budgets. The city school board has made a clear and enthusiastic commitment to having a registered nurse in every city school for the entire school day. During the 2008–2009 school year, student illness and injury visits to school clinics totaled more than 15,000. In that same year, more than 1000 students in the system were documented as having asthma, 215 with severe allergy, 48 with diabetes, 103 with hypertension, 19 with sickle cell disease, 19 with migraine, 69 with seizure disorder, 134 with moderate to profound mental retardation, and 108 with other serious health impairments (Green, 2007).

There are eight schools in the city school system, each with a registered nurse. The nurses are white females who range in age from 28 to 45 years of age. They come from a variety of pediatric practice backgrounds. Their experience in school nursing ranges from 1 year to 10 years.

JUSTIFYING THE INTERVENTION: POTENTIAL FOR CULTURAL MISMATCH, POTENTIAL FOR CULTURAL BROKERAGE

Madeleine Leininger is a nurse anthropologist who began her theory development in the 1960s in the western United States, in response to the growing diversity of the population and the need for nurses to have relevant practice skills. Leininger's theory of transcultural nursing ("culture care, diversity, and universality") posits that caring is the essence of nursing. *Care* is a culturally universal phenomenon that refers to a feeling of compassion, interest, and concern for people. Leininger's (1985, 1987) theory places caring within a context of culture, and defines culture as "the lifeways of an individual or a group with reference to values, beliefs, norms, patterns, and practices . . . that are learned, shared, and handed down" (1997, p. 38). In addition to culture, the environmental context of care includes physical, ecological, and sociopolitical influences that give meaning to human expressions of care. Transcultural nursing care "is congruent with cultural values, beliefs, and practices" (Dayer-Berenson, 2011, p. 16). Caring assists, supports, and enables behaviors that comfort or heal the patient (Leininger, 1985). Culture care is universal, but its expression—in the form of action, pattern, expression, lifestyle, and meaning—may vary (Leininger, 1985).

Leininger's theory requires that the nurse both develop an awareness of his or her own personal style and cultural values and consider the possibility of cultural misunderstandings that may occur when caring for patients—what Leininger (1985) calls *cultural mismatch*. Cultural mismatch causes cultural pain when the receiver feels insulted, hurt, or stressed because of inappropriate words spoken or actions performed by someone who lacks awareness, sensitivity, or understanding of another culture (Leininger, 1985, 1997). If a cultural mismatch occurs within a patient–provider encounter, it must be recognized and addressed; if it is ignored, a critical failure to form a therapeutic alliance may result (Dayer-Berenson, 2011). Majority-culture institutions, such as schools and hospitals, that provide care or service to minority populations are fertile ground for cultural mismatch (Sadler, Samuels, Cleveland, & Tyler, 2009; Villegas, 1988). Indeed, as many as 40% of school health professionals report that their programs are affected by cultural issues (Center for Health and Health Care in Schools, 2004).

School nurses exist with their patients in the intersection of two majority-culture institutions—education and health care—and are uniquely situated to act as cultural brokers. The National Center for Cultural Competence (NCCC, 2010) states that anyone may serve as a cultural broker, even if that person is not a member of the particular community. Cultural brokers must, however, possess the following: trust and respect of the community; knowledge and understanding of the cultures values, beliefs, and health practices; understanding of traditional health networks; and experience navigating health care and other supportive community systems (NCCC, 2010). Coleman (2009) found that culturally congruent care resulted in African American mothers perceiving friendliness, respectfulness, and attentiveness from their nurse. Research has demonstrated that culturally congruent care results in care recipients being more likely to follow healthcare recommendations, whereas recipients who do not feel respected have less confidence in treatment recommendations (Betancourt, Green, Carrillo, & Park, 2005; Blanchard & Lurie, 2004). Others have identified the critical nature of connectedness between nurses and their patients in public health settings as a component of cultural competence (Doutrich & Storey, 2004).

Brooks, Kendall, Bunn, Bindler, and Bruya (2007) confirm that the school nurse may be pivotal as the "only professional concerned with children's wellbeing that traverses all the environments of the child, i.e. the home, the school and the wider community as well as connecting with the multi-sectoral nature of the service provision for young people" (p. 8). The potential for cultural mismatch in the relationship between school nurses and their patients and families, in combination with the pivotal role that school nurses are positioned to fill as cultural brokers, creates a perfect opportunity to improve the provider–patient relationship and to infuse that relationship with compassion. Pacquiao (2008) identifies compassion in the nurse–patient relationship as a means to improve outcomes by reducing the negative influences of cultural differences.

CHARACTERISTICS OF AFRICAN AMERICAN HEALTH AND CULTURE

African Americans make up approximately 13.5% of the total U.S. population (Dayer-Berenson, 2011). The majority of African Americans in the United States are descended from enslaved Africans brought to North America against their will beginning in the seventeenth century. Other African Americans are more recent voluntary immigrants from Africa and the Caribbean. The United States has a long history of institutional and non-institutional racism and discrimination against African Americans. Dayer-Berenson cited this long history as contributing to "the legacy of mistrust of the healthcare system that persists today" (2011, p. 137). Consideration of the health of the African American family would not be complete without the acknowledgment of this dynamic.

Health Issues

Although the top three causes of death for African Americans—heart disease, cancer, and stroke—are the same as those for whites, the Centers for Disease Control and Prevention (CDC) has reported that "the risk factors and incidence, morbidity, and mortality rates for these diseases and injuries often are greater among Africans than whites" (2005, p. 1). In addition, three of the top 10 leading causes of death for African Americans are not leading causes of death for whites—namely, homicide, human immunodeficiency virus (HIV), and septicemia (CDC, 2005). African Americans lose a greater number of potential life years than whites due to perinatal diseases and diabetes (CDC, 2005). Among African American women, the incidence of colorectal cancer, pancreatic cancer, and stomach cancer is substantially higher than that for white women; among African American men, the incidence of prostate, lung, colorectal, and stomach cancer is significantly higher than that for white men (CDC, 2005). African American children also develop asthma at a much higher rate than white children (Gold & Wright, 2005).

Access to Health Care

African Americans also lag behind white Americans in percentage of persons younger than 65 years old with health insurance (CDC, 2005). African Americans are more likely to rely on hospitals and clinics (as opposed to a primary care provider) for health care than are white Americans (U.S. Department of Health and Human Services [HHS], 2000b). Despite the obvious contributors to reduced access to care, lower rates of health insurance, and lower incomes of African Americans, more insidious processes are at work in determining access to care. In one study, researchers found that African Americans received poorer quality of care during hospitalization for congestive heart failure and pneumonia; another showed that African women were less likely than white men to be referred for cardiac catheterization, even when they exhibited similar symptoms (HHS, 2000b). These examples of disparities in health care are only a few of many cited in the literature.

Other cultural factors may also affect access to care for African Americans. The National Minority AIDS Education and Training Center (NMAETC, 2011) identified some of these factors as poor availability of services in certain neighborhoods or communities; economic hardship; stigmatization of certain diseases, such as HIV; cultural avoidance of discussing sex-related and drug- or alcohol-related behaviors; privacy and honor; distrust; and language or communication difficulty.

African adults are also less likely than white adults to be vaccinated against flu and pneumococcus, receive prenatal care in the first trimester of pregnancy, and participate in regular moderate physical activity (CDC, 2005). African children have lower rates of immunization than white children. Both African adults and children are more likely to be obese than their white counterparts (CDC, 2005). Again, these are just a few examples of many differences in healthcare outcomes related to healthcare access.

Other Disparities

Disparities in areas other than health exist between African and white Americans. Some of these include income, educational, and employment disparities, as well as higher rates of incarceration and homelessness (Hopps, Tourse, & Christian, 2002; Utsey, Geisbrecht, Hook, & Stanard, 2008). They also have lower wages and more often live in substandard housing than whites (Brody, Dorsey, Forehand, & Armistead, 2002). In addition, some research has found that African Americans suffer from race-related stress and resultant poorer mental health functioning, and that racism may result in greater psychological distress than even stressful life events (Utsey et al., 2008).

In short, many complex factors influence the disparities experienced by African Americans. Copeland (2005) describes the sources of these disparities as multivariate and complex, with contributing factors including "lack of access to care; barriers to care; increased risk of disability and disease resulting from occupational exposure; biologic, socioeconomic, ethnic and family factors; cultural values and education; social relationships between majority and minority population groups . . . ; and culturally insensitive health care systems" (p. 265). There are, however, many positive cultural influences on the health of African Americans.

Strengths, Protective Factors, and Resilience

The literature suggests that particular strengths and protective factors are associated with African American cultural values. The NMAETC (2011) identified these cultural values as spirituality, meaning "an inner strength that comes from trusting in God"; communalism, or "a strong history of collective group orientation that incorporates personal relationships, social support systems, and collective resources over individualism"; oral tradition, which "speaks to the communal nature of the people that focuses on face-to-face contact and dialogue"; internal strength; resolve; and respect for elders (valuing the wisdom and experience of elder family members).

Seminal work by Hill (1972) refuted much previous research that had identified African American family structure as pathological (when compared with white family structure). According to Hill, successful African American families demonstrate strong kinship bonds, strong work orientation, adaptability in family roles, strong achievement orientation, and strong religious orientation.

Miller-Cribbs and Farber (2008) evaluated the traditional literature identifying close kinship and extended family structures as evidence of resilience in African American families. In the face of limited and unpredictable availability of resources, the African American community has demonstrated adaptive strategies by creating extended kinship care, with shared resources including money, child care, and housing. These authors, however, cited evidence that as the African middle class has grown and as individuals with greater economic choice have moved away from low-income communities, those left behind have tended to become more isolated and less resilient as the kin network became more stretched. The farther kin moved away, the less support they provided to the original kinship network. As a consequence, as support needed increased, support received decreased. In a painful twist, in low-income neighborhoods where shared living may ameliorate financial stress, the same shared living has been demonstrated to increase relationship stress due to overcrowding, lack of privacy, and sharing scarce resources. After their review of the literature of several decades, Miller-Cribbs and Farber (2008) questioned whether it can be assumed that kinship networks remain a source of resilience in African American families.

Sanders, Lim, and Sohn (2008), in their study of African American families with incomes less than 250% of the federal poverty level, suggested that although institutional discrimination and poverty may increase susceptibility to poor social integration, low control, depressive symptoms, and a fatalistic outlook in some African Americans, supportive social networks and church attendance may act as a buffer to these negative effects, thereby enhancing resilience. These authors also piloted a study using tooth loss as a highly quantitative measure of health resilience. Health resilience was determined by evaluating indicators such as housing quality, social support, familial influence, religiosity, and mental health status. The researchers found that resilient adults in this particular African American community were more than three times more likely to retain 20 or more teeth than less resilient adults. Likewise, children who had resilient caregivers had a lower rate of tooth decay.

DESIGN OF THE EDUCATIONAL INTERVENTION

Learning specifics about African American culture, health and health disparities, strengths, and protective factors was a critical component of preparing the educational intervention for school nurses. The Office of Minority Health (OMH) educational module (HHS, 2007a) stresses the importance of both skill and knowledge. A sound knowledge base paved the way for designing the cultural competence educational intervention for school nurses.

There is a wealth of literature available related to models and methods for promoting cultural competence of clinicians, and its importance in the clinical setting and in the education of clinicians (Betancourt, Green, Carrillo, & Aneneh-Firempong, 2003; Briggs & McBeath, 2010; Campinha-Bacote, 1999, 2009; Douglas et al., 2009; Eiser & Ellis, 2007; Jakeway, Cantrell, Cason, & Talley, 2006; Kim-Godwin, Clark, & Barton, 2001; Kleinman & Benson, 2006; Martin et al., 2005; Pacquiao, 2008; Parish, 2003). In an extensive review of these sources and others, the curriculum design of the "Delivering Culturally Competent Nursing Care Course I" training module offered by the U.S. Department of Health and Human Services' (2007a) Office of Minority Health seemed most comprehensive and user-friendly, and carefully aligned with nationally accepted Culturally and Linguistically Appropriate Services (CLAS) standards defined by the OMH (HHS, 2000a). A complete list of the references used in developing this comprehensive curriculum can be found on the OMH's website (HHS, 2007b). Senior Health Policy analyst Darci Graves graciously gave the author permission to use and modify the content of the module as needed (D. Graves, personal communication, September 24, 2010). The OMH module is designed to award 3.0 hours of continuing education (CE) credit; therefore, in addition to receiving professional learning credit through the school system, nurses who participated in the class were able to register on the OHM website, complete the online module, and receive CE credits for completing the module.

The OMH module was modified by the addition of content specific to African American health, based on the author's literature review. Two group activities and three case studies were added, designed to elicit personal, experiential engagement in the topic. The 15-item pre-test and post-test were based on the OMH tests, but included new questions relevant to African American health and one open-ended question related to school nursing.

DESCRIPTION OF THE IMPLEMENTATION

One week prior to the scheduled in-service program, the participants were provided with a letter of explanation and consent requesting that they participate. At that time they were provided with a pre test of the material to complete prior to the in-service session. In the letter, they were advised that completion of the pre-test and participation in the in-service activity implied consent to participate, and that they could freely choose to decline participation at any time. All consented to participate and brought the completed pre-test to the in-service program.

Six school nurses were welcomed to the cultural competence training session held at the Central Office boardroom of the city school system in November 2010. The participants are well acquainted with one another, both professionally and socially. A brief overview of the course was provided, and participants were directed to restrooms and vending areas. Snacks were provided. The training opened with a 10-minute fun and informal group activity designed to serve as an ice-breaker and to highlight the impact of cultural difference in interpersonal and group interactions. The group members were told that each had been chosen to participate in an important group task—building a tower out of marshmallows and spaghetti noodles. Each nurse was privately assigned a hypothetical cultural role she was expected to act out during the activity. Some examples of the purely imaginary cultural roles are as follows:

> You come from a cultural group that practices extended hand-shaking when communicating. Whenever engaged in conversation, you grip the other speaker's hand warmly and shake the hand vigorously for the length of the conversation. You speak a language with variations of the word "google": googly-goo-goo.
>
> You are committed to self-reflection and personal improvement. Whenever you are asked to participate in a group activity, it is important to you to get everyone's opinion about yourself, your strengths, and your weaknesses before beginning work. Personal insight is much more important than the task at hand.
>
> You come from a cultural group in which any physical contact or communication with blondes is expressly forbidden. If a blonde speaks to you, you must squeeze your eyes shut and clap three times to ward off evil.
>
> This group requires strong moral leadership. It is imperative that you take a moral stand and lead this group. You are aware that building marshmallow towers is a dangerous activity, and think that keeping the marshmallows together in the bag is important.

The group activity was followed by a debriefing in which the participants were asked to consider feelings that occurred during the activity, reflect on how the activity mimics what happens in real life, and think about how the activity might have gone more smoothly if participants had understood cultural and personal differences.

The rest of the presentation followed roughly the content of an online educational module for nurses entitled "Delivering Culturally Competent Nursing Care, Course I," which is part of the OMH's (HHS, 2007a) *Think Cultural Health* series (available at https://ccnm.thinkculturalhealth.hhs.gov/). The content of this module was modified for use in a lecture and PowerPoint format, with content specific to African American health added for relevance to the school nurse practice situation.

Culture was defined and cultural competence described as an ongoing process. Participants were asked to identify some cultures different from their own. As a practical point, the Western healthcare system was identified as a culture with its own set of beliefs and values. A discussion of why culture is important in the healthcare setting included a discussion of health disparities in minority populations and identification of the clinician's purpose and role as a provider of patient-centered care. Key terms, such as "ethnocentrism" and "essentialism," were defined as an introduction to becoming more culturally competent. Personal reflection questions were asked that clinicians might consider in their desire to become more culturally competent. These questions were part of the author's modification of the OHM curriculum, and were based on Camphina-Bacote's (2002) ASKED mnemonic self-examination questions. They included "Am I aware of my biases and prejudices towards other cultural groups?"; "Am I knowledgeable about the worldviews of different cultural and ethnic groups?"; and "Do I seek out face-to-face and other types of interactions with individuals who are different from myself?"

Part of this discussion included a group activity (based on a similar exercise described by Wicks, 2003) in which participants were asked to identify a value that they had held since childhood. They were asked who taught them this value, how the value influences them today, how it affects their health and illness behavior, and how their life might be different if they did not hold this value. Some of their responses included "honesty" and "strong work ethic." They were asked to consider how other cultures might hold other, conflicting values, such as family cohesion or fatalism, which might influence them just as strongly and result in different health and illness responses.

Three case studies, based on the OMH curriculum (HHS, 2007a), were presented in a slightly modified format: One was a case study of a Native American toddler brought to the emergency room by his grandmother; a second described a young Vietnamese American gang-affiliated youth receiving treatment from an HIV clinic; and the third involved an elderly Chinese man on a medical–surgical floor following surgery. Each of these cases was reviewed in terms of cultural barriers to care, and discussion ensued regarding how specific cultural mismatches could have been avoided and patient outcomes improved. The importance of avoiding stereotyping was emphasized.

The Western approach to disease and illness was identified as a possible barrier to culturally competent care. Specific cultural beliefs about health and illness were offered as examples of potential conflict. Cultural insights about health and illness from a variety of cultural perspectives were offered, with specific recommendations for clinical practice. A more comprehensive discussion of African American culture as related to health ensued, with particular reference to African American history and institutional racism, extended family support networks, religion and spirituality, and health literacy, as well as factors associated with resilience in African Americans. The content was based on the literature review previously completed by the author. A reference list of these sources was provided to the participants, as well as a particularly salient and interesting article by Russell and Jewell (1992).

Specific interventions for clinicians working with African Americans were suggested. Some of these included encouraging patients to ask their primary care providers about their illness. Specific reference was made to the "Ask Me 3" program described by Michalopoulou, Falzaran, Arfken, and Rosenberg (2010), which has been demonstrated to improve African American patients' knowledge of their illness and increase their satisfaction with the healthcare encounter.

Recommendations were also made for culturally competent communication. These guidelines included approaching patients slowly, greeting them respectfully, asking them how they would like to be addressed, avoiding severe facial expressions and gestures, and asking questions, among others.

Culturally competent care was characterized as effective, restoring the patient to his or her desired health status (not the clinician's goal); understandable, accommodating the patient's language, reading level, and comprehension; respectful, creating a nonjudgmental environment where the values and preferences of the patient are of high priority; and knowledgeable, based on knowledge of a culture gained from unbiased sources, key informants, and the patient, rather than stereotyping. Cultural competence was characterized as requiring desire, self-awareness, and a balance between skill and knowledge. The module was closed with a quote from Campinha-Bacote: "Cultural humility is a quality of seeing the greatness in others and coming into the realization of the dignity and worth of others. As health care professionals, nurses do not have to accept the patient's belief system; however, nurses must treat each person as a unique human being worthy and deserving of love and care" (2009, pp. 49–50).

Time for questions and discussion followed the module, with an opportunity for a course evaluation and post-test. In addition, all of the participants were provided with a Cultural Diversity Self-Assessment (n.d.) from Indiana University as a tool they might use to initiate discussion about cultural competence with friends, families, and coworkers, as well as a fact sheet about African American demographics and health from the OMH (HHS, 2010).

EVALUATION AND RECOMMENDATIONS (WHAT THEY LEARNED, WHAT I LEARNED)

Each participant's test score improved following implementation of the curriculum, demonstrating that the test questions accurately reflected the content of the module. Ten of the test questions were borrowed directly from the OMH *Think Cultural Health* test questions; the other four closed-ended questions were added to test comprehension of the added content related to African American health and culture. Pre-test scores ranged from a low of 29% to a high of 64%. Post-test scores ranged from a low of 86% to a high of 100%.

The following open-ended item was added at the end of the pre-test: "As a school nurse, write briefly about an encounter with a patient or family in which you think race/ethnicity was a significant factor." Some excerpts of the responses were as follows:

- "I was examining a fourth-grade student one day, and she told me she wished she looked like me. When I asked her why, she responded that it was because she wanted to go to college and get a job."
- "I recently called to speak to a parent about her child's health. The child had told me she had for dinner the night before nachos, hot dogs, fried chicken, and pineapple upside-down cake. The mother went on to tell me that that is 'just how we eat' and that her daughter is heavy 'because the whole family is heavy.'"
- "I have a problem with parents constantly changing their phone numbers. Then when they have a working phone, they avoid answering calls from the school."
- "As a school nurse of a predominantly African American school, I have found that the majority of my African American teachers suffer from hypertension. Most have medication but do not follow instructions about how to take them. Daily meds are not taken daily but as the patient feels they need them. I frequently hear about home remedies that a family member has had success with, like drinking vinegar or eating garlic. But I do realize that all races and ethnicities have problems with noncompliance."

- "A mom was unhappy that I called her at work to get her child because he had vomited the night before and the morning of school, and had a stomach ache. She 'smacked and popped' in her attitude toward me. Not a respectful dialogue."
- "I had a father say to me after I tried to explain the importance of getting medical attention for a child's problem that I couldn't understand because I was 'just a white woman.'"
- "I have experienced confusion with terminology that I am not familiar with. For example, I was not familiar with the term 'risen' for a weeping lesion. It surprised me that medical attention was not sought for such a lesion, that it is commonplace."
- "In many cases, the parents are not the primary caregivers; they either live with grandparents, aunts, and uncles. Even though this occurs with other cultural groups, I do see it more in the African American population."

These comments are reflective of the reality that many clinicians have encounters with patients and families in which they feel race or ethnicity is a significant factor either in the health and health practices of the patient or in the patient–clinician communication or perception. It is clear that good intentions and a caring heart, while good starting places for clinicians, are not sufficient in creating cultural competence. Cultural competence requires desire to learn specific skills and knowledge. Cultural competence training and cultural awareness may foster personal insight for clinicians in examining their own biases, convey knowledge for understanding the cultural values of their patients, and provide skills with which they may respond more effectively and sensitively to their patients.

During discussion following the in-service, the nurses reflected on some of their responses to the open-ended test item. They acknowledged the impact they may have in creating a dynamic for children to have a more positive perception of health care in general—not just for the times during the school year in which they encounter the school nurse, but possibly for a lifetime of encounters with healthcare professionals.

For a full suite of assignments and additional learning activities, use the access code located in the front of your book to visit this exclusive website: http://go.jblearning.com/dechesnay. If you do not have an access code, you can obtain one at the site.

REFERENCES

Betancourt, J., Green, A., Carrillo, J., & Aneneh-Firempong, O. (2003). Defining cultural competence: A practical framework for addressing racial/ethnic disparities in health and health care. *Public Health Reports, 118*, 293–302.

Betancourt, J., Green, A., Carrillo, J., & Park, E. (2005). Cultural competence and health care disparities: Key perspectives and trends. *Health Affairs, 24*, 499–505.

Blanchard, J., & Lurie, N. (2004). RESPECT: Patient reports of disrespect in the health care setting and its impact on care. *Journal of Family Practice, 53*, 721.

Briggs, H., & McBeath, B. (2010). Infusing culture into practice: Developing and implementing evidence-based mental health services for African American foster youth. *Child Welfare, 89*(1), 31–60.

Brody, G., Dorsey, S., Forehand, R., & Armistead, L. (2002). Unique and protective contributions of parenting and classroom processes to the adjustment of African American children living in single-parent families. *Child Development, 73*(1), 274–286.

Brooks, F., Kendall, S., Bunn, F., Bindler, R., & Bruya, M. (2007). The school nurse as navigator of the school health journey: Developing the theory and evidence for policy. *Primary Health Care Research, 8*(2), 1–25.

Campinha-Bacote, J. (1999). A model and instrument for addressing cultural competence in health care. *Journal of Nursing Education, 38*(5), 203–207.

Campinha-Bacote, J. (2002). Cultural competency in healthcare delivery: Have I "ASKED" myself the right questions? Retrieved from the Transcultural C.A.R.E Associates website: http://www.transculturalcare.net/Cultural_Competence_Model.htm

Campinha-Bacote, J. (2009). A culturally competent model of care for African Americans. *Urologic Nursing, 29*(1), 49–54.

Centers for Disease Control and Prevention (CDC). (2005). Health disparities experienced by black or African Americans—United States. *Morbidity and Mortality Weekly Report, 54*(1), 1–3. Retrieved from http://www.cdc.gov/mmwr/preview/mmwrhtml/mm5401a1.htm

Center for Health and Health Care in Schools. (2004). Caring across cultures: Achieving competence in a school health setting. Retrieved from http://www.healthinschools.org

Coleman, J. (2009). Culture care meanings of African American parents related to infant mortality and health care. *Journal of Cultural Diversity, 16*(3), 109–119.

Copeland, V. (2005). African Americans: Disparities in health care access and utilization. *Health & Social Work, 30*(3), 265–270.

Cultural Diversity Self-Assessment Inventory. (n.d.). Retrieved from the Indiana University Continuing Education website: http://www.cue.indiana.edu/activitymanual/activities/Cultural%20diversity%20self%20assessment.pdf

Dayer-Berenson, L. (2011). *Cultural competencies for nurses: Impact on health an illness.* Sudbury: MA. Jones & Bartlett Learning.

Douglas, M., Pierce, J., Rosenkoetter, M., Callister, L., Hattar-Pollara, M., Lauderdale, J., . . . Pacquiano, D. (2009). Standards of practice for culturally competent nursing care: A request for comments. *Journal of Transcultural Nursing, 20*(3), 257–269.

Doutrich, D., & Storey, M. (2004). Education and practice: Dynamic partners for improving cultural competence in public health. *Family & Community Health, 27*(4), 298–307.

Eiser, A., & Ellis, G. (2007). Cultural competence and the African American experience with health care: The case for specific content in cross-cultural education. *Academic Medicine, 82*(2), 176–183.

Gold, D., & Wright, R. (2005). Population disparities in asthma. *Annual Review of Public Health, 26*, 89–113.

Green, R. (2007). *Valdosta city schools clinics.* Presented at the Valdosta City School Board meeting on January 28, 2007, Valdosta, GA.

Hill, R. (1972). *The strengths of African families.* New York, NY: Emerson Hall.

Hixon, J. (1998). Developing culturally anchored services: Confronting the challenge of intragroup diversity. In F. Brisbane (Ed.), *Cultural competence for health care professionals working with African American communities: Theory and practice. Cultural Competence Series 7.* DHHS Publication No. 98-3238. Rockville, MD: Substance Abuse and Mental Health Services Administration.

Hopps, J., Tourse, R., & Christian, O. (2002). From problems to personal resilience: Challenges and opportunities in practice with African American youth. *Journal of Ethnic and Cultural Diversity in Social Work, 11*(1–2), 55–77.

Jakeway, C., Cantrell, E., Cason, J., & Talley, B. (2006). Developing population health competencies among public health nurses in Georgia. *Public Health Nursing, 23*(2), 161– 167.

Kim-Godwin, Y., Clarke, P., & Barton, L. (2001). A model for the delivery of culturally competent community care. *Journal of Advanced Nursing, 35*(6), 918–925.

Kleinman, A., & Benson, P. (2006). Anthropology in the clinic: The problem of cultural competency and how to fix it. *PLoS Medicine, 3*(10), 1673–1676.

Leininger, M. (1985). Transcultural care, diversity, and universality: A theory of nursing. *Nursing and Health Care, 6*(4), 209–212.

Leininger, M. (1997). Understanding cultural pain for improved health care. *Journal of Transcultural Nursing, 9*(1), 32–35.

Martin, M., Keys, W., Person, S., Kim, Y., Ashford, R., Kohler, C., & Norton, P. (2005). Enhancing patient–physician communication: A community and culturally based approach. *Journal of Cancer Education, 20*, 150–154.

Master Settlement Agreement 1998. (2002). Washington, DC: National Association of Attorneys General. Retrieved from www.naag.org

Michalopoulou, G., Falzaran, P., Arfken, C., & Rosenberg, D. (2010). Implementing Ask Me 3 to improve African American patient satisfaction and perceptions of physician cultural competency. *Journal of Cultural Diversity, 17*(2), 62–67.

Miller-Cribbs, J., & Farber, N. (2008). Kin networks and poverty among African Americans: Past and present. *Social Work, 53*(1), 43–51.

National Center for Cultural Competence. (2010). Who can fulfill the role of cultural brokers in health care settings? Retrieved from http://www.culturalbroker.info/2_role/4_role.html

National Minority AIDS Education and Training Center (NMAETC). (2011). African- Americans/Africans: Cultural history and beliefs. Retrieved from http://www.nmaetc.org/hiv_impact/african_Americans.php

Pacquiao, D. (2008). Nursing care of vulnerable populations using a framework of cultural competence, social justice and human rights. *Contemporary Nurse, 28*(1–2), 189–196.

Parish, T. (2003). Cultural competence: Do we agree on its meaning and should it be considered a core competency in training programs. *Internet Journal of Academic Physician Assistants, 3*(2). Available at the IJAPA website: http://www.ispub.com/journal/the_internet_journal_of_academic_physician_assistants/volume_6_number_2_23/article/cultural_competence_do_we_agree_on_its_meaning_and_should_it_be_considered_a_core_competency_in_training_programs.html

Russell, K., & Jewell, N. (1992). Cultural impact of health-care access: Challenges for improving the health of African Americans. *Journal of Community Health Nursing, 9*(3), 161–169.

Sadler, S., Samuels, A., Cleveland, R., & Tyler, T. (2009). Cultural competency: A viable approach to health disparities in urban schools. *Journal of Praxis in Multicultural Education, 4*(1). Retrieved from Berkeley Common Press: http://digitalcommons.library.unlv.edu/cgi/viewcontent.cgi?article=1005&context=jpme

Sanders, A., Lim, S., & Sohn, W. (2008). Resilience to urban poverty: Theoretical and empirical considerations of population health. *American Journal of Public Health, 98*(6), 1101– 1106.

U.S. Department of Education. (2010). Guide to U.S. Department of Education programs: Fiscal year 2010. Retrieved from http://www2.ed.gov/programs/gtep/gtep.pdf

U.S. Department of Health and Human Services (HHS), Office of Minority Health. (2000a). Assuring cultural competence in health care: Recommendations for national standards and an outcomes-focused research agenda. *Federal Register, 65*(247), 80865–80879.

U.S. Department of Health and Human Services (HHS). (2000b). *Addressing racial and ethnic disparities in health care fact sheet.* Rockville, MD: Agency for Healthcare Research and Quality. Retrieved from http://www.ahrq.gov/research/disparit.htm

U.S. Department of Health and Human Services (HHS), Office of Minority Health. (2007a). Culturally competent nursing care: A cornerstone of caring. Retrieved from https://ccnm.thinkculturalhealth.hhs.gov

U.S. Department of Health and Human Services (HHS), Office of Minority Health. (2007b). Course I reference library. Retrieved from https://ccnm.thinkculturalhealth.hhs.gov/Content/References/Course1/References15.asp

U.S. Department of Health and Human Services (HHS), Office of Minority Health. (2010). African American profile. Retrieved from http://minorityhealth.hhs.gov/templates/browse.aspx?lvl=3&lvlid=23

Utsey, S., Geisbrecht, N., Hook, J., & Stanard, P. (2008). Cultural, sociofamilial, and psychological resources that inhibit psychological distress in African Americans exposed to stressful life events and race-related stress. *Journal of Counseling Psychology*, *55*(1), 49–62.

Villegas, A. (1988). School failure and cultural mismatch: Another view. *Urban Review*, *20*(4), 253–265.

Wicks, M. (2003). *Seeking professional nursing excellence through cultural competence.* Presentation at the University of Tennessee Health Science Center. Available at the Old Dominion University website: http://hs.odu.edu/nursing/news/Seeking_Professional_Nursing_Excellence_Through_Cultural_Competence.pdf

CHAPTER 38

Clinical Immersion in Family Nursing Practice in Lac du Flambeau

Cheryl Ann Lapp

Objectives

At the end of this chapter, the reader will be able to

1. Describe how a clinical experience conducted on a Native American reservation might differ from a clinical immersion in a foreign country.
2. Identify the cultural characteristics of the Ojibwe population described in the chapter.
3. Describe how the project might be implemented on other reservations.

This chapter describes a clinical immersion project that was piloted on an Indian reservation in northern Wisconsin. Designed for graduate students of nursing, it was developed with the assistance of Family Nurse Practitioner Dana Irmick, Nursing Manager of the Peter Christensen Health Center in Lac du Flambeau, Wisconsin.

INTRODUCTION

Advocacy has been discussed by Lynda Nauright (2008) as a nursing ethic. Given the premise that advocacy is a core nursing value, the question is raised by Nauright: "How then do we prepare students to be patient advocates, to care about advocacy, and to exercise social responsibility?" This question becomes critical when nurses are charged with preparing students for leadership roles in advanced practice with vulnerable populations. When populations are vulnerable due to greater than average risk for developing health problems, the nurse must be prepared for advocacy by being able to assess patients within their operating social context. Simply stated, this means breaking the mold of the individual unit of service in clinic settings, and practicing holistically through considering the many operant forces of family, community, socioeconomic, and cultural features of everyday life.

As a nursing educator, it has been surprising to me how many experienced nurses are resistant to viewing a patient beyond the individual framework. That is, many nurses consider the assessment to be complete when it involves primarily a physical review of systems and perhaps a short interview to "cover" any socioemotional problems. As a consequence, nurse practitioner students are themselves at risk for embracing the constraints of their physician counterparts—being time bound and focused almost exclusively on treatment, diagnosis, and medication disbursement in the most efficient amount of time. The danger for the nurse, of course, is in losing oneself in the medical model and abandoning the nursing identity of loyalty to and advocacy for patients. For example, several of my graduate students—typically those from emergency room (ER), intensive care unit (ICU), or trauma work settings—have admitted in family nursing seminars that they often view the family as an inconvenience. They explain that the families "get in the way of getting my work done" and they would rather not think about routinely incorporating the family into the overall healthcare process. As startling as this position may sound, it is not inconsistent with recent literature (Benzein et al., 2008).

As an educator, it is important to examine with students the structure of the healthcare system and, in their roles as nurses, ways to work with patients within the context of the family and community. One strategy for exploring family nursing practice with students is to work within a culture where family and social context cannot be ignored.

At our university, there is a strategic focus on diversity, cultural competence, and high-impact educational practices. In my own work, I had been regularly visiting the Lac du Flambeau Indian Reservation with the Human Development Center in connection with my school's interdisciplinary undergraduate student activities in the Head Start and School Health program. When I toured the health center and discovered that a former graduate student of family nursing from the University of Wisconsin–Oshkosh was now employed there, I recognized the possibility of a comprehensive and challenging nursing practice experience for my current students. At our university, the educational initiatives for cultural exchange, diversity projects, and other "high impact' experiences are typically located within a funding domain exclusive to undergraduate students because of differential tuition. However, my personal connection with Family Nurse Practitioner and Nursing Manager Dana Irmick gave me the motivation to try to negotiate a clinical contract and "pilot" this opportunity.

BACKGROUND: A DOMESTIC INTERCULTURAL IMMERSION PROJECT

Coincidentally, as this potential practice setting was revealing itself, our Associate Chancellor for Academic Affairs invited proposals for development of a "domestic intercultural immersion project." After consultation with her office, I was enthusiastically encouraged to submit my proposal to benefit graduate students. However, because it did not qualify for differential tuition funding reserved for undergraduates, it was subsequently funded by a local foundation. The budget request was funded to cover six students' shared travel mileage, lodging in a nearby hotel, admission to two cultural heritage centers on the reservation, and miscellaneous educational supplies. Although budgeted food expenses for the students were not funded, a sum of several hundred dollars was reinstated by the funders with the instruction that it be allocated to gifts and food for Ojibwa community members.

The pilot was funded on a one-time basis only, pending the participation of private donors through the Foundation office. This experience has since been repeated twice, in response to ongoing student requests and students' willingness to absorb all of their personal and travel expenses. Community access to this setting was greatly enhanced by the university's Human Development Center (HDC) and its 10-year history of sponsoring the Lac du Flambeau Service-Learning Project, in which interdisciplinary students participate in the Lac du Flambeau Indian School and Head Start Program.

It was through this exposure and taking students to the Indian school and cultural heritage center that I began to explore credit-bearing opportunities for MSN candidates. Our university's essential course content in family nursing (theory and clinical) is designed to develop confidence and beginning expertise in working with families. Students are expected to plan nursing interventions that are appropriate for families within the social and cultural context of their own community. Special attention is paid to learning about vulnerable populations, with a focus on health promotion, risk reduction, and clinical decision making that utilizes population data and research. In addition to integrating healthcare ethics, cultural influences, and social awareness in providing holistic care for families in the advanced practice role, learning outcomes for students include demonstration of an ability to collaborate with families and with other members of an interdisciplinary healthcare team of providers.

On the Lac du Flambeau Reservation, students can rotate through the clinic setting at the Peter Christensen Health Center, the Community Wellness Center to participate in public health programs and family home visits, and the nursing office of the Lac du Flambeau Indian School. In the words of Dr. Mike Axelrod, Director of Human Development Center at University of Wisconsin–Eau Claire, "An immersion experience is perhaps the most practical way to help family health nursing graduate students begin to develop culturally competent clinical skills."

THE COMMUNITY

The Lac du Flambeau Reservation in north central Wisconsin is home to the Lake Superior Chippewa Indians, historically known as the Ojibwa. The year-round population, which expands in the summer season, is estimated to be close to 3000, with at least two-thirds of the population being Native American. The reservation was established in 1854, although by that time the area had been a permanent settlement of the Chippewa Indians for more than a century. The Lac du Flambeau ("Lake of the Torches") area acquired its name from French traders and trappers, for the gathering practices of harvesting fish at night by torchlight. The geographic area is beautiful to this day, characterized by lakes, rivers, and woodlands with abundant wildlife. All contribute to play a major role in the economy, as this is one of Wisconsin's popular recreational centers. The Lac du Flambeau Chippewa operate LDF Industries (pallet manufacturing), the Ojibwa mall, campground, fish hatchery, gas station, smoke shop, and Lake of the Torches hotel and casino.

Using population data from the Wisconsin Department of Health and Family Services (2008), indicators of vulnerability for health risks can be detected. Although Native Americans represent only 0.8% of Wisconsin's total population, 22% live in poverty—more than double the rate for the entire state of Wisconsin. In Wisconsin, 23% of Native Americans aged 25 and older have not graduated from high school, and the percentage of individuals 55 or older meeting this criterion is 13.7%, compared to 23.5% for Wisconsin as a whole. The median age of Native Americans in Wisconsin is 27 years, which suggests that this population is not living as long as other residents of Wisconsin. Indeed, according to the Department of Health, in 2006, for the nation as a whole, the life expectancy of Native American men was 71 years—6 years less than the life expectancy of Caucasian men (Ho, 2009).

In Wisconsin, vital statistics indicate the existence of other disparities related to health. The age-adjusted death rate shows that American Indians have more deaths (1031.5 per 100,000) than the state as a whole (769.4 per 100,000). The leading causes of death among this population are heart disease, cancer, unintentional injury, and diabetes. American Indians are 3.3 times more likely to die from diabetes than whites, 1.9 times more likely to die from unintentional injury than whites, and 3.9 times more likely to die from homicide than whites (Wisconsin Department of Health and Family Services, 2008).

In the area of Lac du Flambeau specifically, according to the U.S. Census Bureau, 86.6% of the population is American Indian, with a median age of 24 years. Approximately 33% of individuals aged 25 or older have not graduated from high school. At least 20% of the Lac du Flambeau American Indians live below poverty level, and according to Irmick, "an individual becomes an elder at age 50" (personal communication, October 2010). Other health disparities observed by the director of the reservation's Indian Child Welfare program include higher rates of drugs and alcohol use, in addition to poverty, all of which have a great impact on the lives of many American Indians. Historically, fur traders and trappers often used alcohol as part of the barter process with Native Americans.

Some features of diet affect the health of today's Native American community. As Dana Irmick points out, these peoples' traditional diet of wild rice, game, berries, and nuts were all relatively low in fat. Along with government assistance to these groups, however, came "commodities"—that is, food subsidies that are inexpensive and high in fat and carbohydrates. The introduction of a Western diet has led to many of the comorbidities seen in this community. At feasts, high-fat food choices such as fry bread are used, but this choice has cultural significance. Prevalent health problems among this population today include diabetes, hypertension, cardiac disease, hyperlipidemia, and obesity.

As health providers trying to gain a beginning understanding of any diverse community, Irmick reminds nurses that they need to attend to not only cultural similarities, but also individual variations within a group. Nurses need to take time to learn about the history of a culture, the socioeconomic realities of an area, verbal and nonverbal communication styles and practices, spirituality, rituals, dietary practices, and family relationships and dynamics within the community. Irmick recalls: "One of the first things I needed to examine prior to starting my clinical rotation were my own beliefs and prejudices. I think in order to understand another culture you must understand your own culture as well." Irmick goes on to recommend self-reflection as a necessary strategy to see which prejudices exist, and to discover what they are based upon. She explains, "It is harder to imagine the lifestyle or decisions of others, if you already accept that your beliefs and practices are better." This approach of assessing preconceived notions is certain to result in barriers to further understanding.

Irmick recommends that students read about a culture beforehand, keeping in mind that there is diversity between and within tribes. She explains that she went to the George Brown, Jr. Museum and Cultural Center and to the Waswagoning Indian Village to learn as much as she could about the area, culture, and people of Lac du Flambeau. Once employed by the tribe, her learning continued as she attended traditional ceremonies, funerals, memorials, and feasts not just to show respect, but to actively build trusting relationships.

Before arriving in the Lac du Flambeau community, Irmick had earlier exposures to other community members through the ER or urgent care settings of an area hospital. She recalls that she was influenced at the time by her lack of knowledge and ideas of noncompliance in relation to patients' and family members' lack of follow-through for appointments, instructions, or medications. She explains:

> Since working within this community, both as a student and a nurse practitioner, I have learned to forgo these prejudices and to work with patients and their family members to understand their view of health and work proactively to maintain or improve it. I no longer think of noncompliance, but rather I see the apparent inability to follow through resulting from a need for better rapport and further trust building. [As a provider,] I need to understand what each patient wants to know, and how I can be a part of their health care . . . it is also vital to understand how a lack of resources (education, money, knowledge) can affect health care and the management of any illnesses that occur.

Most poignantly she states, "As nurses we offer compassion, understanding, and education, while continually reassessing readiness for intervention. This shows respect. Lecturing about noncompliance does not work."

Clearly, this advanced practice nurse is operating within the nursing framework of intentionality (Hartrick Doane & Varcoe, 2005), where a heightened awareness enhances the practitioner's ability to look beyond the surface and join families as they are. Nurses who are intentionally engaged with others in relational moments of practice are actively shaping the health and healing process (Hartrick Doane & Varcoe, 2005).

While it is important to identify how a particular population may be vulnerable to health risks, it is equally important for providers to absorb what the community or culture can teach them. When providers are open to learning, the use of alert and keen listening skills can help them reach a therapeutic level of consciousness that can only enrich their knowledge and enhance their own best practice.

THE IMMERSION EXPERIENCE

Although nursing students may be participating fully in providing health services, an immersion is very much a service–education exchange. In other words, in return for providing service, students gain an education from the community. In the Native American culture, they learn new norms for verbal communication, such as the skill of astute listening to find an answer within a story, while resisting any urge to interrupt or interject. They also encounter new norms for nonverbal communication, such as respecting the importance of silences and pauses in discussion, allowing for a few feet of personal space, and accepting the avoidance of prolonged eye contact (a practice regarded as a sign of respect in Native American culture). In addition, students learn about combining herbal remedies, spiritual practices, and ritual health practices with modern medicine and pharmacology. Moreover, there is much to be learned about family relationships, the parameters of which are very likely to include extended family and even close friends. Native American youth are taught to respect elders; likewise, healthcare providers can learn a great deal from elders through their stories. This reciprocity of service–education exchange is rare and precious. It is also one sure way of building a necessary foundation for advocacy.

The course objective when planning this immersion was to critically examine social, cultural, and community influences that affect advanced nursing practice with families. At our university, the planned activities that met this objective would also directly satisfy the liberal education learning goals of understanding human culture and developing respect for diversity among people. The major participants included six graduate students; the faculty clinical instructor; the designated on-site preceptor with advanced nursing practice skills in family health nursing; the clinic staff, who included several Native American physicians and nurses; the nurse practitioner; a physician's assistant; the school nurse at the Lac du Flambeau public school; the public health nurses and dieticians at the Community Wellness Center; and the families and patients, who were encountered in both clinic and home settings.

In the Peter Christensen Health Center, each student was assigned to rotate between two designated providers, for both chronic and acute care, and these providers also served as cultural guides. Students participated directly with the seasoned providers in completing assessment updates, and collaborated directly with staff and family members on each plan of care. In the Community Wellness Center, students worked directly with public health nurses in facilitating group discussion on smoking cessation programs, sexually transmitted infection (STI) awareness, and in Women's, Infants, and Children (WIC)–funded clinics. Students also accompanied the public health nurses on home visits to families with newborns and to adults for chronic disease management. The school nurse's busy routine provided opportunity for interaction with family members when children were sick or injured and needed to be taken home. There was much to be learned from the school about life on the reservation, including how cultural heritage is promoted and honored in the school, while superimposed on more negative forces such as drug involvement and gang recruitment that are affecting the children outside of school.

The immersion activities for graduate students were designed to be participatory rather than observational. The goals were to encourage students to utilize appropriate assessment skills, actively promote targeted health teaching, and give direct care when needed (e.g., dressing changes) to individuals and families utilizing the health services on the reservation. Additionally, students interacted with cultural guides at the George W. Brown, Jr. Ojibwa Museum and Cultural Center and at the Waswagoning Indian Village. The reservation was a 4-hour drive from the university, and the on-site lodging for the 7-day duration of the immersion was a nearby hotel, located 12 miles from the reservation.

Cultural Immersion

The cultural opportunities of this immersion were rich. Students worked directly with Native American individuals and families, and the experience was designed to inform students of the Native American perspective on health, which could best be described as a journey as opposed to a labeled health status at a given point in time. Students were directed to expand their parameters of health assessment beyond the individual, progressing to family (clan) and community. Through preparatory reading, students were encouraged to develop an awareness of the Native American core connectedness to the earth, and to a greater power that teaches reverence for all life forms. The role of family is especially instructive as it typically extends intergenerationally, and even to collective responsibility for parenting the young within a community. Families who observe traditional ways defer to their elders in matters of decision making, including those pertaining to health.

The providers who worked in this community gladly shared their own knowledge and wisdom gained through their years of service. This kind of immersion as a "lived experience" was a privilege for students, and one that cannot be duplicated in its intensity through classroom content or video presentations. Each student created his or her own experience and gave meaning to it in proportion to depth of preparation, which in turn allowed for purposeful reflection, cultural self-examination, and committed passion.

Immersion Design

A pre-immersion seminar was held on campus prior to travel. A student handbook was prepared for the experience, which included immersion expectations, objectives, historical and population data to provide demographic background of the community, scheduled events, activities, assignment guidelines, driving directions, and restaurant information. The "critical guidance plan" seminar, encompassing 6 to 8 hours of discussion, focused on course expectations, clinical activities, and introduction to Ojibwa heritage and cultural traditions of the present-day Lac du Flambeau band of Lake Superior Chippewa. This session also reviewed the confidentiality protocols for healthcare workers as well as expectations for conduct in etiquette, courtesy, and professionalism. Students were asked to complete exercises that included an assessment of personal background with socioeconomic survival skills, individual communication styles, and personal assessment of listening ability.

The on-site immersion experience consisted of an introductory orientation day; five consecutive working days, exclusive of the on-site pre-immersion preparation; and a post-immersion on-site debriefing. Upon arrival in Lac du Flambeau, an orientation to the physical setting was provided, followed by a guided tour of the museum and cultural heritage center. Arrangements were also made for a guided tour, during the immersion week, of the reservation's Waswagoning Indian Village.

Post-immersion activities were designed to enhance shared reflection and evaluation of the experience. A focus-group format provided opportunity for verbal feedback, both in the assessment of formal learning content and in the self-appraisal of personal growth toward cultural awareness. Although this area cannot necessarily be reflected in the grading process, achieving a greater consciousness is most assuredly transformative. Nursing participants who are able to articulate the personal meaning of the experience will improve their likelihood of becoming more consciously effective in serving future diverse populations.

The immersion experience yielded many benefits for students. Sometimes classroom dialogue and the discussion of reading assignments are not sufficient to achieve a full understanding; rather, a focused experience in a contextual environment is needed for high-impact learning. Another beauty of an on-site immersion is the fact that students can be physically transported and "immersed" into a new setting. With some thoughtful planning and concentrated effort, they can be persuaded to try living somewhat separated from the familiar distractions of "life as usual."

EVALUATION OF THE IMMERSION EXPERIENCE

The immersion experience is based on the premise that meaningful engagement with persons whose shared meanings are different from our own helps us to reflect on the assumptions underlying our own culture, and gives us a way to see the other persons as if for the first time. By becoming more aware of multiple perspectives, we may accomplish the transformative experience of getting to know ourselves in a new way. Guided clinical reflection can be life altering for students who are able to reflect on questions of the human experience, including how experience is created and how it gives meaning to life. With increased understanding of others comes increased understanding of self. Such meaningful engagement can yield greater tolerance and compassion for the well-being of others.

In nursing, the skill of engaged practice is called "relational practice" (Hartrick Doane & Varcoe, 2005). My goal for my students was to experience the best that education could offer. A cultural immersion can open and enrich one's world in ways that cannot be anticipated.

Students were asked to keep a journal of all activities, whether viewed as a participant, observer, or both. This journal was meant to serve as a basis for guided reflection of each student's own journey of exploration and learning, and was shared (to a degree) in the post-immersion group session. In addition, a family assessment paper was completed following guidelines that included socioeconomic and cultural features affecting the health of the family, as the family defined both the meaning of health and "family." Finally, a presentation, poster representation, or artistic interpretation of a selected aspect of the immersion experience was developed by each student and shared with a larger peer group on campus. One student organized a display case for the enjoyment of the college, depicting cultural artifacts and photographs to illustrate her learning about traditional and modern healthcare practices in the immersion community.

In evaluation comments prepared by Dana Irmick, the students revealed to her that they were surprised at the welcoming and friendly nature of staff and patients alike. This experience was their first exposure to a clinic rotation as a nurse practitioner student, and some stated it helped them determine which type of practice or position (e.g., "family practice–type job") they would like to seek after graduation. Some participants also mentioned that "working with a whole family seems to be ideal." Irmick characterized the students' response to the experience as "eye opening" and "enjoyable." She reported that the patients and family members also enjoyed meeting the students and sharing their stories with them. All preceptors were given the opportunity to fill out feedback forms for the students who worked with them, and I later shared this information with each student individually.

Pre- and post-immersion surveys were administered to the students to determine their expectations and to what extent they were met. Students were also asked to describe one learning experience that stood out for them. They were also asked to explain what they had done to contribute to the value of their own learning.

Students reported that the cultural guides on the tours were very helpful. As one student stated, "Our guide welcomed our questions and appreciated the opportunity to talk about his tribe and their culture." Another student elaborated, "I felt that the guided tour at the village and the museum helped me understand how the tribe portrays itself. The two guides explained what the tribe enjoys, how they live now compared to the past, what they have held onto . . . what is important in their lives. The history shaped what and how I saw things." She went on to make an important connection:

> With this understanding, I had a better perspective when observing and working with the healthcare providers and community health staff. It explained why they interacted with their patients/clients the way they did. I also had more respect for the providers themselves, if they did not address certain issues I felt were important. They often did this since they are aware that the tribe's culture did not accept certain things.

In response to the question of whether expectations were met, a student replied: "My week of cultural immersion at Lac du Flambeau will be ever present in my life as I share my experiences with others. I will be reflecting on my own experiences but also use these opportunities to educate others about the Ojibwa culture. I believe this experience will continue to affect my personal life and professional career in ways I am only beginning to comprehend and it will continue to have a profound effect on me."

Under "other comments," a student wrote the following:

> Most Americans know very little about the governments of indigenous people and even less about their diverse cultures, values, and lifeways. . . . instead, they receive information through popular culture, mass communication outlets, and not through personal contact. Academic programs and teachers need to influence students to learn as much as they can about the history and partner with

> tribal people to help eliminate negative stereotypes about Native Americans and address unconscious racism that may be involved. I will be forever grateful to UW–Eau Claire for initiating this cultural immersion experience for graduate students and that I was able to participate.

One student remarked:

> I would highly recommend continuing this experience with future classes; it provided an opportunity I don't believe can necessarily be offered in a traditional once or twice a week clinical experience. I'm *very* thankful I was able to participate.

Another student wrote of an immersion highlight:

> The home visit with a new mom with breastfeeding concerns was an excellent experience. The nurse provided great teaching for the family while providing positive reinforcements. Being welcomed into an Indian home was a humbling experience. I was able to witness their current culture first hand.

Were expectations met? "Yes. My expectations were exceeded daily."

CONCLUSION

The goal of this immersion was to combine required family nursing skills for advanced practice (academic and clinical), with self-growth in areas of cultural sensitivity and awareness (cultural competence). Whether this immersion can fully achieve cultural competence depends on how one defines "cultural competence." However, if this term is taken to mean sensitivity to differences and respect for client values and traditions while performing activities of nursing care, then we are definitely moving closer to the goal. This immersion sought to give students confidence in approaching new situations with increased wisdom and curiosity. With the skills emphasized in such immersion experiences, future nurse leaders will approach challenging patients and vulnerable populations with open minds and greater generosity of spirit.

WWW

For a full suite of assignments and additional learning activities, use the access code located in the front of your book to visit this exclusive website: http://go.jblearning.com/dechesnay. If you do not have an access code, you can obtain one at the site.

REFERENCES

Benzein, E., Johansson, P., Arestedt, K. F., & Saveman, B. I. (2008). Nurses' attitudes about the importance of families in nursing care: A survey of Swedish nurses. *Journal of Family Nursing, 14*(2), 162–180.

Hartrick Doane, G., & Varcoe, C., (2005). *Family nursing as relational inquiry: Developing health-promoting practice.* Philadelphia, PA: Lippincott Williams & Wilkins.

Ho, V. (2009). Native American death rates soar as most people are living longer. Retrieved from http://www.seattlepi.com/local/403196_tribes12.html

Nauright, L. (2008). Preparing nursing professionals for advocacy: Service learning. In M. de Chesnay & B. Anderson (Eds.), *Caring for the vulnerable.* (pp. 473–482). Sudbury, MA: Jones & Bartlett.

Wisconsin Department of Health and Family Services. (2008) Minority health report, 2001–2005. Retrieved from http://www.dhs.wisconsin.gov/Health/MinorityHealth/report20012005.htm

UNIT VII

Policy Implications

The hardest hit, as everywhere, are those who have no choice.
—Adorno, Theodor W. (1974), *Minima moralia. Reflections from damaged life. (First published in German 1951.)* London (NLB), 39.

CHAPTER 39

Public Policy and Vulnerable Populations

Jeri A. Milstead

Objectives

At the end of this chapter, the reader will be able to

1. Identify key concepts of vulnerability that are terms used by policy makers.
2. Describe how agendas are set, implemented, and evaluated by policy makers.
3. Discuss the ways in which nurses can influence legislation.

Government policies that target vulnerable populations may seem like an oxymoron (if we can use that word to explain a phrase). On the one hand, vulnerable populations may be difficult to define. On the other hand, vulnerable populations may not have much of a voice to articulate their plight. How and to whom in government do "populations" direct their pleas––agencies? Programs? This chapter seeks to define vulnerable populations, examine the policy process, and consider issues inherent in linking the two. Examples are provided of how nurses can work within the policy process to the benefit of vulnerable populations.

DEFINITIONS

The term "vulnerable populations" is a latecomer to nursing literature; "special populations" first appeared in 1995 as a descriptor in *The Cumulative Index to Nursing and Allied Health Literature* (CINAHL) in 1995, but "vulnerability" did not appear until 1997. Users of the term "vulnerable populations" often mean to refer to groups of low socioeconomic status (the poor and those out of work), the underserved (i.e., those who lack healthcare insurance or lack access to healthcare delivery), persons with diagnoses in certain disease categories (e.g., diabetes, congestive heart failure), persons with chronic illness (arthritis, AIDS), or those at risk for developing disease or illness. These terms are not really interchangeable, however. For example, all diabetics are not poor, and low socioeconomic status may not indicate the presence of chronic disease. Thus these terms may not accurately reflect either vulnerability or populations.

CINAHL (2002) includes a category of vulnerability that is defined as "the state of being at risk or more susceptible physically, mentally or socially" (p. 405). Flaskerud et al. (2002) define vulnerable populations as "social groups who experience health disparities as a result of a lack of resources and/or increased exposure to risk" (p. 75). The two major concepts incorporated in these definitions appear to be the degree of risk and the experience of health problems without access to resources. However, a full understanding of vulnerable populations requires a deeper look.

Flaskerud et al. (2002) addressed the evolution of knowledge about vulnerable populations from the 1950s to the early 2000s through a study of articles published in *Nursing Research*. Although the study was not comprehensive, in that writings from other journals or other sources were excluded, the researchers chronicled terms that were used in investigating groups or aggregates. Only one study was published in the 1950s, which focused on chronically ill aged adults. Group identity was based in the 1960s on socioeconomic status, education, occupation, gender, or race. The literature of the 1970s noted "race, ethnicity and gender" (p. 76), with research at this time focusing on high-risk parents, infants, women, and immigrants. The concept of culture and its effect on the delivery of health care came into the literature in the 1980s (Leininger & McFarland, 2002). Reported as an "influence" in outcomes of social groups, culture became the context for studying a variety of societal problems that were not limited to either health or health care.

The concept of health disparities did not surface until late in the 1990s, when this term was introduced to reflect differences in health care and outcomes among many groups, such as adolescents and the elderly, women and infants, and low- and middle-income families. Ethnic groups also were studied as groups, often with a focus on the quality (or lack thereof) of health and health care. Quality was approached through professional accountability (vis-à-vis ethics and standards), marketing accountability (as evidenced in informed choices), and regulatory accountability (as reflected in government action) (Taub, 2002). Although the marketing method seemed prominent at that time, the regulatory scheme used the Health Plan Employer Data and Information Set (HEDIS), hospital discharge data from the now-defunct Health Care Financing Administration (HCFA), and information on the quality of managed care organizations from the National Committee for Quality Assurance. Today, Medicare assesses "representatives of aged, disabled, and institutionalized Medicare beneficiaries" through the Medicare Current Beneficiary Survey (MCBS; http://www.cms.hhs.gov/MCBS).

In the early years of the twenty-first century, many terms surfaced that referred to vulnerable populations. "Uninsured" became a blanket term for poor and low-income people, regardless of their gender, ethnicity, or employment status. Researchers discovered that the uninsured, that included the working poor, had more health problems than persons who carried insurance. The homeless, as a group, were uninsured (often because they were also unemployed) and exhibited many physical and mental health problems. The range of health disparities was great. Migrant workers were considered "disadvantaged" (Ward, 2003), and often less attention was paid to their health concerns than the health issues of established workers. African Americans (Plowden & Thompson, 2002; Richards, 2000) and Latinos (Campinha-Bacote, 2002) experienced much inequity related to health care. The disabled were identified as having social and physical barriers to health (Harrison, 2002). Those who lived near hazardous waste sites were considered at increased risk for serious health problems (Gilden, 2003). Finally, the term "vulnerable populations" evolved to include whole populations, not just aggregates of individuals, as identifiable groups.

On an international scale, migration is occurring from rural areas to urban areas. Nurses often are the key care providers in rural areas. Resettlement of individuals and populations from farm to city, although providing greater opportunities for jobs and higher salaries, often results in a serious lack of healthcare services for the rural underserved population (Buchan, 2006).

POLICY PROCESS

Many people think of legislation or laws when they hear the term "policy." Although legislation may be its most recognizable component, the policy process includes many other components. When discussing public policy (as opposed to private-sector policy), the author of this chapter means the process of taking problems to the administration that can or should be addressed by government and obtaining a governmental response. (The author notes her opinion that not all social problems warrant a governmental action.) Within this broad approach, four major aspects are evident: agenda setting, government response, program and policy implementation, and program and policy evaluation.

The policy process is not always linear or sequential. That is, one does not always start with agenda setting and move immediately to government response. A nurse, for example, may initially become involved during program implementation after a law has been signed. A garbage can model of organizations (Cohen, March, & Olsen, 1982) provides a foundation for considering the process of making public policy as the interweaving of streams of problems, policies, and politics. These streams mingle in government circles, often joining and breaking apart as ideas and solutions are considered, rejected, or reconsidered (Kingdon, 1995). At times, a solution hooks up with a problem, and a window of opportunity opens that results in creation of a program that addresses the difficulty. The following brief discussion of each component of the policy process reveals opportunities for becoming involved in these activities.

AGENDA SETTING

The national agenda is a list of items to which the president and his advisors (known as the administration) attend. Agenda setting is the activity in which problems are brought to the attention of the administration. If the president is not interested in a problem, it has little chance of being addressed. The issue is how to get the president's attention (Furlong, 2008). Crises can propel an issue onto the national agenda. For example, the attacks of September 11, 2001, brought immediate attention to the issue of terrorism, and funding was made available for projects and programs such as the establishment of the Department of Homeland Security.

One of the issues in agenda setting is defining a problem so that it is palatable to the administration and to the public. When HIV/AIDS was first discovered, for example, it was defined as a problem of intravenous drug users and homosexuals. The Reagan administration believed that the public would not support funding for research into the cause or treatment of the disease, so little funding was forthcoming. When children like Ryan White and heterosexual non-drug users began to get the disease (most often from infected blood products), the disease was redefined as a community health problem, and funding was made available.

Nurses are experts at choosing words and scenarios to describe problems. Creative use of language may not be necessary in alerting an administration to a problem, but one should know how to use key words to advantage. The point in defining a problem is to pique the interest of the administration so that a solution can be found. Knowing that the public will scrutinize funding options is part of the context of defining the difficulty.

GOVERNMENT RESPONSE

The government may respond to a problem in several ways. The three most common responses are the enactment of a law, a regulation, or a program. Policy experts develop these activities in policy communities. Policy communities are loosely knit groups of people who can provide expertise about an issue and who, for the most part, work in government agencies. Policy experts often know one another through professional associations, the literature or other media exposure, or prior experience. In many situations, legislative aides, who serve as staff in the offices of legislators, are good contacts for nurses who want to connect with "insiders." Experts discuss problems, suggest solutions, and exercise their opinions about the relative political worth of issues. Legislative aides in one legislator's office often talk informally with legislative aides in other legislators' offices and with staff in government agencies, faculty in university settings, and members of special-interest groups to establish a priority list and to consider alternative solutions. Nurses who have cultivated relationships with government policy staff have a golden opportunity to be recognized as experts who are sought out to consider problems (Wakefield, 2008).

Laws are made in legislative sessions that last two years. Bills (potential laws) are introduced throughout the session, but bills introduced early have a better chance of action. The "how a bill becomes a law" page that can be found in nearly every basic government or political science textbook provides a simplified overview of the steps for moving a bill from introduction to signature by the president. Neither legislators nor their aides are expected to know everything about the myriad issues brought to their attention, as these issues range from health to transportation to the economy to defense and beyond. Nurses have a wonderful opportunity to serve as experts about many health issues. A nurse can provide a one-page overview of a problem, a summary of relevant research in ordinary language, and phone or e-mail information to pave the way for a serious contact.

Seasoned nurses understand the importance of informal processes—political processes. Many nurses shun the idea of politics, thinking that it to be a tainted process that skews judgment and biases legislators. On the contrary, the political process is merely the exercise of persuasion and education to one's perspective. What nurse has not spoken informally to others before a decision was made in an effort to gather support, challenge a conclusion, or talk out a problem? The same communication techniques are used with legislators and their staffs or anyone in the policy community. Reflection, active listening, and clarification are therapeutic communication skills that are integral to how nurses approach others. The art of using talents in this way should be natural for nurses.

The legislative process must be followed carefully, and nurses must be vigilant for amendments that may either help or hurt their causes. Developing strong, positive relationships with legislators, staff, and other interested parties results in a network that leads to "inside" information. Working at the subcommittee level is a more efficient use of time than letting a bill get to the committee level, but it is important to stay with a bill through its passage by both houses of Congress and, in many instances, a conference committee where final negotiations are completed. Nurses may recommend language for inclusion in drafting a bill or an amendment and must be cognizant of amendments that could derail or inhibit passage of the legislation.

Once a bill becomes a law that establishes a program, the program is assigned to a government agency for implementation. The choice of which agency is designated as the controller of the program is very political. Not all health programs go to agencies in the Department of Health and Human Services. Some, for example, go to the Department of Defense (for piloting by the military), the Department of Education (school health programs), the Department of the Treasury (drug enforcement programs), or other departments and agencies. The choice may be based on past experience with similar programs, the chance for an infusion of new funding needed by an agency, rejection of a program due to lack of time or expertise, or many other reasons.

Agencies must write regulations or rules that interpret the law and provide for its smooth implementation (Loversidge, 2008). The regulatory process is similar to the legislative process in that legislative action is required. However, the regulatory process is governed by the Administrative Procedures Act, which dictates a specific format and course. All proposed rules require notification of the public, an established period of time for public comment, and public announcement of the final rule. The *Federal Register* is the vehicle for publication of information on federal issues.

Public comment can take the form of letters, e-mail messages, phone calls, or in-person visits to the appropriate agency. All comments must be considered before the final rule is adopted. The comment stage is a particularly easy way for nurses to involve themselves in expressing their opinions about potential rules. Communication should be brief, focused, and identifiable (i.e., specific to the rule on which you are commenting). Arguments should be stated clearly and prefaced by whether you are for or against the issue or section of the rule. Solutions are welcomed.

IMPLEMENTATION

Implementation is a fluid process that involves getting a program up and running. Agency staff may need assistance in determining eligibility. That is, who is entitled to participate? Who is excluded from participation? What are the criteria, and who monitors participation? Nurses can suggest policy tools, such as incentives (waivers, coupons), educational brochures, posters advertising a program, or learning tools (training sessions), to assist staff in operating a program (Smart, 2008).

Nurses should confer with agency personnel, known as street-level bureaucrats, who are putting the programs into operation. These street-level bureaucrats often use ideas from participants in the programs or program staff about how to streamline programs or make them more efficient or user-friendly. Nurses may provide tips about the population being served or thoughts about how a program could be conducted. Sometimes programs can be expanded to include broader involvement or shrunk to remain within the legislative intent and purpose. Nurses can provide concrete assistance and guidance by recommending ideas about how to alter the provision of a program.

In his classic work on implementation, Bardach (1977) identified games that are played by agency personnel during the implementation phase of a program. Many of the games have to do with budget, policy goals, and administrative control. For government agencies, spending funds early and requesting additional funding later is one way to increase a budget. Encouragement of overspending, known as boondoggling, can be seen when consultant fees exceed the budget. Inflation of the estimated cost of a program is a way of padding a budget so that some of the funds can be used later (e.g., as discretionary funds) or in a way different from original intent.

Nurses study implementation to determine to what extent programs meet the original policy goals (Wilken, 2008). They investigate any modifications that were made and seek explanations for changes. Researchers examine the level of difficulty or "tractability" of the initial problem and whether technology was accessible to address the problem. On the one hand, the range of services provided by a program may produce variation in program performance such that many services might dilute operations negatively. On the other hand, successful programs can become a target for piling on additional objectives. The idea is to be part of a thriving program, but to avoid the inclusion of too many extra activities may result in program failure.

EVALUATION

Evaluation is rarely conducted and usually is not part of an original program plan, despite the vast body of literature that recommends appraisal as part of monitoring program success. Such an evaluation should be both formative and summative.

Formative data can help bureaucrats determine progress during implementation, informing decisions about whether the program should continue to function as usual or whether a change in direction should be sought. Formative data can also indicate whether resources are adequate and are being distributed appropriately.

Summative data can be useful for evaluating public programs for effectiveness or outcomes, not just efficiency or outputs. That is, what difference does it make to the public good if thousands of poor women are offered free mammograms? Has this screening method resulted in significant prevention or early treatment of breast cancer? This is not to say that efficiency is not worth assessing, because a poorly run program will waste tax dollars.

Evaluative reports should be provided to agency personnel, legislators, and the public. Charts and other visual media can be used to present aggregate data, identify trends, and track progress. Reports may contain recommendations for adjusting goals and objectives or implementation strategies.

LINKING THE POLICY PROCESS AND VULNERABLE POPULATIONS

Agenda Setting

Nurses can propel issues of vulnerable populations onto the national agenda by defining needy groups, serving as a voice for vulnerable populations, and alerting legislators to problems that affect the public health. For example, the homeless usually are not organized in any formal way and have little voice as a group. Their worries about health care may go unheard unless someone, known as a policy entrepreneur, makes available his or her reputation, money, or other resources on their behalf. A nurse can serve as an entrepreneur or can mobilize the media to take up a cause.

Issues of social justice are political issues. Discrimination against marginalized populations and against people based on health status, income, employment status, or type of disease or disability is unethical and unjust and may be illegal in the United States. The distribution and allocation of resources is also a political process. The choice of which problems get on the national agenda is very political, and nurses are skilled in political interaction because of their expert ability to communicate and think critically. Nurses must take up the mantle of social problems, especially health problems, for those who cannot or do not speak for themselves. In the truest sense of the term "advocacy," nurses also must educate vulnerable populations about how to advocate for themselves. Self-advocacy is empowering for every population.

Nurses can help bureaucrats define problems in ways that help the public understand and value them. Drug users, for example, are often unemployed or financially poor, and may be disenfranchised in the public eye because of related crimes. (In contrast, employed drug users often go undetected by the general public and escape bias [Milstead, 1993].) Legislators ignore or shun known drug users as a group, often because officials perceive that the "druggies" create violence, do not vote, and are not organized politically.

In the 1980s, social activists (including nurses) formed groups such as the Association for Drug Abuse Prevention and Treatment (ADAPT) and the AIDS Coalition to Unleash Power (ACT UP) as vehicles to address drug use and health. Members recognized the link between gay men, intravenous drug users, and HIV/AIDS, and a few created needle exchange programs and served as policy entrepreneurs. These volunteers changed the terminology used from drug "addict" to drug "user," recognizing this transformation as one way to change the public's perception of a vulnerable group. Notably, volunteers in Tacoma, Washington, and New York City educated legislators, bureaucrats, and public health officials about HIV transmission and the need for research on diagnosis and treatment (Milstead, 1993). Communications techniques such as consciousness raising and the use of sound bites were developed to a high level.

Policy entrepreneurs may take years to attain their goals. Indeed, some of the first groups of volunteers related to drug use and health are still staffing needle exchange programs on the streets and working the state legislature to obtain legitimacy for their programs. Most needle exchange programs in the United States are still operating—and are still illegal—despite the sustained efforts of volunteers to change the laws and a legal opinion that "possession of needles [is] a 'medical necessity' that [is] intended to prevent a greater societal harm, AIDS" ("Manhattan Criminal Court," 1991).

Government Response

Laws are composites of language that reflect the wishes and priorities of those who craft them. Laws often are the result of negotiation and compromise among many people with disparate philosophies and values. Nurses can help shape laws by means of their expertise in health care and healthcare delivery. Congressional representatives usually do not know much about diseases such as diabetes or tuberculosis. A nurse who has nurtured relationships with elected officials by becoming a contact for health issues and providing understandable explanations of medical terminology has a great opening to contribute to language as a bill is being constructed. A nurse's knowledge of current issues can be a tremendous help to a legislator or the staff. Nurses also bring anecdotes to the policy community that put a personal face on an issue.

The elderly, for example, are often considered a vulnerable population. This designation may be confusing because the term does not necessarily refer to low socioeconomic status, the underserved, or disease categories for older persons. Instead, "elderly" cuts across all types of categories. As a vulnerable population, there is inference of risk and lack of resources for health care for the elderly, specifically in relation to an increased danger of suffering disease or disability and a lack of resources because of fixed incomes. The elderly have a strong, organized lobby through the American Association of Retired Persons (AARP). During the early years of the twenty-first century, AARP waged a campaign in the U.S. Congress to create protection for members (aged 50 years or older) in the form of a program for funding prescription drugs.

The Medicare Prescription Drug Improvement and Modernization Act of 2003 amended Title XVIII (Medicare) of the Social Security Act to add a new Part D (Voluntary Prescription Drug Benefit Program), under which each individual who is entitled to benefits under Medicare Part A (hospital insurance) or Medicare Part B (supplemental medical insurance) is entitled to obtain qualified prescription drug coverage. The law was passed by both the House of Representatives and the Senate and became public law 108-173 on December 8, 2003 (http://www.thomas.loc.gov). Many people found that prescription costs soared under this law and vulnerable populations who were supposed to have been helped actually suffered when they could not afford needed medications.

Nurses, physicians, and other healthcare providers participated in a focused assault on legislators in an effort to influence the form of the bill before it became law. Senators and representatives held hearings, met with lobbyists and AARP members, talked with constituents, and discussed issues within the policy community. The issue evolved into a hotly debated partisan battle, but compromise language created a bill that was acceptable enough to pass the Republican-dominated House and Senate. Herein lies a caveat: Although the bill has been signed into law, many changes must be made as the program continues to be implemented. Nurses have an occasion to become knowledgeable about the current law and can peruse the law and how it came into being through the website previously noted (http://www.thomas.loc.gov).

The Medicare prescription plan is an example of how the streams of agenda setting, government response, and implementation interconnect. During efforts to move the issue of prescription costs onto the national agenda, work already was in process to determine alternative solutions, and the basic rudiments of a program were already being conceived.

Implementation

An example of a purely symbolic policy action is the Stewart B. McKinney Act of 1987. Vladeck (1990) studied the homeless, including their characteristics, causes of homelessness, and health status of homeless persons. He chronicled the evolution of a joint initiative between the Robert Wood Johnson Foundation and the Pew Charitable Trusts that became a model for a program that would provide federal support for the homeless. Even though there was agreement among policy makers that homelessness was a problem worthy of government intervention, authorization of funding did not eliminate the problem or even address most of the social, economic, healthcare, and other issues. The McKinney Act was symbolic in that legislators could document an attempt to address the issue of homelessness, even if the issue had little probability of being resolved.

A brief search for initiatives about the homeless in the 111th Congress shows a plethora of attempts in which bills were introduced but stalled in committee or subcommittee. (Note that relief for vulnerable populations can be addressed within a variety of committees and through a variety of topics.) These attempts include House of Representatives (H.R.) 2754, the Nurse Managed Clinics Investment Act of 2009, which would provide for medical homes so that medically underserved populations could access primary care and wellness services that would lead to a decrease in health disparities experienced by vulnerable populations. Primary care services would include screenings and diagnostic tests. Wellness services would include health education, case management, smoking cessation, and physical education programs. Both types of services would be funded through grants to nurse-managed clinics. H.R. 2795 and H.R. 2817 were collectively titled Roadmap to End Global Hunger and Promote Food Security Act of 2009. The aim of these bills was to decrease hunger and promote food security throughout the world. H.R. 4321, the Comprehensive Immigration Reform ASAP Act of 2009, included provisions that would combat human smuggling and offer basic protection for vulnerable populations. None of these bills was voted out of the House and sent to the Senate.

Evaluation

Evaluation of health policy that affects vulnerable groups does not occur often at the program level. Rather, policy itself is more typically evaluated through research. Nurse-led studies in the 1990s and the early 2000s reported in *Nursing Research* (Flaskerud et al., 2002), for example, evaluated resources available for Hispanics, Cubans, African Americans, Filipinos, lesbians and other women, men, low-income families and age-related groups, and the homeless. Disease categories included mental illness (including depression), chronic illness, addictive disease, pregnancy, injuries, and specific populations with asthma, hypertension, HIV/AIDS, lung and heart disease, sexually transmitted diseases, and tuberculosis. The discovery of health disparities between vulnerable groups and the general population indicated that the former have higher levels of risk and less access to healthcare providers and resources.

Research has also uncovered problems in defining vulnerable populations, specifically in relation to issues of race and ethnicity. The Institute of Medicine, for instance, challenged the National Institutes of Health (NIH) to replace the term "race" with "ethnic group" (Oppenheimer, 2001). The Office of Management and Budget (OMB) sets policy about which racial and ethnic classes are to be referenced by any federal agency, although OMB recognizes that these terms are based on ill-defined social or political types, not scientific categories. The American Anthropological Association adopted the concept of race/ethnicity as an interim combined term, but the category of "race" was eliminated in the 2010 national census. Thus researchers must take care to define race or ethnicity clearly as they study various groups. Issues related to vulnerable groups will be subject to increased scrutiny in the future, and federal agencies that authorize programs, initiate policies, and appropriate funds must take into consideration the legal, governmental, cultural, and historic implications of terms.

Sudduth (2008) asserts that nurses "are not strangers to evaluation" (p. 194). She urges advanced practice nurses to transfer the skills they use to determine outcomes in a healthcare setting to evaluation of government programs. "Social programs are public policy made visible" (p. 197), and nurses are well equipped to determine the worth, efficacy, and efficiency of many programs.

CONCLUSION

Nurses work with vulnerable populations in the provision, administration, and evaluation of health care. Public officials design policies in response to problems that rise to the agenda-setting attention of the president and his advisors. The policy community is involved in defining problems, prioritizing their value, and seeking and considering alternative solutions. Legislators, their staff, special-interest groups, and others in the community of interest draft government responses to the problems, often in the form of laws, regulations, and programs.

Nurses must integrate their political knowledge and skill into their professional lives. Nurses can identify problems, bring them to the attention of law makers, keep them from fading from public view, suggest redefinitions, and propose alternative solutions. Nurses must persevere throughout this process by using their expertise to help legislators choose policy tools and implement and evaluate programs and policies. Public officials are not used to nurses participating actively in the process of policy making; therefore, nurses must initiate the contacts, provide information that a layperson can understand, and acknowledge those legislators or bureaucrats who respond positively and move government to action.

Nurses are experts in the provision of health care, especially for the vulnerable. Not only do nurses have an ethical obligation to inform policy makers on issues for which at-risk populations have little or no voice, but as professionals they must recognize that they will cede their societal accountability if they do not.

For a full suite of assignments and additional learning activities, use the access code located in the front of your book to visit this exclusive website: http://go.jblearning.com/dechesnay. If you do not have an access code, you can obtain one at the site.

REFERENCES

Bardach, E. (1977). *The implementation game: What happens after a bill becomes a law.* Cambridge, MA: MIT Press.

Buchan, J. (2006). The impact of global nursing migration on health services delivery. *Policy, Politics, & Nursing Practice, 7*(3), 16S–25S.

Campinha-Bacote, J. (2002). The process of cultural competence in the delivery of healthcare services: A model of care. *Journal of Transcultural Nursing, 13*(3), 181–184.

Cohen, M., March, J., & Olsen, J. (1982). A garbage can model of organizational choice. *Administrative Science Quarterly, 17,* 1–25.

Cumulative index to nursing and allied health literature (CINAHL). (2002). Glendale, CA: EBSCO Publishing. Retrieved August 11, 2010, from www.ebscohost.com/cinahl

Flaskerud, J. H., Lesser, J., Dixon, E., Anderson, N., Conde, F., Kim, S., . . . Verzemnieks, I. (2002). Health disparities among vulnerable populations. *Nursing Research, 51*(2), 74–85.

Furlong, E. A. (2008). Agenda setting. In J. A. Milstead (Ed.), *Health policy and politics: A nurse's guide* (3rd ed., pp. 41–60). Sudbury, MA: Jones & Bartlett.

Gilden, R. C. (2003). Community involvement at hazardous waste sites: A review of policies from a nursing perspective. *Policy, Politics, & Nursing Practice, 4*(1), 29–35.

Harrison, T. C. (2002). Has the Americans with Disabilities Act made a difference? A policy analysis of quality of life in the post–Americans with Disabilities Act era. *Policy, Politics, & Nursing Practice, 3*(4), 333–347.

Kingdon, J. W. (1995). *Agendas, alternatives, and public policies* (2nd ed.). New York NY: Harper Collins.

Leininger, M., & McFarland, M. R. (2002). *Transcultural nursing: Concepts, theories, research and practice* (3rd ed.). New York, NY: McGraw-Hill.

Medicare Prescription Drug and Modernization Act of 2003. (2003). Retrieved December 31, 2003, from http://www.thomas.loc.gov

Milstead, J. A. B. (1993). *The advancement of policy implementation theory: An analysis of three needle exchange programs.* PhD dissertation, University of Georgia, Atlanta, GA. Retrieved August 11, 2010, from Dissertations and Theses A&I (Publication Number AAT 9329821).

Oppenheimer, G. M. (2001). Paradigm lost: Race, ethnicity, and the search for a new population taxonomy. *American Journal of Public Health, 91*(7), 1049–1054.

Plowden, K. O., & Thompson, L. S. (2002). Sociological perspectives of black American health disparity: Implications for social policy. *Policy, Politics, & Nursing Practice, 3*(4), 325–332.

Richards, H. (2000). And miles to go before we sleep: Rising to meet the challenges of ending health care disparities among African-Americans. *Journal of National Black Nurses Association, 11*(2), 2.

Smart, P. (2008). Policy design. In J. A. Milstead (Ed.), *Health policy and politics: A nurse's guide* (3rd ed., pp. 129–141). Sudbury, MA: Jones & Bartlett.

Sudduth, A. L. (2008). Policy evaluation. In J. A. Milstead (Ed.), *Health policy and politics: A nurse's guide* (3rd ed., pp. 171–193). Sudbury, MA: Jones & Bartlett.

Taub, L.-F. M. (2002). A policy analysis of access to health care inclusive of cost, quality, and scope of services. *Policy, Politics, & Nursing Practice, 3*(2), 167–176.

Vladeck, B. (1990). Health care and the homeless: A political parable for our time. *Journal of Health Politics, Policy and Law, 15*(2), 305–317.

Wakefield, M. (2008). Government response: Legislation. In J. A. Milstead (Ed.), *Health policy and politics: A nurse's guide* (3rd ed., pp. 65–88). Sudbury, MA: Jones & Bartlett.

Ward, L. S. (2003). Migrant health policy: History, analysis, and challenge. *Policy, Politics, & Nursing Practice, 4*(1), 45–52.

Wilken, M. (2008). Policy implementation. In J. A. Milstead (Ed.), *Health policy and politics: A nurse's guide* (3rd ed., pp. 157–164). Sudbury, MA: Jones and Bartlett.

CHAPTER 40

Advancing Healthcare Policy Through the Use of Political Narratives to Give Voice to a Vulnerable Population

Charles Bobo and Kathie Aduddell

Objectives

At the end of this chapter, the reader will be able to

1. Describe how stories can be sued to influence public policy.
2. Describe how nurses can elevate stories and anecdotes beyond self-interest to improve health.
3. In the case of undocumented immigrants, develop an alternate story to plead their plight.

WWW

This chapter discusses the ways in which nurses can use stories about vulnerable populations to create narratives that influence public opinion and spur political action on healthcare policy. A well-developed political narrative has the potential to change beliefs and facilitate support by linking vulnerable individuals or populations with the public, with policy advocates, and with political policy makers (Bennet & Edelman, 2006). Associating a policy, bill, or law with a particular person or group provides a human connection that can overcome the impersonal aspect of policy development and legislation. In addition to enhancing public and political support, well-crafted narratives can even be persuasive in hindering opposition (Clark, 2008). In this way, creation of narratives that bring about positive change for a vulnerable patient population serves as a powerful tool in the arsenal of political advocacy for nurses.

In examining the political narrative process, the chapter presents a case study of one particular vulnerable group—namely, the American-citizen children of undocumented immigrants. This particular group provides an opportunity to discuss nursing's purpose in shaping health policy as well as the importance of recognizing and understanding policy implications for vulnerable populations. In addition, this case presentation highlights the importance of considering key legal, social, and political components of healthcare policy when developing political narratives. The chapter concludes by describing an opportunity presented by the passage of the 2010 Healthcare Reform Act for nurse advocates to develop and use narratives that influence and advance healthcare policies related to vulnerable populations.

NURSING PRACTICE, HEALTH POLICY, AND THE USE OF NARRATIVES

Creating a politically powerful narrative requires understanding the stories of the vulnerable. By determining the legal, social, and political factors affecting their patients, nurses can create stories powerful enough to move the sentiment of public opinion and apply political pressure to change health care as needed for these vulnerable individuals, families, and communities. The well-crafted political narrative goes beyond simply telling a tale of healthcare woe and need. Contained within that narrative is a story that is not only formative regarding the healthcare deficits, but also provides a foundation for the formulation and implementation of healthcare policy. *Nurses who use political narratives to achieve their healthcare advocacy objectives find the root of the problem in the legal, social, and political arena that the vulnerable individual or group encounters and then frame the political narratives to suggest potential solutions to these problems.*

The American public and political policy makers are familiar with the use of narratives or stories to associate a law with a particular victim or group who personify the intent of the law. In many cases, just naming the law for a victim provides an immediate context, explains the law, and reinforces the need for it. In this way, a connection is created between the public, policy makers, and those benefiting from the laws. For example, consider Megan's Law—named for Megan Kanka, a seven-year-old girl who was murdered by the sex offender living as her neighbor; this law requires the establishment of sexual offender registries and release of that information to protect the public. The Amber Hageman Child Protection Act established a public child abduction alert system ("Amber Alert"); Amber was a nine-year-old child who was abducted and murdered in Texas. The Matthew Shepard and James Byrd, Jr. Hate Crimes Prevention Act expanded the federal hate-crime law to include gender, sexual orientation, gender identity, or disability Matthew Shepard was a 21-year-old man who was tortured and murdered because of his sexual orientation; James Byrd, Jr., was a 49-year-old African American male victim of a racially motivated torture and murder.

An example in health care in which policy makers were able to overcome public resistance and create the political will to pass a socially controversial law was the Ryan White HIV/AIDS Treatment Extension Act (originally the Ryan White Comprehensive AIDS Resources Emergency Act), which provides publicly funded services for patients with HIV/AIDS. The law was named for Ryan White, a teenager who acquired HIV infection through a blood transfusion and later died from AIDS. Perhaps most important to note about this narrative was that even though Ryan White was the public face for the narrative, he was not representative of the overwhelming majority of individuals with HIV/AIDS. Yet, when his story was turned into a narrative for public and political use, it inspired forces to act in this situation. With this narrative, the discussion went from being solely focused on homosexuals and drug users who might have contributed to their own exposure to one focused on a middle-class, white, teenage boy who was blameless in his exposure to the HIV virus.

Some recent examples of the use of narratives involve politicians. As he signed the new healthcare reform bill, President Barack Obama stood next to a young child, Marcelas Owens, whose mother died fighting insurance companies for cancer treatment. When Obama signed the Children's Health Insurance Program Bill into law, he was with Gregory Secrest, a man who lost his job and healthcare coverage for his two children; Secrest's children had offered their piggy-bank with $4 to help pay the costs of insurance (Office of the Press Secretary, 2009). Essential to the power of these narratives is the implicit political and social story that they portray. With both the Marcela Owens and Gregory Secrest narratives, the story helped the president frame the political need for insurance company regulation and the importance of providing access to health care for out-of-work individuals in the new healthcare reform bill. The public opinion focus for both narratives was the pain, suffering, and hardship faced by innocent children due to lack of healthcare access. Not to be underestimated is the narrative's inclusion of the Secrest children's willingness to sacrifice even the last penny in their piggybank. This was not just an incidental fact presented by the president, but rather a critical aspect of the story that addressed the public perception of deservedness and willingness of individuals to self-sacrifice so as to be public healthcare recipients under the healthcare reform bill.

Perhaps the ultimate universal healthcare narrative came from Representative Billy Tauzin, who invoked the idea that he was doing it for his "Momma" when engineering the passage of the Medicare Part D bill. What political or public group would willingly want to take a position against their mothers?

These anecdotes are just a few examples of how narratives have been used to drive public opinion and motivate political policymakers to pass legislation. Many of the laws mentioned previously had their origins in the efforts by individual family members to ensure the loss of their loved ones was not forgotten. Thus the passage of these laws at the state and national levels was not necessarily a result of limitless financial resources. The truly powerful lesson for nurses is that by using a narrative, even individual families and small groups with limited resources may be able to generate widespread public support and political action in creating and passing laws that change policy in various arenas.

IDENTIFYING A PURPOSE FOR SHAPING HEALTH POLICY: RECOGNIZING AND UNDERSTANDING VULNERABLE POPULATIONS

To be true patient advocates, nurses must find a way to move beyond their own individual interests in shaping health policy. It may be important to recognize that, even in the nursing profession's advocacy for health policy, there remains discord among the profession's own members on many of the healthcare-related political and social issues of the day. From personal concerns about providing care to patients having abortions and caring for patients with HIV/AIDS to providing indigent care and publicly funded healthcare services, nursing professionals do not always agree about where their professional ethical obligation ends and their personal opinions begin. Failing to achieve professional agreement on health issues leaves nursing with a somewhat fragmented and weakly supported approach to political advocacy. Ultimately, it wastes the potential political power of the approximately 3 million nurses in the United States that might otherwise be employed to advocate for patients. Finding ways to build consensus within the nursing profession on a particular health issue, or for a specific patient population, is an important part of identifying a nursing purpose in shaping and influencing health policy.

A first step might be to identify the communities and individuals that may benefit the most from the use of a nurse-developed narrative in advancing public policy and healthcare advocacy. Without a defined target population for nursing support, nursing's professional political advocacy efforts are likely to become lost in the greater social and political debates surrounding health care today. Nurses may achieve greater success by selectively advocating for specific vulnerable populations who lack the ability to bring their problems to the public view or who are unable to find a place on the policy-making agenda. The American-citizen children of undocumented immigrants are an isolated and vulnerable group whose situation helps demonstrates this first step. Despite the controversial and divisive debate surrounding immigration and publicly funded health care, efforts can be made to select and support specific issues that are unique to this group, yet still fall within nurses' professional ethical obligations. Ideally, this framing of the issues will provide a basis for agreement as to the advocacy purpose on a professional level that moves nurses beyond their individual social or political preferences.

In developing a narrative to achieve healthcare policy objectives, nurses must be able to identify the unique root problems of health care associated with specific vulnerable populations that create the barriers to healthcare access, affordability, and quality. The U.S. healthcare system is characterized by extremes of excess and deprivation. Some individuals do not have access to the care they need, as in the case presented in this chapter, while others receive more than enough care. As Starfield (2000) indicated, the United States has the least universal, most costly healthcare system in the industrialized world. This costly system of healthcare financing has evolved through a series of social interventions in an attempt to solve a problem, which in turn created their own problems requiring further intervention (Bodenheimer & Grumbach, 2005).

Undoubtedly, many contributing factors have created barriers for groups or individuals in attempting to access quality health care. As we examine the components of high-quality health care, even more disparities become apparent. Bodenheimer and Grumbach (2005) identified the mechanisms for high-quality care as having access to care, adequate scientific knowledge, competent healthcare providers, separation of financial and clinical decisions, and an organization of healthcare institutions that maximize quality. Extensive research has also identified socioeconomic factors, such as language, education level, poverty level, substandard housing, and poor nutrition, as barriers faced by immigrants when accessing quality health care (Rivers & Patino, 2006). The almost overwhelming diversity in actual or potential factors contributing to healthcare disparities makes finding solutions a challenge for society and policy makers.

Because these factors represent such a broad and intransigent societal challenge for many individuals and communities, their use (or overemphasis) in a political narrative may merely lessen the persuasiveness of the narrative. Thus distinguishing a particular vulnerable population from the overwhelming general healthcare need that exists is an important part of developing the effective narrative. Carefully considering and identifying the unique legal, social, and political issues that are faced by the target population will help nurses convey their story in a way that creates empathy, understanding, and support from both the public and policy makers.

American-born children of undocumented immigrants are a vulnerable population who suffer from healthcare access barriers due to two current polarizing public policy issues rooted in legal, social, and political concerns: immigration and publicly funded health care. When considered in the larger context of the national healthcare debate, this group of American-citizen children represents only a small minority of stakeholders. Yet, these small, isolated, and marginalized groups and individuals may be the ones who can benefit the most from having nurse advocates bring their issues to the forefront of the healthcare debate.

CASE PRESENTATION: DISPARITIES FOR AMERICAN-CITIZEN CHILDREN OF UNDOCUMENTED IMMIGRANTS

In developing the parameters of a narrative, nurses must go beyond the familiar healthcare needs that they are trained to identify. This case study briefly explores three major factors that help explain the healthcare disparities for American-citizen children of undocumented immigrants by utilizing a fictitious immigrant family. First, it discusses the legal considerations that frame the healthcare access for this vulnerable population. Second, it considers the social aspects of being a member of an ostracized and isolated ethnic minority immigrant community. Third, it examines the political barriers associated with the healthcare disparities.

The key member of this fictitious immigrant family is David, a five-year-old American-citizen child born in the metro Atlanta, Georgia, area to parents who are undocumented Guatemalan immigrants. David has been diagnosed with diabetes and requires daily injections of insulin. Unfortunately, he has not seen a pediatric endocrinologist except for one emergency room visit for hyperglycemia, during which he received his diagnosis of diabetes. In a visit to a community clinic, the parents indicated to the nurse that they have not established regular primary care visits with a pediatrician due to lack of insurance and lack of appropriate papers to qualify for insurance. The mother does not work; the father works part-time in the housing industry as an unlicensed plumber; he earns less than $10,000 annually, which is used to support this family of four.

Population Background and Healthcare Significance

A 2009 Pew Hispanic Center Research Report estimated that American-citizen children account for 73% of children residing within family units of mixed legal residency status. The same report estimated that the number of American-citizen children in these mixed family households exceeded 4 million as of 2009 (Passel & Cohn, 2009).

Based on current U.S. law, these children are U.S. citizens, with all the rights and protections that accrue to every citizen. Specifically, these children are citizens based on the principle of *jus soli*, which comes from the Latin meaning "right of the soil" and is a broad principle of birthright citizenship based on the country in which a person is born. This right of citizenship is independent of the nationality of the parents or the legal status of parents in the United States, and is granted based on birth in U.S. territory and territories under its jurisdiction. It is expressly granted in the United States Constitution (Fourteenth Amendment, Citizenship Clause), in the federal Immigration and Naturalization Act [INA Title III, sec. 301(a)], and codified in the United States Code (18 USC §1401). When the right of citizenship by birth is written into law, it is referred to as *lex soli*, a Latin term meaning "law of soil." Fundamentally, *lex soli* is current U.S. law and valid for children born in the United States, with a few exceptions, regardless of whether their parents are U.S. citizens or undocumented immigrants.

One aspect of legal status to consider in presenting David's narrative is the label used to describe the group or population. While the underlying issue of unauthorized adult immigrants is a divisive and challenging subject even for nurses, it need not be the focus of a political narrative for the American children's healthcare needs. David, having been born in Atlanta, is a U.S citizen. It is literally and legally correct to describe him as an American, both in the sense of being American born and in the sense of meeting the legal criteria for citizenship. Choosing alternative phrasing such as "children with U.S. citizenship of undocumented immigrant parents" or "children born in the United States of illegal aliens," however, takes the focus off the legal status of the child and elicits the negative connotations resulting from the parents' immigrant status. It needlessly raises the issue of their parents' legal status. As discussed previously, that issue is irrelevant in terms of whether the child is an American: David is an American citizen.

In the example presented here, David is also a member of a family of Guatemalan descent. Members of this small ethnic minority within the larger immigrant population in the United States are frequently included under the broader label of Hispanic. Despite Guatemala's location in Central America, this population differs from that of other Latin countries in ethnicity, culture, and language. More than half of all Guatemalans are of indigenous Indian descent. Even though half of the population speaks Spanish, many speak and understand only one or more of the indigenous population's 24 dialects (http://www.state.gov/r/pa/ei/bgn/2045.htm). In the United States, these differences have kept Guatemalans somewhat isolated from the mainstream social and political support groups available to more visible and larger Central and South American immigrant groups. These factors also reduce their ability to participate in the broader public dialogue and leave Guatemalans with significantly less political clout in their local communities to address healthcare needs.

In a report to the National Conference of State Legislatures, Wilkicki and Spencer (2008) noted that, as of 2005, American-citizen children with noncitizen parents were twice as likely to lack health coverage as other low-income children. Although these children may have potential access to healthcare services through a group of safety-net providers, including publicly supported hospital and community-based systems, private and charitable free clinics, and faith-based organizations, many of these healthcare delivery systems provide only emergency or occasional urgent care services and lack specialist coverage for managing chronic disorders.

In both episodic illness and chronic disorders, delays in seeking treatment can result in the health condition reaching a crisis point, which then requires utilization of emergency services. The community at large pays the price for this crisis care through increased cost and the over-burdening of emergency services (Rivers & Patino, 2006).

In addition, the lack of healthcare services during childhood can have a significant impact on families and communities. For children, lack of access to quality health care during their early years can create health disparities that persist throughout their entire lives. The potential also exists that the health of their surrounding communities will be negatively affected through failure to diagnose and treat communicable diseases. Lack of consistent primary care may result in ongoing health damage throughout life. Over a lifetime, the lack of disease management is likely to result in increased care costs that will be borne by society. In David's situation, lack of appropriate preventive and primary care for his diabetes early in his life may lead to numerous health consequences throughout his life, a potentially shortened life span, and, ultimately, increased public expense.

Legal Issues to Consider

Because he is a U.S. citizen, David's legal status is not in question. This is an important fact to clarify when discussing such volatile issues as immigration and publicly funded services such as health care. Regardless of the public and political debate surrounding the principle of *jus soli*, as of 2010 it remained the immutable law of the United States. The important fact of David's American citizenship status cannot be overemphasized when developing a useful political narrative. The legal rights to and benefits from healthcare services for which a nurse would be advocating find their basis not just in a vague moral obligation, but also in a concrete legal obligation. Legal obligations are concepts that all Americans understand; thus, by emphasizing this fact, David's narrative starts on the path to forming links with the public and policy makers.

Looking at the existing laws regulating this population's access to health care is the second step in developing an effective narrative. Becoming more aware of the specific laws affecting the population of interest and monitoring the implementation and changes in those laws over time are important parts of understanding healthcare access for the vulnerable population of interest. This case study is limited to one publicly supported healthcare service for low-income children—namely, Medicaid. Medicaid is a jointly funded federal and state entitlement program that is intended to fill gaps in the U.S. health insurance system. Established by legislation passed by Congress in 1965, it is a safety-net healthcare program.

Significantly for David and his family, the Centers for Medicare and Medicaid Services (CMS) program overview specifically speaks to the appropriateness of access to Medicaid healthcare services for American-children citizens of undocumented immigrants: "Your child may be eligible for coverage if he or she is a U.S. citizen or a lawfully admitted immigrant, even if you are not . . . Eligibility for children is based on the child's status, not the parent's" (http://www.cms.gov/MedicaidGenInfo/). Yet, actual access to health services for children in the population of interest is a two-pronged test, based not only on the child's eligibility status, but also on the parents' income and resources qualification. Therein lies the dilemma for the population of interest here. While meeting the eligibility requirements by virtue of being American citizens, the case population is excluded from receipt of services in many cases by the inability of their parents to prove qualifying income status. The issue is not a denial of access to healthcare services based on the family exceeding the allowed income level, but rather a disqualification based on the inability of the parents to either prove their poverty level due to lack of employment documentation or fear of providing employment documentation to prove their poverty level due to their undocumented immigration status (Fernandez, 2009; Fuchs, 2007).

With the ongoing public concern and debate about illegal immigration issues, in 1996 Congress passed the Personal Responsibility and Work Opportunity Reconciliation Act (PRWOR), which enacted major welfare reform under the Clinton administration. For undocumented immigrants, the legislation increased barriers to healthcare access by issuing a restrictive definition of a "qualified alien" meeting the eligibility requirements. For David, even though his eligibility for Medicaid is based on his American citizen status, his access continues to rely on the parents' qualifying proof of financial need. The PRWOR had a significant impact on healthcare access and resulted in denial of federal benefits to numerous eligible American-citizen children of mixed-status families (Wasem, 2008). It was a surprisingly regressive development in publicly funded healthcare coverage for children, which was driven by public pressure on politicians to address the ongoing economic impact of illegal migration.

A decade later, with immigration still a national hotly debated social and political issue, Congress passed the Deficit Reduction Act (2005), which tightened the requirement for personal documentation proving citizenship to access Medicaid benefits. This specific provision was included to target a perceived abuse of Medicaid by illegal immigrants. Unfortunately, it continued the trend of legislative efforts to address immigration enforcement through the denial of benefits to citizen children (Calvo, 2008). Since implementation of the proof of citizenship and identity requirements of the Deficit Reduction Act, states have continued to report a negative impact on enrollment and renewal of children in healthcare programs (Shin, Finnega, Hughes & Rosenbaum, 2007).

For a nurse interested in healthcare policy advocacy, it is important to recognize how legislative efforts to address broader social issues can result in negative collateral consequences for other populations, even American children. More importantly for the population described in this case study, government policy makers are not restricted from knowingly making legislative decisions that cause collateral harm to children even though they are not the target of the law. In *Plyler v. Doe* (1982), the U.S. Supreme Court recognized the inherent unfairness of penalizing children based on their parents' illegal migration; even so, it held that the government could restrict benefits to this population, despite the harm to children, as a legitimate government action to achieve immigration enforcement.

Although nurse policy advocates may not be successful in arguing against legislative actions that collaterally cause harm to children based on existing law or unfairness, they may be much more successful in utilizing the political narrative to generate public support and influence political policy makers. A narrative that puts a face on and tells the story of a specific American child as the sufferer of the harm the law is causing may be more persuasive in convincing legislators to find alternative methods to achieve their goals. As an alternative to nurses walking the halls of the legislative capital building talking about broad healthcare issues in general, a nurse advocate utilizing a narrative may have a more persuasive impact on legislators by introducing David, an articulate, bright, playful, English-speaking American child to each legislator and discussing the severe suffering and harm from untreated diabetes, and the future cost to the healthcare system, that may result from their legislation requiring parental qualifiers for David to receive public services.

Another important aspect of Medicaid-funded healthcare coverage for low-income children is the part states play in implementation of programs and services. Within specific parameters, states are given leeway to structure their programs and services to meet the unique needs of their state populations. This is an important consideration for nurse policy advocates, because they must be aware of and guide state Medicaid policy decisions that affect their vulnerable population's access to health care.

One aspect of the current political policy reform relates to the Section 1115 Medicaid waiver process. Section 1115 is intended to encourage states to develop new and innovative programs that help them meet the healthcare needs within their borders. States have used the Section 1115 waiver process to cover individuals who do not meet the categorical requirements, meaning they do not fit within the traditional mandated categories provided by law—that is, pregnant women, children, parents, elderly, and persons with recognized disabilities. States are still eligible to receive Medicaid matching funds if their programs to cover these noncategorical groups are approved under the Section 115 waiver process. For example, six states (Maine, Michigan, New Mexico, New York, Oregon, and Utah), plus the District of Columbia, have received waivers to expand coverage to low-income adults without dependent children—a group not traditionally covered by Medicaid. The important point to note is that when state legislators are moved to expand coverage for particular groups, there is a mechanism to do so and also the political will to successfully modify the state Medicaid programs (Artiga & Mann, 2005).

Each state's implementation of its specific program guidelines is an important consideration when addressing the barriers American-citizen children face in accessing the healthcare services they are entitled to through Medicaid. Using the waiver process, states can expand eligibility requirements and experiment with different models of care delivery. Exploitation of this potentially important avenue for rectifying disparities in American-citizen children's access to health care, separate and apart from their parents' legal status, provides an example of how the nurse advocate can examine the existing laws and provide evidence-based solutions when developing an effective narrative.

Social Issues to Consider

Social and community dynamics affecting a diverse and vulnerable population are also important to understand when developing a narrative. Understanding the social barriers that specific populations face requires nurses to explore the ethnic, cultural, and language differences inherent in a particular group or individual. Collection of data at the community and individual levels, therefore, is an essential component of developing and improving health care for diverse and vulnerable populations (The Joint Commission, 2009).

Finding a way to create a link between a diverse population or individual and the general public is an important part of narrative development. Creating connections between an isolated or marginalized population and the general population establishes a bond that reveals the chosen individual or group on a personal level. Although other sections of this text provide more detail on cultural issues, an example that illustrates the beginning of this process is understanding the religious affiliations that are important to groups and communities. As part of the narrative for David, it may be important to know and emphasize that the Guatemalan population has assimilated Western religious beliefs and its members are predominantly Roman Catholic and Protestant (http://www.state.gov/r/pa/ei/bgn/2045.html). While this fact may not necessarily be significant for healthcare delivery, it is an important factor for establishing familiarity, connectedness, and inclusiveness between a marginalized individual or community and the general public.

It is also important to consider the barriers to healthcare access that may arise from these social differences. As discussed earlier, David's community is not only isolated from the national population, but their language and culture also keep members even further isolated within the larger Hispanic immigrant population. The changing legal landscape of immigration enforcement and heightened requirements for documentation of parental status to access Medicaid services also serve to isolate this community. Even the news and reporting in a state or community that focuses on undocumented immigrant issues fosters an atmosphere of social isolation. When discussing broader immigration issues, the immigration status of adults serves as the general basis for debate. In contrast, the children of immigrant parents and the effects that immigration policy has on their welfare receive limited media coverage and are rarely the focus of public concern (Population Reference Bureau, 2009).

Collectively, these forces create an atmosphere of fear. From a healthcare perspective, this type of community fear results in delays in seeking care and treatment (Clark, 2008). In some cases, the undocumented immigrant parents of American-citizen children must either expose their own illegal status and risk incarceration and deportation or deny and delay their child's health care. The reality of a parent's struggle to balance family welfare with the need for a child's health care is not unique or unknown. President Obama specifically addressed the fact that parents can be put into situations where they must decide between the child's welfare and that of the family when signing the Children's Health Insurance Program Bill: "It's hard to overstate the toll this takes on our families: the sleepless nights worrying that someone's going to get hurt, or praying that a sick child gets better on her own. The decisions that no parent should ever have to make—how long to put off that doctor's appointment, whether to fill that prescription . . ." (Office of the Press Secretary, 2009).

The social fabric of the community faced with such dilemmas becomes interwoven with fear and distrust. Note that the issue here for the nurse advocate is not the moral, ethical, or legal issues surrounding the fear caused by enforcement of the U.S. laws on immigration, but rather the resulting denial of, or failure to access, healthcare services for which American-citizen children are legally eligible. The narrative need not address the parent's plight in suffering the consequences of illegal migration; instead, its sole focus should be the American-citizen children's inability to obtain the healthcare services to which they are entitled.

Political Action and Politicians

In U.S. government, political policy making is as much a function of public pandering as it is problem solving. The feelings, moods, and personal biases of constituents are important considerations for politicians, who rely on their constituents' vote to gain and remain in office. Politicians' ability to vacillate with the mood of the electorate and change to reflect the wishes of their constituents is actually an important part of a representative government model. Recognizing this dynamic as part of the political process helps ensure the nurse develops a narrative that both reflects the public's changing sentiments and lays foundation for politicians' support of the nursing goals.

As a reflection of society's growing discontent with the immigration issue, state legislatures are becoming more active in passing laws that target the illegal immigrant population. These laws, which are designed to reach into the everyday lives of immigrants, range from specific restrictions on healthcare access to laws that regulate employment, housing, travel education, and law enforcement. While not all negative or punitive in nature, they signal the mood of an increasingly polarized society that is focused on immigration and immigrants themselves. For instance, state laws related to immigration increased from 570 introduced, 84 laws enacted, and 12 resolutions adopted in 2006 to 1180 immigration bills introduced, 107 laws enacted, and 87 resolutions adopted in the first quarter of 2010 (National Conference of State Legislatures, 2010).

Understanding how politicians approach allocation of public resources is important in framing the political narrative. The concept of worthiness, for example, plays out in how public policy is developed and in how public resources are allocated to serve and treat the needy in our society (Clemen-Stone, McGuire, & Eigsti, 2002). LaFrance (2007) identified the concept of *worthy poor* as integral to Congressional decision making. In examining the specific needs addressed by legislative action, politicians may evaluate and label individuals, groups, and communities as *worthy* or *unworthy* of public assistance. Being *unworthy* may be the basis for denial of benefits and a lack of Congressional or political attention.

Policy makers may justify a lack of distributive justice in their allocation of resources by this process of evaluation and labeling. For example, in public debates, restrictions and heightened requirements on publicly funded health care are often explicitly tied to illegal immigrants' potential abuse of the healthcare services that they have no legitimate right to and to which they did not contribute. These individuals are deemed essentially *unworthy* and seen as not deserving to access the public supported healthcare services. Thus the debate does not deal with moral or ethical human rights and healthcare services; rather, the policy decision may be based on the simple perception of whether or not the individuals or populations deserve the public support.

In the *CRS Report for Congress: Unauthorized Aliens' Access to Federal Benefits: Policy and Issues* (2008), the Congressional Research Services (CRS) reported to Congress that the PRWOR legislation did result in denial of benefits to U.S.-citizen children. However, before explicitly stating what should be a troubling fact for political policy makers and making a call to action to correct this result, CRS referenced a study by a policy researcher that estimated "The U.S. citizen children of unauthorized aliens account for much of the costs associated with illegal migration" (Wasem, 2008, p. 2). It is an amazingly broad placement of blame on such a specific small group. With an understanding of Congressional need to determine worthiness, it becomes clear that if this statement is true, it is easier to justify a policy that results in denial of benefits for a group who already represent such a huge expense for the United States. In turn, these American-citizen children can comfortably be determined *unworthy* to receive the public benefits to which they are entitled.

Ensuring that the political narrative contains the supporting information regarding why the individual or population is deserving or worthy of support is essential in influencing political action. Think back to the political narrative regarding the Secrest family. President Obama included the detail of the Secrest children's willingness to self-sacrifice and give up their last piggybank pennies. In such a staged and tightly controlled environment as a legislative bill signing, it is not likely that this miscellaneous fact was added randomly. Rather, it enhanced the narrative, and thereby the message conveyed to the public, and supported these recipients' *worthiness* to receive publicly funded health benefits. They were willing to give all they had, and do all they could, on their own, and so were deemed worthy of federal assistance.

Linking Legal, Social, and Political Factors to Develop a Narrative

For nurses, the goal is to reframe the narrative about specific vulnerable populations to remove or reduce barriers to healthcare access. In this case, framing the discussion as involving illegal immigrants will not change the agenda. However, transforming the narrative into an issue of access for American-citizen children will bring an essential focus to the discussion instead of viewing these children's dilemma through the lens of immigration, which tends to generate both social and political resistance. These American-citizen children have all the rights and privileges of every other American citizen. The goal in developing the narrative to emphasize their situation is not to ignore all of the other illegal immigrants' plight; instead, the goal is to highlight true characteristics about the vulnerable population for public and political support. The narrative would reinforce the principle that these American citizens should have access to healthcare services equal to that of every other American citizen. The nurse advocate engenders empathy and understanding by associating a person like David with the narrative and conveying his story of healthcare eligibility, need for health care, and worthiness. The narrative creates a way for the nurse to move public opinion and supplies the needed support for policy changes. This process may be an invaluable tool nurses must use in achieving policy goals.

In 2009, Congress passed the Children's Health Insurance Program Reauthorization Act (CHIPRA), which represented a sweeping reaffirmation of the importance of children's health care as a priority for the future. The bill expanded coverage for an estimated 4 million children. Although legal immigration status is still required to be eligible for coverage, the law specifically revoked the 1995 law requiring a five-year waiting period for eligibility for new immigrants (Kaiser Commission on Medicaid and the Uninsured, 2010). Additionally, the law included incentives for outreach efforts to enroll low-income uninsured children (CMS, National CHIP Policy Overview, http://www.cms.gov/NationalCHIPPolicy). Because it did not change the practice of establishing eligibility based on a parent's legal status, the population of American-citizen children lost an opportunity to seek relief from the government's use of their vulnerability as an immigrant enforcement effort. Was there an opportunity for nurses to use a story like David's to raise awareness of these American children's healthcare situation?

Developing Narratives to Influence Public Opinion and Political Action

The case study presented here illustrates how nurses must think creatively to develop narratives that will help society redefine how a particular vulnerable population and their healthcare issues are perceived—here, the population of American-citizen children. Is there a way to separate their status from the gatekeeping aspect of parental qualifications? Medicare allows unusual disassociation of benefits that a child may receive from his or her living arrangements in qualifying. For instance, the case example that CMS provides in its Medicaid Program Overview document is a non–family member child living with a nonqualifying family. According to the CMS guidelines, "[I]f someone else's child lives with you, the child may be eligible even if you are not because your income and resources will not count for the child" (https://www.cms.gov/MedicaidGenInfo/). Is there a way to frame the narrative so as to move the perception of these American-citizen children under this type of exclusion? In the case example provided by CMS, it would be irrelevant if the family taking care of the child were millionaires. The eligibility and qualification rest solely on the child's own status; the adult household income is not a consideration for access to services.

A powerful way to overcome resistance is to develop the narrative so that similarities between the vulnerable population and existing exceptions are established. As nurses help policy makers see the justification for the change, present examples of vulnerable individuals and populations, and convey the worthiness of their access to public benefits, they will help overcome the barriers that these individuals and populations face, give them a voice in the policy arena, and advance healthcare policy to the benefit of all. **Table 40–1** summarizes recommended steps in developing effective narratives to advance public policy and healthcare advocacy.

Table 40–1 Developing Effective Narratives in Advancing Public Policy and Healthcare Advocacy

Step 1	Identify the communities and individuals that may benefit the most from the use of narratives.
Step 2	Examine existing laws regulating the population's access to health care to define the problems and find solutions.
Step 3	Create connections and links between the vulnerable populations and the general population by understanding the social and community dynamics affecting the diverse and vulnerable population.
Step 4	Ensure that the narrative reflects the public's sentiments and supports the dynamics of the political process, including information regarding why the individual or population is deserving or worthy of support of healthcare eligibility, need for health care, and worthiness.

Link all of these factors together to show healthcare eligibility, need for the health care, and worthiness to receive the care.

For a full suite of assignments and additional learning activities, use the access code located in the front of your book to visit this exclusive website: http://go.jblearning.com/dechesnay. If you do not have an access code, you can obtain one at the site.

REFERENCES

Artiga, S., & Mann, C. (2005). Kaiser Commission on Medicaid and the uninsured: New directions for Medicaid Section 1115 waivers: Policy implications of recent waiver activity. Retrieved from http://www.kff.org/medicaid/upload/New-Directions-for-Medicaid-Section-1115-Waivers-Policy-Implications-of-Recent-Waiver-Activity-Policy-Brief.pdf

Bennet, L. & Edelman, M. (2006). Toward a new political narrative. *Journal of Communication, 35*(4), 156–171.

Bodenheimer, T. S., & Grumbach, K. (2005). *Understanding health policy: A clinical approach* (5th ed.). New York, NY: McGraw-Hill.

Calvo, J. (2008). The consequences of restricted health care access for immigrants: Lessons from Medicaid and SCHIP. In *Annual Health Law, 17* (p. 175). Chicago: Loyola University School of Law, and Beazley Institute for Health, Law, and Policy.

Clark, B. (2008, Summer). The immigrant health care narrative and what it tells us about the U.S. health care system. In *Annual Health Law, 17* (p. 229). Chicago: Loyola University School of Law, and Beazley Institute for Health, Law, and Policy.

Clemen-Stone, S., McGuire, S. & Eigsti, D. (2002). *Comprehensive community health nursing: Family, aggregate, and community practice* (6th ed.). St. Louis, MO: Mosby.

Fernandez, V. (2009). Fearing new law, Arizona immigrants forego health services. Retrieved from http://news.newamericamedia.org/news/view_article.html?article_id=fe28b22400495055eeedd7627bc58332

Fuchs, E. (2007). Medical needs of Hispanics targeted. *Chattanooga Times/Free Press.* Retrieved from http://www.timesfreepress.com/news/2007/jul/28/Medical-needs-of-Hispanics-targeted

The Joint Commission. (2009, October). Executive summary: Hospitals, language, and culture study. Retrieved from http://www.jointcommission.org/NR/rdonlyres/C4694C27-D5A1-4D08-AC97-4CB9A8B6CECA/0/HLC_One_Size_Exec_Summary.pdf

Kaiser Commission on Medicaid and the Uninsured. (2010, June). Medicaid: A primer: Key information on our nation's health coverage program for low-income people. Retrieved from http://www.kff.org/medicaid/upload/7334-04.pdf

LaFrance, A. (2007). Healthcare reform in the United States: the role of the states. *Canterbury Law Review, 13*, 227. Retrieved from http://www.austlii.edu.au/nz/journals/CanterLawRw/2007/8.html

National Conference of State Legislatures. (2010, January–March). Immigration-related bills and resolutions in the states. Retrieved from http://www.ncsl.org/default.aspx?tabid=20244

Office of the Press Secretary. (2009, February 4). Remarks by President Barack Obama on Children's Health Insurance Program bill signing. Retrieved from http://www.whitehouse.gov/the_press_office/RemarksbyPresidentBarackObamaOnChildrensHealthInsuranceProgramBillSigning

Passel, J., & Cohn, D. (2009, April 14). *A portrait of unauthorized immigrants in the United States.* Pew Research Center Publications. Retrieved from http://pewhispanic.org/files/reports/107.pdf

Personal Responsibility and Work Opportunity Reconciliation Act of 1996, H.R.3734, 104th Cong. (1996).

Population Reference Bureau. (2009, February). *Children in immigrant families chart new path* (PRB Reports On America). Washington, DC: Mather, M.

Rivers, P., & Patino, F. (2006). Barriers to health care access for Latino immigrants in the USA. *International Journal of Social Economics, 33*(3/4): 207.

Shin, P., Finnega, B., Hughes, L. & Rosenbaum, S. (2007). *An initial assessment of the effects of Medicaid documentation requirements on health centers and their patients.* Retrieved from http://www.gwumc.edu/sphhs/departments/healthpolicy/CHPR/downloads/Medicaid_Doc_Requirements.pdf

Starfield, B. (2000). Is U.S. health really the best in the world? *Journal of the American Medical Association, 284*, 483.

Wasem, R. E. (2008, May 21). CRS report for Congress: Unauthorized aliens' access to federal benefits: Policy and issues. Retrieved from http://fpc.state.gov/documents/organization/106160.pdf

Wilkicki, K. & Spencer, A. (2008). *Health care access for children in immigrant families: A primer for state legislators.* Washington DC: National Conference of State Legislatures.

CHAPTER 41

Health Policy and Advocacy for Vulnerable Populations

Kathryn Osborne

Objectives

At the end of this chapter, the reader will be able to

1. Compare and contrast the Healthy People Outcomes for 2010 and 2020 in terms of vulnerable populations.
2. Make the case for continued national healthcare reform.
3. Describe the implications for nursing of the passage of the bills described in the chapter.

INTRODUCTION

The creation of health policy as a mechanism to improve health outcomes for vulnerable populations has been a part of the national agenda in the United States for more than a century. Current efforts to improve health outcomes in the United States are occurring at the local, state, and national levels. This chapter focuses on federal health policy and healthcare reform. Readers are encouraged to investigate the impact of health policy on vulnerable populations in their individual states and local communities.

VULNERABLE POPULATIONS FROM A HEALTH POLICY PERSPECTIVE

The U.S. Department of Health and Human Services (HHS, 2009) defines members of vulnerable populations as individuals "who tend to have poorer health status and more medical needs than the general population" (p. 22). In 1998, the federal Agency for Health Care Policy and Research (AHCPR) defined vulnerable populations as "groups of people made vulnerable by their financial circumstances or place of residence; health, age, or functional or developmental status; or ability to communicate effectively . . . [and] personal characteristics, such as race, ethnicity, and sex" (1998, para. 1). AHCPR—which is now known as the Agency for Healthcare Research and Quality (AHRQ)— has shifted its focus to "*priority populations* – groups with unique healthcare needs that require special focus" (2008a, para. 1). The definition of these groups was specified with passage of the Healthcare Research and Quality Act of 1999 to include "minority groups; low-income groups; women; children (age 0–17); older adults (age 65 and over); residents of rural areas; and individuals with special healthcare needs, including individuals with disabilities and individuals who need chronic care or end-of-life care" (AHRQ, 2008a, AHRQ's Priority Populations, para. 1).

Healthy People 2010 and the *Healthy People 2020* provide national objectives relative to improving the health status of the United States. The two overarching goals of the program are to "increase quality and years of healthy life, and eliminate health disparities" (*Healthy People 2010*, n.d., para. 1). These disparities include differences in health outcomes and health status that occur as a result of race or ethnicity, gender, sexual orientation, education, income, disability, or geographic location (Centers for Disease Control and Prevention [CDC], 2009). While the goals of *Healthy People 2010* are aimed at improving the overall health of the U.S. population, it is clear that the health policy agenda of this government-sponsored program places a high priority on reducing disparities for vulnerable populations.

HISTORICAL BACKGROUND

The origins of health policy aimed at improving the health status of vulnerable populations in the United States can be traced as far back as the late nineteenth century. Early public policy attempts often focused on "upstream" interventions—meaning policy that dealt with root causes of poor health such as overcrowded housing, poor sanitation, waste management, poor working conditions, and other social and economic determinants of health (Lantz, Lichtenstein, & Pollack, 2007). The enactment of the Sheppard-Towner Act in 1921 was an early example of health policy aimed at altering the healthcare delivery system. The Sheppard-Towner Act was passed in response to research conducted by the Federal Children's Bureau, which revealed alarmingly high rates of maternal and infant mortality in the United States. The Act allocated funds to individual states for the purpose of establishing maternal and child health services (Rooks, 1997).

Despite the efforts of several U.S. presidents during the first half of the twentieth century, health policy in the form of national healthcare reform did not come about until the 1965 passage of Title XVIII and Title XIX of the Social Security Act, during the Lyndon Johnson administration (Morone, 2010). Title XVIII and Title XIX called for the establishment of Medicare and Medicaid. Medicare provided healthcare coverage for most Americans at or older than age 65, while the purpose of Medicaid was to expand the healthcare coverage for low-income populations that was available under existing federal–state welfare programs (Centers for Medicare and Medicaid Service [CMS], 2010a). In 1972, passage of the Federal Supplemental Security Income (SSI) program extended Medicare eligibility to persons younger than age 65 with long-term disabilities (and to persons of any age with end-stage renal disease), and allowed states to expand Medicaid eligibility to elderly, blind, and disabled individuals (CMS, 2010a).

Over the next three decades, several modifications to Medicare and Medicaid were adopted. Perhaps most notable were the creation of the State Children's Health Insurance Program (SCHIP) in 1997, which expanded Medicaid coverage for children, and passage of the Medicare Prescription Drug, Improvement, and Modernization Act (MMA) in 2003, which was intended to improve drug benefits for senior citizens. Included in MMA was a provision to implement Medicare Part D, which further expanded drug benefits for senior citizens (CMS, 2010a).

THE CASE FOR NATIONAL REFORM

Despite implementation of these programs, the overall health status of Americans has been relatively dismal. In 2008, total health expenditures in the United States rose to more than $2.3 trillion ($7681 per capita), representing slightly more than 16% of the country's gross domestic product (CMS, 2010b). Per capita spending on health care in the United States is higher than the equivalent rate in any other country (World Health Organization [WHO], 2010), yet the United States has the lowest life expectancy at birth among industrialized nations, and ranks twenty-ninth in the world in terms of infant mortality rates (Organization for Economic Cooperation and Development [OECD], 2009). In 2007, the United Nations Children's Fund report card ranked the United States next to last, among 21 developed nations, for overall child well-being, and last on measures of child health and safety (United Nations Children's Fund, 2007). In 2010, Amnesty International referred to maternal health outcomes in the United States as a "human rights crisis," citing increased rates of maternal mortality (higher than those in 40 other countries), especially among African American women.

Increased Access to Care: Is It Really the Answer?

Access to health care is defined by AHRQ as having "the timely use of personal health services to achieve the best health outcomes" (AHRQ, 2008b, Components of Health Care Access, para. 1). Access to care is measured in three distinct ways: identification of resources (such as insurance or a usual source of care) that facilitate health care; patient assessment of the ease with which access to care was gained; and identification of utilization measures (AHRQ, 2008b). Given that the acquisition of health insurance facilitates entry into the U.S. healthcare system, the degree to which Americans are covered by health insurance is often used as a key indicator of access to care. Clearly, individuals without health insurance experience disparities in health outcomes and overall health status (AHRQ, 2008a; National Center for Health Statistics, 2007). It is with this understanding that current measures to improve disparities in health outcomes for vulnerable populations have focused on improving access to health insurance as a way to increase access to care.

Improved access to care was clearly an outcome of the implementation of Medicare and Medicaid. Yet even many years after the introduction of these programs, Americans continue to have some of the poorest health outcomes in the world. For example, despite advances in perinatal care, racial and ethnic disparities persist with regard to death and disease related to pregnancy, preterm birth, and infant and fetal mortality in the United States. Reasons for these disparities remain largely unexplained (Healy et al., 2006; MacDorman & Kirmeyer, 2009), although limited access to quality health care has been cited as one of the contributing factors (MacDorman & Kirmeyer, 2009). During the past decade, expansion of statewide Medicaid programs has significantly improved access to care for pregnant women, but yielded little or no change in disparate perinatal outcome measures. Nonetheless, efforts to eliminate disparities in perinatal outcomes continue to focus on increasing access to early and adequate prenatal care.

According to the most recent statistics, 83.9% of pregnant women in the United States receive prenatal care in the first trimester, 3.5% receive prenatal care only in the third trimester or not at all, and racial disparities in the utilization of early prenatal care persist (National Center for Health Statistics, 2008). Recognizing that early and adequate prenatal care is associated with an improvement in several perinatal outcome measures, the federal government identified increased access to early and adequate prenatal care as one of the objectives of *Healthy People 2010* in an attempt to eliminate disparities in perinatal outcomes. However, the fact that access to early prenatal care has vastly improved over the last decade without a corresponding reduction in racially disparate outcomes (Amnesty International, 2010; Paul, Lehman, Suliman, & Hillemeier, 2007) may suggest that simply improving access to care falls short when it comes to reducing racial disparities in health outcomes (Healy et al., 2006; Mainous, Hueston, Love, & Griffith, 1999; Schempf, Kroelinger, & Guyer, 2007).

The passage of the Patient Protection and Affordable Care Act (PPACA), described in the next section, vastly increases access to affordable health insurance coverage for Americans. It lays the groundwork for improvements in the healthcare delivery system so that issues such as the availability of appropriate healthcare providers and the delivery of culturally sensitive health care become priorities.

The Patient Protection and Affordable Care Act (H.R. 3590)

On March 23, 2010, President Barack Obama signed the Patient Protection and Affordable Care Act (H.R. 3590) into law. Depending on how one defines vulnerability or vulnerable populations, it is possible to find provisions on any one of the 2000-plus pages of the PPACA that relate to one vulnerable population or another. This legislation is so comprehensive that it focuses on vulnerable populations in a number of ways, many of which are embedded within larger provisions in which vulnerable populations are not explicitly mentioned. For example, one of the provisions in the PPACA creates state-based American Health Benefit Exchanges through which individuals will be able to purchase more affordable healthcare coverage. Farmers, who because of their geographic location are considered a vulnerable population, and who because of the dangerous nature of their work have had difficulty purchasing affordable health insurance policies, will have access to more affordable healthcare coverage through these Exchanges.

Another provision of the PPACA increases Medicare reimbursement to certified nurse–midwives from 65% to 100% of the reimbursed rate for physicians. This provision increases access to primary care providers for women age 65 and older, as well as young disabled women who qualify for Medicare. Under yet another provision of the legislation, dependent children up to age 26—many of whom are members of vulnerable populations—will now qualify for coverage under their parent's private health insurance plans.

A complete review of the PPACA is beyond the scope of this chapter. Key provisions of the law, as identified by the Kaiser Family Foundation (2010), are summarized in **Table 41–1**, with an emphasis on provisions that directly affect vulnerable populations. Although the PPACA was signed into law in early 2010, plans for its implementation include a phasing in of many of the provisions over the next eight years. Full implementation will not occur until 2018. Readers are encouraged to visit http://www.kff.org/healthreform/8061.cfm for a full summary of the PPACA, including a timeline for implementation.

Table 41–1 Key Provisions of the Patient Protection and Affordable Care Act with Direct Implications for Vulnerable Populations

Provisions That Became Effective 90 Days Following Enactment

Establishment of a temporary high-risk pool to provide healthcare coverage for individuals with preexisting medical conditions (effective only until January 1, 2014)

Provision of dependent coverage for adult children up to age 26 for private individual and group insurance policies

A prohibition of individual and group health plans from placing lifetime limits on total health spending prior to 2014

A requirement for qualified health plans to provide coverage for preventive services rated A or B by the U.S. Preventive Services Task Force, recommended immunizations, and preventive care and screening for women, infants, and children without cost sharing

A requirement for Medicare to provide a $250 rebate to beneficiaries who reach the Part D coverage gap ("the doughnut hole") in 2010 and to eliminate the Part D coverage gap by 2020

A requirement for states to create an option for coverage of childless adults through Medicaid expansion

A requirement for states to cover family planning services for low-income individuals through Medicaid expansion

Establishment of a Patient-Centered Outcomes Research Institute to conduct comparative effectiveness research

A reauthorization and amendment of the Indian Health Care Improvement Act

An increase in the workforce supply of primary care providers, which includes increased funding for scholarships and loans for the education and training of these providers

Provisions That Must Be Implemented in 2011

Establishment of a national, voluntary long-term care insurance program

Elimination of cost sharing for Medicare-covered preventive services that are recommended by the U.S. Preventive Services Task Force

A requirement for Medicare to provide comprehensive risk assessment and personalized preventive health plans for beneficiaries

Continued

Table 41–1 Continued

A requirement for Medicare and Medicaid to provide incentives for behavior modification programs for beneficiaries

A requirement for pharmaceutical companies to provide a 50% discount on brand-name drugs filled in the Medicare Part D coverage gap

A prohibition on Medicare Advantage Plans from imposing higher cost-sharing requirements for covered benefits

Creation of state Medicaid plans that allow an option for some beneficiaries to designate a healthcare provider as a health home

Establishment of the Community First Choice Option under Medicaid to provide community-based attendant support services for certain disabled individuals

Development of a national quality improvement program that includes priorities to improve healthcare delivery, patient outcomes, and population health

Establishment of the Community-Based Collaborative Care Network Program to support healthcare providers in the coordination and integration of health services for low-income uninsured and underinsured individuals

Increased funding by $11 billion for community health centers and by $1.5 billion for a National Health Service Corps over five years

Establishment of new programs to support school-based health centers and nurse-managed clinics

Provisions That Must Be Implemented in 2012

Implementation of several programs that remove disincentives and provide incentives for healthcare providers and institutions to offer services to Medicare and Medicaid beneficiaries

A mandate for the collection and reporting of data on race, ethnicity, gender, primary language, and disability status, and the collection and reporting of data on underserved and frontier populations

Phase-in of federal monies to subsidize brand-name prescriptions filled in the Medicare D coverage gap

An increase in Medicaid payments for primary care services (delivered by primary care *physicians*) to 100% Medicare rates for 2013 and 2014

Provisions That Must Be Implemented in 2014

A requirement for every U.S. citizen and legal resident to have health coverage; tax penalties will be phased in for those without coverage

The creation of state-based American Health Benefit Exchange and Small Business Health Options Program (SHOP) Exchanges that will be administered by a government agency or nonprofit organization; individuals and small businesses will be able to purchase qualified coverage through these Exchanges

A reduction in the out-of-pocket spending limits for individuals with incomes up to 400% of the federal poverty level (FPL)

Limitation of waiting periods to no more than 90 days

Limitation of deductibles for small-group and individual health plans

A requirement for qualified health plans to meet operating standards and reporting requirements

The provision of cost-sharing subsidies for the purchase insurance through the Exchanges to qualified families and individuals at 133% to 400% of FPL

A reduction in out-of-pocket expenses required for Medicare enrollees to become eligible for catastrophic coverage

Expansion of Medicaid to all individuals younger than age 65 who are not eligible for Medicare and who have incomes up to 133% of FPL

IMPLICATIONS FOR NURSING

For many years, the American Nurses Association (ANA) has been a leading advocate for healthcare reform, including the availability of universal health care. In 2008, this organization published *The ANA's Health System Reform Agenda*, which identified four critical issues that must be considered during the reformation of the healthcare delivery system: access, cost, quality, and workforce (ANA, 2008). A comparative analysis of the PPACA and *The ANA's Health System Reform Agenda* reveals that all four critical issues identified in the ANA agenda were addressed in the PPACA. Further, most of the recommendations included in the *Health System Reform Agenda* will be addressed with the implementation of the PPACA provisions between 2010 and 2018 (ANA, 2010a).

With regard to *access*, provisions in the PPACA ensure access to care in all geographic locations to all American citizens regardless of age, gender, ethnicity, and socioeconomic status. Other provisions call for health care to be delivered in a way that is acceptable to recipients—that is, delivered with respect for patient autonomy, cultural sensitivity, and in a way that is patient centered. The PPACA also focuses on ensuring the affordability of health care for U.S. citizens, whether that care consists of a standard package of essential health services (including mental health parity). The legislation falls short with regard to the provision of health care for undocumented immigrants, however, and it fails to recognize health care as a basic human right (ANA, 2010a).

Recognizing the importance of improving both access to care and *quality* of care, the ANA identified six quality indicators to be addressed as the healthcare delivery system is reformed. Included in the PPACA are provisions to improve the quality of health care on all six measures: safety, effectiveness, patient-centeredness, timeliness, efficiency, and equitability. Consistent with the framework within which nursing research is often conducted, the PPACA establishes the Patient-Centered Outcomes Research Institute. Also in keeping with the recommendations of the ANA, it includes provisions that support continuity of care and address chronic disease management. Moreover, the new law includes provisions that promote health and that will, over time, lead to disease prevention. Finally, the PPACA contains provisions that will establish a national quality improvement strategy as well as the adoption of quality indicators for nursing (ANA, 2010a).

While the PPACA does not call for the public funding (including creation of a single-payer system) that was supported by the ANA, it does contain provisions that will control *costs* and protect the financial well-being of families with high medical expenses. The PPACA also contains provisions for cost sharing between individuals and payers (based on income level) while recognizing the importance of personal responsibility on the part of the healthcare recipient. Finally, it include measures to enhance the delivery of primary care and recognize the economic value of nurses, including the recognition of advanced practice nurses as primary care providers (ANA, 2010a).

Although the provisions related to *workforce* development may not be explicitly stated in terms of vulnerable populations, it is important to remember that by 2014 an estimated 32 million U.S. citizens, most of whom have been without any form of health insurance, will gain access to the healthcare system as a result of the PPACA (Goodson, 2010). Further, only 30% of the physicians practicing in the United States are providing primary care services (Goodson, 2010). In recognition of the shortage of primary care providers, the PPACA supports expansion of the primary care workforce, including recognition of nurse practitioners and certified nurse–midwives as primary care providers. It also establishes grant programs for school-based health clinics and authorizes funds to support nurse-managed health centers operated by advanced practice nurses (ANA, 2010b). Both of these provisions will expand opportunities for nurses at all levels of practice. It is further anticipated that the mandate for expanded funding of nursing education will increase the size of the nursing workforce—both the number of practicing nurses and the faculty necessary to prepare new nurses.

CONCLUSION

The United States has a lengthy history of policy aimed at improving the health outcomes for vulnerable populations. Recent passage of the PPACA is anticipated to narrow the gap between health outcomes for affluent Americans and health outcomes for vulnerable populations. Nurses are poised to play a key role in implementation of the PPACA, through their continued advocacy for the vulnerable populations whom they serve. In light of the fact that much of the implementation of the healthcare reform legislation will occur on state and local levels, it will be important for nurses to become involved in state and local government, including individual state legislative proceedings. The full effect of the PPACA on health disparities for vulnerable populations will not be felt until well into the next decade. Even so, the future looks bright, both for the profession of nursing and for vulnerable populations served by nurses.

WWW

For a full suite of assignments and additional learning activities, use the access code located in the front of your book to visit this exclusive website: http://go.jblearning.com/dechesnay. If you do not have an access code, you can obtain one at the site.

REFERENCES

Agency for Healthcare Research and Quality (AHRQ). (2008a). 2008 national healthcare quality and disparities reports, Chapter 4: Priority populations. Retrieved from http://www.ahrq.gov/qual/nhdr08/Chap4.htm

Agency for Healthcare Research and Quality (AHRQ). (2008b). 2008 national quality and disparities reports, Chapter 3: Access to health care. Retrieved from http://www.ahrq.gov/qual/nhdr08/Chap3.htm

Agency for Health Care Policy and Research (AHCPR). (1998). AHCPR seeks proposals to develop quality of care measures for vulnerable Populations. Retrieved from http://www.ahrq.gov/news/press/vulnpr.htm

American Nurses Association (ANA). (2008). *Health system reform agenda.* Silver Spring, MD: American Nurses Association.

American Nurses Association (ANA). (2010a). ANA policy and provisions of health reform law. Retrieved from http://www.rnaction.org/site/DocServer/PPACAProvisions_April2010.pdf?docID=1261

American Nurses Association (ANA). (2010b). Health care reform: Key provisions related to nursing. Retrieved from http://www.rnaction.org/site/DocServer/KeyProvisions_Nursing-PublicLaw.pdf?docID=1241&verID=1

Amnesty International. (2010). Deadly delivery: The maternal health care crisis in the US. Retrieved from http://www.amnestyusa.org/dignity/pdf/DeadlyDelivery.pdf

Centers for Disease Control and Prevention (CDS). (2009). Eliminating racial and ethnic health disparities. Retrieved from http://www.cdc.gov/omhd/About/disparities.htm

Centers for Medicare and Medicaid Services (CMS). (2010a). Key milestones in CMS programs. Retrieved from https://www.cms.gov/History

Centers for Medicare and Medicaid Services (CMS). (2010b). National health expenditure data. Retrieved from http://www.cms.gov/NationalHealthExpendData

Goodson, J. (2010). Patient Protection and Affordable Care Act: Promise and peril for primary care. *American College of Physicians, 152,* 742–744.

Healthy People 2010. (n.d.). What are its goals. Retrieved from http://www.healthypeople.gov/About/goals.htm

Healthy People 2020-Improving the health of Americans (n.d.) Retrieved from http://www.healthypeople.gov

Healy, A., Malone, F., Sullivan, L., Porter, F., Luthy, D., Comstock, C., . . . D'Alton, M. E. (2006). Early access to prenatal care: Implications for racial disparity in perinatal mortality. *Obstetrics and Gynecology, 107(3),* 625–631.

Kaiser Family Foundation. (2010). Summary of new health reform law. Retrieved from http://www.kff.org/healthreform/8061.cfm

Lantz, P., Lichtenstein, R., & Pollack, H. (2007). Health policy approaches to population health: The limits of medicalization. *Health Affairs, 26(5),* 1253–1257.

MacDorman, M., & Kirmeyer, S. (2009). National vital statistics reports: Fetal and perinatal mortality, United States, 2005. Retrieved from http://www.cdc.gov/nchs/data/nvsr/nvsr57/nvsr57_08.pdf

Mainous, A., Hueston, W., Love, M., & Griffith, C. (1999). Access to care for the uninsured: Is access to a physician enough? *American Journal of Public Health, 89(6),* 910–912.

Morone, J. (2010). Presidents and health reform: From Franklin D. Roosevelt to Barack Obama. *Health Affairs, 29(6),* 1096–1100.

National Center for Health Statistics. (2008). Prenatal care. Retrieved from http://www.cdc.gov/nchs/fastats/prenatal.htm

National Center for Health Statistics. (2007). Health, United States, 2007: With chartbook on trends in the health of Americans. Retrieved from http://www.cdc.gov/nchs/data/hus/hus07.pdf

Organization for Economic Cooperation and Development (OECD). (2009). Health at a glance 2009. Retrieved from http://www.oecd-ilibrary.org/social-issues-migration-health/health-at-a-glance-2009_health_glance-2009-en

Patient Protection and Affordable Care Act, H.R. 3590. (2010). Retrieved from http://www.opencongress.org/bill/111-h3590/text

Paul, I., Lehman, E., Suliman, A., & Hillemeier, M. (2007). Perinatal disparities for black mothers and their newborns. *Maternal Child Health Journal, 12*, 452–460.

Rooks, J. (1997). *Midwifery and childbirth in America*. Philadelphia: Temple University.

Schempf, A., Kroelinger, C., & Guyer, B. (2007). Rising infant mortality in Delaware: An examination of racial difference in secular trends. *Maternal Child Health Journal, 11*, 475–483.

United Nations Children's Fund. (2007). Child poverty in perspective: An overview of child well-being in rich countries. Retrieved from http://www.unicef-irc.org/publications/pdf/rc7_eng.pdf

U.S. Department of Health and Human Services (HHS). (2009). Data sources, definitions, and notes: Community health status indicators. Retrieved from http://communityhealth.hhs.gov/HomePage.aspx?GeogCD=&PeerStrat=&state=&county

World Health Organization (WHO). (2010). Spending on health: A global overview. Retrieved from http://www.who.int/mediacentre/factsheets/fs319/en/index.html

CHAPTER 42

The Nursing Workforce Shortage: The Vulnerability of the Healthcare System

Barbara A. Anderson

Objectives

WWW

At the end of this chapter, the reader will be able to

1. Describe the global nursing workforce shortage and the implications for health care around the world.
2. Explain how the nursing faculty shortage exacerbates the nursing workforce shortage.
3. Provide a solution in terms of how resources can be allocated to reduce the shortage of faculty and nurses.

INTRODUCTION

The World Health Organization (WHO) estimates there is a shortage of more than 4 million healthcare professionals globally. Half of the shortfall is in the nursing profession. This shortage is most acute in 57 low-income nations (WHO, 2006a). For example, sub-Saharan Africa, with 11% of the world's population, carries 24% of the global burden of illness, but has only 3% of the world's health professionals. Moreover, there is widespread migration of these essential workers to more affluent regions. Out-migration from low-resource areas—a trend seen across the world—contributes to critical shortages for healthcare and public health programs in poor countries (Chaguturu & Vallabhaneni, 2003; Garrett, 2007; International Council of Nurses [ICN], 2006; "Poaching Nurses," 2006; Ross, Polsky, & Sochalski, 2003).

WHO's Millennium Development Goals (MDGs), which were adopted globally in 2000, target the stabilization of the healthcare professional workforce shortage as essential to improving world health (WHO, 2005, 2006b). In the document, "Why the Workforce Is Important," the WHO calls for nations to plan and manage collaboratively to address these critical shortages. A WHO roadmap guides capacity building through preservice preparation of healthcare workers, competency maintenance, and prevention of attrition (WHO, 2006c).

The effects of the workforce shortage, especially the nursing shortage, are being felt globally, not just in low-resource nations (Khaliq, Broyles, & Mwachofi, 2008; Potempa, Redman, & Landstrom, 2009). There are 126,000 vacant nursing positions in the United States, with a projected deficit of 1 million nurses by 2020. The anticipated impact of the nursing workforce shortage on the health of the U.S. population is an issue of major concern (Buchan, 2006; Buerhaus, Staiger, & Auerbach, 2000, 2008; Chaguturu & Vallabhaneni, 2003; Kuehn, 2007; Spacracio, 2003).

Nursing plays a key role in protecting and promoting the nation's health as well as sustaining the healthcare system. Factors such as inadequate nursing staffing ratios, the high acuity and aging of the general population, and the aging and attrition of the nursing workforce are all contributing to the nursing shortage (Aiken, Clarke, Cheung, Sloane, & Silber, 2003; American Association of Colleges of Nursing [AACN], 2008b; Buerhaus, Donelan, Ulrich, Norman, DesRoches, & Dittus, 2007; Institute of Medicine [IOM], 2001; The Joint Commission, 2008). It is a "perfect storm" (Hinshaw, 2008, p. 4).

Vulnerability is a term that is generally applied to individuals or aggregates; rarely is it applied to communities, nations, or systems. Yet, systems are vulnerable when they fail to address deficiencies and dissatisfactions as well as factors contributing to resiliency.

The nursing workforce shortage in the United States is a critical vulnerability within the healthcare system. This chapter addresses how this vulnerability undermines the healthcare system and how current policy efforts are striving to increase the resiliency of the system by addressing a root cause of the nursing workforce shortage—namely, the nursing faculty shortage.

THE STATE OF NURSING IN THE UNITED STATES

The 2.4 million nurses in the United States represent the largest group of health professionals in the nation (AACN, 2008b). The shortage in the nursing workforce, however, points to deep problems in the healthcare system. Job satisfaction is low (Christmas, 2008; Clark, 2010; *Employee and Nurse Check-up Report*, 2008; Hinshaw, 2008; The Joint Commission, 2008) and attrition is a major issue (Oulton, 2006). Faculty shortages are acute (Allen, 2008; Malone, 2007; National League for Nursing–Carnegie Foundation, 2008). Currently, the pipeline of new graduates is inadequate to meet the escalating healthcare needs of the U.S. population, putting the health of the nation at risk, especially the country's most vulnerable groups (AACN, 2010a; Reinhard & Hassmiller, 2009). At the center of the nursing workforce shortage is the severe shortage of prepared and available nursing faculty (Aiken, 2007; Allen, 2008; The Joint Commission, 2008). This shortage, which directly affects the number of U.S. nurses, has inspired the aggressive recruitment of nurses in low-income nations, thereby leading to declines in healthcare services in low-income nations (Anderson & Issacs, 2007; Proto & Dzurec, 2009).

The faculty shortage is fueled by the low salaries paid to nurses compared to clinicians, by the late age at which many nurses obtain the higher levels of education necessary for entry into academia, the limited number of doctoral-prepared faculty, cost-cutting measures decreasing faculty sizes in universities, and the aging of the U.S. nursing workforce (Allen, 2008; American Academy of Nursing, 2006; AACN, 2008a, 2008c, 2010b; ICN, 2006; Kuehn, 2007; Potempa et al., 2009; Ross et al., 2003; Yordy, 2006).

The faculty shortage creates a highly competitive admissions process for nursing programs. In fact, there is a high level of rejection for *qualified* applicants because of faculty and institutional limitations (Ross et al., 2003). In 2005, 150,000 qualified applicants were denied admission (Dugger, 2006; ICN, 2006: Yordy, 2006). In 2007, 40,285 qualified applicants were denied admission to graduate and baccalaureate programs (AACN, 2008c). The denial of applicants from U.S. nursing programs has an escalating effect on the workforce shortage, the outsourcing of preservice education to other nations, and the aggressive recruitment of nurses from other nations, usually low-income countries (ICN, 2006; "Migration Threatens Health Systems," 2003; "Poaching Nurses," 2006; Spacracio, 2003). It is projected that the growing nursing shortage in the United States will further be intensified by ongoing healthcare reform efforts to improve services to the population (Donelan, Buerhaus, DesRoches, & Burke, 2010). This shortage is a major vulnerability threatening to further fracture an already fragile, fragmented healthcare system.

BUILDING RESILIENCY IN A FRAGILE HEALTHCARE SYSTEM

The United States needs to strengthen its capacity in building the nursing workforce for a number of reasons. On the global front, there is continued ethical concern about aggressive recruitment of nurses from low-income nations, which essentially sabotages viable healthcare systems in poor nations (Clark, Stewart, & Clark, 2006; Eastwood, Conroy, Naicker, West, Tutt, & Plange-Rhule, 2003; Green, 2006; ICN, 2006; McElmurry, Solheim, Kishi, Coffia, Woith, & Janepanish, 2006; "Poaching Nurses," 2006; Spacracio, 2003; Xu & Zhang, 2003). Across the globe, low-income nations have been forced to ramp up their preservice nursing education to compensate for aggressive U.S. recruitment of nurses. For the most part, these efforts to increase preservice nursing education have come at the expense of Ministries of Health in poor nations that are trying to ensure an adequate workforce for their own primary care and public health programs (Anderson & Issacs, 2007). Justice concerns compel that the United States recognize this vulnerability of poor nations and advocate for a domestic policy that builds its own nursing workforce.

Building capacity for an adequate workforce is essential for the health of the United States, especially for those of its groups who are most vulnerable, such as the elderly; the uninsured; members of rural, underserved communities; and young families (Cramer, Duncan, Megel, & Pitkin, 2009; Ganley & Sheets, 2009). A key strategy in building the cadre of nurses needed is to reach youth with the message of career opportunities in nursing (Gormley, Frerick, & Dean, 2009). This is, however, an empty promise unless the faculty shortage is resolved and schools of nursing have enough places for qualified aspirants.

A hopeful policy sign in addressing the nursing shortage is the recent release of the landmark report by the Institute of Medicine and the Robert Wood Johnson Foundation (2010),

The Future of Nursing: Leading Change, Advancing Health. This report advances the profession of nursing by supporting four key messages:

- Full utilization of the training and education of nurses
- Support for higher levels of education in seamless progression from the bachelor's level to the doctoral level
- Full partnership with physicians and other healthcare professionals in healthcare reform and redesign
- Improved nursing workforce policy and planning (AACN, 2010c)

This document describes nursing as an essential catalyst in healthcare reform, calling for doubling the number of doctoral-prepared nurses by 2020 faculty (American Academy of Nursing, 2010). A key focus is prioritizing doctoral education through educational stipends and seamless academic programming from the bachelor's level to the doctoral level. These strategies promise to attack a root cause of the nursing shortage in the United States—the dearth of doctoral-prepared nursing faculty. Such an approach addresses one of the key vulnerabilities in today's highly fragile healthcare system—namely, the inability of qualified applicants to access nursing education due to the limited number of faculty available to teach them.

In a winding, circuitous fashion, prioritizing doctoral preparation in this country has the capacity to affect the health of both the United States and the world. It will increase the number of nurses qualified to serve in a faculty role and strengthen national efforts directed toward healthcare reform by ensuring an adequate pipeline of nurse leaders. Having sufficient nursing faculty has the potential to effect the transformation of a fragile and sick healthcare system by providing a safety net of nurses for vulnerable populations in the United States, decrease U.S. dependence on nurses from low-resource nations, and enhance global health by decreasing demand for nurses from low-resource nations.

In a welcome change, U.S. national policy is now supporting greater investment in nursing leadership. Nursing has an unprecedented opportunity to care for and participate in the healing of the broken U.S. healthcare system. This is the moment in history for nursing to step forward and accept this challenge.

WWW

For a full suite of assignments and additional learning activities, use the access code located in the front of your book to visit this exclusive website: http://go.jblearning.com/dechesnay. If you do not have an access code, you can obtain one at the site.

REFERENCES

Aiken, L. (2007). U.S. nurse labor market dynamics are key to global nurse sufficiency. *Health Services Research, 42*, 1299–1320.

Aiken, L., Clarke, S., Cheung, R., Sloane, D., & Silber, J. (2003) Educational levels of hospital nurses and surgical patient mortality. *Journal of the American Medical Association, 290*, 1617–1623.

Allen, L. (2008). The nursing shortage continues as faculty shortage grows. *Nursing Economics: Journal for Health Care Leaders, 26*(1), 35–40.

American Academy of Nursing, Expert Panel on Global Nursing and Health. (2006). White paper on global nursing and health: A brief. *Nursing Outlook, 32*, 111–113.

American Academy of Nursing. (2010). IOM report provides vision for future of health care. Retrieved October 5, 2010, from www.aannet.org

American Association of Colleges of Nursing (AACN). (2008a, September). *Addressing the nursing shortage: A focus on nurse faculty*. Washington, DC: Author.

American Association of Colleges of Nursing (AACN). (2008b, September). *Ensuring access to safe, quality, and affordable health care through a robust nursing workforce*. Washington, DC: AACN Policy Brief.

American Association of Colleges of Nursing (AACN). (2008c, September). *Nursing faculty shortage fact sheet*. Washington, DC: Author.

American Association of Colleges of Nursing (AACN). (2010a). Joint statement from the Tri-Council for nursing on recent registered nurse supply and demand projects. Retrieved October 8, 2010, from http://www.aacn.nche.edu/Education/pdf/Tricouncilrnsupply.pdf

American Association of Colleges of Nursing (AACN). (2010b, September 17). Shortage of faculty and resource constraints hinder growth in U.S nursing schools according to the latest AACN report. Retrieved October 9, 2010, from http:www.aacn.nche.edu/IDS/pdf/vacancy10.pdf

American Association of Colleges of Nursing (AACN). (2010c, October). AACN applauds the new Institute of Medicine report calling for transformational change in nursing education and practice. Retrieved October 5, 2010, from http://www.aacn.nce.edu/Media/NewsReleases/2010/futurenursing.html

Anderson, B., & Isaacs, A. (2007). Simply not there: The impact of international migration of nurses and midwives—Perspectives from Guyana. *Journal of Midwifery and Women's Health, 52*, 392–397.

Buchan, J. (2006). The impact of global nursing migration on health services delivery. *Policy, Politics and Nursing Practice, 7*(suppl), 16S–25S.

Buerhaus, P., Donelan, K., Ulrich, B., Norman, L., DesRoches, C., & Dittus, R. (2007). Impact of the nurse shortage on hospital patient care: Comparative perspectives. *Health Affairs, 26*, 853–862.

Buerhaus, P., Staiger, D., & Auerbach, D. (2000). Implications of an aging registered nurse workforce. *Journal of the American Medical Association, 281*, 2928–2932.

Buerhaus, P., Staiger, D., & Auerbach, D. (2008). *The future of the nursing workforce in the United States: Data, trends and implications*. Sudbury, MA: Jones & Bartlett.

Chaguturu, S., & Vallabhaneni, B. (2003). Aiding and abetting: Nursing crises at home and abroad. *New England Journal of Medicine, 131*, 1761–1761.

Christmas, K. (2008). How work environment impacts retention. *Nursing Economics, 26*, 316–318.

Clark, C. (2010). The nursing shortage as a community transformational opportunity: An update. *Advances in Nursing Science, 33*(1), 35–52.

Clark, P., Stewart, J., & Clark, D. (2006).The globalization of the labor market for health-care professionals. *International Labor Review, 145*, 37–64.

Cramer, M., Duncan, K., Megel, M., & Pitkin, S.(2009). Partnering with rural communities to meet the demand for a qualified nursing workforce. *Nursing Outlook, 57*(3), 148–157.

Donelan, K., Buerhaus, P., DesRoches, C., & Burke, S. (2010). Health policy thoughtleaders' views of the health workforce in an era of health reform. *Nursing Outlook. 58*, 175–180.

Dugger, C. (2006, May 24). U.S. plan to lure nurses may hurt poor nations. *New York Times*. Retrieved February 12, 2007, from http://topics.nytimes.com/top/reference/timestopics/people/d/celia_w_dug ger/index.html?inline=nyt-per

Eastwood, J., Conroy, R., Naicker, W., West, P., Tutt, R., & Plange-Rhule, J. (2003). Loss of health professionals from sub-Sahara Africa: The pivotal role of the UK. *Lancet, 163*, 1891–1900.

Employee and nurse check-up report: Employee and nurse perspectives on American health care organizations. (2008). South Bend, IN: Press Ganey Associates, pp. 1–18.

Ganley, B., & Sheets, I. (2009). A strategy to address the nursing shortage. *Journal of Nursing Education, 48*(7), 401–405.

Garrett, L. (2007). The challenge of global health. *Foreign Affairs.* Retrieved October 28, 2008, from http://www,foreignaffairs.org/20070101faessay86103

Gormley, D., Frerick, J., & Dean, A. (2009). Pathways to nursing: An innovative program to encourage high school students to enter nursing. *Kentucky Nurse, 57*(4), 7–8.

Green, A. (2006). Nursing and midwifery: Millennium development goals and the global human resource crisis. *International Nursing Review, 31*, 11–13.

Hinshaw, A. (2008). Navigating the perfect storm: Balancing a culture of safety with workforce challenges. *Nursing Research, 57*, S4–S9.

Institute of Medicine (IOM). (2001). *To err is human: Building a safer health system.* Washington, DC: National Academies Press.

Institute of Medicine (IOM) & Robert Wood Johnson Foundation. (2010). *The future of nursing: Leading change, advancing health.* Washington, DC: National Academies Press. Retrieved October 5, 2010, from http://ww.nap.edu/catlog.php?record_id=12956

International Council of Nurses (ICN). (2006). *The global nursing shortage: Priority areas for intervention.* Geneva, Switzerland: Author.

Khaliq, A., Broyles, R., & Mwachofi, A. (2008). Global nurse migration: Its impact on developing countries and prospects for the future. *World Health and Population, 19*(3), 55–73.

Kuehn, B. (2007). No end in sight to nursing shortage: Bottleneck at nursing schools is key factor. *Journal of the American Medical Association, 298*, 1623.

Malone, B. (2007, November 30). Job satisfaction in nursing. *Chronicle of Higher Education*, A35.

McElmurry, B., Solheim, K., Kishi, R., Coffia, M., Woith, W., & Janepanish, P. (2006). Ethical concerns in nurse migration. *Journal of Professional Nursing, 22*, 226–235.

Migration threatens health systems in developing countries [Editorial]. (2003). *Australian Nursing Journal, 11*, 10.

National League for Nursing–Carnegie Foundation. (2008, September 20). Nationwide Foundation study examines nurse faculty workload. Retrieved October 10, 2007, from http://www.nln.org/nlnjournal/index.htm

Oulton, J. (2006). The global nursing shortage: An overview of issues and actions. *Policy, Politics, and Nursing Practice, 7*(suppl), 34S–39S.

Poaching nurses from the developing world [Editorial]. (2006). *Lancet, 167*, 1791.

Potempa, K., Redman, R., & Landstrom, G (2009). Human resources in nursing education: A worldwide crisis. *Collegian, 16*(1), 19–23.

Proto, M., & Dzurec, L. (2009). Strategies for success management and oversight of nurse faculty workforce initiatives: Lessons from the field. *Journal of Professional Nursing, 25*(2), 87–92.

Reinhard, S., & Hassmiller, S. (2009). Partners in solutions to the nurse faculty shortage. *Journal of Professional Nursing, 25*(6), 335–339.

Ross, S., Polsky, D., & Sochalski, J. (2003). Nursing shortages and international nurse immigration. *International Nursing Review, 32*, 231–262.

The Joint Commission. (2008). Health care at the crossroads: Guiding principles for the development of the hospital of the future. Retrieved December 10, 2008, from http:www.aramarkhealthcare.com

Spacracio, D. (2003). Winged migration: International nurse recruitment—Friend or foe to the nursing crisis? *Journal of Nursing Law, 10*, 97–111.

World Health Organization (WHO). (2005). Health and the Millennium Development Goals. Retrieved October 9, 2010, from http://www.who.int/hdp/publications/mdg_en.pdf

World Health Organization (WHO). (2006a) Global Health Workforce Alliance: List of 57 countries facing human resources for health crisis. Retrieved October 9, 2010, from http://www.who.int/workforcealliance/countries/57crisiscountries.pdf

World Health Organization (WHO). (2006b). *Working together for health: The world health report 2006.* Geneva, Switzerland: Author. Retrieved October 9, 2010, from http://www.who.whr06_en.pdf

World Health Organization (WHO). (2006c). Why the workforce is important. Retrieved November 12, 2006, from www.who.int/whr/2006/overview/en/print.html

Yordy, K. (2006). *The nursing faculty shortage: A crisis for health care.* Princeton, NJ: Robert Wood Johnson Foundation.

Xu, Y., & Zhang, J. (2003). One size doesn't fit all: Ethics of international nurse recruitment from the conceptual framework of stakeholder interests. *Nursing Ethics, 12*, 371–381.

Index

Figures and tables are indicated by f and t following the page number.

B

C

D

E

F

G

J

K

L

T

X

Y

Z

www.ingramcontent.com/pod-product-compliance
Lightning Source LLC
Chambersburg PA
CBHW081123180926
51611CB00004B/39
* 9 7 8 1 2 8 4 1 3 3 5 2 3 *